New Frontiers in Thyroid Surgery

New Frontiers in Thyroid Surgery

Edited by Selena Brooks

hayle medical

New York

Hayle Medical,
750 Third Avenue, 9th Floor,
New York, NY 10017, USA

Visit us on the World Wide Web at:
www.haylemedical.com

ISBN: 978-1-64647-519-3

Cataloging-in-Publication Data

New frontiers in thyroid surgery / edited by Selena Brooks.
p. cm.
Includes bibliographical references and index.
ISBN 978-1-64647-519-3
1. Thyroid gland--Surgery. 2. Thyroid gland--Diseases. I. Brooks, Selena.
RD599.5.T46 N49 2023
617.539--dc23

Table of Contents

Preface

Thyroid is a tiny butterfly-shaped gland, located just below the voice box in the lower front part of the neck. Thyroid surgery involves removal of the thyroid gland partially or completely. The presence of tumors or nodules on the thyroid gland is the most frequent reason for thyroid surgery. The majority of nodules are benign but some are precancerous or cancerous. Thyroid surgery can be categorized into different types such as total thyroidectomy, lobectomy and subtotal thyroidectomy. Thyroid surgery carries various risks such as negative reaction to general anesthesia, infection and excessive bleeding. After the surgery, the patient may also experience permanent, transient or superior laryngeal nerve injury, seromas, permanent or temporary hypoparathyroidism, and hematomas. This book aims to understand the various aspects of thyroid surgery. It will help the readers in keeping pace with the rapid changes in this field. Medical professionals and students actively engaged in this field will find it full of crucial and unexplored concepts.

The researches compiled throughout the book are authentic and of high quality, combining several disciplines and from very diverse regions from around the world. Drawing on the contributions of many researchers from diverse countries, the book's objective is to provide the readers with the latest achievements in the area of research. This book will surely be a source of knowledge to all interested and researching the field.

In the end, I would like to express my deep sense of gratitude to all the authors for meeting the set deadlines in completing and submitting their research chapters. I would also like to thank the publisher for the support offered to us throughout the course of the book. Finally, I extend my sincere thanks to my family for being a constant source of inspiration and encouragement.

Editor

1

Evaluation of Autofluorescence in Identifying Parathyroid Glands by Measuring Parathyroid Hormone in Fine-Needle Biopsy Washings

Zhen Liu[1], *Run-sheng Ma*[1], *Jun-li Jia*[2], *Tao Wang*[1], *Dao-hong Zuo*[1] *and De-tao Yin*[1*]

[1] *Department of Thyroid Surgery, The First Affiliated Hospital of Zhengzhou University, He'nan, China,* [2] *Department of Respiratory, The First Affiliated Hospital of Zhengzhou University, He'nan, China*

***Correspondence:**
De-tao Yin
detaoyin@zzu.edu.cn*

Background: Near-infrared autofluorescence imaging has potentially great value for assisting endocrine surgeons in identifying parathyroid glands and may dramatically change the surgical strategy of endocrine surgeons in thyroid surgery. This study is designed to objectively evaluate the role of near-infrared autofluorescence imaging in identifying parathyroid glands during thyroid surgery by measuring intraoperative parathyroid hormone in fine-needle aspiration biopsy washings.

Methods: This study was conducted at a tertiary referral teaching hospital in China from February 2020 to June 2020. Patients undergoing total thyroidectomy with or without neck lymph node dissection were consecutively included. The surgeon used near-infrared autofluorescence imaging to identify parathyroid glands during thyroid surgery and confirmed suspicious parathyroid tissues by measuring their intraoperative parathyroid hormone. Nanocarbon was injected into the thyroid gland if the thyroid autofluorescence intensity was too strong. The sensitivity and accuracy of near-infrared autofluorescence imaging and vision for identifying parathyroid glands, and the difference in autofluorescence intensity in various tissues were the main outcomes.

Results: Overall, 238 patients completed the trial. Based on the pathological and aIOPTH results, the sensitivity of near-infrared autofluorescence imaging for detecting parathyroid glands (568 of 596 parathyroid glands; 95.30%)was significantly higher than that of vision (517 of 596 parathyroid glands; 86.74%, *P*<.001). The accuracy of near-infrared autofluorescence imaging (764 of 841 tissues; 90.84%) was significantly higher than that of vision (567 of 841 tissues; 67.42%, *P*<.001) when the evaluations of certain tissues were inconsistent. There was a significant difference between the autofluorescence intensity of the parathyroid glands and that of the lymph nodes (74.19 ± 17.82 *vs* 33.97 ± 10.64, *P*<.001).

Conclusion: The use of near-infrared autofluorescence imaging, along with intraoperative parathyroid hormone and nanocarbon for the identification of parathyroid glands in thyroid surgery may increase the number of confirmed parathyroid glands. Using near-infrared autofluorescence imaging can effectively distinguish lymph nodes and parathyroid glands during lymph node dissection.

Keywords: autofluorescence, parathyroid, thyroid surgery, nanocarbon, lymph node

INTRODUCTION

Hypocalcemia after thyroid surgery is a problem that has long plagued endocrine surgeons. In a statistical analysis of 14,540 patients undergoing thyroidectomies in the United States from 2013 to 2015, 450 cases of severe postoperative hypocalcemia occurred (3.3% overall, 0.6% after partial, and 4.7% after subtotal or total thyroidectomy) (1). Severe postoperative hypocalcemia can be life-threatening and seriously impair quality of life. Accurate identification of parathyroid glands (PGs) is the first step to reduce postoperative hypocalcemia. At present, the recognition of PGs mainly depends on visual identification by the surgeon. However, due to their small size and unstable location, as well as the difficulty in distinguishing them in color and shape from lymph nodes and adipose tissue, highly subjective visual identification is often unreliable. Therefore, any technologies that might assist the visual identification of PGs can be of great clinical application value.

There have been a few reported studies relating to parathyroidectomy or thyroidectomy combined with autofluorescence, fluorescent methylene blue, 5-aminolevulinic acid, indocyanine green, optical coherence tomography, laser speckle contrast imaging, dynamic optical contrast imaging and Raman spectroscopy (2). These optical technologies could become complementary to the surgeon's eyes and thus may reduce the hypocalcemia rate after thyroid surgery. Among them, near infrared-induced autofluorescence (NIRAF) technology based on the spontaneous auto fluorescent signal of the PG is most widely reported (3). Studies have shown that NIRAF can reduce the risk of postoperative hypocalcemia (4–6). However, reduction in hypocalcemia is only an indirect proof since it is also highly related to the further protection of recognized PGs.

The exact number of PGs identified by NIRAF is crucial to its clinical evaluation. In previous studies, NIRAF showed good sensitivity and specificity in the identification of PGs (7–9). However, all identified PGs during thyroid surgery need to be retained. Therefore, the pathological examination based on the study's purpose is against ethical requirements since it would cause permanent damage. Visual identification by the surgeon has been used in most trials as a confirmation method for PGs (10). The subjective visual identification itself lacks accuracy and is less persuasive to be used as the criterion. Although some of the trials used pathological examination to confirm PGs, the included patients mostly had parathyroid tumors or hyperparathyroidism (7). Many studies have shown that the NIRAF of diseased PGs is completely different from that of normal PGs, so it is better to exclude these patients in the study to explain the value of NIRAF in thyroid surgery (11, 12).

The intraoperative parathyroid aspiration for parathyroid hormone assay (aIOPTH) technology is considered to have high sensitivity (80%-100%) for the confirmation of PGs and has a high specificity close to 100% (13). Meanwhile, aIOPTH, as a minimally invasive examination method, causes minimal damage to PGs; consequently, evaluating suspected parathyroid tissues with aIOPTH completely meets the ethical requirements. Thus, aIOPTH is very suitable as an alternative to parathyroid pathology to evaluate the value of NIRAF.

This study was a large sample case series study including patients undergoing thyroidectomies. The purpose was to use aIOPTH to evaluate the value of NIRAF in thyroid surgery. We introduced several new methods to improve the effect of NIRAF during the study and tried to find a new strategy using NIRAF and aIOPTH to improve the identification of PGs.

METHODS

The study was approved by the institutional review board of the First Affiliated Hospital of Zhengzhou University (2019-KY-283) and registered on Chictr.org.cn (ChiCTR2000030025)and all patients gave written informed consent. Patients undergoing thyroidectomy with or without neck lymph node dissection between February 2020 to June 2020 were consecutively included in a prospective cohort. Previous thyroid or parathyroid surgery, parathyroid tumor and parathyroid dysfunction, including primary and secondary hyperparathyroidism, were exclusion criteria.

The equipment used in this study was a commercially available, handheld NIR camera (PDE-Neo II; Hamamatsu Photonics). The camera emits infrared light at a wavelength of 760 nm and captures NIR wavelengths of 790–830 nm. Since the light from an LED lamp has little influence on the imaging process, we were able to keep the routine lighting of the operating room and simply move the surgical light away from the surgical field, which reduced the impact of frequent light switching (**Supplementary Figure 1**).

Surgical Process

After routine dissection of the band muscles and exposure of the thyroid gland, the first fluorescence imaging was performed. If the thyroid autofluorescence intensity was too strong, then nanocarbon (Chongqing Laimei Pharmaceutical Co) was slowly injected into the thyroid gland until the gland was black-stained. While the surgeon used NIRAF to identify PGs, he also identified PGs through routine visual observation (**Supplementary Video 1**). The fluorescent images using NIRAF to identify the PGs were saved, and the assistant took pictures with a high-resolution camera of the same operative field for subsequent image comparison. The tissues co-identified by vision and NIRAF as PGs were considered as confirmed PGs. If NIRAF revealed PGs in areas that had been visually neglected, it was considered that NIRAF first discovered them. If the judgment of tissue was inconsistent, the measurement of aIOPTH was used for confirmation (**Supplementary Video 2**). The specific method was to puncture the suspicious tissue with a 1 ml syringe containing 0.1 ml saline and then to drip the 0.1 ml saline through the needle onto the reaction area of the test strip and culture for 10 minutes according to the instructions of the parathyroid hormone (PTH) detection kit (Bioda Diagnosis Co) (**Supplementary Figure 2**). If the saline contained PTH, it would combine with PTH antibodies in the reaction zone to form a complex. The strip included the distal control band and the proximal test band. When the liquid containing the complex flowed from the reaction zone to the test band, the complex bound to the anti-PTH antibody in the test band, making it appear red. Furthermore, the detector was used to calculate the PTH level according to the color depth of the band, which ranged from 10 pg/mL to 1,000 pg/mL. A PTH dose greater than 130 pg/mL was regarded as the standard to justify the node as a parathyroid gland (**Figure 1**).

Finally, all tissues not identified as PGs during the procedure were examined pathologically. Among them, nonparathyroid tissues confirmed by aIOPTH were classified into two groups (the visually suspected parathyroid group and the NIRAF suspected parathyroid group) and submitted for pathology separately. The pathologist composed a report for each punctured tissue and carefully searched for the presence of PGs in all tissues.

Lymph Node Fluorescence Imaging

To observe the fluorescence intensity of the lymph nodes, we separated the specimens of lateral neck lymph node dissection into a high fluorescence intensity group and a low fluorescence

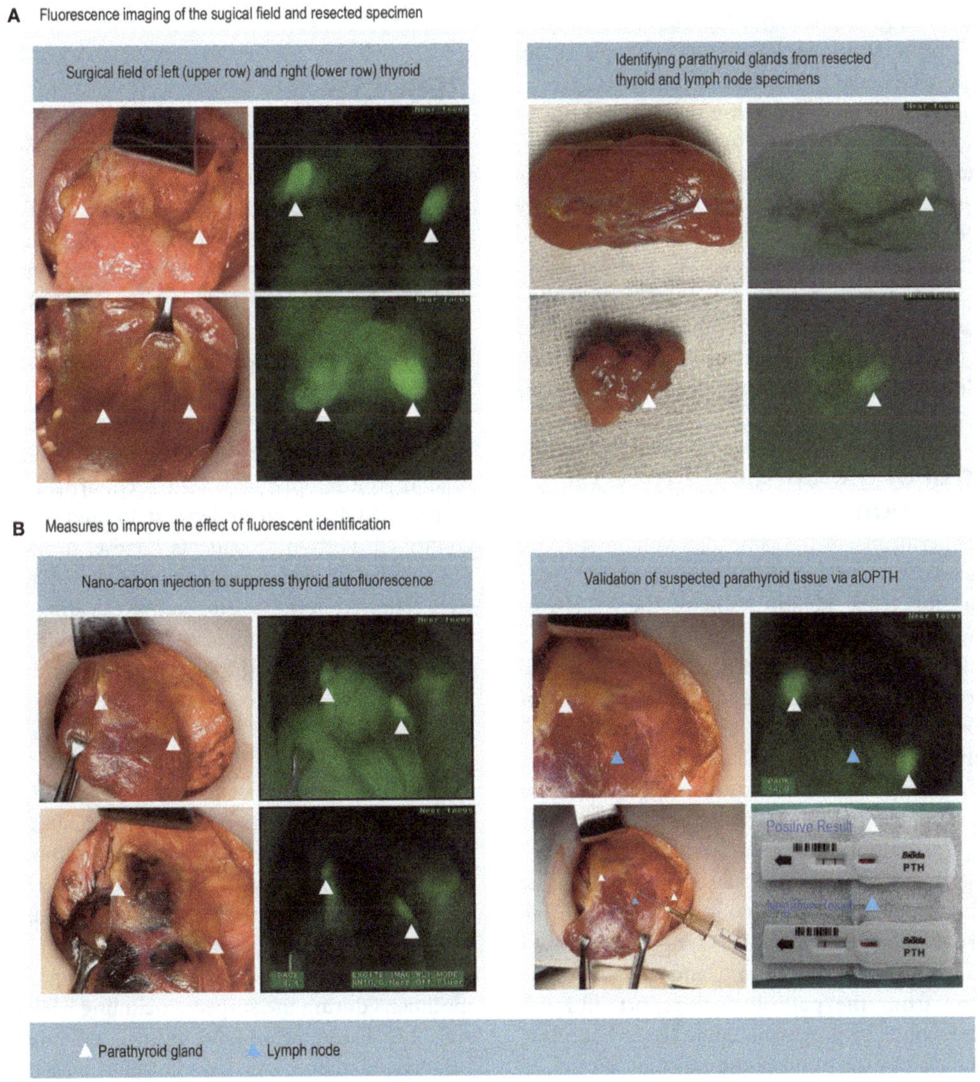

FIGURE 1 | We used fluorescence imaging of the surgical field and resected thyroid and lymph nodes specimens to locate the parathyroid gland. Parathyroid tissues can be highlighted as green in the images **(A)**. Nano-carbon can suppress the fluorescence of the thyroid gland and thus make it easier to recognize parathyroid glands. The lymph node (blue triangle) was visually recognized as the parathyroid gland, but it had weak fluorescence and was finally excluded via aIOPTH **(B)**.

intensity group under the fluorescence image and sent them separately for pathological examination. The number of lymph nodes in both groups was collected.

Data Collection

The following variables were collected during the trial: sex, age, body mass index (BMI; calculated as weight in kilograms divided by height in meters squared), preoperative calcium level, preoperative PTH level, type of surgery, number of patients who used nanocarbon during surgery, number of PGs first identified by NIRAF, number of identified PGs during total thyroidectomy and thyroid lobectomy separately, number of autotransplanted PGs, number of inadvertently resected PGs, PTH in fine-needle aspiration washout fluids from the PG, final diagnosis, postoperative hypocalcemia at postoperative day 1 or 2, nadir of postoperative calcium (considered in the normal range when it was >8.0 mg/dL; to convert to mmol/L, multiply by 0.25), PTH level at postoperative day 1 (considered in the normal range when it was ≥15 pg/mL; to convert to ng/L, multiply by 1.0), number of lymph nodes in lateral neck lymph nodes dissection and hypocalcemia at postoperative month 1.

Because the fluorescence intensity in the image could not be quantified in the imaging system, we used ImageJ software (National Institutes of Health, Bethesda, MD) to measure the fluorescence intensity of different tissues after surgery. First, we confirmed the type of certain tissue in the image and then used the ROI tool in ImageJ software to circle the boundaries of different tissues in the image and measure the average fluorescence intensity of the tissue within the boundary. When multiple identical tissues existed in one image, these tissues were continuously circled, and then the overall average fluorescence intensity was measured.

Quality Control of the Surgical Process and Data Collection

All operations were performed by the same high-volume surgeon and his assistant, who completed over 800 thyroidectomies a year together. Opinions for visual identification of the PGs were obtained from the surgeon. Before the end of the operation, the assistant checked to ensure that the necessary images and photos were correctly retained and that all specimens sent for pathological examination were correctly labeled.

The image analysis process was completed by the surgeon and his assistant after obtaining the postoperative pathological report. The first step was to compare the image with the operation record and pathological report and then to mark the corresponding tissue type in the fluorescent image. The confirmation of the thyroid and lymph nodes was based on the pathological report, confirmation of the PGs was obtained from aIOPTH results and the pathology report, and adipose tissue confirmation came from the pathological report and the judgment of the surgeon. The process of circle tissue boundary in ImageJ was completed by the surgeon and assistant. To reduce the error in the circle selection process, the arithmetic mean of the measurement results from both of them was used as the final result.

Statistical Analysis

Non-Gaussian distribution continuous variables (BMI, Preoperative calcium, Parathyroid hormone) are reported using medians and interquartile ranges (IQRs); autofluorescence intensity of tissues was tested to be normally distributed and thus reported as Mean±SD; categorical variables are reported using counts, percentages, and 95% CIs. Pearson's chi-square analysis was performed to compare the sensitivity and accuracy of NIRAF with vision in identifying parathyroid glands. The sensitivity was calculated by dividing the detected PGs by the final confirmed PGs. The accuracy was calculated by dividing the number of correctly judged tissues by the number of all suspicious tissues in this study. A paired-sample t-test was performed to compare the fluorescence intensity of PGs and other tissues separately. All analyses were 2-tailed, with $p \leq 0.05$ set as the criterion for statistical significance. All data were analyzed using SPSS statistical software, version 24.0 (SPSS, Inc.).

RESULTS

Overall, 250 patients were enrolled in this study, 122 patients used nanocarbon tracers due to strong thyroid autofluorescence during initial imaging, of whom 12 patients had contaminated the surgical field after injecting nanocarbon into the thyroid gland, which made subsequent NIRAF difficult to perform and thus were excluded from the study. The remaining 238 patients completed the trial; 145 patients underwent thyroid lobectomy, and 93 patients underwent total thyroidectomy. Most of them (198 of 238 patients; 83.2%) were diagnosed with malignant tumors. A total of 186 patients (186 of 238 patients; 78.2%) underwent lymph node dissection. Fifty-seven of 93 patients (61.3%) who underwent total thyroidectomy had 4 PGs confirmed, while 118 of 145 patients (81.4%) who underwent thyroid lobectomy had 2 PGs confirmed. Forty-nine patients (20.6%) developed hypocalcemia on the first or second postoperative day. A total of 234 patients were followed up for postoperative calcium, 2 of whom still had hypocalcemia one month after surgery, but these two patients had recovered in the second follow-up at 3 months (**Table 1**).

Overall, 841 suspicious parathyroid tissues were identified; 490 tissues were co-confirmed by vision and NIRAF as PGs, of which 88 PGs were first identified by NIRAF. A total of 351 tissues showed inconsistency between vision and NIRAF, and fine-needle aspiration was performed. Of the 128 tissues recognized as PGs only by NIRAF, 78 were eventually confirmed. Correspondingly, of 223 tissues only visually recognized, only 27 were confirmed as PGs. The mean PTH in fine-needle aspiration washout fluids of the parathyroid was 264 pg/mL.

Pathological examinations were performed on all the resected specimens during the surgery, including 246 labeled tissues with aIOPTH lower than 130 pg/ml. Of the 246 tissues, no parathyroid tissue was found, which was consistent with the aIOPTH results. There were 167 lymph nodes, 28 adipose tissues and 1 thyroid tissue among the tissues misidentified as PGs visually. Forty-nine tissues misidentified by NIRAF were adipose

TABLE 1 | Clinical Characteristic of Participants.

Characteristic	Patients No. (%) (N=238)	
Preoperative Variables		
Sex, No. (%)		
Male	54 (22.7)	
Female	184 (77.3)	
Age, median (IQR), y	45.0 (36.0-54.0)	
BMI, median (IQR)	25.4 (22.3-27.4)	
Preoperative calcium, median (IQR), pg/mL	9.20 (8.91-9.56)	
Preoperative parathyroid hormone, median (IQR), pg/mL	33.9 (27.6-43.6)	
Operative Variables		
Type of surgery.		
Total thyroidectomy with lymph nodes dissection	89 (37.4)	
Total thyroidectomy without lymph nodes dissection	4 (1.69)	
Thyroid lobectomy with lymph nodes dissection	97 (40.8)	
Thyroid lobectomy without lymph nodes dissection	48 (20.2)	
Patients who used nano-carbon during surgery	110 (46.2)	
Identified parathyroid glands during total thyroidectomy, No.		
1	1 (1.1)	n=93
2	1 (1.1)	
3	34 (36.6)	
4	57 (61.3)	
Identified parathyroid glands during thyroid lobectomy, No.		
0	1 (0.7)	n=145
1	26 (17.9)	
2	118 (81.4)	
Autotransplanted parathyroid glands, No.		
0	215 (90.3)	
1	21 (8.8)	
2	2 (0.8)	
Inadvertently resected parathyroid glands	1 (0.4)	
Parathyroid hormone[a] in fine-needle aspiration washout fluids of parathyroid, median (IQR), mg/dL	264 (198-367)	
Postoperative Variables		
Final diagnosis		
Benign condition	47 (19.7)	
Malignant condition	198 (83.2)	
Postoperative hypocalcemia at postoperative day 1 or 2	49 (20.6)	
Nadir of postoperative calcium, median (IQR), mg/dL	8.54 (8.21-9.07)	
Parathyroid hormone at postoperative day 1, median (IQR), pg/ml	24.6 (17.8-34.5)	
Hypocalcemia at postoperative 1 month	2[b]	

BMI, body mass index (calculated as weight in kilograms divided by height in meters squared); IQR, interquartile range. SI conversion factor: To convert calcium to mmol/L, multiply by 0.25; to convert parathyroid hormone to ng/L, multiply by 1. [a]Parathyroid hormone was tested by the rapid parathyroid hormone detection based on immune colloidal gold technique. [b]There were 4 losses in the follow-up period.

in pathology, and 1 tissue was thyroid (**Figure 2**). An inadvertently resected PG was found in the regular specimens sent for the final pathological examination.

Based on the pathological and aIOPTH results, the sensitivity of NIRAF to detect PGs (568 of 596 PGs; 95.30%) was significantly higher than that of vision (517 of 596 PGs; 86.74%, $P<.001$). Out of 841 suspected parathyroid tissues, there were 595 PGs, 167 lymph nodes, 77 adipose tissues and 2 thyroid tissues (**Figure 2**). The accuracy rate of NIRAF (764 of 841 tissues; 90.84%) was significantly higher than that of vision (567 of 841 tissues; 67.42%, $P<.001$) (**Supplementary Table 1**).

Combined with the final parathyroid identification results, a retrospective analysis was performed on the selected 331 fluorescent images. The mean fluorescence intensity was 74.19 ± 17.82 for parathyroid tissue in 331 images, 63.24 ± 17.53 for thyroid tissue in 331 images, 48.22 ± 15.31 for adipose tissue in 266 images, and 33.97 ± 10.64 for lymph nodes in 167 images (**Figure 3**). The fluorescence intensity of the parathyroid was significantly higher than that of other tissues in paired samples. The mean increase in parathyroid fluorescence intensity was 10.96 (95% CI, 9.18-12.73) with thyroid tissue ($P<.001$), 26.49 (95% CI, 24.63-28.36) with adipose tissue ($P<.001$), and 40.30

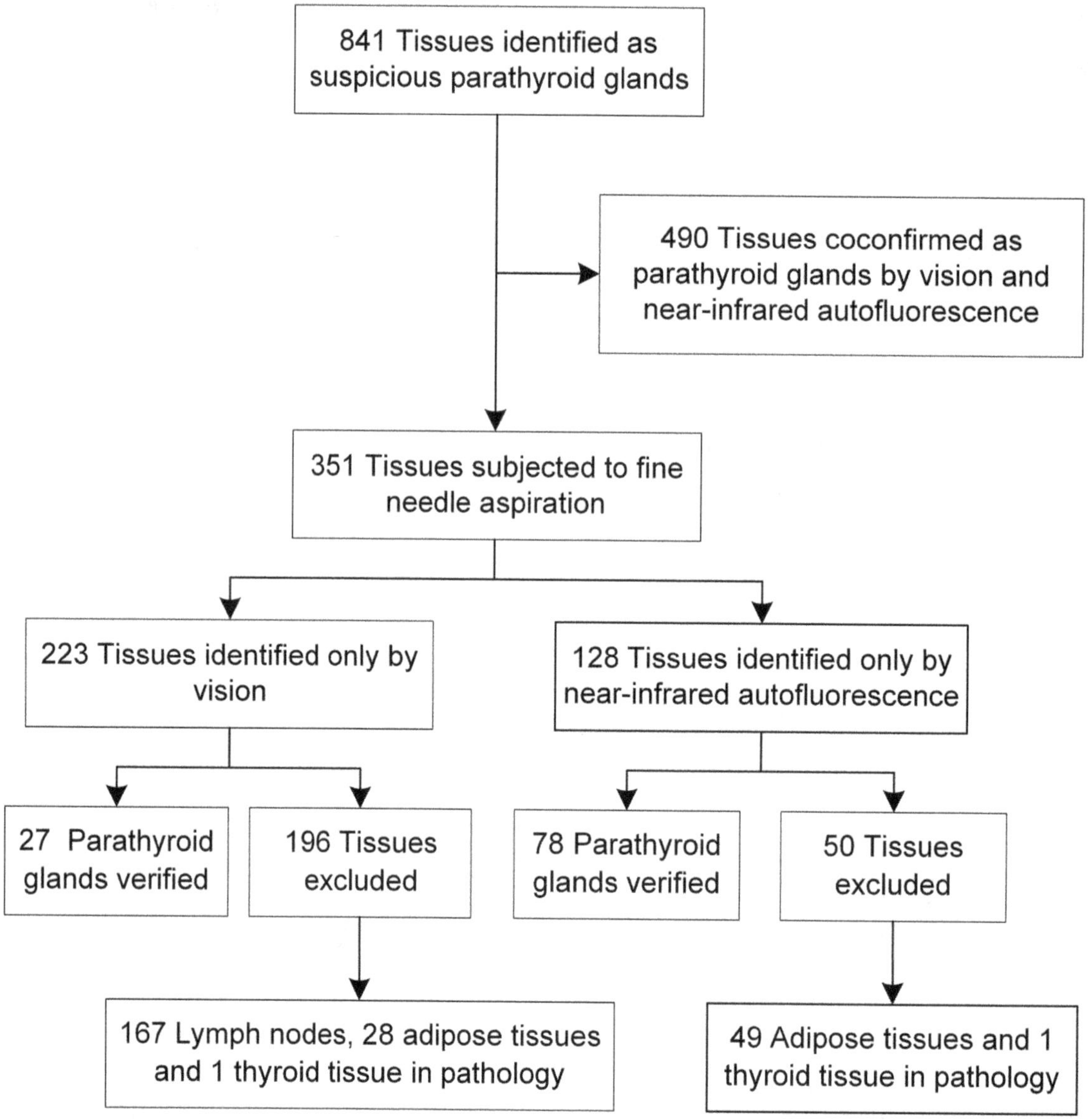

FIGURE 2 | The verification process of 841 suspicious parathyroid tissues.

(95% CI, 38.00-15.02) with lymph node tissue ($P<.001$) (**Supplementary Table 2**).

The lateral neck dissection specimens of 22 patients were sorted according to the autofluorescence intensity. The final pathological results showed that there were 536 lymph nodes in the tissues with low fluorescence intensity. No lymph nodes were found in the tissues with high fluorescence intensity (**Figure 4**).

DISCUSSION

To date, the highest quality of evidence on the effect of NIRAF comes from a multicenter randomized controlled study published by Benmiloud et al. (4), which showed that the rate of postoperative low calcium was significantly lower than that of the control group (from 26% to 11%). The rate of postoperative hypocalcemia after using NIRAF in our study was 20.6%. Our study included a higher proportion of patients with malignant tumors (83.2% *vs* 25.6%), and lymph node dissection was performed in most patients (186 of 238 patients, 78%), which led to a higher rate of postoperative hypocalcemia. However, the mean number of PGs found on each side of the thyroid in their study was 1.61 (390 PGs of 242 patients), compared to 1.80 (595 PGs of 331 patients) in our study. We found more PGs benefiting from the use of nanocarbon but the incidence of postoperative hypocalcemia increased, which indicated that the scope of the operation and protection of the parathyroid blood supply also had a crucial impact (14, 15). The effect of NIRAF is limited to the identification of PGs. Therefore, in evaluating the effect of

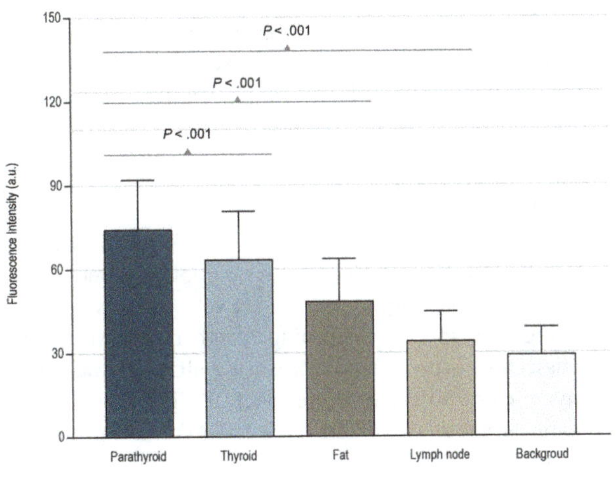

FIGURE 3 | Paired-samples t-test of fluorescence intensity in different tissues.

this technique, the number of identified PGs during surgery is a more direct variable.

The innovation of this study is the introduction of aIOPTH as a confirmatory method for PGs. The application of aIOPTH may provide an alternative to frozen section examination, dodging the injurious effect of the bioptic process and achieving similar or even more accurate results (16–18). However, the application of aIOPTH is not widespread, many endocrine surgeons are not familiar with this technology, and traditional PTH detection methods take much time (19). The rapid PTH detection method used in this study only takes approximately 10 minutes. In actual use, the test strip can turn red in an even shorter time with a positive result. When the cut-off value is 130 pg/mL, this method has proven to be highly consistent with pathological results in identifying PGs (20, 21). It has already been widely used in China and written in the 2018 perioperative parathyroid function protection guidelines for thyroid surgery by the Chinese Thyroid Association. Comparing the pathological results, aIOPTH achieved 100% specificity in our study.

To date, most studies have used visual recognition to confirm PGs due to ethical limitations. The results showed that NIRAF had extremely high sensitivity in identifying PGs (from 76% to 100%) (5, 8, 22). Most studies found that NIRAF could detect PGs before vision in nearly two-thirds of cases (4, 8, 23). Our study concluded that the sensitivity of NIRAF for identifying PGs was 95% by combining aIOPTH results and pathological results, and in the inconsistent cases between vision and NIRAF, the accuracy of NIRAF was 90.84%, while the accuracy of vision was only 67%, indicating that NIRAF was more trustworthy. Among the co-confirmed PGs, 88 PGs were first detected by NIRAF, and 78 PGs were found only by NIRAF. Therefore, of the 596 PGs found in the trial, the surgeon benefited from NIRAF in identifying 166 (28%) PGs.

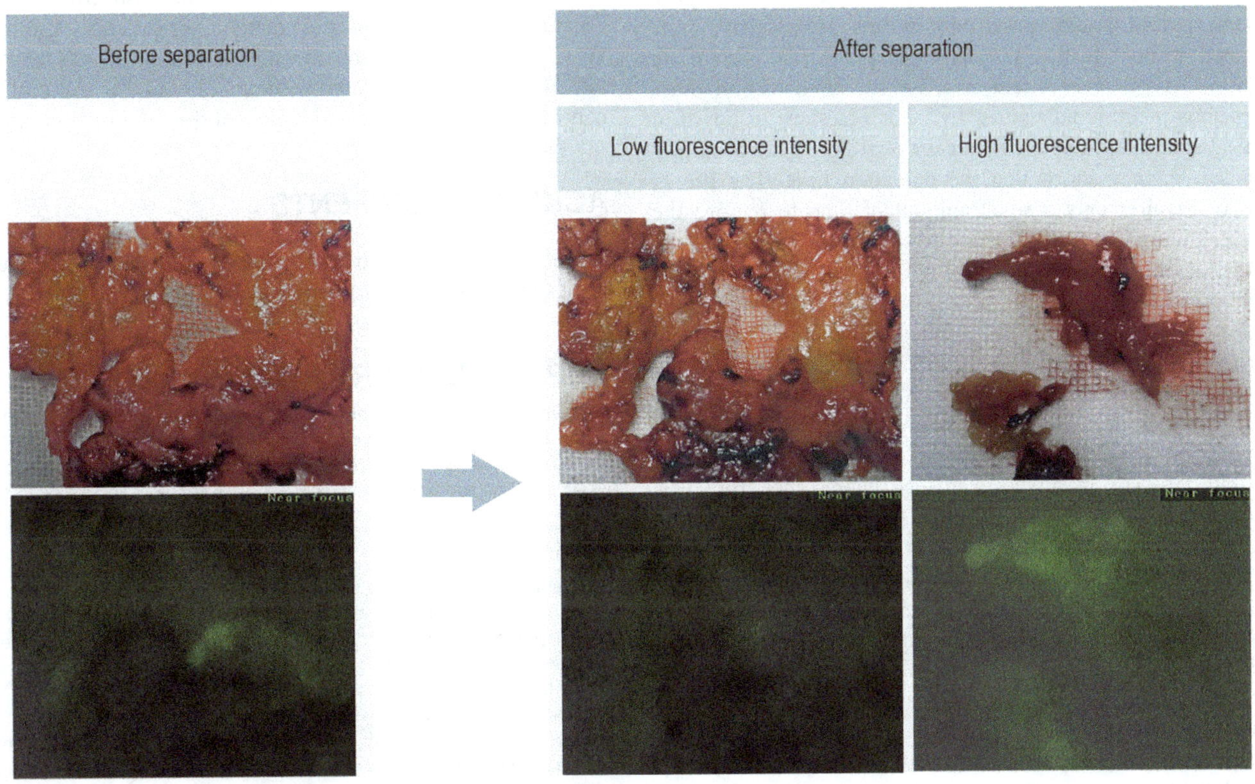

FIGURE 4 | Fluorescence imaging of lateral neck lymph node dissection specimens.

By comparing the fluorescence intensity of different tissues, we found that the autofluorescence intensity of the thyroid gland was closest to that of the PG (74.19 ± 17.82 *vs* 63.24 ± 17.53). This is concordant with a study by Falco et al. (22). The phenomenon that the autofluorescence intensity of the thyroid gland occasionally approaches or even exceeds the PG during surgery often affects the detection of PGs, and we suppressed the autofluorescence of the thyroid by injecting nanocarbon into the thyroid gland, thereby improving the fluorescence contrast of the PGs.

Of note, there was a significant difference in the autofluorescence intensity of the parathyroid and lymph nodes (74.19 ± 17.82 *vs* 33.97 ± 10.64), which is consistent with the result from Shinden et al. (24). Therefore, no lymph nodes were found in the 50 NIRAF false-positive tissues. Furthermore, we used NIRAF to sort out the tissues with no obvious fluorescence in lateral neck lymph node dissection, in which 536 lymph nodes were found pathologically. Meanwhile, no lymph nodes were found in the tissues with strong fluorescence intensity. We conclude from this result that the fluorescence intensity of lymph nodes is pretty weak compared to that of PGs. Lymph nodes are often misidentified as PGs during thyroid surgery. Of the 196 visual false-positive tissues in this study, 167 were lymph nodes. The surgical strategy of retaining all tissues with strong fluorescence intensity will help ensure a thorough dissection of lymph nodes, thereby reducing the tumor residue caused by misidentifying lymph nodes as PGs.

A total of 351 fine-needle aspirations were performed in 238 patients. According to the final result, the tissues with strong fluorescence intensity are mostly parathyroid and adipose tissues, thyroid tissues appear only in rare cases, which can be retained without further testing. During the trial, even if we identified a PG in a certain area, we still tried to find other suspicious parathyroid tissues. It is not necessary to do so in clinical applications, so the frequency of aIOPTH can be largely reduced, thereby shortening the operation time. The use of NIRAF requires only a small amount of time to remove the surgical lamp. Therefore, the use of NIRAF and aIOPTH technology in thyroid surgery will not significantly increase the duration of surgery.

To date, NIRAF has satisfied but not perfect sensitivity and specificity in published studies (10, 25). However, the strong fluorescence of thyroid sometimes may cover the fluorescence of PGs and thus decrease the sensitivity of NIRAF. The use of nanocarbon can solve the problem. Meanwhile, aIOPTH can separate false-positive tissues with high fluorescence from PGs and enhance the specificity. All these measures are time-saving and easy to implement. These methods along with NIRAF form a perfect complement in thyroid surgery, which can effectively find atypical PGs and prevent them from being inadvertently resected.

This case series study, despite its careful experimental design, strict quality control, and a large number of patients, is still not enough to show that this new surgical strategy can improve the number of identified PGs. Therefore, we plan to conduct a further randomized controlled study to illustrate this issue. Another drawback is that we did not puncture the PGs identified by both vision and NIRAF, which is mainly based on the purpose of reducing parathyroid damage. Although fine-needle biopsy poses minimal damage to the tissue, there is still a report that such puncture may cause secondary lesions of the PGs (26).

CONCLUSIONS

In conclusion, we evaluated the effect of NIRAF in identifying PGs in thyroid surgery through a large-sample case series. Using NIRAF in thyroid surgery can effectively assist surgeons in identifying PGs and distinguishing lymph nodes when lymph node dissection is performed. Measuring aIOPTH was an ideal objective method to evaluate the effect of NIRAF. It may work with nanocarbon as complements to NIRAF and thus improves the sensitivity and specificity.

ETHICS STATEMENT

The studies involving human participants were reviewed and approved by The institutional review board of the First Affiliated Hospital of Zhengzhou University. The patients/participants provided their written informed consent to participate in this study.

AUTHOR CONTRIBUTIONS

Conception and design: ZL and D-tY. Administrative support: ZL and D-tY. Provision of study materials or patients: ZL and D-tY. Collection and assembly of data: ZL, R-sM, J-lJ, TW, and D-hZ. Data analysis and interpretation: ZL and J-lJ. All authors contributed to the article and approved the submitted version.

ACKNOWLEDGMENTS

The authors would like to acknowledge the support of colleagues from the operation department.

SUPPLEMENTARY MATERIAL

Supplementary Table 1 | Comparing the sensitivity and accuracy of NIRAF with vision in identifying parathyroid glands. PGs parathyroid glands; [a]The sensitivity of NIRAF was significantly higher than vision in 596 parathyroid glands, *P*<.001. [b]The accuracy of NIRAF was significantly higher than vision in 841 suspected parathyroid tissues. *P*<.001

Supplementary Table 2 | Paired-samples t-test of fluorescence intensity in different tissues.

Supplementary Figure 1 | Fluorescence imaging device and operating environment. The operating room illuminated by LED light sources does not need to turn off the light, only needs to remove the operating lamp, but the operating room illuminated by a halogen lamp needs to turn off the light source. During the NIRAF imaging process, it is necessary to avoid the camera shooting of the surgery field, which will cause the flicker of the fluorescent image. The electrocautery should be used with caution during the operation to reduce the generation of eschar, which has extremely strong autofluorescence under fluorescent imaging.

Supplementary Figure 2 | Test strip and parathyroid hormone detector for measuring intraoperative parathyroid hormone in fine-needle aspiration biopsy washings. **(A)** Control line **(B)** Test line **(C)** Reaction zone. The test line requires a 10-minute incubation time to reach a stable final result, but in most cases, the test line can turn red in a shorter time with a positive result. Parathyroid hormone detector is not needed if exact values are not required

Supplementary Video 1 | Intraoperative near-infrared autofluorescence imaging of parathyroid glands. The NIRAF probe is wrapped with a sterile lens cover, and the surgeon holds the NIRAF probe with one hand to perform fluorescence imaging of the surgical field. The operating room lighting can be kept after removing the surgical lamp from the surgical field.

Supplementary Video 2 | Measuring intraoperative parathyroid hormone in fine-needle aspiration biopsy washings of the suspicious parathyroid gland. The suspicious tissue with strong fluorescence intensity was punctured with a 1 ml syringe containing 0.1 ml saline and then drip the 0.1 ml saline through the needle onto the reaction area of the test strip.

REFERENCES

1. Liu JB, Sosa JA, Grogan RH, Liu Y, Cohen ME, Ko CY, et al. Variation of Thyroidectomy-Specific Outcomes Among Hospitals and Their Association With Risk Adjustment and Hospital Performance. *JAMA Surg* (2018) 153:1–10. doi: 10.1001/jamasurg.2017.4593
2. Abbaci M, De Leeuw F, Breuskin I, Casiraghi O, Lakhdar AB, Ghanem W, et al. Parathyroid Gland Management Using Optical Technologies During Thyroidectomy or Parathyroidectomy: A Systematic Review. *Oral Oncol* (2018) 87:186–96. doi: 10.1016/j.oraloncology.2018.11.011
3. Rudin AV, Berber E. Impact of Fluorescence and Autofluorescence on Surgical Strategy in Benign and Malignant Neck Endocrine Diseases. *Best Pract Res Clin Endocrinol Metab* (2019) 33:101311. doi: 10.1016/j.beem.2019.101311
4. Benmiloud F, Godiris-Petit G, Gras R, Gillot JC, Turrin N, Penaranda G, et al. Association of Autofluorescence-Based Detection of the Parathyroid Glands During Total Thyroidectomy With Postoperative Hypocalcemia Risk: Results of the PARAFLUO Multicenter Randomized Clinical Trial. *JAMA Surg* (2019) 155:106–12. doi: 10.1001/jamasurg.2019.4613
5. Benmiloud F, Rebaudet S, Varoquaux A, Penaranda G, Bannier M, Denizot A. Impact of Autofluorescence-Based Identification of Parathyroids During Total Thyroidectomy on Postoperative Hypocalcemia: A Before and After Controlled Study. *Surg (United States)* (2018) 163:23–30. doi: 10.1016/j.surg.2017.06.022
6. Dip F, Falco J, Verna S, Prunello M, Loccisano M, Quadri P, et al. Randomized Controlled Trial Comparing White Light With Near-Infrared Autofluorescence for Parathyroid Gland Identification During Total Thyroidectomy. *J Am Coll Surg* (2019) 228:744–51. doi: 10.1016/j.jamcollsurg.2018.12.044
7. Kose E, Rudin AV, Kahramangil B, Moore E, Aydin H, Donmez M, et al. Autofluorescence Imaging of Parathyroid Glands: An Assessment of Potential Indications. *Surg (United States)* (2019) 228:744–51. doi: 10.1016/j.surg.2019.04.072
8. Kahramangil B, Dip F, Benmiloud F, Falco J, de la Fuente M, Verna S, et al. Detection of Parathyroid Autofluorescence Using Near-Infrared Imaging: A Multicenter Analysis of Concordance Between Different Surgeons. *Ann Surg Oncol* (2018) 25:957–62. doi: 10.1245/s10434-018-6364-2
9. McWade MA, Sanders ME, Broome JT, Solórzano CC, Mahadevan-Jansen A. Establishing the Clinical Utility of Autofluorescence Spectroscopy for Parathyroid Detection. *Surg (United States)* (2016) 159:193–203. doi: 10.1016/j.surg.2015.06.047
10. Wang B, Zhu C-R, Liu H, Yao X-M, Wu J. The Accuracy of Near Infrared Autofluorescence in Identifying Parathyroid Gland During Thyroid and Parathyroid Surgery: A Meta-Analysis. *Front Endocrinol (Lausanne)* (2021) 12:701253. doi: 10.3389/fendo.2021.701253
11. Squires MH, Shirley LA, Shen C, Jarvis R, Phay JE. Intraoperative Autofluorescence Parathyroid Identification in Patients With Multiple Endocrine Neoplasia Type 1. *JAMA Otolaryngol - Head Neck Surg* (2019) 145:897–902. doi: 10.1001/jamaoto.2019.1987
12. Kose E, Kahramangil B, Aydin H, Donmez M, Berber E. Heterogeneous and Low-Intensity Parathyroid Autofluorescence: Patterns Suggesting Hyperfunction at Parathyroid Exploration. *Surg (United States)* (2019) 165:431–7. doi: 10.1016/j.surg.2018.08.006
13. Trimboli P, D'Aurizio F, Tozzoli R, Giovanella L. Measurement of Thyroglobulin, Calcitonin, and PTH in FNA Washout Fluids. *Clin Chem Lab Med* (2017) 55:914–25. doi: 10.1515/cclm-2016-0543
14. Giordano D, Valcavi R, Thompson GB, Pedroni C, Renna L, Gradoni P, et al. Complications of Central Neck Dissection in Patients With Papillary Thyroid Carcinoma: Results of a Study on 1087 Patients and Review of the Literature. *Thyroid* (2012) 22:911–7. doi: 10.1089/thy.2012.0011
15. Wang X, Xing T, Wei T, Zhu J. Completion Thyroidectomy and Total Thyroidectomy for Differentiated Thyroid Cancer: Comparison and Prediction of Postoperative Hypoparathyroidism. *J Surg Oncol* (2016) 113:522–5. doi: 10.1002/jso.24159
16. Shawky MS. Quick Parathyroid Hormone Assays: A Comprehensive Review of Their Utility in Clinical Practice. *Hormones* (2016) 15:355–67. doi: 10.14310/horm.2002.1689
17. Ketha H, Lasho MA, Algeciras-Schimnich A. Analytical and Clinical Validation of Parathyroid Hormone (PTH) Measurement in Fine-Needle Aspiration Biopsy (FNAB) Washings. *Clin Biochem* (2016) 49:16–21. doi: 10.1016/j.clinbiochem.2015.09.006
18. Pelizzo MR, Losi A, Boschin IM, Toniato A, Pennelli G, Sorgato N, et al. Rapid Intraoperative Parathyroid Hormone Assay in Fine Needle Aspiration for Differential Diagnosis in Thyroid and Parathyroid Surgery. *Clin Chem Lab Med* (2010) 48:1313–7. doi: 10.1515/CCLM.2010.247
19. Coan KE, Yen TWF, Carr AA, Evans DB, Wang TS. Confirmation of Parathyroid Tissue: Are Surgeons Aware of New and Novel Techniques? *J Surg Res* (2020) 246:139–44. doi: 10.1016/j.jss.2019.08.006
20. James BC, Nagar S, Tracy M, Kaplan EL, Angelos P, Scherberg NH, et al. A Novel, Ultrarapid Parathyroid Hormone Assay to Distinguish Parathyroid From Nonparathyroid Tissue. *Surg (United States)* (2014) 156:1638–43. doi: 10.1016/j.surg.2014.08.081
21. Wei H, Huang M, Fan J, Wang T, Ling R. Intraoperative Rapid Aspiration Cytological Method for Parathyroid Glands Identification and Protection. *Endocr J* (2019) 66:135–41. doi: 10.1507/endocrj.EJ18-0363
22. Falco J, Dip F, Quadri P, de la Fuente M, Prunello M, Rosenthal RJ. Increased Identification of Parathyroid Glands Using Near Infrared Light During Thyroid and Parathyroid Surgery. *Surg Endosc* (2017) 31:3737–42. doi: 10.1007/s00464-017-5424-1
23. Kim SW, Lee HS, Ahn YC, Park CW, Jeon SW, Kim CH, et al. Near-Infrared Autofluorescence Image-Guided Parathyroid Gland Mapping in Thyroidectomy. *J Am Coll Surg* (2018) 226:165–72. doi: 10.1016/j.jamcollsurg.2017.10.015
24. Shinden Y, Nakajo A, Arima H, Tanoue K, Hirata M, Kijima Y, et al. Intraoperative Identification of the Parathyroid Gland With a Fluorescence Detection System. *World J Surg* (2017) 41:1506–12. doi: 10.1007/s00268-017-3903-0
25. Solórzano CC, Thomas G, Baregamian N, Mahadevan-Jansen A. Detecting the Near Infrared Autofluorescence of the Human Parathyroid: Hype or Opportunity? *Ann Surg* (2020) 272:973–85. doi: 10.1097/SLA.0000000000003700
26. Kim J, Horowitz G, Hong M, Orsini M, Asa SL, Higgins K. The Dangers of Parathyroid Biopsy. *J Otolaryngol - Head Neck Surg* (2017) 46:2–5. doi: 10.1186/s40463-016-0178-7

2

Intraoperative Management of the Recurrent Laryngeal Nerve Transected or Invaded by Thyroid Cancer

Hiroo Masuoka and Akira Miyauchi*

Department of Surgery, Kuma Hospital Center for Excellence in Thyroid Care, Kobe, Japan

***Correspondence:**
Hiroo Masuoka
masuoka@kuma-h.or.jp

Thyroid cancer often invades the recurrent laryngeal nerve (RLN), causing vocal cord paralysis. In such patients, the invaded portion of the RLN usually needs to be resected through curative surgery. We attempt to preserve the nerve by performing sharp dissection in such cases. During nerve dissection, an intraoperative nerve monitoring system helps identify the course of the RLN in the fibrous tissue around the tumor or even within the tumor, and also helps evaluate the nerve integrity. Because of extensive dissection, the preserved RLN may become much thinner than its original thickness. We refer to this procedure as "partial layer resection" of the RLN. In our cases, although the dissected RLNs became thinner, we found that vocal cord function recovered in most patients. If the RLN is fully involved by thyroid cancer or response of the vocal cord against electric stimulation to the RLN is lost, we resect the portion of the RLN together with the tumor and repair it using one of the reconstruction techniques. When a unilateral RLN is resected, the vocal cord on that side is paralyzed. Symptoms include hoarseness, mis-swallowing, and short phonation. RLN reconstruction using one of the reconstruction techniques leads to the recovery of phonatory and swallowing function, although the normal motion of the vocal cord on the side of the anastomosis is not restored. We used direct anastomosis, free nerve grafting, ansa cervicalis-RLN anastomosis, and vagus-RLN anastomosis to reconstruct the RLN. Thyroid cancer often invades the RLN near the Berry's ligament. In such patients, surgeons might assume that reconstruction of the RLN may not be possible because the peripheral stump of the RLN cannot be observed. However, if we divide the inferior pharyngeal constrictor muscles along the lateral edge of the thyroid cartilage, the peripheral RLN can be identified, and nerve reconstruction can be performed. We refer to this procedure as "laryngeal approach".In summary, of the patients with thyroid cancer who required resection of the RLN, RLN reconstruction led to the recovery of phonatory function. We suggest that all thyroid surgeons familiarize themselves with these reconstruction techniques.

Keywords: Recurrent Laryngeal Nerve, reconstruction, Intraoperative neural monitoring (IONM), laryngeal approach, partial layer resection

INTRODUCTION

Thyroid cancer often invades the recurrent laryngeal nerve (RLN), causing vocal cord paralysis (VCP). In such patients, the invaded portion of the RLN usually needs to be resected through curative surgery. Even in patients with functional vocal cords preoperatively, RLN may be involved when performing thyroid surgery for thyroid cancer. We attempt to preserve the nerve by performing sharp dissection in such cases. Nishida et al. reported that preservation of the RLN invaded by differentiated thyroid cancer with sharp dissection rarely causes local recurrence (1). Our results are in accordance with those of their report.

In recent years, we have routinely used an intraoperative neural monitoring system to evaluate the integrity of the inferior laryngeal nerve (RLN) and external branches of the superior laryngeal nerve during thyroid surgery (2). This system helps assess the electrophysiological response of the RLN prior to dissection. If the response is normal, we try preserving the RLN by shaving off the tumor (3). During nerve dissection, an intraoperative nerve monitoring system helps identify the course of the RLN in the fibrous tissue around the tumor or even within the tumor and also helps evaluate the nerve integrity. If the response is weakened or lost, we resect the portion of the RLN together with the tumor and repair it using one of the reconstruction techniques described below.

In the personal case series of one of the authors (Miyauchi A.), among 721 primary thyroid cancer cases treated between 1998 to 2008, 4.3% of the patients presented with VCP preoperatively, and even in patients with functioning vocal cords preoperatively, 2.2% required resection of the RLN because of cancer invasion. Therefore, in total, 6.4% of the patients required resection of the RLN (**Table 1**). If a unilateral RLN is severed or fully injured, the vocal cord on that side is paralyzed. It remains fixed in a paramedian position, becomes atrophied, and loses its tension during phonation. Symptoms include hoarseness, mis-swallowing, and short phonation due to the waste of exhaled air during phonation. Aspiration can be a dangerous symptom, particularly among elderly patients.

We reported vocal improvement after various methods of RLN reconstruction, although normal vocal cords movements were not restored (4, 5).

Here, we describe how to manage the RLN invaded by thyroid cancer.

PARTIAL LAYER RESECTION OF THE RLN

Because of extensive dissection, the preserved RLN may become much thinner than its original thickness (**Figure 1**). We refer to this procedure as "partial layer resection" of the RLN. In our case, although the dissected RLNs became thinner, we found that vocal cord function recovered in most patients. We reviewed our medical records and found that 18 patients underwent partial layer resection of the RLN to remove thyroid cancer. Postoperatively, two (11%) patients had no VCP, 13 (72%) patients had temporary VCP followed by full recovery of vocal cord function, and only three (17%) patients had permanent VCP (6). These unexpected outcomes prompted us to study the anatomy of the RLN. We studied the histology of the cross-sections of the normal portions of RLNs resected due to thyroid cancer invasion. We found that the true nerve component was surrounded by thick perineural tissue (**Figure 2**). This anatomy may explain the favorable outcomes obtained after partial layer resection of RLNs (6). Even in cases where the preserved RLN becomes thinner than its original thickness following extensive shaving, we concluded that it is worth preserving the nerve if it was functioning well preoperatively.

RECONSTRUCTION OF THE TRANSECTED OR RESECTED RLN

Methods of Reconstruction of the RLN

In 2009, Miyauchi A., one of the co-authors in this paper, reported improvement in phonation following RLN reconstruction performed during thyroid surgery in 88 patients with thyroid cancer invading the nerve in his personal series from 1984 to 2007 at Kuma Hospital or Kagawa Medical University Hospital (7). The patients included 72 women and 16 men aged 18–78 years with a mean age of 55.6 years. Of the patients, 51 (58%) underwent preoperative VCP. Seven patients underwent a second surgery for recurrent disease, while the others were primary cases. We used direct anastomosis (DA), free nerve grafting (FNG), ansa cervicalis-RLN anastomosis (ARA), and vagus-RLN anastomosis (VRA) to reconstruct the RLN (**Figure 3**). ARA was performed in most patients (n=65; 74%). DA was performed in only seven patients, FNG was performed in 14 patients, and VRA was attempted in two patients in whom both the unilateral RLN and its ipsilateral vagus nerve required resection due to cancer invasion. In 3 FNG cases and 31 ARA cases, anastomosis was performed behind the thyroid cartilage. In 8 ARA cases, anastomosis was performed using the contralateral ansa cervicalis. Surgical loupes at 2.5 × magnification were used in 51 patients. The operating microscope was used in 10 patients, and no magnifier was used in 27 patients. The thickness of the thread used for anastomosis ranged from 6-0 to 9-0, with 8-0 being the most common thickness. He generally used three stitches for end-to-end anastomosis of the nerves and used microsurgical instruments to construct the anastomosis. At Kuma Hospital, we use 8-0 monofilament thread and microsurgery instruments and encouraged the use of surgical loupes at 2.5 × magnification.

TABLE 1 | Number (%) of patients who required resection of the recurrent laryngeal nerve in A.M.'s personal series from 1998 to 2008 consisting of primary thyroid cancer cases.

	VCP preoperatively		
	No	Yes	Total
No. of patients	690 (95.7%)	31 (4.3%)	721 (100.0%)
Patients with RLN resection	16 (2.2%)	30 (4.2%)	46 (6.4%)

VCP, vocal cord paralysis.

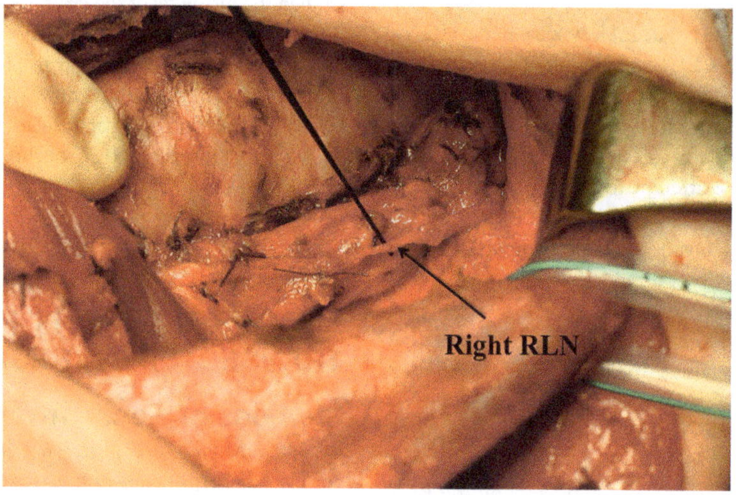

FIGURE 1 | The recurrent laryngeal nerve after partial layer resection. Due to extensive resection, the recurrent laryngeal nerve became much thinner than its original thickness.

In patients with extensive node metastases, the ansa cervicalis on the same side may not be available. In such cases, the contralateral ansa cervicalis can be used for reconstruction. In cases, we inserted a suction tube between the trachea and the esophagus, sucked the contralateral ansa cervicalis into the tube, and then brought it to the side of the defect, where we made a contralateral ansa cervicalis-to-RLN anastomosis (**Figure 4**) (8). This route appears to be the shortest for performing the anastomosis. If the contralateral ansa cervicalis is too short, the FNG technique can be combined for safe anastomosis. However, this would require a longer time for reinnervation of the vocal cords and recovery during phonation. Furthermore, avoiding tension on anastomoses is key to this procedure.

Evaluation of the Reconstructed RLN

Although we examined all patients using a fiberoptic laryngoscope after surgery, a laryngoscopic examination is not suitable for evaluating the recovery of vocal cord function because vocal cords do not return to normal motion after reconstruction of the RLN. Serial measurements of maximum phonation time (MPT) are the easiest and most practical method for evaluating recovery in phonation. We used the MPT one year after surgery to evaluate the outcomes. Thirty-four healthy subjects (26 women and eight men) and 27 patients (18 women and nine men) with unilateral VCP served as controls. Serial measurements of the MPT showed a sudden increase in MPT, usually around 3 months after surgery, when the patient's voice improved. The MPTs were significantly

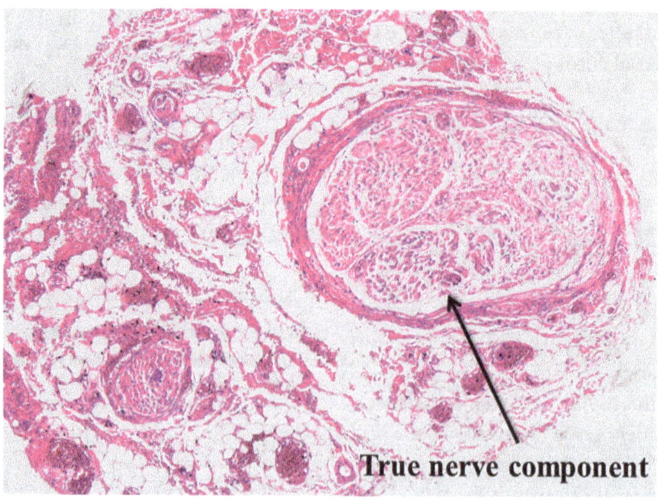

FIGURE 2 | Microscopic cross-section of the normal portion of the recurrent laryngeal nerve resected due to invasion by thyroid cancer. The true nerve component is surrounded by thick peri-neural tissue.

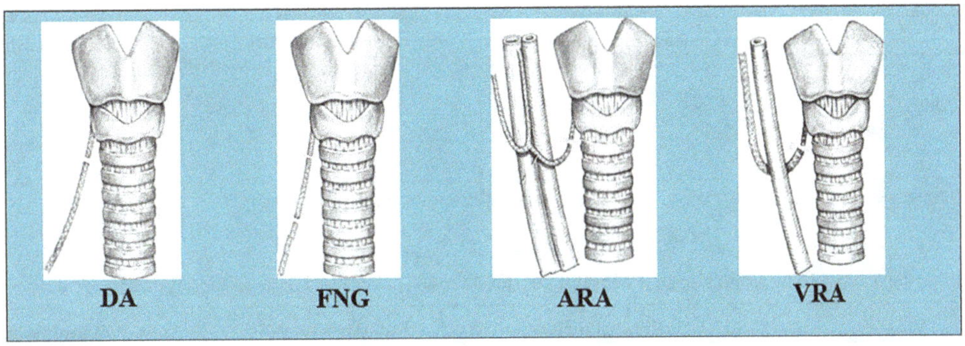

FIGURE 3 | Methods of reconstruction of the RLN used in this series: DA, direct anastomosis; FNG, free nerve grafting; ARA, ansa cervicalis-RLN anastomosis; VRA, vagus-RLN anastomosis.

shorter in patients with VCP than in healthy subjects. Normal MPT values were achieved in patients who underwent RLN reconstruction (**Table 2**) (7).

There were significant sex-specific differences in MPT in healthy subjects and in patients with VCP (**Table 2**). The MPT divided by the VC ratio (sec/L) indicates the vocal cord function of converting a unit volume of exhaled air to a certain length of phonation. This value is called the phonation efficiency index (PEI) (7). When PEIs were calculated, the sex-specific differences in healthy subjects and patients with VCP disappeared completely. It was noted that patients with VCP had significantly smaller PEIs than the healthy subjects. Nearly normal PEI values were achieved in patients who underwent RLN reconstruction (**Table 3**) (7) . Since PEI did not differ based on sex, this value is considered suitable for evaluating vocal cord function regardless of the patient's sex. We analyzed factors that might be related to PEI one year after surgery, such as age at surgery, presence or absence of VCP preoperatively, method of RLN reconstruction, use of magnifier, and thread thickness. None of these factors significantly affected PEI one year after surgery. In general, insignificant data points did not add any value to analysis. However, in this case, they highlighted a very crucial idea. These data indicated that regardless of age or the presence/absence of VCP preoperatively, reconstruction of the transected RLN using any method/technique can help recover the patients' voices to nearly normal levels.

Laryngeal Approach

Thyroid cancer often invades the RLN near the Berry's ligament. In such patients, surgeons might assume that reconstruction of the RLN may not be possible because the peripheral stump of the RLN cannot be observed. However, if we divide the inferior pharyngeal constrictor muscles along the lateral edge of the thyroid cartilage, the peripheral RLN can be identified, and nerve reconstruction can

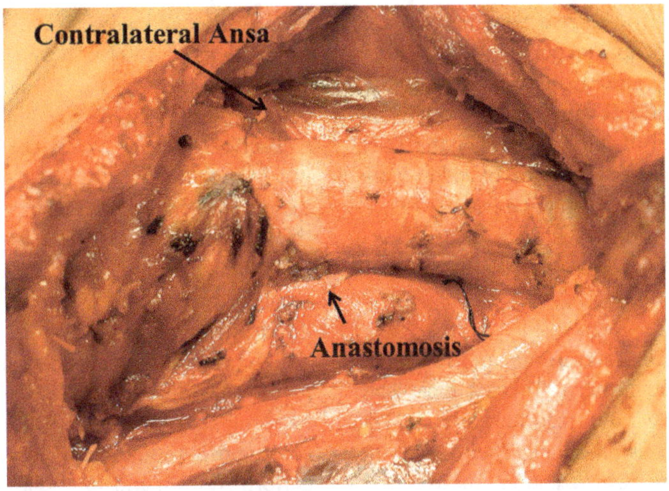

FIGURE 4 | Contralateral ansa cervicalis-to-RLN anastomosis: The contralateral ansa-cervicalis was brought to the side of the defected RLN between the trachea and the esophagus to make contralateral ansa cervicalis-to-RLN anastomosis.

TABLE 2 | Maximum phonation time in healthy subjects, patients with vocal cord paralysis, and patients who underwent reconstruction of the recurrent laryngeal nerve (9).

		Healthy subjects	Patients with VCP	Patients with RLN reconstruction
Male	No. of patients	8	9	16
	MPT	28.6±10.8	10.1±4.3	20.9±11.7
Female	No. of patients	26	18	72
	MPT	16.7±5.1	6.3±2.9	18.8±6.6

MPT, maximum phonation time; values are mean ± SD (seconds). VCP, vocal cord paralysis; RLN, recurrent laryngeal nerve.

TABLE 3 | Phonation efficiency index in healthy subjects, patients with vocal cord paralysis, and patients who underwent reconstruction of the recurrent laryngeal nerve (9).

		Healthy subjects	Patients with VCP	Patients with RLN reconstruction
Male	No. of patients	8	9	16
	PEI	6.79±2.52	3.24±1.49	5.53±2.72
Female	No. of patients	26	18	72
	PEI	6.73±2.04	3.29±1.48	7.59±2.82

PEI: phonation efficiency index; values are mean ± SD (seconds/L). VCP, vocal cord paralysis; RLN, recurrent laryngeal nerve.

be performed (10). The anterior branch should be selected for anastomosis if possible since it usually goes to the adductor muscles. Subsequently, ARA or FNG can be performed behind the thyroid cartilage. However, finding the peripheral portion of the RLN behind the thyroid cartilage after resection of the invaded portion is challenging. We modified the surgical approach to overcome this challenge by identifying the peripheral portion of the RLN by dividing the inferior pharyngeal constrictor muscle before dissecting the nerve. We refer to this procedure as "laryngeal approach (11)". This procedure is illustrated in **Figure 5**. Briefly, we made a small hole in the inferior pharyngeal constrictor muscle using electrocautery at the edge of the thyroid cartilage (**Figure 5A**). Next, we elevated the muscle using the jaws of a mosquito hemostat (**Figure 5B**) and cut the muscle with a pair of bipolar coagulators (**Figure 5C**). Next, we identified the peripheral portion of the RLN behind the thyroid cartilage (**Figure 5D**). This procedure makes dissection of the RLN invaded by thyroid cancer much easier because the RLN can be dissected from the central and peripheral sides. If only a portion of the RLN requires resection, the nerve can be readily reconstructed since the peripheral portion of the nerve is already identified and secured, and ansa cervicalis-to-RLN anastomosis can then be performed (**Figure 5E**) (5). For some special reasons, FNG can be used to fill the defect of the RLN, although this procedure requires two anastomoses. In addition, the divided pharyngeal muscle ends do not need to be fixed.

DISCUSSION

In cases where RLN is transected, surgeons can attempt its repair by direct anastomosis of the cut ends of the nerve. This is a remarkably simple idea for surgeons and was tried more than 100 years ago. The first investigators who performed this procedure reported that the movements of vocal cords were restored after anastomosis. However, other investigators later argued that this was incorrect and that recovery of vocal cord movement did not occur. As a result, anastomosis of the cut ends of the transected RLN was abandoned. However, Ezaki et al. reported that voices of seven patients recovered after direct anastomosis of the transected RLN, although their vocal cords were fixed at the median. They explained the reason behind the recovery of these patients' voices as follows (9).

The RLN includes adductor and abductor nerve fibers without special segregation of these nerve fibers within the RLN. Following anastomosis, even if the anastomosis was performed under an operating microscope, the nerves regenerated in a mixed fashion, which is called misdirected regeneration (**Figure 6**). Therefore, the adductor and abductor muscles contract simultaneously during inspiration and phonation. In the RLN, the number of adductor nerve fibers is three times the number of abductor nerve fibers. The adductor muscles in the larynx are generally much stronger than the abductor muscles. Therefore, the normal motion of the vocal cord on the side of the anastomosis was not restored. While the cord is fixed at the median, it is not paralyzed. This condition is better expressed as synkinesis, simultaneous contraction of the adductor and abductor muscles. Following reinnervation, the vocal cord recovers from atrophy and restores tension during phonation. For good phonation, a narrow gap between the vocal cords, good tension between the vocal cords, and symmetrical volume and weight of the vocal cords are necessary. Following anastomosis, all these conditions seem to be achieved. Consequently, this improves the patient's voice, increases phonation times, and reduced aspiration. However, paradoxical movements of the reinnervated vocal cord may occur in rare cases of extreme misdirection during the regeneration process.

DA is a simple procedure. However, this method can only be performed when the portion of the nerve defect is short or in cases of accidental transection of the RLN. Tension on the anastomosis should be avoided, and the anastomosis should be performed in an end-to-end fashion. If the defect portion is long, it can be repaired using a free nerve graft; however, this method requires two anastomoses. The graft can be harvested from the

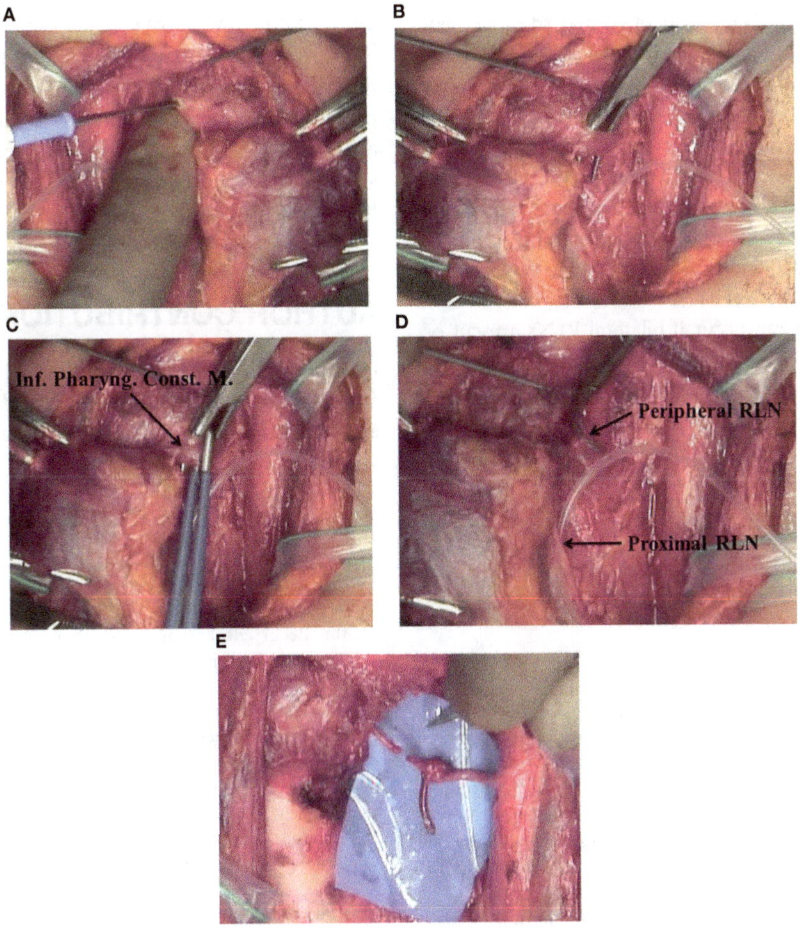

FIGURE 5 | **(A)** Laryngeal approach: Marking a hole in the inferior pharyngeal constrictor muscle at the lateral edge of the thyroid cartilage using electrocautery. **(B)** Laryngeal approach: Dissection of the inferior pharyngeal constrictor muscles along the lateral edge of the thyroid cartilage. **(C)** Laryngeal approach: Cutting the inferior pharyngeal constrictor muscles along the lateral edge of the thyroid cartilage using a pair of bipolar coagulators. **(D)** Laryngeal approach: Locating the peripheral RLN behind the thyroid cartilage. **(E)** Laryngeal approach: Performing ARA with the distal portion of the RLN that was found behind the thyroid cartilage.

supraclavicular cutaneous nerves, transcervical nerves, auricular nerves, and ansa cervicalis, irrespective of the motor or sensory nerves. If the defect extends to the mediastinum, anastomosis at the mediastinal site may be challenging or practically impossible.

In 1990, Miyauchi et al. reported ARA as their own idea (5). However, this method was previously reported by Crumley et al. in 1986 (12). The ansa cervicalis forms a loop in front of the internal jugular vein and branches into the sternothyroid, sternohyoid, and

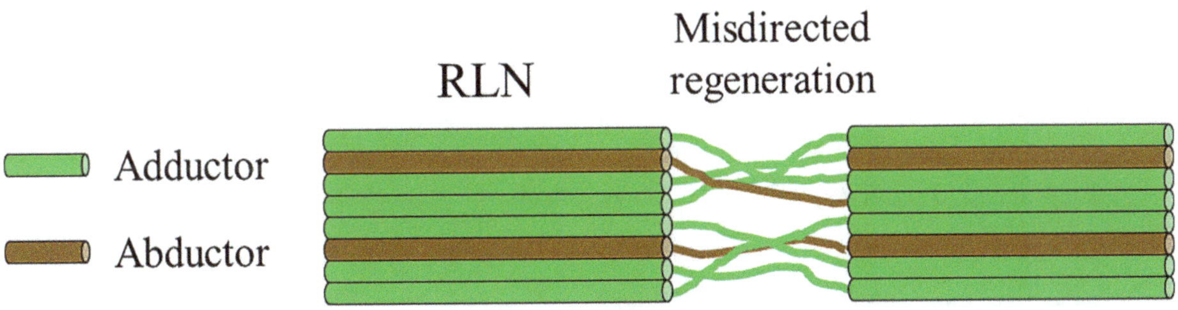

FIGURE 6 | Misdirected regeneration of the recurrent laryngeal nerve. The RLN contains adductor and abductor nerve fibers without special segregation of these nerve fibers within the RLN. Following the anastomosis, the nerve fibers regenerate in a mixed fashion.

omohyoid muscles. It is a motor nerve that is activated during phonation and respiration. The results of ARA are quite similar to those of DA of the RLN, with no recovery of vocal cord movement but recovery of phonation. Paradoxical movements of the vocal cords following ARA have never been observed. ARA requires only one anastomosis, which can be performed in an easy-to-access position of the neck near the larynx. Therefore, the time necessary for nerve regeneration and voice recovery following nerve reconstruction should also be shorter than that required for FNG. VRAs were performed in only two exceptional cases in which thyroid cancer invaded the RLN and ipsilateral vagus nerve, thus requiring resection of both nerves.

Dyspnea on inspiration can occur if bilateral RLNs are cut or injured. Depending on the degree of dyspnea, the airway may have to be opened *via* tracheostomy. Reconstruction of the RLN is not indicated for this disastrous condition because this procedure does not help restore the normal motion of the vocal cords; instead, the cords become fixated at the median position.

CONCLUSION

Of the patients with thyroid cancer who needed resection of the RLN, RLN reconstruction led to the recovery of phonatory function in nearly 90% of patients. Recovery was achieved in all patients regardless of patient characteristics, presence or absence of VCP preoperatively, reconstruction method, or surgical aid. Therefore, we suggest that all thyroid surgeons familiarize themselves with these reconstruction techniques and attempt reconstructing the RLN if necessary.

AUTHOR CONTRIBUTIONS

HM and AM designed the study. HM reviewed clinical records, and prepared the article, tables, and figures. AM revised the article. All authors contributed to the article and approved the submitted version.

REFERENCES

1. Nishida T, Nakao K, Hamaji M, Kamiike W, Kurozumi K, Matsuda H. Preservation of Recurrent Laryngeal Nerve Invaded by Differentiated Thyroid Cancer. *Ann Surg* (1997) 226:85–91. doi: 10.1097/00000658-199707000-00012
2. Randolph GW, Dralle H, Abdullah H, Barczynski M, Bellantone R, Brauckhoff M, et al. Electrophysiologic Recurrent Laryngeal Nerve Monitoring During Thyroid and Parathyroid Surgery: International Standards Guideline Statement. *Laryngoscope* (2011) 121(Supplement 1): S1–16. doi: 10.1002/lary.21119
3. Wu CW, Dionigi G, Barczynski M, Chiang FY, Dralle H, Schneider R, et al. International Neuromonitoring Study Group Guidelines 2018: Part II: Optimal Recurrent Laryngeal Nerve Management for Invasive Thyroid Cancer-Incorporation of Surgical, Laryngeal, and Neural Electrophysiologic Data. *Laryngoscope* (2018) 128(Supplement 3):S18–27. doi: 10.1002/lary.27360
4. Miyauchi A, Ishikawa H, Matsusaka K, Maeda M, Matsuzuka F, Hirai K, et al. Treatment of Recurrent Laryngeal Nerve Paralysis by Several Types of Nerve Suture. *J Jap Surg Soc* (1993) 94:550–5.
5. Miyauchi A, Matsusaka K, Kihara M, Matsuzuka F, Hirai K, Yokozawa T, et al. The Role of Ansa-to-Recurrent-Laryngeal Nerve Anastomosis in Operations for Thyroid Cancer. *Eur J Surg* (1998) 164:927–33. doi: 10.1080/110241598750005093
6. Kihara M, Miyauchi A, Yabuta T, Higashiyama T, Fukushima M, Ito Y, et al. Outcome of Vocal Cord Function After Partial Layer Resection of the Recurrent Laryngeal Nerve in Patients With Invasive Papillary Thyroid Cancer. *Surgery* (2014) 155:184–9. doi: 10.1016/j.surg.2013.06.052
7. Miyauchi A, Inoue H, Tomoda C, Fukushima M, Kihara M, Higashiyama T, et al. Improvement in Phonation After Reconstruction of the Recurrent Laryngeal Nerve in Patients With Thyroid Cancer Invading the Nerve. *Surgery* (2009) 146:1056–62. doi: 10.1016/j.surg.2009.09.018
8. Miyauchi A, Yokozawa T, Kobayashi K, Hirai K, Matsuzuka F, Kuma K, et al. Opposite Ansa Cervicalis to Recurrent Laryngeal Nerve Anastomosis to Restore Phonation in Patients With Advanced Thyroid Cancer. *Eur J Surg* (2001) 167:540–1. doi: 10.1080/110241501316914939
9. Ezaki H, Ushio H, Harada Y, Takeichi N. Recurrent Laryngeal Nerve Anastomosis Following Thyroid Surgery. *World J Surg* (1982) 6:342–6. doi: 10.1007/BF01653553
10. Miyauchi A. *Surgical Techniques in Reconstruction of Injured RLN for Voice Rehabilitation*. Tokyo: Intermerc Co. (2001).
11. Miyauchi A, Masuoka H, Tomoda C, Takamura Y, Ito Y, Kobayashi K, et al. Laryngeal Approach to the Recurrent Laryngeal Nerve Involved by Thyroid Cancer at the Ligament of Berry. *Surgery* (2012) 152:57–60. doi: 10.1016/j.surg.2011.12.033
12. Crumley RL, Izdebski K. Vocal Quality Following Laryngeal Reinnervation by Ansa Hypoglossi Transfer. *Laryngoscope* (1986) 96:611–6. doi: 10.1288/00005537-198606000-00004

3

Safety Parameters of Quantum Molecular Resonance Devices During Thyroid Surgery: Porcine Model using Continuous Neuromonitoring

Hsin-Yi Tseng[1], *Tzu-Yen Huang*[1], *Yi-Chu Lin*[1], *Jia Joanna Wang*[1,2], *How-Yun Ko*[1], *Cheng-Hsun Chuang*[1], *I-Cheng Lu*[3], *Pi-Ying Chang*[4], *Gregory W. Randolph*[5], *Gianlorenzo Dionigi*[6,7], *Ning-Chia Chang*[1,2*] *and Che-Wei Wu*[1]

[1] Department of Otorhinolaryngology-Head and Neck Surgery, International Thyroid Surgery Center, Kaohsiung Medical University Hospital, Kaohsiung Medical University, Kaohsiung, Taiwan, [2] Department of Otorhinolaryngology-Head and Neck Surgery, Kaohsiung Municipal Siaogang Hospital, Faculty of Medicine, College of Medicine, Kaohsiung Medical University, Kaohsiung, Taiwan, [3] Department of Anesthesiology, Kaohsiung Municipal Siaogang Hospital, Kaohsiung Medical University Hospital, Faculty of Medicine, College of Medicine, Kaohsiung Medical University, Kaohsiung, Taiwan, [4] Department of Anesthesiology, Kaohsiung Municipal Tatung Hospital, Kaohsiung Medical University Hospital, Faculty of Medicine, College of Medicine, Kaohsiung Medical University, Kaohsiung, Taiwan, [5] Division of Thyroid and Parathyroid Endocrine Surgery, Department of Otolaryngology—Head and Neck Surgery, Massachusetts Eye and Ear Infirmary, Harvard Medical School, Boston, MA, United States, [6] Division of General Surgery, Endocrine Surgery Section, Istituto Auxologico Italiano (IRCCS), Milan, Italy, [7] Department of Pathophysiology and Transplantation, Faculty of Medicine and Surgery, University of Milan, Milan, Italy

***Correspondence:**
Ning-Chia Chang
ncchang1972@gmail.com

Objectives: Quantum molecular resonance (QMR) devices have been applied as energy-based devices in many head and neck surgeries; however, research on their use in thyroid surgery is lacking. This study aimed to investigate the safety parameters of QMR devices during thyroidectomy when dissection was adjacent to the recurrent laryngeal nerve (RLN).

Methods: This study included eight piglets with 16 RLNs, and real-time electromyography (EMG) signals were obtained from continuous intraoperative neuromonitoring (C-IONM). QMR bipolar scissor (BS) and monopolar unit (MU) were tested for safety parameters. In the activation study, QMR devices were activated at varying distances from the RLN. In the cooling study, QMR devices were cooled for varying time intervals, with or without muscle touch maneuver (MTM) before contacting with the RLN.

Results: In the activation study, no adverse EMG change occurred when QMR BS and MU were activated at distances of 2 mm or longer from the RLNs. In the cooling study, no adverse EMG change occurred when QMR BS and MU were cooled in 2-second intervals or immediately after MTM.

Conclusion: QMR devices should be carefully used when performing RLN dissection during thyroid surgery. According to the activation and cooling safety parameters in this study, surgeons can avoid RLN injury by following standard procedures when using QMR devices.

Keywords: thyroid surgery, intraoperative neuromonitoring (IONM), recurrent laryngeal nerve (RLN), quantum molecular resonance (QMR) devices, porcine model safety parameters

INTRODUCTION

Hemostasis of the blood-rich thyroid gland is an important issue during thyroid surgery, and postoperative hematoma is a life-threatening complication that should be avoided as much as possible (1). As an equipment to assist hemostasis, many energy-based devices (EBDs) have been developed in the past 30 years and are widely used in thyroid surgery (2). High temperatures are unavoidable when using EBDs, and direct or indirect thermal energy can transfer to the recurrent laryngeal nerve (RLN) and result in thermal injury (3–5). RLN thermal injury causes more irreversible impairment of vocal cord movement than RLN mechanical injury, resulting in more voice disturbance (6, 7).

The quantum molecular resonance (QMR) device is an innovative EBD that has been safely and effectively applied in otolaryngology-head and neck surgeries such as phonomicrosurgery (8), tonsillectomy (9–11), oral surgery (12), and adenoidectomy (13). QMR devices are powered using electron energy quanta, which is generated by alternate current and high-frequency electron waves, and it is characterized by a well-defined dominant wave at 4 MHz, followed by waves at 8, 12 and 16 MHz with reduced amplitude (13, 14). As the electron energy quanta is delivered, cell molecular bonds in human tissue resonate, followed by subsequent bond breakage and a minimal temperature increase (13–16). The hemostasis of the QMR device is completed by triggering the denaturation of the protein fibrinogen to coagulate after breaking cell molecular bindings. The process also activates the physiological coagulation cascade without the need for necrotic plugs, which is contrary to methods that use other cauterization methods (13, 14). Vesalius Quantum (Telea Engineering, Vicenza, Italy) is a popular QMR system and was adopted in the current study. Two surgical instruments were most commonly used in head and neck surgery, including the QMR bipolar scissor (BS) and the QMR monopolar unit (MU). Details about Vesalius Quantum can be found at https://teleamedical.com/en/vesalius-quantum).

QMR devices have been applied as energy-based devices in many head and neck surgeries; however, research on their use in thyroid surgery and dissection adjacent to the recurrent laryngeal nerve (RLN) is lacking. The purpose of this study was to investigate real-time electromyographic (EMG) data for the RLN to define safety parameters for using a QMR device in thyroidectomy. For this purpose, we recorded the dynamic laryngeal EMG signals under continuous intraoperative neuromonitoring (C-IONM), when the QMR device was activated at various distances from the RLN in the activation study, and when the QMR device was cooled after activation for various durations with or without a muscle touch maneuver (MTM) in the cooling study.

MATERIALS AND METHODS

Animal Preparation and Anesthesia

This prospective porcine experimental study was performed by the IONM research team at Kaohsiung Medical University, Taiwan, which has a well-established C-IONM protocol for RLN research. The animal-use protocols comply with national/international regulations. Guidelines for animal experiments, including principles of replacement, reduction, and refinement, were strictly followed. This experimental study was also approved by the Institutional Animal Care and Use Committee of Kaohsiung Medical University, Taiwan (IACUC Approval No. 110129).

Anesthesia was initiated by intramuscular administration of 2 mg/kg tiletamine/zolazepam 30 minutes before the experiment. No muscle relaxants were used during anesthesia to avoid neuromuscular blockade, which could interfere with EMG signals during neuromonitoring. Endotracheal tube surface electrodes were used to record EMG signals. After the piglets were intubated, the tidal volume was set at 8–12 mL/kg, and the respiratory rate was set at 15 to 20 breaths per minute. General anesthesia was maintained with 1% to 2% sevoflurane.

IONM Equipment Setting and Operation

All piglets were placed in the supine position and intubated with a nerve integrity monitor size #6 EMG endotracheal tube (NIM Trivantage Tube, Medtronic, Jacksonville, Florida, USA). The EMG endotracheal tube as the recording electrode was applied to the piglets in the same conventional manner that it is applied to humans. The C-IONM monitoring system was performed by the Nerve Integrity Monitoring system (NIM 3.0, Medtronic, Jacksonville, Florida, USA) (**Figure 1A**). The automatic periodic stimulation (APS) as the stimulation electrode was placed on the vagus nerve (VN) (**Figure 1B**), and the nerve was stimulated continuously at 1 mA every second. The dynamic EMG signal changes during RLN injury were recorded efficiently and in real time.

The animal operation procedure began with a long transverse cervical incision, and the subcutaneous tissue and muscles were retracted away from the midline. The lateral border of the sternocleidomastoid (SCM) muscle was dissected and retracted medially. The thyroid gland, VNs, and RLNs were adequately exposed (**Figure 1B**). Next, RLNs were dissected and freed from

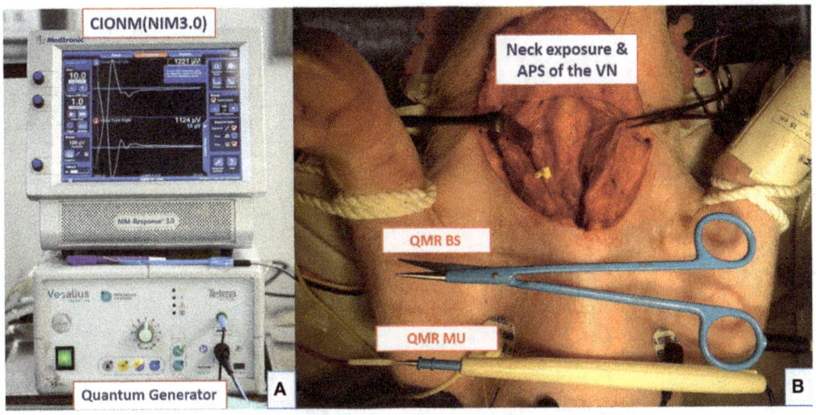

FIGURE 1 | Equipment setting and animal setting. **(A)** Setup of the continuous intraoperative neuromonitoring (C-IONM) system with the Nerve Integrity Monitor (NIM 3.0) system and Quantum generator system (MX 90, Telea Engineering, Vicenza, Italy). **(B)** Neck wound exposure with automated periodic stimulation (APS) placed on the vagus nerve (VN). The quantum molecular resonance (QMR) bipolar scissor (BS) and monopolar unit (MU) are shown.

fascia and kept dry for further experimental procedures. The APS was also set up at the fifth tracheal ring level with optimal stability. The amplitude and latency of the evoked response from VNs were calibrated to baseline values. Adverse EMG changes were defined as a 50% decrease in amplitude or a 10% increase in latency. Loss of signal (LOS) was defined as the amplitude of the RLN signal decreasing to less than 100 μV.

Study Design

There are two studies in this experiment. The activation study determined the distance from the RLN at which the QMR devices could be safely activated. The cooling study determined the time intervals and procedures required to cool the QMR devices before further use for hemostasis and dissection near the RLN. **Figure 1A** shows the QMR Generator system (MX 90, Telea Engineering, Vicenza, Italy), and the power was set at 5 in this study. The QMR BS and MU instruments are shown in **Figure 1B**.

Activation Study

Figures 2A, 2B, 3A, 3B describe the designs of the QMR BS and QMR MU activation studies, respectively. Both devices were applied to soft tissue in a single activation for 3 seconds. The QMR device activations began with a distance of 5 mm from the RLN. If there was no adverse EMG event (e.g., significant adverse decrease in amplitude or increase in latency) after 3 repetitions,

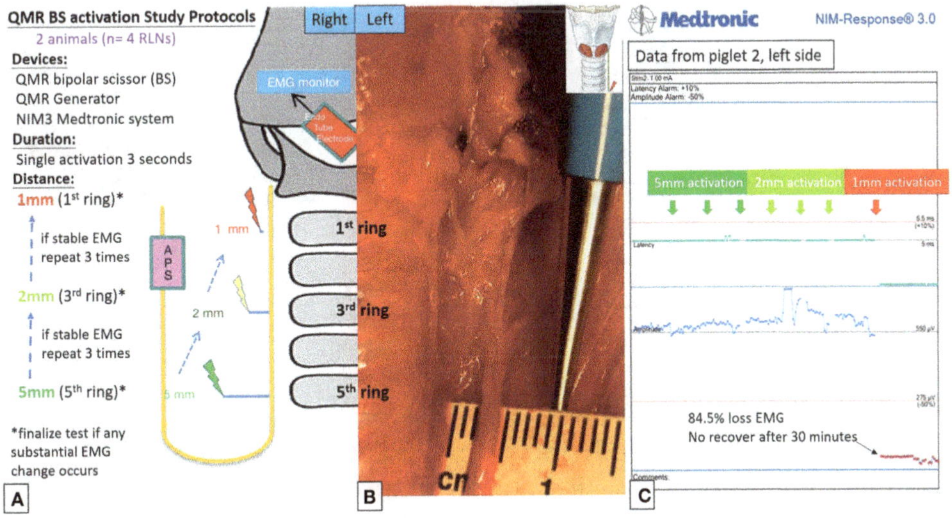

FIGURE 2 | QMR BS activation study protocols. **(A)** Flowcharts of the QMR BS activation study. **(B)** QMR BS was tested at a distance of 5 mm from the left RLN. **(C)** EMG recording of the left side RLN in Piglet 2 under C-IONM. The QMR BS was activated at distances of 5, 2, and 1 mm. After activation at 1 mm, the EMG showed sudden 84.5% EMG signal loss without recovery after 30 minutes of observation.

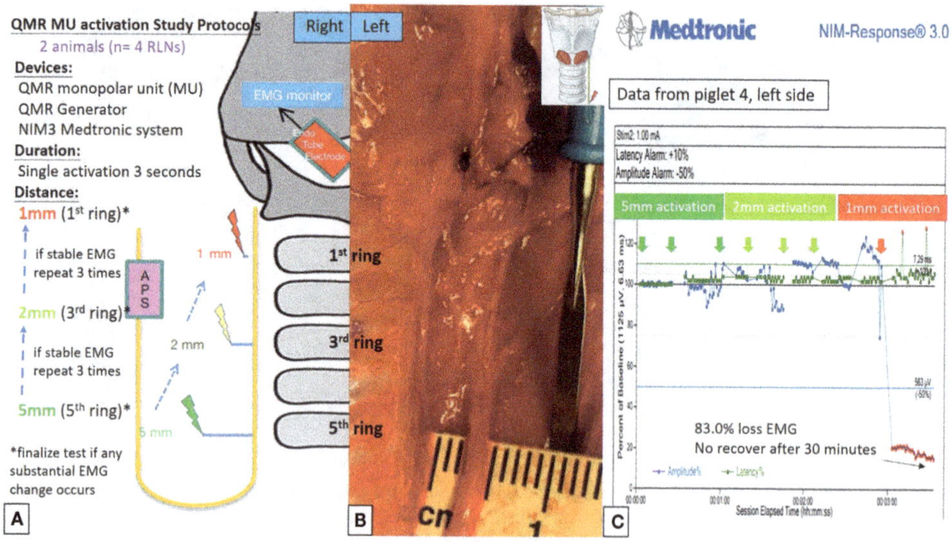

FIGURE 3 | QMR MU activation study protocols. **(A)** Flowcharts of the QMR MU activation study. **(B)** QMR MU was tested at a distance of 5 mm from the left RLN. **(C)** EMG recording of the left side RLN in Piglet 4 under C-IONM. The QMR MU was activated at distances of 5, 2, and 1 mm. After activation at 1 mm, the EMG showed a sudden 83.0% EMG signal loss without recovery after 30 minutes of observation.

the distance was progressively decreased to 2 mm (3 repetitions) and then to 1 mm (3 repetitions). Real-time EMG information under C-IONM was continuously recorded during each QMR device activation. If an adverse EMG event occurred, the RLN was interpreted as injured, and the procedure ended. Dynamic EMG changes were continuously recorded for at least 30 minutes to observe any recovery of the electrophysiological response.

Cooling Study

Figures 4A, 4B, 5A, 5B describe the designs of the QMR BS and QMR MU cooling studies, respectively. The QMR device was applied to the SCM muscle in a single activation of 5 seconds followed by cooling for 5 seconds at room temperature. The blade of the QMR MU or the open blade of the QMR BS was then touched to the RLN for 3 seconds. If there was no

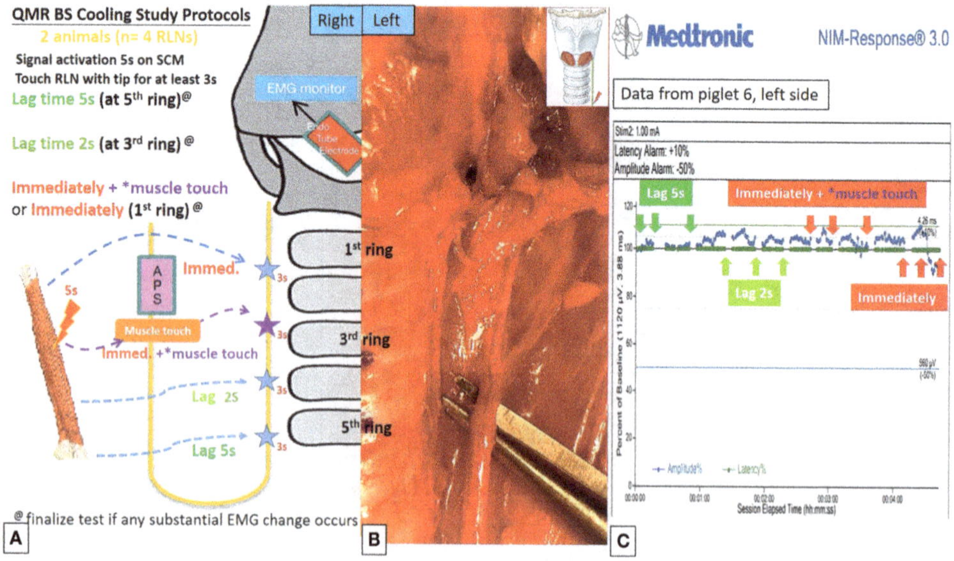

FIGURE 4 | QMR BS cooling study protocols. **(A)** Flowchart of the QMR BS cooling study. **(B)** The open blade of QMR BS touched the left RLN. **(C)** EMG recording of the left side RLN in Piglet 6 under C-IONM. After a single activation on sternocleidomastoid (SCM) muscle, the cooling study was performed with 5 seconds, 2 seconds, immediately without muscle touch maneuver (MTM), and immediately with MTM. The EMG results showed no adverse effects. The EMG signal remained stable in repeated tests.

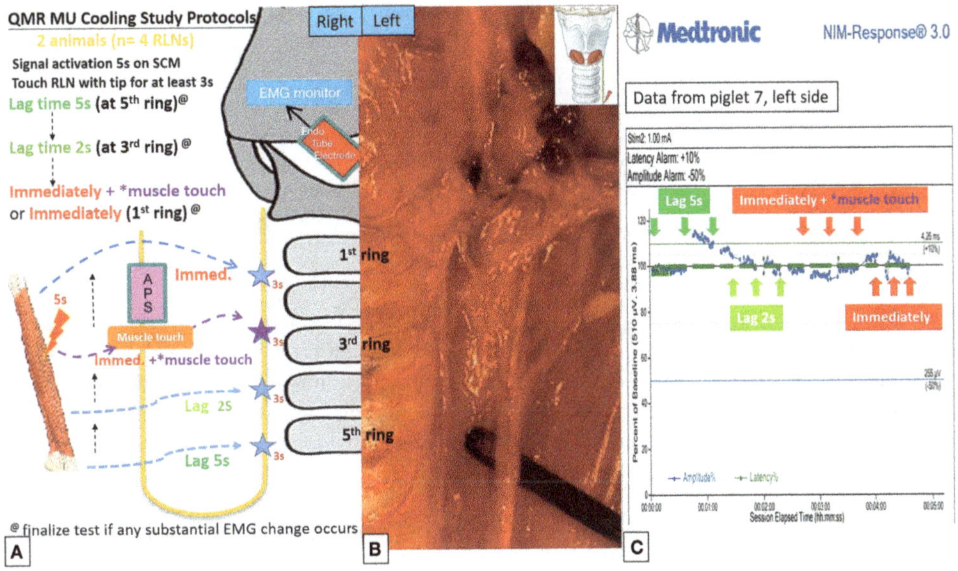

FIGURE 5 | QMR MU cooling study protocols. **(A)** Flowchart of the QMR MU cooling study. **(B)** The blade of the QMR MU touched the left RLN. **(C)** EMG recording of the left side RLN in Piglet 7 under C-IONM. After a single activation of the SCM muscle, the cooling study was performed for 5 seconds, 2 seconds, immediately without MTM, and immediately with MTM. The EMG results showed no adverse effects. The EMG signal remained stable in repeated tests.

adverse EMG event after 3 repetitions, the cooling time was decreased to 2 seconds, then immediately with "muscle touch maneuver (MTM)", and then immediately without MTM. MTM means that after a single activation of the SCM muscle and before contact with the RLN, the operator quickly contacts the QMR device (blade of QMR MU and open blade of QMR BS) with the ipsilateral strap muscle to achieve a contact cooling effect. Real-time EMG information under C-IONM was continuously recorded during the cooling procedure of each QMR device. If an adverse EMG event occurred, the RLN was interpreted as injured, and the procedure ended. Dynamic EMG changes were continuously recorded for at least 30 minutes to observe any recovery of the electrophysiological response.

RESULTS

The animal anesthesia, surgical approach, and C-IONM of the RLNs were successfully performed in all studies.

Activation Study

Activation study was performed in 8 RLNs of 4 piglets (animal No. 1-4). No adverse EMG events (amplitude decrease or latency increase) were observed when the QMR BS and QMR MU were activated at distances of 5 and 2 mm. With the QMR BS activated at a distance of 1 mm, all RLNs showed a signal decrease (63.0%, 60.0%, 84.5% loss and LOS) after a 30-minute observation (**Table 1**). The left RLN in piglet 2 showed 84.5% loss without recovery (**Figure 2C**). With the QMR MU activated at a distance of 1 mm, 3 of 4 RLNs showed a signal decrease (83.0% loss and 2 LOS) after a 30-minute observation (**Table 1**). The left RLN in piglet 4 showed 83.0% loss without recovery (**Figure 3C**).

Cooling Study

Cooling study was performed in 8 RLNs of 4 piglets (animal No. 5-8). In the QMR BS cooling study, no adverse EMG events were noted at any cooling time (5 seconds, 2 seconds, immediately with MTM, and immediately without MTM) (**Table 2**). The left RLN in piglet 6 showed a stable EMG signal without amplitude decrease or latency increase (**Figure 4C**).

TABLE 1 | Activation study: real-time EMG changes after QMR BS and QMR MU activation at varying distances to the RLN.

Animal No.	Side	5mm, amplitude [times]	2mm, amplitude [times]	1mm, amplitude [times]
1 (QMR BS)	Left	Stable [3]	Stable [3]	63.0% loss [1]
	Right	Stable [3]	Stable [3]	60.0% loss [1]
2 (QMR BS)	Left	Stable [3]	Stable [3]	84.5% loss [1]
	Right	Stable [3]	Stable [3]	LOS [1]
3 (QMR MU)	Left	Stable [3]	Stable [3]	Stable [3]
	Right	Stable [3]	Stable [3]	LOS [1]
4 (QMR MU)	Left	Stable [3]	Stable [3]	83.0% loss [1]
	Right	Stable [3]	Stable [3]	LOS [1]

EMG, electromyographic; QMR, Quantum molecular resonance; BS, bipolar scissor; MU, monopolar unit; RLN, recurrent laryngeal nerve; LOS, loss of signal.

TABLE 2 | Cooling study: real-time EMG changes after QMR BS and QMR MU activation and varying cooling time.

Animal No.	Side	5 seconds, amplitude [times]	2 seconds, amplitude [times]	Immediately with MTM, amplitude [times]	Immediately without MTM, amplitude [times]
5 (QMR BS)	Left	Stable [3]	Stable [3]	Stable [3]	Stable [3]
	Right	Stable [3]	Stable [3]	Stable [3]	Stable [3]
6 (QMR BS)	Left	Stable [3]	Stable [3]	Stable [3]	Stable [3]
	Right	Stable [3]	Stable [3]	Stable [3]	Stable [3]
7 (QMR MU)	Left	Stable [3]	Stable [3]	Stable [3]	Stable [3]
	Right	Stable [3]	Stable [3]	Stable [3]	LOS [1]
8 (QMR MU)	Left	Stable [3]	Stable [3]	Stable [3]	Stable [3]
	Right	Stable [3]	Stable [3]	Stable [3]	LOS [1]

EMG, electromyographic; QMR, Quantum molecular resonance; BS, bipolar scissor; MU, monopolar unit; LOS, loss of signal.

In the QMR MU cooling study, there were no adverse EMG events when the cooling time was more than 2 seconds or immediately with MTM. When the cooling time was immediately without MTM, 2 of 4 RLNs with LOS after 30 minutes of observation (**Table 2**). The left RLN in piglet 7 showed a stable EMG signal (**Figure 5C**).

DISCUSSION

The current study is the first to provide RLN safety parameters when using QMR devices in thyroid surgery. In the activation study, activation of the QMR BS and QMR MU at a distance longer than 2 mm from the RLN showed no adverse EMG events. In the cooling study, cooling of the QMR BS and QMR MU for 2 seconds or with MTM showed no adverse EMG events.

The application of EBDs during thyroid surgery has increased worldwide due to significantly reduced intraoperative blood loss, operating time, and postoperative hematoma rates (2, 17). In addition, the risk of thermal injury to nerves during thyroid surgery continues to increase (18). Sixty degree Celsius is a critical temperature, and exceeding this temperature will cause functional damage to the endoneurium (19, 20). Thermal injuries to nerves often occur suddenly and unexpectedly, and they are difficult to recognize visually and difficult to recover. Therefore, in addition to referring to the data provided by the manufacturer before using the new EBDs for thyroid surgery, a well-established C-IONM animal experimental model is helpful for safe application in clinical settings. Several animal studies have reported commonly used EBDs and their safety parameters during thyroidectomy. The safety parameters for devices such as the bipolar electrocautery, LigaSure, Harmonic scalpel, THUNDERBEAT, and FM devices were more than 2 mm to the nerve when activated, and a with 5 mm distance was best for monopolar electrocautery (21–27). All devices should be cooled by the MTM before contact with the RLN. The QMR MU and QMR BS are suggested to activate at 2 mm or longer from the RLN. Although the QMR BS showed a faster cooling time than QMR MU (less than the time the instrument required to move from the SCM muscle to the RLN), considering that the instruments are usually closed to the RLN during dissection, a MTM and an adequate cooling time (at least two seconds) are still essential cooling procedures that cannot be omitted.

The first experimental study of QMR energy involved performing a thoracotomy in rats and evaluating its effect histologically in 2007 (28). By resonating and breaking molecular boundaries, QMR devices are said to cut tissue while maintaining a low temperature around the tissue (29), and tissue dissection is not facilitated through thermal vaporization as it is with traditional electrocautery or lasers (13, 15). Some literature (13, 14) and the manufacturer's website report that the temperature can be lower than 50 degrees Celsius with minimal thermal spread depth. D'Eredità et al. reported a mean 43 ± 9 μm depth of injury with QMR, while the depth of injury was 126 ± 11 μm with coblation in the histopathological evaluation of tonsillectomy specimens (11). For hemostasis, unlike electro and radiosurgery devices that produce a relatively large-area of burnt vessel collapse, QMR devices deploy a special waveform (with a slight loss of resonance) that elevates the temperature to 45-65°C (12, 28). This waveform triggers the denaturation process of fibrinogen, which turns into fibrin and clots the blood without causing thermal damage to the blood vessels. The above contents fully illustrate the potential benefits of QMR devices used in thyroid surgery, such as low temperature, effective hemostasis, and a small range of lateral thermal spread. However, in the dry environment, the QMR device reached a maximum temperature of 72°C after a single activation (3 seconds), and need approximately 2 seconds to decrease the temperature below 60°C in our preliminary thermographic study. It must be emphasized that, according to the results of this study, thyroid surgeons must still maintain adequate activation distance and cooling time to ensure the safety of their clinical application.

For the application of QMR devices in thyroid surgery, the interchangeability between QMR BS and QMR MU is an advantage worth mentioning. Thyroid surgeons can choose appropriate instruments according to the requirements of the thyroid dissection. In some relatively dense structures, such as Berry's ligaments, the scissor structure of QMR BS can have advantages during dissection compared with the sealer structure of other EBDs. Hence, QMR instruments are more likely to be dissected when they are directly adjacent to the RLN, and knowledge of the neural safety parameters of QMR devices is even more necessary for thyroid surgeons.

Several limitations in the study need to be mentioned. First, this study only had a 30-minute observation period after an adverse EMG event, and nerves with incomplete signal loss may not predict postoperative neural function. However, because of the difficult-to-repair nature of thermal injury, the occurrence of adverse EMG events is a well-established way to assess the neural safety parameters of a new EBD (21–27). Second, some aspects in this prospective porcine model study may not be applicable to human surgery. Several factors can affect heat transfer from the QMR devices to the RLNs, including the difference in body temperature between human and experimental animals and the temperature of the surrounding environment. However, animal studies still provide useful and reliable data for human surgery. Finally, to have stable contact between the QMR devices and RLNs to avoid motion-affected C-IONM recordings, the part of the QMR devices that make direct contact with RLNs is closed but not the exact same as that in clinical surgery, especially the QMR BS cooling study. Therefore, although this study showed that QMR requires a very short cooling time, it is still recommended that the MTM or a 2-second cooling time should be performed before neural dissection.

CONCLUSION

QMR devices should be carefully used when performing RLN dissection during thyroid surgery. Safety recommendations regarding the use of QMR MU and QMR BS are as follows: activation should be at least 2 mm from the RLN and cooling procedures should include the MTM or an adequate cooling time (at least two seconds). According to the activation and cooling safety parameters in this study, surgeons can avoid RLN injury by following standard procedures when using QMR devices.

ETHICS STATEMENT

The animal study was reviewed and approved by Institutional Animal Care and Use Committee of Kaohsiung Medical University, Taiwan (IACUC Approval No. 110129).

AUTHOR CONTRIBUTIONS

Supervision – GR, GD, N-CC, and C-WW; Materials – H-YT, T-YH, Y-CL, JW, H-YK, C-HC, and C-WW; Data Collection and Processing – H-YT, T-YH, N-CC, and C-WW; Analysis and Interpretation- H-YT, T-YH, I-CL, and P-YC; Literature Search - H-YT, T-YH, Y-CL, JW, H-YK, and C-HC; Writing Manuscript – All authors. All authors have read and agreed to the published version of the manuscript. All authors contributed to the article and approved the submitted version.

ACKNOWLEDGMENTS

The authors are grateful to Hui-Chun Chen (clinical nurse specialist, Department of Nursing, Kaohsiung Medical University Hospital [KMUH], Kaohsiung Medical University [KMU], Taiwan) and Hsiu-Ya Chen (nurse anesthetist, Department of Anesthesiology, KMUH, KMU, Taiwan) for their excellent technical assistance.

REFERENCES

1. Lang BH-H, Yih PC-L, Lo C-Y. A Review of Risk Factors and Timing for Postoperative Hematoma After Thyroidectomy: Is Outpatient Thyroidectomy Really Safe? *JWjos* (2012) 36(10):2497–502. doi: 10.1007/s00268-012-1682-1
2. Wang JJ, Huang T-Y, Wu C-W, Lin Y-C, Tseng H-Y, Liu C-H, et al. Improving Voice Outcomes After Thyroid Surgery–Review of Safety Parameters for Using Energy-Based Devices Near the Recurrent Laryngeal Nerve. *Front Endocrinol* (2021) 12. doi: 10.3389/fendo.2021.793431
3. Dionigi G, Boni L, Rausei S, Frattini F, Ferrari CC, Mangano A, et al. The Safety of Energy-Based Devices in Open Thyroidectomy: A Prospective, Randomised Study Comparing the LigaSure™(LF1212) and the Harmonic® FOCUS. *Langenbecks Arch Surg* (2012) 397(5):817–23. doi: 10.1007/s00423-011-0898-0
4. Dionigi G, Wu C-W, Kim HY, Rausei S, Boni L, Chiang F-Y. Severity of Recurrent Laryngeal Nerve Injuries in Thyroid Surgery. *World J Surg* (2016) 40(6):1373–81. doi: 10.1007/s00423-011-0898-0
5. Dionigi G, Alesina P, Barczynski M, Boni L, Chiang F, Kim H, et al. Recurrent Laryngeal Nerve Injury in Video-Assisted Thyroidectomy: Lessons Learned From Neuromonitoring. *Surg Endosc* (2012) 26(9):2601–8. doi: 10.1007/s00464-012-2239-y
6. Huang T-Y, Yu W-HV, Chiang F-Y, Wu C-W, Fu S-C, Tai A-S, et al. How the Severity and Mechanism of Recurrent Laryngeal Nerve Dysfunction During Monitored Thyroidectomy Impact on Postoperative Voice. *Cancers* (2021) 13 (21):5379. doi: 10.3390/cancers13215379
7. Huang T-Y, Yu W-HV, Chiang F-Y, Wu C-W, Fu S-C, Tai A-S, et al. Prognostic Indicators of Non-Transection Nerve Injury and Vocal Fold Motion Impairment After Thyroid Surgery–Correlation Between Intraoperative Neuromonitoring Findings and Perioperative Voice Parameters. *Front Endocrinol* (2021) 12. doi: 10.3389/fendo.2021.755231
8. Demirhan E, Çukurova İ, Arslan İB, Ozkan ET, Mengi E, Yigitbasi OG. Quantum Molecular Resonance-Assisted Phonomicrosurgery: Preliminary Experience. *Otolaryngology–Head Neck Surg* (2015) 152(1):189–92. doi: 10.1177/0194599814549729
9. Lorusso F, Gallina S, Modica D, Di Salvo N, Riggio F. Bipolar Quantum Molecular Resonance Versus Blunt Dissection Tonsillectomy. *B-ent* (2015) 11 (02):101–8.
10. Chang H, Hah JH. Comparison of Post-Tonsillectomy Pain With Two Different Types of Bipolar Forceps: Low Temperature Quantum Molecular Resonance Device Versus High Temperature Conventional Electrocautery. *Acta Oto-Laryngol* (2012) 132(sup1):S130–3. doi: 10.3109/00016489.2012.659752
11. D'Eredità R, Bozzola L. Molecular Resonance vs. Coblation Tonsillectomy in Children. *Laryngoscope* (2009) 119(10):1897–901. doi: 10.1002/lary.20210
12. Vescovi P, Manfredi M, Merigo E, Fornaini C, Rocca J-P, Nammour S, et al. Quantic Molecular Resonance Scalpel and its Potential Applications in Oral Surgery. *Br J Oral Maxillofacial Surg* (2008) 46(5):355–7. doi: 10.1016/j.bjoms.2007.09.014
13. Tarantino V, D'Agostino R, Melagrana A, Porcu A, Stura M, Vallarino R, et al. Safety of Electronic Molecular Resonance Adenoidectomy. *Int J Pediatr Otorhinolaryngol* (2004) 68(12):1519–23. doi: 10.1016/j.ijporl.2004.07.013
14. Sebben JE. Electrosurgery Principles: Cutting Current and Cutaneous Surgery—Part I. *J Dermatol Surg Oncol* (1988) 14(1):29–31. doi: 10.1111/j.1524-4725.1988.tb03338.x
15. D'Agostino R, Tarantino V, Calevo MG. Blunt Dissection Versus Electronic Molecular Resonance Bipolar Dissection for Tonsillectomy: Operative Time and Intraoperative and Postoperative Bleeding and Pain. *Int J Pediatr Otorhinolaryngol* (2008) 72(7):1077–84. doi: 10.1016/j.ijporl.2008.03.018
16. Pozzato G, Vignato G. Teoria Della Risonanza Quantica Molecolare Nella Realizzazione Del Bisturi Elettronico "Vesalius". *Quintessence Int* (2003) 5 (6):153–5.
17. Dionigi G, Wu C-W, Kim H-Y, Liu X, Liu R, Randolph GW, et al. Safety of

Energy Based Devices for Hemostasis in Thyroid Surgery. *Gland Surg* (2016) 5 (5):490. doi: 10.21037/gs.2016.09.01

18. Liu C-H, Wang C-C, Wu C-W, Lin Y-C, Lu I, Chang P-Y, et al. Comparison of Surgical Complications Rates Between LigaSure Small Jaw and Clamp-and-Tie Hemostatic Technique in 1,000 Neuro-Monitored Thyroidectomies. *Front Endocrinol* (2021) 12:313. doi: 10.3389/fendo.2021.638608
19. Wu C-W, Dionigi G, Sun H, Liu X, Kim HY, Hsiao P-J, et al. Intraoperative Neuromonitoring for the Early Detection and Prevention of RLN Traction Injury in Thyroid Surgery: A Porcine Model. *Surgery* (2014) 155(2):329–39. doi: 10.1016/j.surg.2013.08.015
20. Lin YC, Dionigi G, Randolph GW, Lu IC, Chang PY, Tsai SY, et al. Electrophysiologic Monitoring Correlates of Recurrent Laryngeal Nerve Heat Thermal Injury in a Porcine Model. *Laryngoscope* (2015) 125(8): E283–90. doi: 10.1002/lary.25362
21. Wu C-W, Huang T-Y, Chen H-C, Chen H-Y, Tsai T-Y, Chang P-Y, et al. Intra-Operative Neural Monitoring of Thyroid Surgery in a Porcine Model. *JoVE* (2019) (144):e57919. doi: 10.3791/57919
22. Wu CW, Chai YJ, Dionigi G, Chiang FY, Liu X, Sun H, et al. Recurrent Laryngeal Nerve Safety Parameters of the H Armonic F Ocus During Thyroid Surgery: Porcine Model Using Continuous Monitoring. *Laryngoscope* (2015) 125(12):2838–45. doi: 10.1002/lary.25412
23. Dionigi G, Chiang FY, Kim HY, Randolph GW, Mangano A, Chang PY, et al. Safety of LigaSure in Recurrent Laryngeal Nerve Dissection-Porcine Model Using Continuous Monitoring. *Laryngoscope* (2017) 127(7):1724–9. doi: 10.1002/lary.26271
24. Huang TY, Lin YC, Tseng HY, Dionigi G, Kim HY, Chai YJ, et al. Safety Parameters of Ferromagnetic Device During Thyroid Surgery: Porcine Model Using Continuous Neuromonitoring. *Head Neck* (2020) 42(10):2931–40. doi: 10.1002/hed.26334
25. Huang T-Y, Lin Y-C, Tseng H-Y, Dionigi G, Kim H-Y, Lu I-C, et al. Safety of Ligasure Exact Dissector in Thyroidectomy With Continuous Neuromonitoring: A Porcine Model. *Gland Surg* (2020) 9(3):702. doi: 10.21037/gs.2020.03.17
26. Kim HK, Chai YJ, Lee HY, Kim HY, Dionigi G. Comparing the Safety of Harmonic ACE and ACE+ Around the Recurrent Laryngeal Nerve in Swine Models. *JAoST Res* (2018) 94(6):285–90. doi: 10.4174/astr.2018.94.6.285
27. Kwak HY, Dionigi G, Kim D, Lee HY, Son GS, Lee JB, et al. Thermal Injury of the Recurrent Laryngeal Nerve by THUNDERBEAT During Thyroid Surgery: Findings From Continuous Intraoperative Neuromonitoring in a Porcine Model. *J Surg Res* (2016) 200(1):177–82. doi: 10.1016/j.jss.2015.06.066
28. Schiavon M, Calabrese F, Nicotra S, Marulli G, Pozzato G, Giacometti C, et al. Favorable Tissue Effects of Quantum Molecular Resonance Device (Vesalius®) Compared With Standard Electrocautery. *Eur Surg Res* (2007) 39(4):222–8. doi: 10.1159/000101745
29. Ricciardiello F, Pisani D, Viola P, Pellini R, Russo G, Longo G, et al. The Role of Quantic Molecular Resonance (QMR) in the Treatment of Inferior Turbinate Hypertrophy (ITH): Our Experience With Long-Term Follow-Up in Allergic and Nonallergic Rhinitis Refractory to Medical Therapy Preliminary Results. *Ear Nose Throat J* (2021) 01455613211001599. doi: 10.1177/01455613211001599

4

Papillary Thyroid Microcarcinoma: A Nomogram Based on Clinical and Ultrasound Features to Improve the Prediction of Lymph Node Metastases in the Central Compartment

Jing Ye[1], *Jia-Wei Feng*[1], *Wan-Xiao Wu*[1], *Jun Hu*[1], *Li-Zhao Hong*[1], *An-Cheng Qin*[2], *Wei-Hai Shi*[3] *and Yong Jiang*[1*]

[1] *Department of Thyroid Surgery, The Third Affiliated Hospital of Soochow University, Changzhou First People's Hospital, Changzhou, China,* [2] *The Affiliated Suzhou Hospital of Nanjing Medical University, Suzhou Municipal Hospital, Suzhou, China,* [3] *The Affiliated Hospital of Nanjing Medical University, Changzhou Second People's Hospital, Changzhou, China*

Correspondence:
Yong Jiang
yjiang8888@hotmail.com

Background: Accurate preoperative identification of central lymph node metastasis (CLNM) is essential for surgical protocol establishment for patients with papillary thyroid microcarcinoma (PTMC). We aimed to develop a clinical and ultrasound characteristics-based nomogram for predicting CLNM.

Methods: Our study included 399 patients who were pathologically diagnosed with PTMC between January 2011 and June 2018. Clinical and ultrasound features were collected for univariate and multivariate analyses to determine risk factors of CLNM. A nomogram comprising the prognostic model to predict the CLNM was established, and internal validation in the cohort was performed. The Cox regression model was used to determine the risk factors for recurrence-free survival (RFS) and cumulative hazard was calculated to predict prognosis.

Results: Three variables of clinical and US features as potential predictors including sex (odd ratio [OR] = 1.888, 95% confidence interval [CI], 1.160-3.075; P =0.011), tumor size (OR = 1.933, 95% CI, 1.250-2.990; P =0.003) and ETE (OR = 6.829, 95% CI, 3.250-14.350; P <0.001) were taken into account. The predictive nomogram was established by involving all the factors above used for preoperative prediction of CLNM in patients with PTMC. The nomogram showed excellent calibration in predicting CLNM, with area under curves (AUC) of 0.684 (95% CI, 0.635 to 0.774). Furthermore, tumor size, multifocality, presence of ETE, vascular invasion, and CLNM were the significant factors related to the RFS.

Conclusion: Through this easy-to-use nomogram by combining clinical and US risk factor, the possibility of CLNM can be objectively quantified preoperatively. This prediction model may serve as a useful clinical tool to help clinicians determine an individual's risk of CLNM in PTMC, thus make individualized treatment plans accordingly.

Keywords: thyroid cancer, microcarcinoma, nomogram, central lymph node metastases, recurrence-free survival

INTRODUCTION

Papillary thyroid carcinoma (PTC) has become one of the most common malignancies of the endocrine system, with an average annual incidence growth rate of 6% worldwide (1). If the maximum size of PTC is ≤ 1.0 cm, it is defined as papillary thyroid microcarcinoma (PTMC) by the World Health Organization (2). Although most thyroid cancer usually grows slowly and has a good prognosis, some PTMC tend to metastasize to regional lymph nodes (3). As previous reported (4–6), the incidence of central lymph node metastasis (CLNM) was the highest among the neck compartment, ranging from 19% to 76%. Once diagnosed with CLNM, especially with large macroscopic lymph node metastases, patients were at high risk for poor prognosis and regional recurrence (7).

With the application of routine ultrasonography (US) and the necessary fine-needle aspiration biopsy (FNAB), the diagnostic rate of PTMC has been greatly improved (8). However, the preoperative detection rate of CLNM still remains quite low due to the limitations of current imaging technology (9). A recent meta-analysis showed that the sensitivity of preoperative US to diagnose CLNM of PTC was only 0.33 (10). Considering the high prevalence of CLNM, prophylactic central lymph node dissection (CLND) is usually performed in Asian countries such as Japan and China. As a result, this may cause more complications after thyroid surgery, such as recurrent laryngeal nerve injury, hypoparathyroidism, and chyle leakage (11–14). Hence, an effective and noninvasive tool that could evaluate the invasion of tumors and determine the extent of operation before surgery may help to develop the best treatment plan for PTMC patients.

Unlike other researchers who simply identified the risk factors for CLNM (3), we developed a clinical and US characteristics-based nomogram to evaluate the probability of CLNM in patients with PTMC. With our accurate and convenient evaluation system, clinicians would be able to quantify the possibility of CLNM preoperatively and make better clinical decisions. Moreover, risk factors of recurrence-free survival (RFS) and cumulative hazards were calculated for individualized treatment plan formulation and patient outcomes would be improved eventually.

MATERIALS AND METHODS

Patient Recruitment

This research was performed according to the Declaration of Helsinki. The multi-center retrospective cohort research was approved by the Ethical Committee of the Third Affiliated Hospital of Soochow University and Suzhou Municipal Hospital. All patients provided written informed consent and agreed to use their clinical data for this study. From January 2011 to June 2018, all pathologically proven PTMC cases who were treated at this two hospitals were reviewed retrospectively. In our research, the inclusion criteria were: (1) All patients received surgery for the first time; (2) The primary lesion was located in the thyroid gland; (3) No family history of thyroid cancer; (4) No other malignant tumors; (5) No head and neck radiation exposure history; (6) No distant metastasis; (7) Postoperative pathology confirmed PTC; (8) Complete clinical data. The exclusion criteria were: (1) patients who also had other types of TC; (2) patients who did not undergo radical surgery or CLND; (3) reoperation; (4) diagnosed tumors of other organs previously; (5) history of neck radiation exposure or hereditary malignancy; (6) clinically and/or pathologically detected distant metastasis; (7) patients who were lost to follow-up midway or with incomplete clinical information. In the end, we included and assessed a total of 399 patients in the research.

Preoperative Examination and Surgical Procedures

A thorough examination would be conducted once a thyroid nodule was discovered. In addition to routine testing of serum thyroid hormones, neck US was usually carried out to assess the characteristics of thyroid nodules and lymph nodes in the central compartment. Moreover, FNAB was performed preoperatively to diagnose benign or malignant nodules and pathological types. The BRAF V600E mutation was only conducted since 2017. In our research, the preoperative US variables of thyroid nodules mainly included: tumor size (the largest dimension of primary tumor), multifocality (two or more PTC lesions), and extrathyroidal extension (ETE).

Considering FNAB and imaging findings, if PTMC patients were in any of the following conditions (isthmus lesion, bilateral lesions, or presence of gross ETE), a total thyroidectomy (TT) with bilateral CLND would be performed. Otherwise, only lobectomy with CLND on the affected side would be performed (2). The central compartment (CC) means level VI of neck lymph node partition. The histological analysis of all surgical specimens was routinely conducted in the department of pathology.

Histopathological Examination

Pathological sections and further immunohistochemistry of the specimens were performed by at least two experienced pathologists. Vascular invasion was confirmed by pathologists through the microscope. Disease recurrence was categorized as local (regional cervical lymph nodes or thyroid bed) or distant (other organs) and confirmed by cyto-histopathology or imaging. RFS was identified as the length of time between the date of completion of the thyroid surgery and dates of recurrence. RFS and cumulative hazards were used to evaluate the outcomes.

Postoperative Strategies and Follow-up

The postoperative patients were treated with levothyroxine suppression therapy. Serum thyroglobulin (Tg) and Tg antibodies, US scan of the neck area and physical examinations were conducted every 3 to 6 months for high-risk patients and every 6 to 12 months for middle- and low-risk patients according to the 2015 ATA guidelines. When detected serum Tg and/or Tg antibody levels were significantly elevated, imaging examinations like CT or MRI or further histological confirmation would be performed. Follow-up information was acquired through telephone contact or outpatient consultations.

Statistical Analysis

Clinical data analysis in our study was conducted by utilizing software SPSS for Windows (version 25.0) and the R software (version 3.6.0). Categorical data were presented as numbers and percentages, while continuous data were presented as means ± standard deviations. Pearson's chi-square test or Fisher's exact test was applied for categorical data depending on the situation. Univariate analysis of CLNM-related risk factors in PTMC patients was also performed by using Pearson's chi-square test or Fisher's exact test. The statistically significant variables in the univariate analysis were further included in the multivariate logistic regression analysis to identify independent risk factors of CLNM. Next, the rms/pROC package in the R software was used to construct a predictive nomogram of risk factors based on the results of multivariate logistic regression, which could convert each variable coefficient into a score from 0 to 100. The receiver operating characteristic (ROC) curve was employed to quantify and compare the ability of predicted cases and observed cases to predict CLNM in PTMC. The R software was also used to evaluate the accuracy of the best cut-off value. In order to assess the performance of the nomogram, a calibration chart containing 1,000 bootstrap samples was further performed to compare the predicted probabilities with the actual probabilities of CLNM. Univariate Cox regression analysis was used to identify the risk factors of RFS. The Kaplan-Meier method and the Log rank test were performed to calculate cumulative hazard to assess the differences between groups.

RESULTS

Base Clinical and US Features of PTMC Patients

The clinical data of 399 patients with PTMC were collected in our study. 103 (25.8%) men and 296 (74.2%) women at a mean age of 46.0 ± 11.3 years (range 21-77 years) were included in our study. According to our US findings, the average maximum tumor diameter was 0.60 ± 0.25 cm; 212 (53.1%) were larger than 0.5 cm and 187 (46.9%) were 0.5 cm or smaller. One hundred and four (26.1%) patients had multifocal lesions. ETE were detected in 49 (12.3%) patients. Among 39 patients undergoing BRAF mutation analysis, 34 (87.2%) were positive for the gene mutation. Vascular invasion was evident in 12 (3.0%) cases.

In our study, all 399 PTMC patients underwent CLND, of which 156 (39.1%) patients were detected with CLNM after surgery. Pathology after surgery confirmed that the mean number of central lymph nodes resected was 5.8 ± 4.6 (range 2-26), while the mean number of metastases was 2.3 ± 1.2 (range 0-13). According to postoperative pathology, the average size of positive central lymph node was 0.6 ± 0.3 cm. The post-operative median follow-up was 25 months (range 3-89 months). During the follow-up, 18 patients (4.5%) developed recurrent disease, including 12 patients (3.0%) who had cervical lymph node recurrence, 3 patients (0.7%) who had contralateral lobe recurrence, 2 patients (0.5%) who had both lymph node and contralateral lobe recurrence and 1 patient (0.3%) who had lung recurrence.

Correlation Between Clinical and US Features and CLNM in PTMC Patients

In 399 PTMC cases, clinical variables that significantly related to CLNM were age, sex, tumor size, ETE and vascular invasion. In our univariate analysis, compared with non-CLNM, the incidence of CLNM in patients with age <55 years, male, tumor size >0.5 cm, ETE, and vascular invasion was substantially higher (*P*=0.027, *P*=0.001, *P*=0.001, *P*<0.001, and *P*=0.010, respectively). Further, the multivariate analysis indicated that male (OR: 1.888, 95% CI: 1.160-3.075, *P*=0.011), tumor size >0.5 cm (OR: 1.933, 95% CI: 1.250-2.990, *P*=0.003) and ETE (OR: 6.829, 95% CI: 3.250-14.350, *P*<0.001) were independent predictive factors associated with CLNM in PTMC (**Table 1**).

Development and Performance of the Nomogram

As mentioned above, a nomogram was created from previous independent risk factors (sex, tumor size, and ETE) to assess the CLNM incidence of PTMC preoperatively (**Figure 1**). According to the analysis, ETE contributes the most to the prediction model, followed by tumor size. These variables were finally rated on a scale of 0-100, and the risk rate of CLNM would be calculated by summing up all total scores. The usage of nomogram (**Figure 2**) is as follows: locate the patient's sex on the sex axis. Draw a line straight upward to the point axis to establish how many points toward the probability of CLNM the patient may get. Repeat the process for each of the other variables. Calculate total points for each of the predictors. Pinpoint the final score on the total point axis. Draw a line straight down to determine the patient's predicted probability of CLNM. For example, the nomogram predicted a PTC male (33 points) patient with the tumor more than 0.5cm (34 points). The tumor had the ETE (100 points). The total point was 167 for this patient. This patient had more than 80.0% chance of CLNM.

The ROC curve was also constructed, and an area under curves (AUC) of 68.4% (95% CI: 0.635-0.774) with specificity and sensitivity as 0.885 and 0.391 respectively showed good

TABLE 1 | Univariate and multivariate analyses of factors associated with CLNM and score in patients with PTMC.

Characteristics	CLNM, No. (%)			Multivariate analysis	*P* value	Score
	Presence (n = 156)	Absence (n = 243)	*P* value	Adjusted OR (95% CI)		
Age (Y)						
≥55	69 (44.2%)	135 (55.6%)		1		
<55	87 (55.8%)	108 (44.4%)	0.027	1.408 (0.911-2.177)	0.123	
Sex						
Female	102 (65.4%)	194 (79.8%)		1		0
Male	54 (34.6%)	49 (20.2%)	0.001	1.888 (1.160-3.075)	0.011	33
Tumor size (cm)						
≤0.5	57 (36.5%)	130 (53.5%)		1		0
>0.5	99 (63.5%)	113 (46.5%)	0.001	1.933 (1.250-2.990)	0.003	34
Multifocality						
Absence	107 (68.6%)	188 (77.4%)				
Presence	49 (31.4%)	55 (22.6%)	0.051			
ETE						
Absence	117 (75.0%)	233 (95.9%)		1		0
Presence	39 (25.0%)	10 (4.1%)	<0.001	6.829 (3.250-14.350)	<0.001	100
Vascular invasion						
Absence	147 (94.2%)	240 (98.8%)		1		
Presence	9 (5.8%)	3 (1.2%)	0.010	1.092 (0.201-5.923)	0.919	
BRAF V600E mutation*						
Negative	2 (10.5%)	3 (15.0%)				
Positive	17 (89.5%)	17 (85.0%)	0.676			

Y, year; SD, standard deviation; ETE, extrathyroidal extension; CLNM, central lymph node metastasis.
**BRAF mutation analysis was started in 2017 and it was performed in 39 patients with PTMC.*

calibration (**Figure 3**). Additionally, the optimal cut-off value of the nomogram was 1.437, which was considered good in the differential diagnosis of CLNM. The calibration chart graphically showed an excellent agreement between the actual probability of CLNM and the metastasis probability predicted by the nomogram, with a mean absolute error of 0.028 (**Figure 4**).

Risk Factors for RFS

We performed univariate analysis related to RFS to identify variables that affect the risk of recurrence (**Table 2**). Risk factors such as tumor size, multifocality, ETE, vascular invasion, and CLNM showed statistically significance associated with RFS (P=0.003, P=0.024, P=0.015, P=0.003, P=0.005, respectively). However, RFS was not significantly related to other factors studied. The risk of recurrence was 3.700, 8.831, 2.934, and 4.340 times higher in patients with tumor size > 0.5 cm, multifocality, ETE and vascular invasion, respectively. It was also found that patients with CLNM had a 3.730 times higher risk of recurrence than that of whom without CLNM. Furthermore, with the extension of follow-up time, the cumulative risk of CLNM patients was substantially higher than that of whom without CLNM (*P*<0.001) (**Figure 5**).

DISCUSSION

The prevalence of PTMC has increased rapidly in the past few years thanks to the development and application of US and necessary FNAB (15). According to Chinese Guidelines for Diagnosis and Treatment of Differentiated Thyroid Cancer (2012), lobectomy and prophylactic CLND was recommended for patients with tumors <1 cm in size. However, previous studies had shown that preventive CLND does not significantly benefit patients with low-risk PTC (16, 17). It was suggested that active surveillance rather than surgery could be taken for low-risk PTMC by the guidelines of the American Thyroid Association (2015) (2). However, some previously considered low-risk PTMCs still progressed during surveillance (18, 19). Therefore, surgical treatment options are more often taken by patients diagnosed with PTMC in China (20–22). Nevertheless, considering the uncertain efficacy and high risk of complications, it was still controversial whether to perform preventive CLND while no obvious evidence of CLNM was found before surgery (23). Thus, careful assessment of cervical lymph node status and determination of risk factors related to CLNM before surgery could guide PTMC patients to adopt appropriate surgical methods and avoid unnecessary complications (24).

According to our study, a logistic regression model based on US and clinical variables was set up to predict the probability of CLNM in patients with PTMC. Factors associated with CLNM of PTMC patients were studied in depth through univariate and multivariate analyses. As previously reported, the occurrence rate of CLNM confirmed by pathologists was between 29.3% and 60.9% in cN0 PTC patients (25–28). In present study, the occurrence rate of CLNM was 39.1%, which was in accordance with the results of previous studies. The incidence of CLNM was higher in patients of male, age <55 years, tumor size >0.5 cm, ETE, and vascular invasion respectively according to our research. Further, multivariate analysis revealed that male, tumor size and ETE were independent risk factors for CLNM. These were similar to the results of some previous studies (29, 30). In addition, tumor size, multifocality, ETE, vascular invasion, and CLNM were found to be significantly correlated

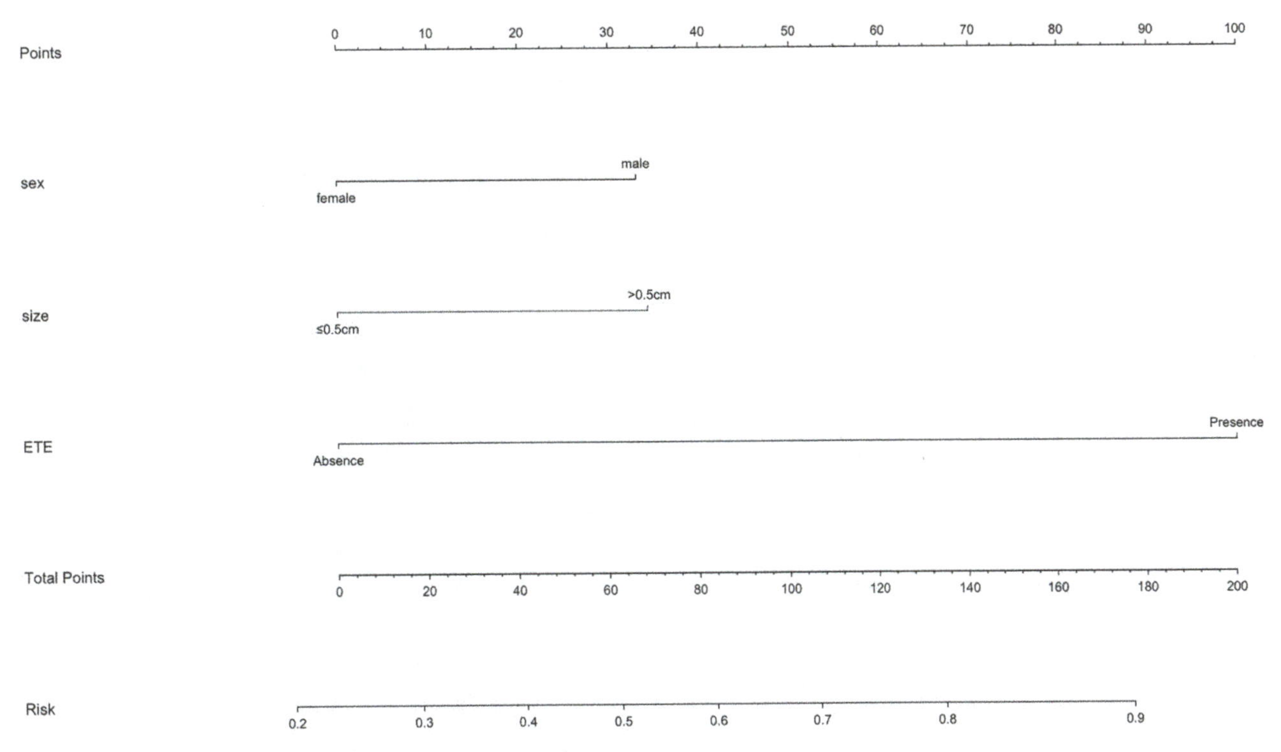

FIGURE 1 | Nomogram for predicting CLNM in patients with PTMC.

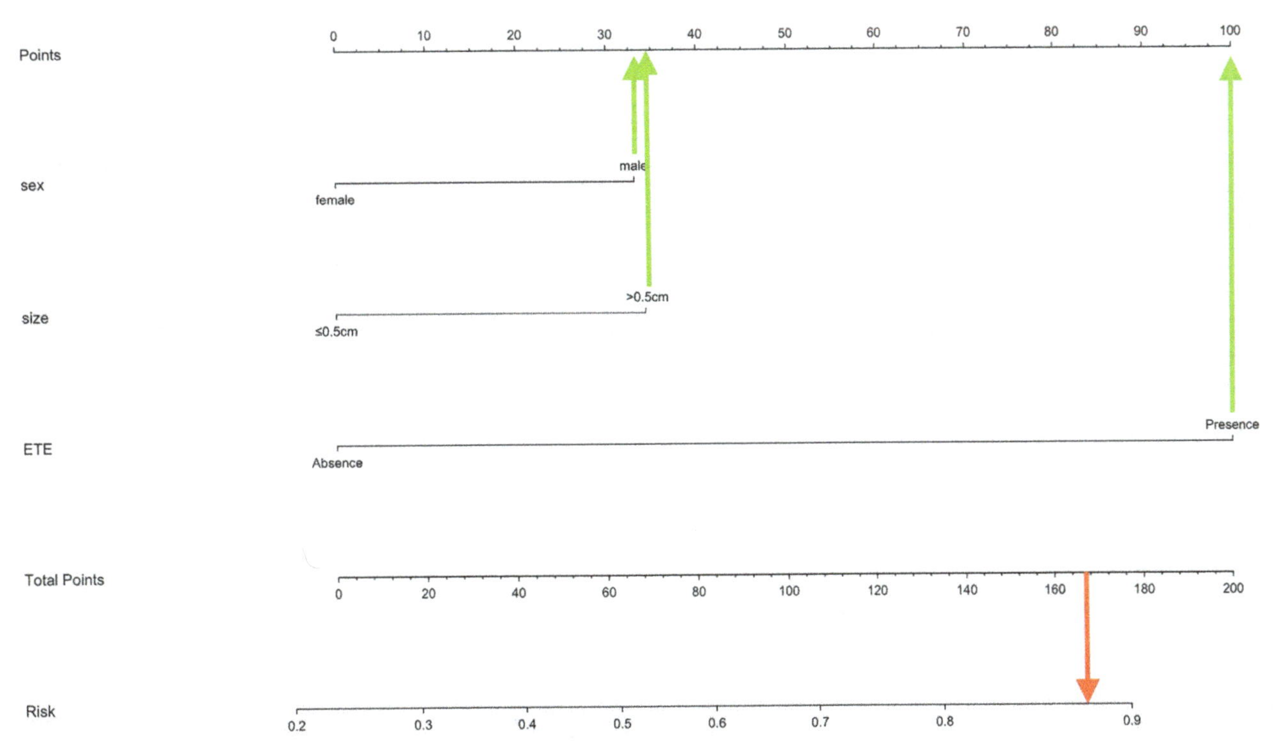

FIGURE 2 | Demonstration of the usage of our nomogram.

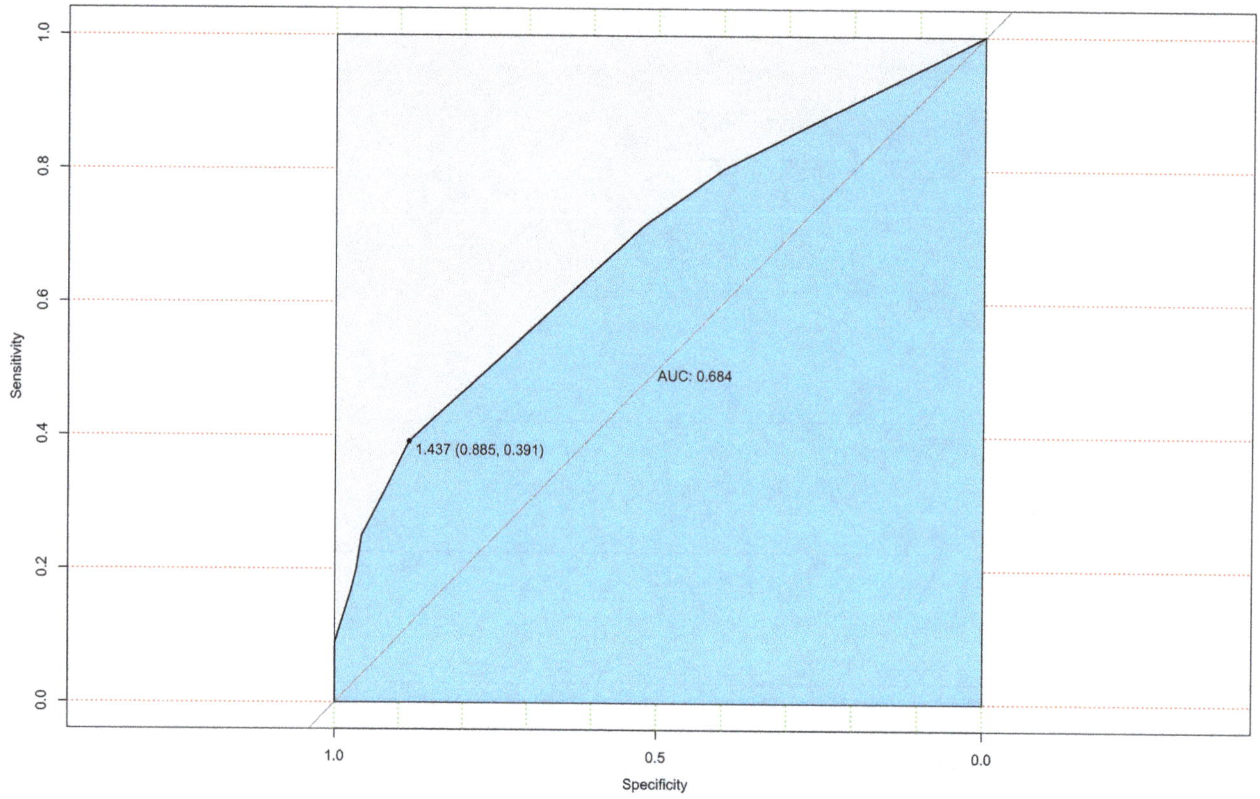

FIGURE 3 | ROC curve for predicting model.

TABLE 2 | Cox proportional hazards model demonstrating factors associated with recurrence-free survival in PTMC patients.

Characteristics	HR	95% CI	*P* value	Cumulative risk
Age (Y)				
≥55	1			
<55	1.601	0.654-3.924	0.303	
Sex				
Female	1			
Male	1.474	0.549-3.959	0.442	
Tumor size (cm)				
≤0.5	1			
>0.5	3.700	1.543-8.875	0.003	
Multifocality				
Absence	1			
Presence	3.111	1.165-8.306	0.024	
ETE				
Absence	1			
Presence	2.934	1.238-6.955	0.015	
Vascular invasion				
Absence	1			
Presence	4.340	1.648-11.432	0.003	
CLNM				
Absence	1			
Presence	3.730	1.482-9.388	0.005	<0.001

Y, year; SD, standard deviation; ETE, extrathyroidal extension; CLNM, central lymph node metastasis.

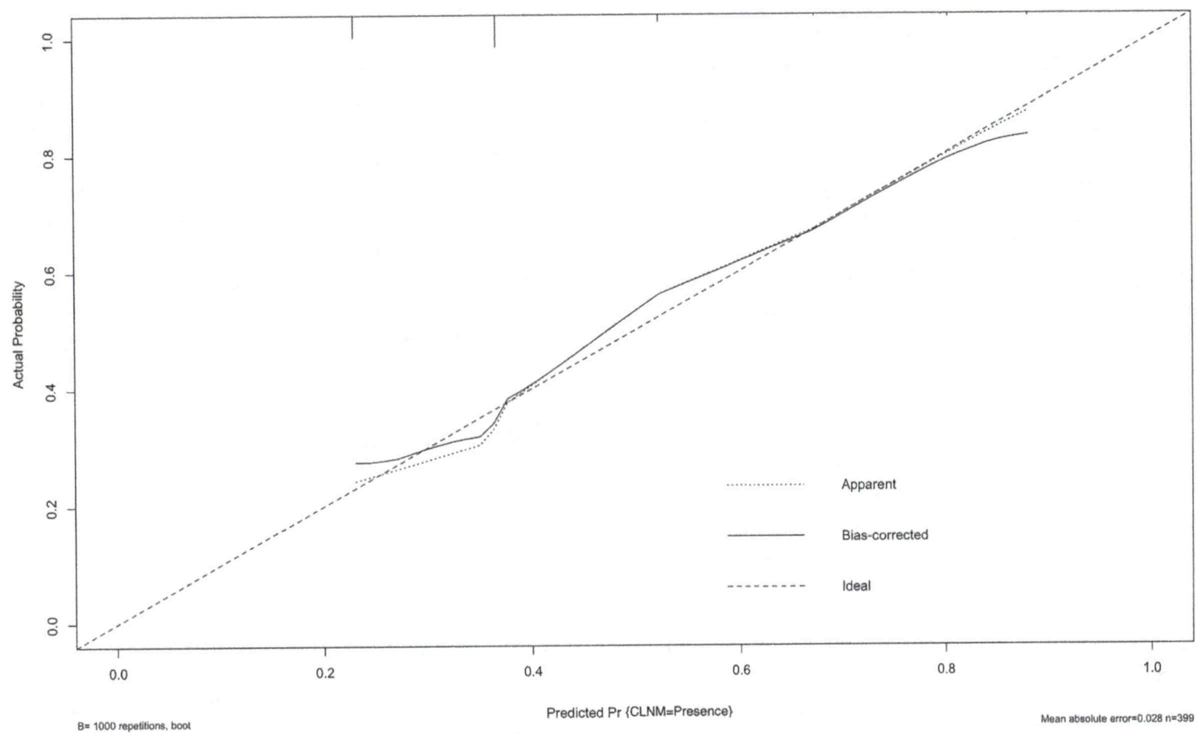

FIGURE 4 | Calibration curve of the model. The diagonal dashed line represents the ideal prediction by the perfect nomogram; the solid line represents the calibration estimate from internally validated model; the dotted line indicates the apparent predictive accuracy. The closer the solid line is to the dotted line, the stronger the predictive ability of the model.

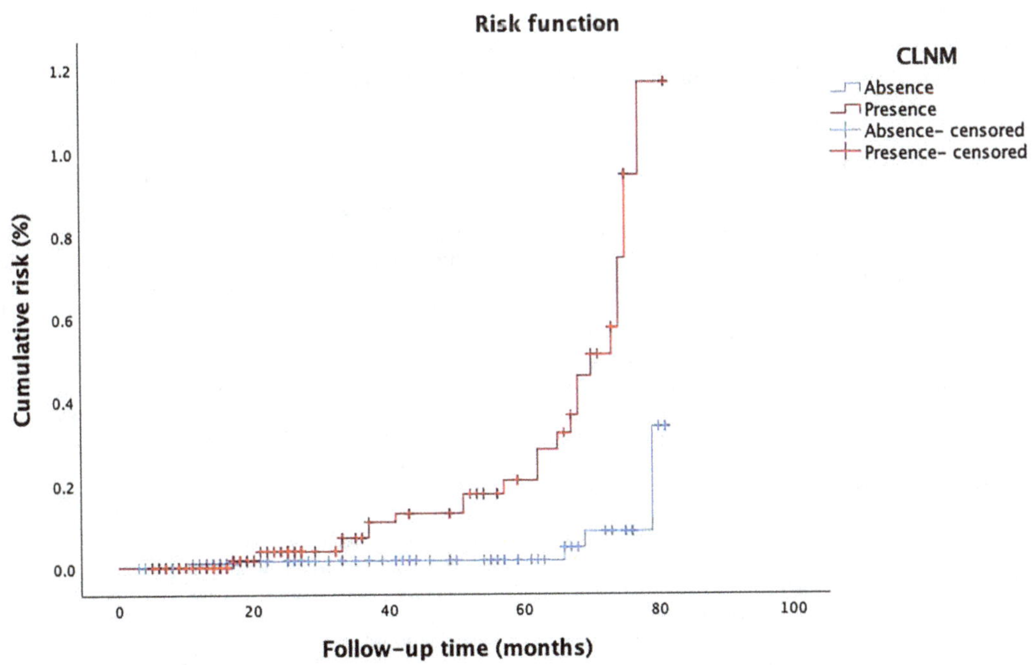

FIGURE 5 | The cumulative risk in patients with CLNM and patients without CLNM.

with RFS in patients with PTMC, and the cumulative hazard of CLNM patients was closely related to the postoperative follow-up time. Therefore, we urgently need a prediction system for individual CLNM probability to determine the extent of surgery and ultimately improve the prognosis.

To further predict the probability of CLNM, our study utilized the previous variables based on the multivariate analysis to construct a nomogram system (**Figure 2**). According to the point scale, we assigned a score to each variable. Next, the CLNM risk for each subject was determined by adding up all the total scores and identifying them on the total point scale. The nomogram incorporates all related clinical and US features to provide an individual risk assessment of CLNM preoperatively, which may avoid unnecessary expansion of extent of surgery. The AUC of the nomogram in our study was 0.684 (95%CI, 0.635-0.774), suggesting good discrimination. Surgeons could make individualized treatment plans accordingly, which is in conformity with the present tendency of personalized precision healthcare (31–34).

Our research still has some potential limitations which we hope to address in the following research. First, this was a retrospective observational research. Biases and errors in retrospective studies are often higher than in prospective studies (35). Hence, the prediction performance may be affected by the retrospective design of the study. Second, although we gathered cases from two hospitals, the sample size and the number of variables studied was not sufficiently large. Therefore, future studies involving more sample sizes and variables are needed, and further multicenter external validation are also needed to develop high-level evidence. More latent variables that are significant for CLNM prediction may be discovered, which can make the nomogram more complete. Third, the performance of the nomogram may be partially affected by different US instruments and operators with different experience. Because of the limitations of US, occult metastasis may not be detected during follow-up and cumulative risk calculation may also be affected (10, 36). Furthermore, we did not discuss whether prophylactic CLND in high-risk patients would reduce the risk of recurrence and improve patient outcomes. We plan to conduct prospective studies in the future, including setting up a comparison group of patients who will not receive prophylactic CLND to explore the impact of prophylactic CLND on postoperative complications and recurrence.

In summary, sex, tumor size, and ETE were significantly related to CLNM of PTMC in our research. By using above variables, we were able to construct a nomogram to evaluate CLNM risk of PTMC and provide a reference for clinicians to make individualized treatment decisions. For patients with high-risk factors for RFS, active surgical strategies are especially important.

ETHICS STATEMENT

Written informed consent was obtained from the individual(s) for the publication of any potentially identifiable images or data included in this article.

AUTHOR CONTRIBUTIONS

JY and J-WF: Writing - Original Draft, Software, Data Curation. W-XW and L-ZH: Validation, Formal analysis, Data Curation. JH: Conceptualization. W-HS and A-CQ: Validation, Investigation. YJ: Writing - Review & Editing, Visualization, Supervision. All authors contributed to the article and approved the submitted version.

ACKNOWLEDGMENTS

Lei Qin, the English language editor, was responsible for correcting language and grammar issues.

REFERENCES

1. Siegel RL, Miller KD, Fuchs HE, Jemal A. Cancer Statistics, 2021. *CA Cancer J Clin* (2021) 71(1):7–33. doi: 10.3322/caac.21654
2. Haugen BR, Alexander EK, Bible KC, Doherty G, Mandel SJ, Nikiforov YE, et al. 2015 American Thyroid Association Management Guidelines for Adult Patients With Thyroid Nodules and Differentiated Thyroid Cancer: The American Thyroid Association Guidelines Task Force on Thyroid Nodules and Differentiated Thyroid Cancer. *Thyroid* (2016) 26(1):1–133. doi: 10.1089/thy.2015.0020
3. Liu C, Xiao C, Chen J, Li X, Feng Z, Gao Q, et al. Risk Factor Analysis for Predicting Cervical Lymph Node Metastasis in Papillary Thyroid Carcinoma: A Study of 966 Patients. *BMC Cancer* (2019) 19(1):622. doi: 10.1186/s12885-019-5835-6
4. Yu XM, Wan Y, Sippel RS, Chen H. Should All Papillary Thyroid Microcarcinomas be Aggressively Treated? An Analysis of 18,445 Cases. *Ann Surg* (2011) 254(4):653–60. doi: 10.1097/SLA.0b013e318230036d
5. Chow SM, Law S, Chan J, Au SK, Yau S, Lau WH. Papillary Microcarcinoma of the Thyroid-Prognostic Significance of Lymph Node Metastasis and Multifocality. *Cancer* (2003) 98(1):31–40. doi: 10.1002/cncr.11442
6. Zheng X, Peng C, Gao M, Zhi J, Hou X, Zhao J, et al. Risk Factors for Cervical Lymph Node Metastasis in Papillary Thyroid Microcarcinoma: A Study of 1,587 Patients. *Cancer Biol Med* (2019) 16(1):121–30. doi: 10.20892/j.issn.2095-3941.2018.0125
7. Jiang LH, Yin KX, Wen QL, Chen C, Ge MH, Tan Z. Predictive Risk-Scoring Model For Central Lymph Node Metastasis and Predictors of Recurrence in Papillary Thyroid Carcinoma. *Sci Rep* (2020) 10(1):710. doi: 10.1038/s41598-019-55991-1
8. Burgess JR, Tucker P. Incidence Trends for Papillary Thyroid Carcinoma and Their Correlation With Thyroid Surgery and Thyroid Fine-Needle Aspirate Cytology. *Thyroid* (2006) 16(1):47–53. doi: 10.1089/thy.2006.16.47
9. Kim E, Park JS, Son KR, Kim JH, Jeon SJ, Na DG. Preoperative Diagnosis of Cervical Metastatic Lymph Nodes in Papillary Thyroid Carcinoma: Comparison of Ultrasound, Computed Tomography, and Combined Ultrasound With Computed Tomography. *Thyroid* (2008) 18(4):411–8. doi: 10.1089/thy.2007.0269
10. Zhao H, Li H. Meta-Analysis of Ultrasound for Cervical Lymph Nodes in Papillary Thyroid Cancer: Diagnosis of Central and Lateral Compartment Nodal Metastases. *Eur J Radiol* (2019) 112:14–21. doi: 10.1016/j.ejrad.2019.01.006
11. Sancho JJ, Lennard T, Paunovic I, Triponez F, Sitges-Serra A. Prophylactic Central Neck Disection in Papillary Thyroid Cancer: A Consensus Report of

the European Society of Endocrine Surgeons (ESES). *Langenbecks Arch Surg* (2013) 399(2):155–63. doi: 10.1007/s00423-013-1152-8
12. Park I, Her N, Choe JH, Kim JS, Kim JH. Management of Chyle Leakage After Thyroidectomy, Cervical Lymph Node Dissection, in Patients With Thyroid Cancer. *Head Neck* (2018) 40(1):7–15. doi: 10.1002/hed.24852
13. Polistena A, Monacelli M, Lucchini R, Triola R, Conti C, Avenia S, et al. Surgical Morbidity of Cervical Lymphadenectomy for Thyroid Cancer: A Retrospective Cohort Study Over 25 Years. *Int J Surg (London England)* (2015) 21:128–34. doi: 10.1016/j.ijsu.2015.07.698
14. Orloff LA, Wiseman SM, Bernet VJ, Fahey TJ3rd, Shaha AR, Shindo ML, et al. American Thyroid Association Statement on Postoperative Hypoparathyroidism: Diagnosis, Prevention, and Management in Adults. *Thyroid* (2018) 28(7):830–41. doi: 10.1089/thy.2017.0309
15. Yoon JH, Lee HS, Kim EK, Youk JH, Kim HG, Moon HJ, et al. Short-Term Follow-Up US Leads to Higher False-Positive Results Without Detection of Structural Recurrences in PTMC. *Medicine* (2016) 95(1):e2435. doi: 10.1097/MD.0000000000002435
16. Alsubaie KM, Alsubaie HM, Alzahrani FR, Alessa MA, Abdulmonem SK, Merdad MA, et al. Prophylactic Central Neck Dissection for Clinically Node-Negative Papillary Thyroid Carcinoma. *Laryngoscope* (2021). doi: 10.1002/lary.29912
17. Yuan J, Li J, Chen X, Lin X, Du J, Zhao G, et al. Identification of Risk Factors of Central Lymph Node Metastasis and Evaluation of the Effect of Prophylactic Central Neck Dissection on Migration of Staging and Risk Stratification in Patients With Clinically Node-Negative Papillary Thyroid Microcarcinoma. *Bull Cancer* (2017) 104(6):516–23. doi: 10.1016/j.bulcan.2017.03.005
18. Oh HS, Ha J, Kim HI, Kim TH, Kim WG, Lim DJ, et al. Active Surveillance of Low-Risk Papillary Thyroid Microcarcinoma: A Multi-Center Cohort Study in Korea. *Thyroid* (2018) 28(12):1587–94. doi: 10.1089/thy.2018.0263
19. Jeong SY, Baek JH, Choi YJ, Lee JH. Ethanol and Thermal Ablation for Malignant Thyroid Tumours. *Int J Hyperthermia* (2017) 33(8):938–45. doi: 10.1080/02656736.2017.1361048
20. Zhang H, Zheng X, Liu J, Gao M, Qian B. Active Surveillance as a Management Strategy for Papillary Thyroid Microcarcinoma. *Cancer Biol Med* (2020) 17(3):543–54. doi: 10.20892/j.issn.2095-3941.2019.0470
21. Ze Y, Zhang X, Shao F, Zhu L, Shen S, Zhu D, et al. Active Surveillance of Low-Risk Papillary Thyroid Carcinoma: A Promising Strategy Requiring Additional Evidence. *J Cancer Res Clin Oncol* (2019) 145(11):2751–9. doi: 10.1007/s00432-019-03021-y
22. Du L, Wang Y, Sun X, Li H, Geng X, Ge M, et al. Thyroid Cancer: Trends in Incidence, Mortality and Clinical-Pathological Patterns in Zhejiang Province, Southeast China. *BMC Cancer* (2018) 18(1):291. doi: 10.1186/s12885-018-4081-7
23. Raffaelli M, Tempera SE, Sessa L, Lombardi CP, De Crea C, Bellantone R. Total Thyroidectomy Versus Thyroid Lobectomy in the Treatment of Papillary Carcinoma. *Gland Surg* (2020) 9(Suppl 1):S18–27. doi: 10.21037/gs.2019.11.09
24. Xue S, Zhang L, Pang R, Wang P, Jin M, Guo L, et al. Predictive Factors of Central-Compartment Lymph Node Metastasis for Clinical N0 Papillary Thyroid Carcinoma With Strap Muscle Invasion. *Front Endocrinol* (2020) 11:511. doi: 10.3389/fendo.2020.00511
25. Wada N, Duh QY, Sugino K, Iwasaki H, Takanashi Y. Lymph Node Metastasis From 259 Papillary Thyroid Microcarcinomas: Frequency, Pattern of Occurrence and Recurrence, and Optimal Strategy for Neck Dissection. *Ann Surg* (2003) 237(3):399–407. doi: 10.1097/01.SLA.0000055273.58908.19
26. Lim YC, Choi EC, Yoon YH, Kim EH, Koo BS. Central Lymph Node Metastases in Unilateral Papillary Thyroid Microcarcinoma. *Br J Surg* (2010) 96(3):253–7. doi: 10.1002/bjs.6484
27. Jin K, Li L, Liu Y, Wang X. The Characteristics and Risk Factors of Central Compartment Lymph Node Metastasis in Cn0 Papillary Thyroid Carcinoma Coexistent With Hashimoto's Thyroiditis. *Gland Surg* (2020) 9(6):2026–34. doi: 10.21037/gs-20-699
28. Li M, Zhu XY, Lv J, Lu K, Shen MP, Xu ZL, et al. Risk Factors for Predicting Central Lymph Node Metastasis in Papillary Thyroid Microcarcinoma (CN0): A Study of 273 Resections. *Eur Rev Med Pharmacol Sci* (2017) 21(17):3801–7.
29. Qu N, Zhang L, Ji QH, Chen JY, Zhu YX, Cao YM, et al. Risk Factors for Central Compartment Lymph Node Metastasis in Papillary Thyroid Microcarcinoma: A Meta-Analysis. *World J Surg* (2015) 39(10):2459–70. doi: 10.1007/s00268-015-3108-3
30. Kim SK, Park I, Woo JW, Lee JH, Choe JH, Kim JH, et al. Predictive Factors for Lymph Node Metastasis in Papillary Thyroid Microcarcinoma. *Ann Surg Oncol* (2016) 23(9):2866–73. doi: 10.1245/s10434-016-5225-0
31. Balachandran VP, Gonen M, Smith JJ, Dematteo RP. Nomograms in Oncology: More Than Meets the Eye. *Lancet Oncol* (2015) 16(4):e173–80. doi: 10.1016/S1470-2045(14)71116-7
32. Huang GQ, Lin YT, Wu YM, Cheng QQ, Cheng HR, Wang Z. Individualized Prediction Of Stroke-Associated Pneumonia For Patients With Acute Ischemic Stroke. *Clin Interv Aging* (2019) 14:1951–62. doi: 10.2147/CIA.S225039
33. Chen S, Liu Y, Yang J, Liu Q, You H, Dong Y, et al. Development and Validation of a Nomogram for Predicting Survival in Male Patients With Breast Cancer. *Front Oncol* (2019) 9:361. doi: 10.3389/fonc.2019.00361
34. Choudhury P, Gupta M. Personalized & Precision Medicine in Cancer: A Theranostic Approach. *Curr Radiopharm* (2017) 10(3):166–70. doi: 10.2174/1874471010666170728094008
35. Sessler DI, Imrey PB. Clinical Research Methodology 2: Observational Clinical Research. *Anesth Analg* (2015) 121(4):1043–51. doi: 10.1213/ANE.0000000000000861
36. Ha SM, Baek JH, Kim JK. Detection of Malignancy Among Suspicious Thyroid Nodules Less Than 1 Cm on Ultrasound With Various Thyroid Image Reporting and Data Systems. *Thyroid* (2017) 27(10):1307–15. doi: 10.1089/thy.2017.0034

5

Ambulatory Endoscopic Thyroidectomy *via* a Chest-Breast Approach has an Acceptable Safety Profile for Thyroid Nodule

Zeyu Zhang, Fada Xia and Xinying Li**

Department of Thyroid Surgery, Xiangya Hospital, Central South University, Changsha, China

Correspondence:
Xinying Li
lixinyingcn@protonmail.com
Fada Xia
xiafadaCSU@protonmail.com

Introduction: With the growing esthetic requirements, endoscopic thyroidectomy develops rapidly and is widely accepted by practitioners and patients to avoid the neck scar caused by open thyroidectomy. Although ambulatory open thyroidectomy is adopted by multiple medical centers, the safety and potential of ambulatory endoscopic thyroidectomy via a chest-breast approach (ETCBA) is poorly investigated.

Material and Methods: Patients with thyroid nodules who received conventional or ambulatory ETCBA at Xiangya hospital, Central South University from January 2017 to June 2020 were retrospectively included. The incidence of postoperative complications, 30-days readmission rate, financial cost, duration of hospitalization, mental health were mainly investigated.

Results: A total of 260 patients were included with 206 (79.2%) suffering from thyroid carcinoma, while 159 of 260 received ambulatory ETCBA. There was no statistically significant difference in the incidence of postoperative complications (P=0.249) or 30-days readmission rate (P=1.000). In addition, The mean economic cost of the ambulatory group had a 29.5% reduction compared with the conventional group (P<0.001). Meanwhile, the duration of hospitalization of the ambulatory group was also significantly shorter than the conventional group (P<0.001). Patients received ambulatory ETCBA showed a higher level of anxiety (P=0.041) and stress (P=0.016). Subgroup analyses showed consistent results among patients with thyroid cancer with a 12.9% higher complication incidence than the conventional ETCBA (P=0.068).

Conclusion: Ambulatory ETCBA is as safe as conventional ETCBA for selective patients with thyroid nodules or thyroid cancer, however with significant economic benefits and shorter duration of hospitalization. Extra attention should be paid to manage the anxiety and stress of patients who received ambulatory ETCBA.

Keywords: ambulatory surgery, endoscopic thyroidectomy, thyroid nodule, postoperative complication, mental health

INTRODUCTION

Thyroid nodule is a very common disease and often discovered by accident mainly because of the asymptomatic feature (1).Although there is an increasing incidence of thyroid malignancy, most of thyroid nodules are benign without the need for invasive therapies (2). For patients who reach the indication of surgery, a traditional open thyroidectomy is the primary choice. However, with the growing esthetic requirements, endoscopic thyroidectomy develops rapidly and is widely accepted by practitioners and patients to avoid the neck scar caused by open thyroidectomy (3). Increasing evidences have shown that endoscopic thyroidectomy has the same efficacy and safety profiles as the open thyroidectomy (4–6).

Ambulatory surgery has become more and more common in recent years, offering various advantages (7). At present, ambulatory open thyroidectomy is adopted by multiple medical centers, showing no difference in readmissions and complications compared with conventional thyroidectomy (8). Moreover, with the development of instruments and techniques, many surgical procedures with a higher complexity are subsequently allowed to be performed with an ambulatory management (9).

Endoscopic thyroidectomy is usually carried out with multiple-day hospitalization, while few medical centers perform ambulatory endoscopic thyroidectomy. In addition, as far as we know, there is no study focusing on the potential of ambulatory endoscopic thyroidectomy. In our medical center, both conventional and ambulatory endoscopic thyroidectomy via a chest-breast approach (ETCBA) is routinely performed. Thus, in this study, we retrospectively evaluated the efficacy and safety of ambulatory ETCBA.

MATERIAL AND METHODS

Study Cohort

Patients with thyroid nodules who received conventional or ambulatory ETCBA at Xiangya hospital, Central South University from January 2017 to June 2020 were retrospectively included. The exclusion criteria were as follows: (1) signs of extrathyroidal tissue invasion; (2) previously received neck surgery or radiation; (3) suffering from infectious diseases or parathyroid disease; (4) lack of essential clinical data, including results of ultrasound, parathyroid hormone, complication data, and assessment of mental health. Patients were divided into conventional group and ambulatory group according to the surgery they received. This study was approved by the Institutional Ethics Committee of Xiangya Hospital, Central South University (No.202011960) and met the guidelines of governmental ethics agency in accordance with the precepts established by the Helsinki Declaration.

Surgical Procedures and Postoperative Management

The preoperative examination, surgeons, and procedures of ETCBA were identical between the two groups. The operative position and the location of operating and observing ports were as same as in the previous report (10). Patients with benign nodules would receive a thyroidectomy, while a central lymph node dissection was additionally performed among patients with malignant nodules. For patients with an undetermined result of fine-needle aspiration (FNA) biopsy, intraoperative frozen section histological examination was performed to determine the further procedures. Generally, ETCBA was not administrated for patients with lateral lymph node metastasis detected by preoperative examinations. However, lateral lymph node dissection was still performed endoscopically when suspicious lateral lymph node metastasis was intraoperatively detected. Patient status and vital signs were carefully monitored after surgery, and discharge assessment included vital signs, consciousness, airway status and sound, incision condition, and serum calcium. Calcium and analgesics were given as appropriate. The removal of the drainage tube and dressing change were performed the next morning. Patients in the conventional group were usually discharged on the third day after ETCBA, while the ambulatory group within 24 hours after ETCBA.

Outcomes and Follow-Up

Medical records and pathological reports were investigated for clinical data and patient characteristics. Every patient was followed up with examinations including ultrasound, thyroid function, and parathyroid hormone (PTH) every 3-6 months after discharge. The outcomes of this study were mainly incidence of postoperative complications, 30-days readmission rate, financial cost, duration of hospitalization. Hypoparathyroidism was recognized as PTH level <15 pg/ml, and hypoparathyroidism and the voice change recovered in six months was considered as transient. An independent surgeon was assigned to record these data.

Furthermore, the mental health of patients was also investigated within one month, using the Depression Anxiety Stress Scales-21 (DASS-21), a screening tool to measure three comorbid depression, anxiety and stress disorders (**Supplement Table 1**) (7).

Statistical Analysis

SPSS 23.0 was used for statistical analyses. The continuous variables were expressed as mean ± standard deviation and analyzed using the independent-sample t-test or Mann-Whitney U test according to its distribution pattern. Categorical variables were expressed as frequency (percentage) and analyzed using Chi-square or Fisher exact test as appropriate. An independent analyst was assigned to assess the statistics, and statistical significance was recognized with $P < 0.05$.

RESULTS

Patient and Tumor Characteristics

Among a total of 260 included patients, 159 received ambulatory ETCBA, while 101 received conventional one (**Table 1**). The mean age of the two groups was 35.74 ± 8.26 and 34.93 ± 9.13 years, and the patients who received ETCBA were mostly female (92.7%). There was no difference in ASA classification between the two groups (P=0.094). 125 (78.6%) and 81 (80.2%) patients

TABLE 1 | Patients and nodules characteristics.

Characteristic	Ambulatory group (n=159)	Conventional group (n=101)	*P*
Age (years)	35.74 ± 8.26	34.93 ± 9.13	0.459
Gender			0.090
Female	151 (95.0)	90 (89.1)	
Male	8 (5.0)	11 (10.9)	
Ethnicity			
Asian	159 (100.0)	101 (100.0)	1.000
ASA classification			0.094
I	61 (38.4)	50 (49.5)	
II	98 (61.6)	51 (50.5)	
Malignant nodules	125 (78.6)	81 (80.2)	0.876
Number of lesion			0.878
Single	124 (78.0)	80 (79.2)	
Multiple	35 (22.0)	21 (20.8)	
Largest tumor size (cm)	1.22 ± 1.19	1.25 ± 1.31	0.840
Surgical procedure			0.246
Unilateral thyroidectomy	27 (17.0)	13 (12.9)	
Unilateral thyroidectomy with CLND	62 (39.0)	49 (48.5)	
Bilateral thyroidectomy	5 (3.1)	7 (6.9)	
Bilateral thyroidectomy with CLND	62 (39.0)	31 (30.7)	
Thyroidectomy with LLND	3 (1.9)	1 (1.0)	

Data are expressed as mean ± standard deviation or n (%). ASA, American Society of Anaesthesiology; CLND, central lymph node dissection; LLND, lateral lymph node dissection.

were diagnosed as malignancy in the ambulatory group and conventional group, respectively. 56 (21.5%) patients suffered from multiple lesions. The largest tumor size was 1.22 ± 1.19 cm and 1.25 ± 1.31 cm in ambulatory group and conventional group, respectively. Moreover, no difference was shown in surgical procedures between the two groups (P=0.246), indicating an identical degree of difficulty of surgery. Overall, there was no difference in the patient and tumor characteristics between two groups.

Surgical Outcomes and Prognosis

As shown in **Table 2**, surgical outcomes and patient prognosis were compared between ambulatory and conventional ETCBA. No difference was shown in the duration of surgery and blood loss. The ambulatory group showed a higher incidence of complications (30.8%) than the conventional group (23.8%), however with no statistically significant difference. Notably, all four patients who suffered from permanent hypoparathyroidism were in the ambulatory group. Two patients failed in the ambulatory management due to seroma or hematoma, and were transferred to the conventional ward for surveillance without re-operation. Furthermore, only one patient in the ambulatory group was readmitted due to hypocalcemia. Till the last follow-up, one patient with a malignant nodule suffered from a recurrence in the ambulatory group and conventional group, respectively. There was no patient suffering from re-operation or death in this study.

Economic Cost and Duration of Hospitalization

Economic cost and duration of hospitalization were also investigated (**Table 3**). The mean economic cost of the ambulatory group had a 29.5% reduction compared with the conventional group. Meanwhile, the duration of hospitalization

TABLE 2 | Surgical outcomes and prognosis.

Characteristic	Ambulatory group (n=159)	Conventional group (n=101)	*P*
Duration of surgery (min)	186.19 ± 31.77	183.78 ± 30.12	0.544
Blood loss (ml)	18.79 ± 10.79	18.84 ± 8.78	0.964
Postoperative complications	49 (30.8)	24 (23.8)	0.258
Transient hypoparathyroidism	39 (24.5)	20 (19.8)	
Permanent hypoparathyroidism	4 (2.5)	0 (0.0)	
Hypoglycemia	0 (0.0)	1 (1.0)	
Transient voice change	5 (3.1)	2 (2.0)	
Seroma	1 (0.6)	0 (0.0)	
Pulmonary infection	0 (0.0)	1 (1.0)	
Hematoma	1 (0.6)	0 (0.0)	
Transfer to the conventional ward	2 (1.3)	–	–
30-days readmission	1 (0.6)	0 (0.0)	1.000
Recurrence of malignancy	1 (0.6)	1 (1.0)	0.627

Data are expressed as mean ± standard deviation or n (%).

TABLE 3 | Economic cost and duration of hospitalization.

Characteristic	Ambulatory group (n=159)	Conventional group (n=101)	P
Economic cost (yuan)	14278.57 ± 2194.22	20261.26 ± 4399.18	<0.001
Duration of hospitalization (day)	1.03 ± 0.29	5.51 ± 1.43	<0.001

Data are expressed as mean ± standard deviation.

of the ambulatory group was also significantly shorter than the conventional group.

Mental Health

Table 4 showed the results of DASS-21. While there was no significant difference in the level of depression (P=0.731), higher levels of anxiety (P=0.041) and stress (P=0.016) were shown in the ambulatory group than the conventional group.

Subgroup Analyses for Patients With Thyroid Cancer

To further investigate the role of ambulatory ETCBA in patients with thyroid cancer, subgroup analyses were performed excluding patients with benign nodules (**Table 5**). The difference between two groups remained insignificant in duration of surgery, blood loss, 30-day readmission, and tumor recurrence. Meanwhile, significant reductions in economic cost and the duration of hospitalization were shown in the ambulatory group than the conventional group, which was consistent with the main results. The results of DASS-21 were also consistent with the main results. Notably, though with no significance, the complication incidence of the ambulatory group was 12.9% higher than the conventional group among patients with thyroid cancer.

DISCUSSION

For the very first time, this study summarized the data of patients undergoing ambulatory or conventional ETCBA in our medical center, and evaluated the safety, economic benefits, and mental health of patients, which showed that ambulatory ETCBA was as safe as the conventional ETCBA, but with great economic benefits and shorter duration of hospitalization regardless of patients with thyroid nodules or thyroid cancer. The results also highlighted that extra attention should be paid to manage the anxiety and stress of patients who received ambulatory ETCBA.

Many studies have proven the safety of ambulatory open thyroidectomy. A meta-analysis by Lee et al. consisting of 10 observational studies with 3427 patients suggested identical safety of outpatient thyroidectomy compared with inpatient thyroidectomy (11). More recently, a propensity score-matched study indicated outpatient thyroidectomy was not associated with a higher rate of readmission or complications (8). Furthermore, the safety of endoscopic thyroidectomy, including ETCBA, was well studied compared with open thyroidectomy. Jiang et al. included 20 publications with 5664 patients to perform a meta-analysis, and the results showed endoscopic thyroidectomy was similar to open thyroidectomy in terms of safety (12). This study stepped further to firstly investigate the safety of ambulatory ETCBA, which may provide the evidence for the adoption and development of ambulatory ETCBA. Meantime, the present study also showed significant economic benefits and a shorter duration of hospitalization in ambulatory ETCBA, which was solid but not surprising because the ambulatory management was administrated to achieve these purposes. Additionally, multiple studies on ambulatory surgery reported similar patient benefits (7, 13–16).

We noticed that included patients were mainly female, which might be caused by the low-level of aesthetic demands of male patients and could be noticed in papers focusing on endoscopic thyroid surgery as well (10, 17). Rare complications, such as seroma and hematoma, all occurred in-hospital within 24 hours after ETCBA, and did not need an invasive treatment or re-operation. However, though with no significance, the present study did show a higher complication rate of ambulatory ETCBA than conventional ETCBA (28.3% vs. 21.8%). Among patients with thyroid cancer, the complication incidence of the ambulatory group was even 12.9% higher than the conventional group. Thus, a prospective study with a larger cohort is needed to validate the safety of ambulatory ETCBA, especially among patients with thyroid cancer, and to investigate the reasons of it.

Nevertheless, this study also had some limitations. Firstly, we failed to investigate the role of ambulatory ETCBA due to the ambulatory ETCBA was currently not allowed in most medical centers. However we considered this study could serve as an important foundation from the conventional ETCBA to outpatient ETCBA. Secondly, patients with permanent hypoparathyroidism still had a chance to recover even after

TABLE 4 | Results of DASS-21.

Characteristic	Ambulatory group (n=159)	Conventional group (n=101)	P
Depression	3.77 ± 2.06	3.86 ± 1.91	0.731
Anxiety	7.79 ± 2.55	7.12 ± 2.64	0.041
Stress	6.91 ± 2.61	6.07 ± 2.89	0.016

Data are expressed as mean ± standard deviation.

TABLE 5 | Subgroup analyses among patients with thyroid cancer.

Characteristic	Ambulatory group (n=125)	Conventional group (n=81)	P
Duration of surgery (min)	193.21 ± 30.44	187.04 ± 28.92	0.149
Blood loss (ml)	19.27 ± 11.07	18.25 ± 8.15	0.446
Postoperative complications	47 (37.6)	20 (24.7)	0.068
Transient hypoparathyroidism	39 (24.5)	17 (21.0)	
Permanent hypoparathyroidism	4 (2.5)	0 (0.0)	
Hypoglycemia	0 (0.0)	0 (0.0)	
Transient voice change	3 (2.4)	2 (2.0)	
Seroma	1 (0.6)	0 (0.0)	
Pulmonary infection	0 (0.0)	1 (1.0)	
Hematoma	1 (0.6)	0 (0.0)	
Transfer to the conventional ward	2 (1.6)	–	–
30-days readmission	1 (0.8)	0 (0.0)	1.000
Recurrence of malignancy	1 (0.8)	1 (1.2)	0.633
Economic cost (yuan)	14778.09 ± 2092.45	20568.27 ± 4476.33	<0.001
Duration of hospitalization (day)	1.04 ± 0.32	5.54 ± 1.50	<0.001
Depression	3.82 ± 2.03	4.00 ± 1.83	0.528
Anxiety	7.92 ± 2.52	7.07 ± 2.65	0.022
Stress	6.95 ± 2.68	6.04 ± 2.91	0.022

Data are expressed as mean ± standard deviation or n (%).

six months, which might cause inaccurate complication data. Thirdly, the follow-up time was too short to fully investigate the long-term outcomes, which would be focused on in the future report with continuous follow-up. Lastly, this study preliminarily showed the mental health assessment of patients undergone ETCBA. However, although no patient was reported to have a history of psychotropic drugs, the correlation may exist between the mental health and the diagnosis of disease. We failed to investigate it because the mental changes may happen before the diagnosis of thyroid nodules, and it is hard to access patients for such assessments before the diagnosis. Future studies will be performed to deal these questions for a more comprehensive assessment of patient mental health.

CONCLUSION

Ambulatory ETCBA is as safe as conventional ETCBA for selective patients with thyroid nodules or thyroid cancer, however with significant economic benefits and shorter duration of hospitalization. Extra attention should be paid to manage the anxiety and stress of patients who received ambulatory ETCBA.

ETHICS STATEMENT

The studies involving human participants were reviewed and approved by Institutional Ethics Committee of Xiangya Hospital, Central South University. Written informed consent for participation was not required for this study in accordance with the national legislation and the institutional requirements.

AUTHOR CONTRIBUTIONS

All authors made substantive intellectual contributions to this study to qualify as authors. XL conceived of the design of the study. FX modified the design of the study. ZZ and FX performed the study, collected the data, and contributed to the design of the study. ZZ analyzed the data. ZZ drafted Result, Discussion, and Conclusion sections. FX drafted Methods sections. FX and XL edited the manuscript. All authors read and approved the final manuscript. All authors have agreed to be accountable for all aspects of the work in ensuring that questions related to the accuracy or integrity of any part of the work are appropriately investigated and resolved.

REFERENCES

1. Singh Ospina N, Maraka S, Espinosa De Ycaza AE, Ahn HS, Castro MR, Morris JC, et al. Physical Exam in Asymptomatic People Drivers the Detection of Thyroid Nodules Undergoing Ultrasound Guided Fine Needle Aspiration Biopsy. *Endocrine* (2016) 54(2):433–9. doi: 10.1007/s12020-016-1054-y
2. Valderrabano P, Khazai L, Thompson ZJ, Leon ME, Otto KJ, Hallanger-Johnson JE, et al. Cancer Risk Stratification of Indeterminate Thyroid Nodules: A Cytological Approach. *Thyroid: Off J Am Thyroid Assoc* (2017) 27(10):1277–84. doi: 10.1089/thy.2017.0221
3. Wang C, Feng Z, Li J, Yang W, Zhai H, Choi N, et al. Endoscopic Thyroidectomy *via* Areola Approach: Summary of 1,250 Cases in a Single Institution. *Surg Endoscopy* (2015) 29(1):192–201. doi: 10.1007/s00464-014-3658-8
4. Park KN, Jung C, Mok JO, Kwak JJ, Lee SW. Prospective Comparative Study of Endoscopic *via* Unilateral Axillobreast Approach Versus Open Conventional Total Thyroidectomy in Patients With Papillary Thyroid Carcinoma. *Surg Endoscopy* (2016) 30(9):3797–801. doi: 10.1007/s00464-015-4676-x
5. Wu G, Fu J, Lin F, Luo Y, Lin E, Yan W. Endoscopic Central Lymph Node Dissection *via* Breast Combined With Oral Approach for Papillary Thyroid Carcinoma: A Preliminary Study. *World J Surg* (2017) 41(9):2280–2. doi: 10.1007/s00268-017-4015-6
6. Chai YJ, Chung JK, Anuwong A, Dionigi G, Kim HY, Hwang KT, et al. Transoral Endoscopic Thyroidectomy for Papillary Thyroid Microcarcinoma: Initial Experience of a Single Surgeon. *Ann Surg Treat Res* (2017) 93(2):70–5.

doi: 10.4174/astr.2017.93.2.70

7. Zhang Z, Xia F, Wang W, Jiang B, Yao L, Huang Y, et al. Ambulatory Thyroidectomy is Safe and Beneficial in Papillary Thyroid Carcinoma: Randomized Controlled Trial. *Head Neck* (2020) 43(4):1116–21. doi: 10.1002/hed.26557
8. Hu QL, Livhits MJ, Ko CY, Yeh MW. Same-Day Discharge Is Not Associated With Increased Readmissions or Complications After Thyroid Operations. *Surgery* (2020) 167(1):117–23. doi: 10.1016/j.surg.2019.06.054
9. Prabhakar A, Helander E, Chopra N, Kaye AJ, Urman RD, Kaye AD. Preoperative Assessment for Ambulatory Surgery. *Curr Pain Headache R* (2017) 21(10):43. doi: 10.1007/s11916-017-0643-7
10. Qu R, Li J, Yang J, Sun P, Gong J, Wang C. Treatment of Differentiated Thyroid Cancer: Can Endoscopic Thyroidectomy *via* a Chest-Breast Approach Achieve Similar Therapeutic Effects as Open Surgery? *Surg Endoscopy* (2018) 32(12):4749–56. doi: 10.1007/s00464-018-6221-1
11. Lee DJ, Chin CJ, Hong CJ, Perera S, Witterick IJ. Outpatient Versus Inpatient Thyroidectomy: A Systematic Review and Meta-Analysis. *Head Neck* (2018) 40(1):192–202. doi: 10.1002/hed.24934
12. Jiang W, Yan PJ, Zhao CL, Si MB, Tian W, Zhang YJ, et al. Comparison of Total Endoscopic Thyroidectomy With Conventional Open Thyroidectomy for Treatment of Papillary Thyroid Cancer: A Systematic Review and Meta-Analysis. *Surg Endoscopy* (2020) 34(5):1891–903. doi: 10.1007/s00464-019-07283-y
13. Nordin AB, Shah SR, Kenney BD. Ambulatory Pediatric Surgery. *Semin Pediatr Surg* (2018) 27(2):75–8. doi: 10.1053/j.sempedsurg.2018.02.003
14. Thompson NB, Calandruccio JH. Hand Surgery in the Ambulatory Surgery Center. *Orthopedic Clinics North America* (2018) 49(1):69–72. doi: 10.1016/j.ocl.2017.08.009
15. Rider CM, Hong VY, Westbrooks TJ, Wang J, Sheffer BW, Kelly DM, et al. Surgical Treatment of Supracondylar Humeral Fractures in a Freestanding Ambulatory Surgery Center is as Safe as and Faster and More Cost-Effective Than in a Children's Hospital. *J Pediatr Orthopedics* (2018) 38(6):e343–8. doi: 10.1097/BPO.0000000000001171
16. Ford MC, Walters JD, Mulligan RP, Dabov GD, Mihalko WM, Mascioli AM, et al. Safety and Cost-Effectiveness of Outpatient Unicompartmental Knee Arthroplasty in the Ambulatory Surgery Center: A Matched Cohort Study. *Orthopedic Clinics North Am* (2020) 51(1):1–5. doi: 10.1016/j.ocl.2019.08.001
17. Guo Y, Qu R, Huo J, Wang C, Hu X, Chen C, et al. Technique for Endoscopic Thyroidectomy With Selective Lateral Neck Dissection *via* a Chest-Breast Approach. *Surg Endoscopy* (2019) 33(4):1334–41. doi: 10.1007/s00464-018-06608-7

6

A Novel and Effective Model to Predict Skip Metastasis in Papillary Thyroid Carcinoma Based on a Support Vector Machine

Shuting Zhu[1†], Qingxuan Wang[2†], Danni Zheng[3†], Lei Zhu[4], Zheng Zhou[5], Shiying Xu[6], Binbin Shi[7], Cong Jin[3], Guowan Zheng[8,9] and Yefeng Cai[2,8,9*]*

[1] Department of Ultrasound, The First Medical Center of Chinese People's Liberation Army (PLA) General Hospital, Beijing, China, [2] Department of Thyroid Surgery, The First Affiliated Hospital of Wenzhou Medical University, Wenzhou, China, [3] Department of Breast Surgery, The First Affiliated Hospital of Wenzhou Medical University, Wenzhou, China, [4] Thyroid Surgery Department, The Fifth Hospital Affiliated to Wenzhou Medical University, Lishui Central Hospital, Lishui, China, [5] Department of Head and Neck Surgery, Bengbu Medical College Graduate School, Anhui, China, [6] Zhejiang Chinese Medical University, The Second Clinical Medical, Hangzhou, China, [7] Department of Medical Ultrasound,the First Affiliated Hospital of Wenzhou Medical University, Wenzhou, China, [8] Department of Head and Neck Surgery, Otolaryngology & Head and Neck Center, Cancer Center, Zhejiang Provincial People's Hospital (Affiliated People's Hospital, Hangzhou Medical College), Hangzhou, China, [9] Key Laboratory of Endocrine Gland Diseases of Zhejiang Province, Hangzhou, China

***Correspondence:**
Guowan Zheng
0818331@163.com
Yefeng Cai
Cyfoncology@gmail.com

[†]These authors have contributed equally to this work

Introduction: Skip metastasis, referred to as lymph node metastases to the lateral neck compartment without involvement of the central compartment, is generally unpredictable in papillary thyroid carcinoma (PTC). This study aims to establish an effective predictive model for skip metastasis in PTC.

Meterials and Methods: Retrospective analysis was performed of clinical samples from 18192 patients diagnosed with thyroid cancer between 2016 to 2020. The First Affiliated Hospital of Wenzhou Medical University. The lateral lymph node metastasis was occureed in the training set (630 PTC patients) and validation set (189 PTC patients). The univariate and multivariate analyses were performed to detect the predictors of skip metastasis and the support vector machine (SVM) was used to establish a model to predict skip metastasis.

Results: The rate of skip metastasis was 13.3% (84/631). Tumor size (≤10 mm), upper location, Hashimoto's thyroiditis, extrathyroidal extension, absence of BRAFV600E mutation, and less number of central lymph node dissection were considered as independent predictors of skip metastasis in PTC. For the training set, these predictors performed with 91.7% accuracy, 86.4% sensitivity, 92.2% specificity, 45.2% positive predictive value (PPV), and 98.9% negative predictive value (NPV) in the model. Meanwhile, these predictors showed 91.5% accuracy,71.4% sensitivity, 93.1% specificity, 45.5% PPV, and 97.6% NPV in validation set.

Conclusion: This study screened the predictors of the skip lateral lymph node metastasis and to establish an effective and economic predictive model for skip metastasis in PTC. The model can accurately distinguish the skip metastasis in PTC using a simple and affordable method, which may have potential for daily clinical application in the future.

Keywords: predict model, skip lymph node metastasis, papillary thyroid carcinoma, support vector, BRAF mutation

INTRODUCTION

The incidence of thyroid cancer has remarkably increased in the last 40 years worldwide primarily because of the increase in the incidence of papillary thyroid carcinoma (PTC) (1). Papillary thyroid carcinoma, a common endocrine malignancy, accounts for 90% of thyroid cancer (2, 3). The dissemination of PTC cells follows a predictable stepwise pattern, metastasizing from the central lymph node (CLN) compartment to the lateral lymph node (LLN) compartment (4, 5). Thus, CLN is considered as the first step of lymphatic drainage of PTC in most previous studies (6, 7). However, lateral lymph node metastasis (LLNM) of PTC without central lymph node metastasis (CLNM) is also found (8). This unpredictable pattern of LNM is known as skip metastasis of PTC.

Skip metastasis is not unique to PTC. This metastatic form without stepwise spread also exists in gastric, colorectal, lung, and breast carcinoma (9–12). Giving inadequate attention to any tumor may adversely affect treatment outcomes and cause poor prognosis. In addition, skip metastasis is not a rare phenomenon. For example, skip metastasis of gastrointestinal cancer is frequent because the location of the lymphatic drainage tract is complicated (13). Skip metastasis is also common in PTC, and its incidence ranges from 5% to 25% (the data are obtained from different samples) (14).

Some studies have suggested that regional lymph node metastasis (LNM) is a vital factor in poor prognosis of patients with PTC (15). In addition, LLNM has shown stronger connection with locoregional recurrence and unfavorable prognosis than CLNM in patients with PTC (16). However, whether skip LNM is associated with a relatively poor prognosis remains unclear (14). Some studies show that LNM can increase the risk of lymph node recurrence, and the reoperation of recurrence can increase operative complications and medical costs to some degree (17–19). Therefore, skip metastasis in clinical diagnosis and treatment must be given importance to avoid risks as much as possible.

Preoperative ultrasonographic evaluation and biopsy results of cervical lymph nodes primarily determined the operative mode of PTC. Suspicious and/or biopsy-proven nodal metastases should be treated with a formal compartmental resection (20). Therefore, the neglect of skip metastasis may lead to incomplete surgical resection. However, few effective methods to predict skip metastasis in PTC were identified. Therefore, our study investigated the frequency and risk factors for skip metastasis and established a model to predict skip metastasis, make a reasonable surgical project or follow-up plan, and achieve treatment effectiveness.

Abbreviations: PTC, papillary thyroid carcinoma; SVM, support vector machine; CLN, central lymph node; LLN, lateral lymph node; CLNM, central lymph node metastasis; LLNM, lateral lymph node metastasis; CLND, central lymph node dissection; LLND, lateral lymph node dissection; CI, confidence interval; OR, odds ratio; PPV, positive predictive value; NPV, negative predictive value.

MATERIALS AND METHODS

Patients

Two sets of patients were included in the training set and validation set. Patients in the training set were used to investigate the predictors of skip metastasis and to establish predictive models, whereas patients in the validation set were used to examine the efficacy of the predictive models. A total 631 patients with PTC who received initial thyroidectomy with central lymph node dissection (CLND) plus lateral lymph node dissection (LLND) at the First Affiliated Hospital of Wenzhou Medical University during January 2016 to September 2019 were included in the training set. Meanwhile, 189 external patients who received the same surgical procedure during October 2019 to June 2020 were included in the validation set (**Figure 1**). All of the patients were identified as PTC with LLNM by postoperative pathological report. Each set was further divided into the skip metastasis group and non-skip metastasis group.

The exclusion criteria were as follows: insufficient data or unknown clinicopathologic profile, undetermined histology, history of neck surgery or irradiation, negative lateral lymph node metastases, and other types of thyroid cancer (follicular thyroid cancer, medullary thyroid cancer, anaplastic thyroid cancer, etc.). The study obtained approval from the Ethics Committee of the First Affiliated Hospital of Wenzhou Medical University.

Operational Approach

The operation was performed by the same experienced surgical team and the same standard procedure. The scope of CLND was up to the thyroid cartilage notch, down to the carotid sheath, posterior to the prevertebral fascia, and final to the innominate vein. In this study, the lateral lymph node compartment included levels II, III, IV, and V. The area was drawn up to the posterior belly of the digastric muscle, down to the subclavian vein, and next to the anterior border of the trapezius muscle.

Parameter Analysis

Our study collected information through electronic clinical records, pathological records, and preoperative ultrasonographic images. Patient's baseline information (gender and age) and

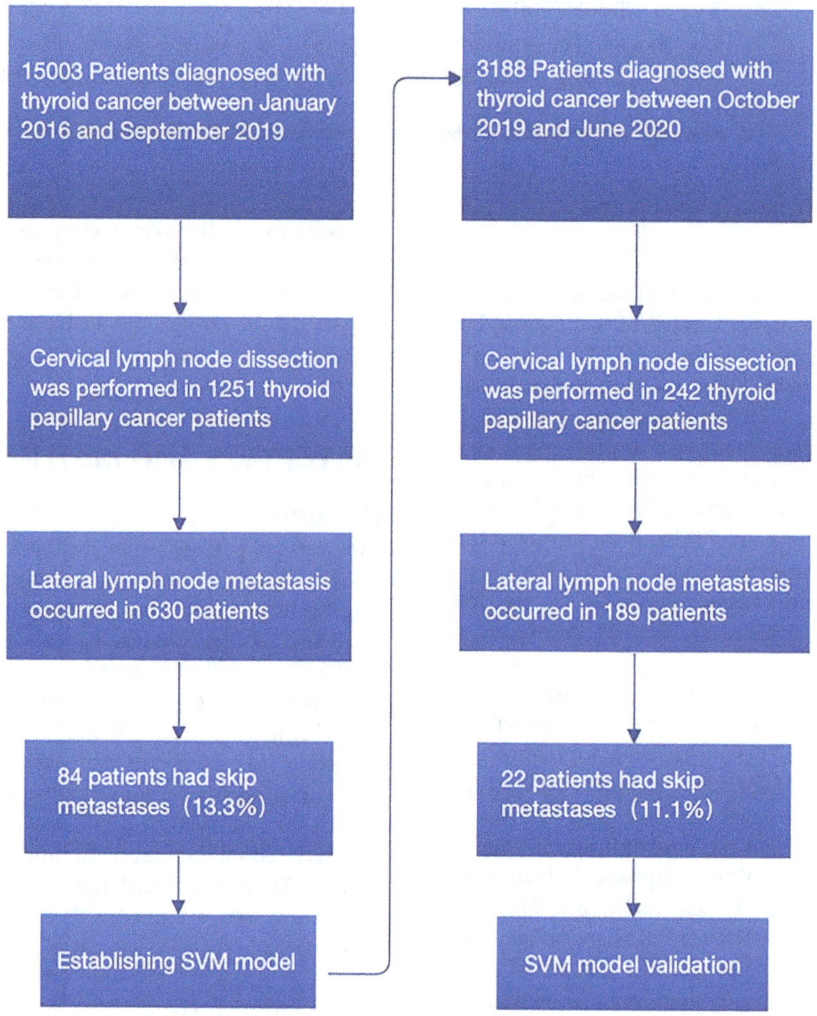

FIGURE 1 | Flowchart for the process of establishment and validation of skip metastasis prediction model of PTC.

clinical data (hashimoto's thyroiditis, body mass index [BMI], metabolic syndrome, hypertension, and diabetes) were analyzed. In addition, the thyroid nodule sonographic features were evaluated and analyzed, by three experienced sonographers, on the basis of the size of tumor, location, margin, taller-than-wide shape, calcification, vascularization, multifocality, extrathyroidal extension, and the information about cervical lymph node. The information about $BRAF^{V600E}$ mutation was collected as well.

We analyzed the largest tumor or the most suspicious dominant nodule of the thyroid, when multiple nodules were found. Standard preoperative sonography of PTC tumor boundaries was performed to determine the size, and taller-than-wide shape. Moreover, the thyroid gland was trisected vertically, dividing it into three locations (upper, middle, and lower) to determine the location of tumors. Calcification was defined as the hyperechoic spots with or without acoustic shadows or as simple fine acoustic shadows in ultrasound (21). The multifocality of a tumor was confirmed when more than one mass was found based on the preoperative ultrasound examination or the intraoperative pathological diagnose (22). Extrathyroidal extension was defined as the tumor perimeter in contact with >25% of the thyroid capsule in a malignant lesion or the loss of the capsule line (23). The diagnosis of hashimoto's thyroiditis relies on the demonstration of circulating antibodies to thyroid antigens (mainly anti-thyroglobulin >30U/ml (normal range is 0-4U/ml); anti-thyroperoxidase (anti-TPO) >30U/ml) (normal range is 0-9U/ml) and reduced echogenicity and prominent heterogeneous thyroid parenchyma on thyroid sonogram in a patient with proper clinical features (24). The information of cervical lymph node was obtained from the final pathological reports.

Model Development

A support vector machine (SVM) was used for establishing skip metastasis prediction models. The prediction models were established by Libsvm 3.20 with the modeling platform of MATLAB 2019a. The C-SVC, RBF kernel functions and grid search method were used to debug the model. The grid c bound, grid c step, grid g bound, and grid g step were −8 to 8, 0.5, −8 to 8, and 0.5, respectively. The fold number of cross-validation was 5. As we divided patients into two groups, the positive value indicated skip metastasis, and the negative value indicated non-skip metastasis.

$$P(label) = \mathbf{sgn}(\textstyle\sum_{n=1}^{\infty} ni = (\mathbf{0wi}\ \ \mathbf{exp}(-\mathbf{ganma}|\mathbf{xi} - \mathbf{x}|\mathbf{2} + \mathbf{b})))$$

Statistics

The data showed a normal distribution through an independent two-sample Student's t-test. Statistical analysis was performed using SPSS version 26.0 (SPSS, Chicago, IL, USA). Categorical variables were compared with the results of Chi-square test or Fisher's exact test. The difference between two sides was statistically significant, when *P* value ≤ 0.05. All factors with significant associations based on univariate analysis were included for multivariate analysis using forward stepwise selection.

RESULTS

The Baseline Information in the Training and Validation Set

1. Gender: The female percent is 67.6% (426/630) in the training set and 61.9% (117/189) in the validation set.
2. Age: The average age of training set is 45.28 ± 12.48 years (range, 17–84 years), and that of the validation set is 46.69 ± 12.11 years (range, 21–74 years).
3. The size of a primary tumor: the mean size is 14.25 ± 8.88 mm (range, 1–67mm) and 12.25 ± 7.74 mm (range, 1–40mm) in the training set and validation set, respectively.
4. The mean number of total harvested CLN is 7.57 ± 5.71 (range, 1–28) in the training set and 6.95 ± 5.18 (range, 1–35) in the validation set.
5. The rate of skip metastasis is 13.3% (84/630) in the training test and 11.6% (22/189) in the validation set.
6. The rate of $BRAF^{V600E}$ mutation is 75.1% (473/630) in the training test and 82.0% (155/189) in the validation set (**Table S1**).

Predictors of Skip Metastasis of PTC in the Training Set

Data from the training set were used to investigate the predictors of skip metastasis in PTC. The first step of analysis was comparing the clinicopathological factors between the skip metastasis group and non-skip metastasis by univariate analysis. The following characteristics of patients were more likely observed in the skip metastasis group (**Table 1**): age>45 (*P*=0.008), tumor size ≤ 10 mm (*P*=0.001), Hashimoto's thyroiditis (*P*=0.009), upper tumor location (*P*<0.001), well-defined margin (*P*=0.05), extrathyroidal extension (*P*=0.002), absence of $BRAF^{V600E}$ mutations (*P*=0.006), BMI≥25 (*P*=0.024), and less number of CLND (the mean number of the skip metastasis was 5.17 ± 3.81, *P*=0.001).

Further multivariate analysis showed that tumor size (≤10 mm; OR 2.331; *P*=0.003; 95% CI 1.342–4.049), upper location (OR 2.595; *P*<0.001; CI 1.535–4.388), Hashimoto's thyroiditis (OR 3.968; *P*<0.001; CI 2.178–7.229), extrathyroidal extension (OR 3.506; *P*<0.001; CI 1.962–6.265), absence of $BRAF^{V600E}$ mutation (OR 0.373; *P*<0.001; CI 0.212–0.658), and less number of CLND (OR 1.304; *P*<0.001; CI 1.193–1.423) were independent predictors of skip metastasis in PTC (**Table 2**). As mentioned previously, a difference in BMI values and well-defined margin was found between the skip metastasis group and non-skip metastasis group in univariate analysis. No further evidence indicated that such characteristics were independent predictors of skip metastasis in PTC.

Information about LLN Between the Skip Metastasis Group and Non-skip Metastasis Group

In addition, the information about LLN between the skip metastasis group and non-skip metastasis group was compared (**Table 3**). We found that the number of LLNM of skip metastasis was less than that of non-skip metastasis (mean 2.04 ± 1.71 and 3.30 ± 2.59, respectively; *P*<0.001). No contralateral LLNM was found in 84 patients with skip metastasis, whereas 26 patients in the non-skip metastasis group showed contralateral LLNM. Therefore, the difference in contralateral LLNM was found between the two groups (*P*=0.037). By contrast, no difference was found in the number of LLND between the two groups (*P*=0.509).

Training Set: Establishing a Model to Predict Skip Metastasis

The predictive panel was built using SVM, which combined the six independent predictors (tumor size, location, Hashimoto's thyroiditis, extrathyroidal extension, $BRAF^{V600E}$ mutation, and number of CLND). In addition, skip metastasis in the training set was predicted by this panel (**Table 4**). These predictors performed with high 91.7% accuracy in the panel (sensibility: 86.4%, specificity: 92.2%, positive predictive value [PPV]: 45.2%, negative predictive value [NPV]: 98.9%), albeit the accuracy of each individual factor was low (**Table 5**). Parameters c, g, and b were 16, 0.0884, and −0.5531, respectively, which were used to make the 3D view (**Figure 2**).

Validation Set: Validating the Model in External Independent Samples

The 189 (22 skip metastasis and 167 non-skip metastasis) external independent samples were used to validate panel performance. The panel also achieved high accuracy in the validation set, with 91.5% accuracy (173/189 samples correctly classified, **Table 4**). Moreover, the specificity and NPV maintained a highly level, 93.1% and 97.6, respectively, in the validation set. On the contrary, the sensitivity and PPV were slightly decreased (71.4% and 45.5%, respectively). The AUC (Area under the curve) of SVM model in ROC Curve is 0.721 (**Figure 3**).

TABLE 1 | Comparison of clinicopathological factors between skip metastasis and non-skip metastasis with PTC. .

Characteristics	Skip metastasis		F	P value
	Present (n=84)	Absent (n=546)		
Sex			2.412	0.12
Male (n, %)	21 (25.0%)	183 (33.5%)		
Female (n, %)	63 (75.0%)	363 (66.5%)		
Age at diagnosis (years)	49.55 ± 11.73	44.62 ± 12.48	6.995	0.008*
≤45 (n, %)	33 (39.3%)	299 (54.8%)		
>45 (n, %)	51 (60.7%)	247 (45.2%)		
Tumor size (mm)	12.83 ± 8.85	14.47 ± 8.87	10.859	0.001*
≤10 (n, %)	50 (59.5%)	217 (39.9%)		
>10 (n, %)	34 (40.5%)	329 (60.1%)		
Multifocality (n,%)			3.249	0.071
Yes (n, %)	21 (25%)	191 (35.0%)		
No (n, %)	63 (75%)	355 (65.0%)		
Hashimoto's thyroiditis			6.784	0.009*
Yes (n, %)	29 (34.5%)	118 (21.6%)		
No (n, %)	55 (65.5%)	428 (78.4%)		
Tumor location			15.066	<0.001*
Upper (n, %)	41 (48.8%)	152 (27.8%)		
Lower/middle/isthmus (n, %)	43 (51.2%)	394 (72.2%)		
Taller than wide			0.74	0.39
Yes (n, %)	17 (20.2%)	134 (24.5%)		
No (n, %)	67 (79.7%)	412 (73.4%)		
Calcification			0.873	0.35
Calcification (n, %)	68 (81.0%)	462 (84.6%)		
Absence (n, %)	16 (19.0%)	84 (15.4%)		
Margin			3.369	0.05*
Well-defined (n, %)	63 (73.8%)	333 (61.0%)		
Without well-defined margin (n, %)	21 (26.2%)	213 (38.5%)		
Shape			1.365	0.243
Regular (n, %)	20 (23.8%)	164 (30.0%)		
Irregular (n, %)	64 (76.2%)	382 (70.0%)		
Extrathyroidal extension			10.077	0.002*
Yes (n, %)	35 (41.7%)	137 (25.1%)		
No (n, %)	49 (58.3%)	409 (74.9%)		
Vascularization			1.715	0.19
Present (n, %)	13 (15.5%)	58 (10.6%)		
Absence (n, %)	71 (84.5%)	488 (89.4%)		
$BRAF^{V600E}$			7.44	0.006*
Mutation (n, %)	53 (63.1%)	420 (76.9%)		
No mutation (n, %)	31 (26.7%)	126 (23.1%)		
BMI			5.065	0.024*
<25 (n, %)	50 (59.5%)	391 (71.6%)		
≥25 (n, %)	34 (40.5%)	155 (28.4%)		
hypertension			0.963	0.326
Yes (n, %)	19 (22.6%)	99 (18.3%)		
No (n, %)	65 (77.3%)	447 (81.9%)		
diabetes			0.856	0.355
Yes (n, %)	6 (7.1%)	26 (4.8%)		
No (n, %)	78 (92.9%)	520 (95.2%)		
Metabolic syndrome			2.097	0.148
Yes (n, %)	18 (21.4%)	83 (15.2%)		
No (n, %)	66 (78.6%)	463 (84.8%)		
Cervical lymphadenopathy			0.826	0.363
Yes (n, %)	54 (64.3%)	378 (69.2%)		
No (n, %)	30 (35.7%)	168 (30.8%)		
Central lymph nodes dissected number	5.17 ± 3.81	6.73 ± 3.79	3.269	0.001*

**P value ≤ 0.05.*

DISCUSSION

To date, PTC in 30%–80% of patients was accompanied by other forms of LNM (6). PTC with LNM was linked to local recurrence and cancer-specific mortality in certain patients (5, 25). The complications from re-operation of PTC, for example, hemorrhage, hypothyroidism, laryngeal nerve injury, and lymphatic leakage, were increased compared with the initial operation. Therefore, predicting LNM is important for surgeons to precisely determine neck dissections.

TABLE 2 | Multivariate analysis between the clinicopathologic factors and skip metastasis.

Characteristic	OR	95% CI	P value
Tumor size (≤10 mm)	2.331	1.342-4.049	0.003*
Extrathyroidal extension	3.506	1.962-6.265	<0.001*
Hashimoto's thyroiditis	3.968	2.178-7.229	<0.001*
BRAFV600E mutation	0.373	0.212-0.658	0.001*
locating in the upper pole	2.595	1.535-4.388	<0.001*
Less CLND number	1.304	1.193-1.423	<0.001*

**P value ≤ 0.05.*

TABLE 3 | Comparison of LLN between skip metastasis and non-skip metastasis with PTC.

	Skip metastasis		F/t value	P Value
	Present (n = 84)	Absent (n = 546)		
The number of LLND (Mean ± SD)	10.79 ± 7.34	11.43 ± 8.49	-0.611	0.509
The number of LLNM (Mean ± SD)	2.04 ± 1.71	3.30 ± 2.59	-5.816	<0.001*
Contralateral LLNM			Fish Test	0.037*
Yes	0	26		
No	84	526		

**P value ≤ 0.05.*

TABLE 4 | The predictive model and pathological diagnosis for skip metastasis in both training and validation set.

		Predicting Model		
		Positive	Negative	Total
Pathological diagnosis in Train set	positive	38	46	84
	negative	6	540	546
	total	44	586	630
Pathological diagnosis in Test set	positive	10	12	22
	negative	4	163	167
	total	14	175	189

TABLE 5 | The predictive value for the model and independent predictors.

Independent predictors	sensitivity	Specificity	PPV*	NPV*	accuracy
Size	13.8%	87.0%	41.7%	60.1%	57.6%
Location	21.2%	90.2%	48.8%	72.2%	69.0%
Number of central lymph node	20.1%	94.3%	79.8%	51.3%	55.1%
Extrathyroidal extension	20.3%	89.3%	41.7%	74.9%	70.5%
$BRAF^{V600E}$ mutation	19.7%	88.8%	36.9%	76.9%	71.6%
Hashimoto's thyroiditis	19.7%	88.6%	34.5%	78.4%	72.5%
The model	86.4%	92.2%	45.2%	98.9%	91.7%

**PPV, positive predictive value; NPV, negative predictive value.*

The underestimation of skip metastasis of PTC will result in incomplete lymph node dissection during the operation and ultimately lead to a poor prognosis in patients with PTC. However, when the CLN is negative, no further LLND will be performed unless lateral cervical lymphadenopathy is proven by preoperative biopsy and imaging modalities (26). However, a high false negative rate of LLNM by preoperative examination is found (27, 28). For example, about 30% of metastatic lymph nodes in level 3 could not be detected by preoperative examination in previous studies (27). Therefore, accurate assessment of the characteristics and mechanisms of the occurrence of skip metastasis to provide clinical guidance, such as close follow-up or more aggressive surgery, will improve the prognosis of thyroid cancer. In this research, the incidence and detailed characteristics associated with skip metastasis were evaluated by our group.

The reported rate of skip metastasis varies considerably, ranging from 5% to 25% (14). The difference in the frequency

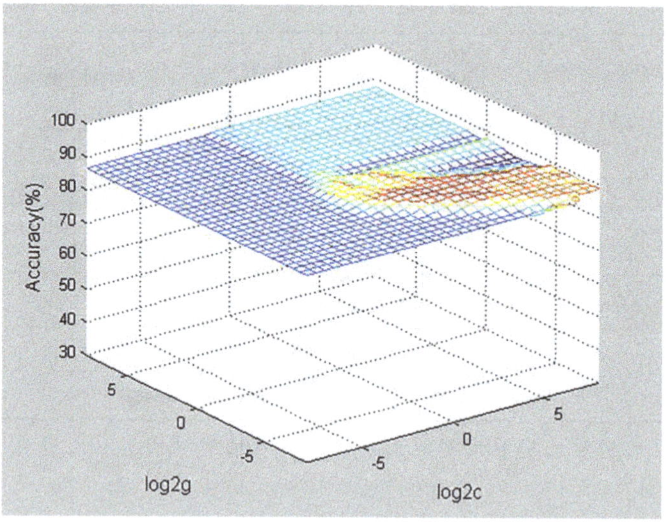

FIGURE 2 | D view of the predictive value for the model (the best parameter c is 16, the parameter g is 0.0884, the parameter b is -0.5531).

of skip metastasis might be due to the different regions and sample sizes. Given the small sample data in most previous studies, the accuracy of data is limited. In our study, we found that the frequency of skip metastasis was 13.3% (84/630), which was the largest sample analysis in skip metastasis. The high rate of skip metastasis indicates that we do not ignore the presence of skip metastasis in the clinical work, although the prognostic relationship between skip metastasis and PTC remains unknown. This form of metastatic spread to regional lymph nodes is also found in other cancer. The non-small-cell lung cancer and colorectal cancer were reported as a prognostic benefit (29, 30). On the contrary, the presence of metastases confers a poor prognosis when synchronous skip metastases are present in osteosarcoma (31). In previous studies, no significant difference in PTC-tumor-free survival was observed between the skip metastasis and non-skip metastasis groups (32). However, these results remain to be verified.

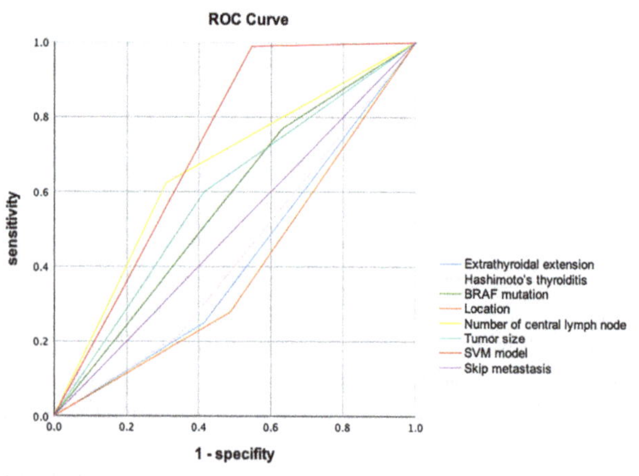

FIGURE 3 | The ROC Curve of the SVM model (The AUC is 0.721).

Machine learning (ML) is type of classifier learning from past date to predict future data. SVM is one of many ML methods (33). Compared to the other ML methods, SVM has very powerful ability to recognize subtle patterns in complex datasets (34). Moreover, Golub et al. had demonstrated the superior performance of SVM in classifying high-dimensional and low sample size data (35). Since 2000, the SVM has been used in many complex classification of cancer study, such as the cancer subtypes, the outcome prognosis, drug benefit prediction, tumorigenesis drivers, or a tumor-specific biological process (36–40). Therefore, in this study, the artificial intelligence of SVM was used to recognize many important factors in a variety of risk characteristics and establish a model to predict skip metastasis in PTC.

In this study, we found six independent predictors (tumor size ≤10 mm, located in the upper pole, Hashimoto's thyroiditis, no $BRAF^{V600E}$ mutation, extrathyroidal extension, and less number of CLND) for skip metastasis in PTC. Some of these clinicopathological or sonographic features were considered as risk factors for skip metastasis in previous studies, but the results were disputed. For example, the positive correlation between upper location and skip metastasis has been shown in many earlier studies (14, 32, 41). This connection may be interpreted by the anatomical structure, which could migrate along the superior thyroid artery to LLN and leap over CLN. Some studies have reported that the skip area in level II or/and III is a predictor of skip metastasis (41, 42). In addition, tumor size ≤ 10 mm, well-defined margin and

extrathyroidal extension were recognized as predictors of skip metastasis (28, 41–43). Furthermore, we observed that skip metastasis could easily occur in PTC patients with Hashimoto's thyroiditis and without $BRAF^{V600E}$ mutation. What's more, the less number of CLND as a predictor was found in both this study and previous studies (44).

To date, the leading causes of skip metastasis are not completely clarified yet. Skip metastasis may be due to the following reasons: first, nodal metastasis bypasses, without normal anatomical lymphatic channels, were observed (14, 45). Thus, less aggressive nodules (tumor size <10 mm) are more easily characterized by skip metastasis as they passes through the metastasis bypasses before invading the central lymph node compartment. Previous reports have suggested that the absence of $BRAF^{V600E}$ mutation and Hashimoto's thyroiditis-positive PTC were associated with a less aggressive disease (43). Second, extrathyroidal extension or neck treatment alters the normal lymphatic channels and induces skip metastasis; In addition, inadequate CLND sampling may cause false negative findings. For example, metastatic lymph node missed during LND could cause a negative finding. Therefore, a less number of CLND is a risk factor of skip metastasis.

A predictive model for skip metastasis was first established in this research. This model has a good performance and high accuracy, indicating its strong clinical feasibility. In addition, the model has high specificity and NPV, which indicates that the model has a high ability to exclude patients with non-skip metastasis. If the model predicts a non-skip metastasis, then the probability that this result is correct is 98.9%. Therefore, patients with non-skip metastasis can be basically excluded when they are predicted negative by this model. Furthermore, although the sensitivity decreased in the validation set (71.4%) compared with the training set (86.4%). The predictive sensitivity of model was significantly higher than that of each single factor. However, the disadvantage of the model's PPV (45.2%) is not obvious. Since there were few guidelines to support perform prophylactic LLND in the cN0 thyroid cancer with high risk of skip metastasis, this model focused on identifying the non-skip metastasis patients and ensure the higher specificity and NPV. Therefore, if the model predicts a high risk of skip metastasis, close follow-up or more aggressive surgery could be considered according to the status of disease.

The current study has several limitations. First, this study is a single-center retrospective study; hence, the results may have some differences from other studies. For further research, we are undertaking a multicenter prospective study. Second, although the model can be more convenient and accurate to guide the operation, whether the model has survival benefits remains unknown. Therefore, more follow-up studies will be conducted in the future.

In conclusion, we found that the rate of skip metastasis was 13.3% (84/631), which was the largest sample analysis so far. We screened six predictors of the skip lateral lymph node metastasis: tumor ≤10 mm, locating in the upper pole, Hashimoto's thyroiditis, extrathyroidal extension, less number of CLND and without $BRAF^{V600E}$ mutation. This study is the first to explore the association of Hashimoto's thyroiditis and $BRAF^{V600E}$ mutation with skip metastasis. Moreover, we established an effective predictive model for skip metastasis in PTC. This model can accurately distinguish the skip metastasis in PTC using a simple and affordable method, which may have the potential for daily clinical application in the future.

ETHICS STATEMENT

The studies involving human participants were reviewed and approved by The Ethics Committee of the First Affiliated Hospital of Wenzhou Medical University. The patients/participants provided their written informed consent to participate in this study.

AUTHOR CONTRIBUTIONS

GZ and YC contributed to the conception and design of the research. BS and CJ contributed to collected the clinical information. SZ, QW and DZ contributed to performed the statistical analysis and make the charts. YC, ZZ and SX contributed to establish the model. All authors contributed to manuscript revision, and all authors read and approved the submitted version.

REFERENCES

1. Bray F, Ferlay J, Soerjomataram I, Siegel RL, Torre LA, Jemal A. Global Cancer Statistics 2018: Globocan Estimates of Incidence and Mortality Worldwide for 36 Cancers in 185 Countries. *CA Cancer J Clin* (2018) 68 (6):394–424. doi: 10.3322/caac.21492
2. Seib CD, Sosa JA. Evolving Understanding of the Epidemiology of Thyroid Cancer. *Endocrinol Metab Clin North Am* (2019) 48(1):23–35. doi: 10.1016/j.ecl.2018.10.002
3. Pellegriti G, Frasca F, Regalbuto C, Squatrito S, Vigneri R. Worldwide Increasing Incidence of Thyroid Cancer: Update on Epidemiology and Risk Factors. *J Cancer Epidemiol* (2013) 2013:965212. doi: 10.1155/2013/965212
4. Machens A, Hinze R, Thomusch O, Dralle H. Pattern of Nodal Metastasis for Primary and Reoperative Thyroid Cancer. *World J Surg* (2002) 26(1):22–8. doi: 10.1007/s00268-001-0176-3
5. Machens A, Holzhausen HJ, Dralle H. Skip Metastases in Thyroid Cancer Leaping the Central Lymph Node Compartment. *Arch Surg* (2004) 139(1):43–5. doi: 10.1001/archsurg.139.1.43
6. Lee YM, Sung TY, Kim WB, Chung KW, Yoon JH, Hong SJ. Risk Factors for Recurrence in Patients With Papillary Thyroid Carcinoma Undergoing Modified Radical Neck Dissection. *Br J Surg* (2016) 103(8):1020–5. doi: 10.1002/bjs.10144
7. Noguchi S, Noguchi A, Murakami N. Papillary Carcinoma of the Thyroid. I. Developing Pattern of Metastasis. *Cancer* (1970) 26(5):1053–60. doi: 10.1002/1097-0142(197011)26:5<1053::aid-cncr2820260513>3.0.co;2-x
8. Gimm O, Rath FW, Dralle H. Pattern of Lymph Node Metastases in Papillary Thyroid Carcinoma. *Br J Surg* (1998) 85(2):252–4. doi: 10.1046/j.1365-2168.1998.00510.x
9. Ilic N, Petricevic A, Arar D, Kotarac S, Banovic J, Ilic NF, et al. Skip Mediastinal Nodal Metastases in the Iiia/N2 Non-Small Cell Lung Cancer. *J Thorac Oncol* (2007) 2(11):1018–21. doi: 10.1097/JTO.0b013e318158d471
10. Zhang C, Zhang L, Xu T, Xue R, Yu L, Zhu Y, et al. Mapping the Spreading Routes of Lymphatic Metastases in Human Colorectal Cancer. *Nat Commun* (2020) 11(1):1993. doi: 10.1038/s41467-020-15886-6
11. Maruyama K, Gunven P, Okabayashi K, Sasako M, Kinoshita T. Lymph Node Metastases of Gastric Cancer. General Pattern in 1931 Patients. *Ann Surg* (1989) 210(5):596–602. doi: 10.1097/00000658-198911000-00005
12. Rosen PP, Lesser ML, Kinne DW, Beattie EJ. Discontinuous or "Skip" Metastases in Breast Carcinoma. Analysis of 1228 Axillary Dissections. *Ann Surg* (1983) 197(3):276–83. doi: 10.1097/00000658-198303000-00006
13. Tangoku A, Seike J, Nakano K, Nagao T, Honda J, Yoshida T, et al. Current Status of Sentinel Lymph Node Navigation Surgery in Breast and Gastrointestinal Tract. *J Med Invest* (2007) 54(1-2):1–18. doi: 10.2152/jmi.54.1

14. Qiu Y, Fei Y, Liu J, Liu C, He X, Zhu N, et al. Prevalence, Risk Factors and Location of Skip Metastasis in Papillary Thyroid Carcinoma: A Systematic Review and Meta-Analysis. *Cancer Manag Res* (2019) 11:8721–30. doi: 10.2147/CMAR.S200628
15. Chow SM, Law SC, Chan JK, Au SK, Yau S, Lau WH. Papillary Microcarcinoma of the Thyroid-Prognostic Significance of Lymph Node Metastasis and Multifocality. *Cancer* (2003) 98(1):31–40. doi: 10.1002/cncr.11442
16. Sywak M, Cornford L, Roach P, Stalberg P, Sidhu S, Delbridge L. Routine Ipsilateral Level Vi Lymphadenectomy Reduces Postoperative Thyroglobulin Levels in Papillary Thyroid Cancer. *Surgery* (2006) 140(6):1000–5; discussion 5-7. doi: 10.1016/j.surg.2006.08.001
17. Wada N, Duh QY, Sugino K, Iwasaki H, Kameyama K, Mimura T, et al. Lymph Node Metastasis From 259 Papillary Thyroid Microcarcinomas: Frequency, Pattern of Occurrence and Recurrence, and Optimal Strategy for Neck Dissection. *Ann Surg* (2003) 237(3):399–407. doi: 10.1097/01.SLA.0000055273.58908.19
18. Nixon IJ, Wang LY, Ganly I, Patel SG, Morris LG, Migliacci JC, et al. Outcomes for Patients With Papillary Thyroid Cancer Who Do Not Undergo Prophylactic Central Neck Dissection. *Br J Surg* (2016) 103 (3):218–25. doi: 10.1002/bjs.10036
19. Shaha AR. Complications of Neck Dissection for Thyroid Cancer. *Ann Surg Oncol* (2008) 15(2):397–9. doi: 10.1245/s10434-007-9724-x
20. Niu XH. [Interpretation of 2020 Nccn Clinical Practice Guidelines in Oncology-Bone Cancer]. *Zhonghua Wai Ke Za Zhi* (2020) 58(6):430–4. doi: 10.3760/cma.j.cn112139-20200204-00061
21. Solbiati L, Cioffi V, Ballarati E. Ultrasonography of the Neck. *Radiol Clin North Am* (1992) 30(5):941–54.
22. Al Afif A, Williams BA, Rigby MH, Bullock MJ, Taylor SM, Trites J, et al. Multifocal Papillary Thyroid Cancer Increases the Risk of Central Lymph Node Metastasis. *Thyroid* (2015) 25(9):1008–12. doi: 10.1089/thy.2015.0130
23. Moon HJ, Kim EK, Yoon JH, Kwak JY. Differences in the Diagnostic Performances of Staging Us for Thyroid Malignancy According to Experience. *Ultrasound Med Biol* (2012) 38(4):568–73. doi: 10.1016/j.ultrasmedbio.2012.01.002
24. Caturegli P, De Remigis A, Rose NR. Hashimoto Thyroiditis: Clinical and Diagnostic Criteria. *Autoimmun Rev* (2014) 13(4-5):391–7. doi: 10.1016/j.autrev.2014.01.007
25. Zhang L, Wei WJ, Ji QH, Zhu YX, Wang ZY, Wang Y, et al. Risk Factors for Neck Nodal Metastasis in Papillary Thyroid Microcarcinoma: A Study of 1066 Patients. *J Clin Endocrinol Metab* (2012) 97(4):1250–7. doi: 10.1210/jc.2011-1546
26. Haugen BR. 2015 American Thyroid Association Management Guidelines for Adult Patients With Thyroid Nodules and Differentiated Thyroid Cancer: What Is New and What Has Changed? *Cancer* (2017) 123(3):372–81. doi: 10.1002/cncr.30360
27. Fraser S, Zaidi N, Norlen O, Glover A, Kruijff S, Sywak M, et al. Incidence and Risk Factors for Occult Level 3 Lymph Node Metastases in Papillary Thyroid Cancer. *Ann Surg Oncol* (2016) 23(11):3587–92. doi: 10.1245/s10434-016-5254-8
28. Lim YS, Lee JC, Lee YS, Lee BJ, Wang SG, Son SM, et al. Lateral Cervical Lymph Node Metastases From Papillary Thyroid Carcinoma: Predictive Factors of Nodal Metastasis. *Surgery* (2011) 150(1):116–21. doi: 10.1016/j.surg.2011.02.003
29. Li X, Li X, Fu X, Liu L, Liu Y, Zhao H, et al. Survival Benefit of Skip Metastases in Surgically Resected N2 Non-Small Cell Lung Cancer: A Multicenter Observational Study of a Large Cohort of the Chinese Patients. *Eur J Surg Oncol* (2020) 46(10 Pt A):1874–81. doi: 10.1016/j.ejso.2019.12.015
30. Shiozawa M, Akaike M, Yamada R, Godai T, Yamamoto N, Saito H, et al. Clinicopathological Features of Skip Metastasis in Colorectal Cancer. *Hepatogastroenterology* (2007) 54(73):81–4.
31. Yang P, Gilg M, Evans S, Totti F, Stevenson J, Jeys L, et al. Survival of Osteosarcoma Patients Following Diagnosis of Synchronous Skip Metastases. *J Orthop* (2020) 18:121–5. doi: 10.1016/j.jor.2019.10.003
32. Feng JW, Qin AC, Ye J, Pan H, Jiang Y, Qu Z. Predictive Factors for Lateral Lymph Node Metastasis and Skip Metastasis in Papillary Thyroid Carcinoma. *Endocr Pathol* (2020) 31(1):67–76. doi: 10.1007/s12022-019-09599-w
33. Cruz JA, Wishart DS. Applications of Machine Learning in Cancer Prediction and Prognosis. *Cancer Inform* (2007) 2:59–77. doi: 10.1177/117693510600200030
34. Huang S, Cai N, Pacheco PP, Narrandes S, Wang Y, Xu W. Applications of Support Vector Machine (Svm) Learning in Cancer Genomics. *Cancer Genomics Proteomics* (2018) 15(1):41–51. doi: 10.21873/cgp.20063
35. Golub TR, Slonim DK, Tamayo P, Huard C, Gaasenbeek M, Mesirov JP, et al. Molecular Classification of Cancer: Class Discovery and Class Prediction by Gene Expression Monitoring. *Science* (1999) 286(5439):531–7. doi: 10.1126/science.286.5439.531
36. Alexander EK, Kennedy GC, Baloch ZW, Cibas ES, Chudova D, Diggans J, et al. Preoperative Diagnosis of Benign Thyroid Nodules With Indeterminate Cytology. *N Engl J Med* (2012) 367(8):705–15. doi: 10.1056/NEJMoa1203208
37. Furey TS, Cristianini N, Duffy N, Bednarski DW, Schummer M, Haussler D. Support Vector Machine Classification and Validation of Cancer Tissue Samples Using Microarray Expression Data. *Bioinformatics* (2000) 16 (10):906–14. doi: 10.1093/bioinformatics/16.10.906
38. Moler EJ, Chow ML, Mian IS. Analysis of Molecular Profile Data Using Generative and Discriminative Methods. *Physiol Genomics* (2000) 4(2):109–26. doi: 10.1152/physiolgenomics.2000.4.2.109
39. Segal NH, Pavlidis P, Antonescu CR, Maki RG, Noble WS, DeSantis D, et al. Classification and Subtype Prediction of Adult Soft Tissue Sarcoma by Functional Genomics. *Am J Pathol* (2003) 163(2):691–700. doi: 10.1016/S0002-9440(10)63696-6
40. Shen Y, Lai Y, Xu D, Xu L, Song L, Zhou J, et al. Diagnosis of Thyroid Neoplasm Using Support Vector Machine Algorithms Based on Platelet Rna-Seq. *Endocrine* (2021) 72(3):758–83. doi: 10.1007/s12020-020-02523-x
41. Zhao H, Huang T, Li H. Risk Factors for Skip Metastasis and Lateral Lymph Node Metastasis of Papillary Thyroid Cancer. *Surgery* (2019) 166(1):55–60. doi: 10.1016/j.surg.2019.01.025
42. Nie X, Tan Z, Ge M. Skip Metastasis in Papillary Thyroid Carcinoma Is Difficult to Predict in Clinical Practice. *BMC Cancer* (2017) 17(1):702. doi: 10.1186/s12885-017-3698-2
43. Lei J, Zhong J, Jiang K, Li Z, Gong R, Zhu J. Skip Lateral Lymph Node Metastasis Leaping Over the Central Neck Compartment in Papillary Thyroid Carcinoma. *Oncotarget* (2017) 8(16):27022–33. doi: 10.18632/oncotarget.15388
44. Jin WX, Jin YX, Ye DR, Zheng ZC, Sun YH, Zhou XF, et al. Predictive Factors of Skip Metastasis in Papillary Thyroid Cancer. *Med Sci Monit* (2018) 24:2744–9. doi: 10.12659/MSM.907357
45. Lim YC, Koo BS. Predictive Factors of Skip Metastases to Lateral Neck Compartment Leaping Central Neck Compartment in Papillary Thyroid Carcinoma. *Oral Oncol* (2012) 48(3):262–5. doi: 10.1016/j.oraloncology.2011.10.006

7

Endoscopic Lateral Neck Dissection: A New Frontier in Endoscopic Thyroid Surgery

Zeyu Zhang, Botao Sun, Hui Ouyang, Rong Cong, Fada Xia* and Xinying Li

Department of Thyroid Surgery, Xiangya Hospital, Central South University, Changsha, China

***Correspondence:**
Fada Xia
xiafadaCSU@protonmail.com

Background: Endoscopic thyroidectomy and robotic thyroidectomy are effective and safe surgical options for thyroid surgery, with excellent cosmetic outcomes. However, in regard to lateral neck dissection (LND), much effort is required to alleviate cervical disfigurement derived from a long incision. Technologic innovations have allowed for endoscopic LND, without the need for extended cervical incisions and providing access to remote sites, including axillary, chest–breast, face-lift, transoral, and hybrid approaches.

Methods: A comprehensive review of published literature was performed using the search terms "lateral neck dissection", "thyroid", and "endoscopy OR endoscopic OR endoscope OR robotic" in PubMed.

Results: This review provides an overview of the current knowledge regarding endoscopic LND, and it specifically addresses the following points: 1) the surgical procedure, 2) the indications and contraindications, 3) the complications and surgical outcomes, and 4) the technical advantages and limitations. Robotic LND, totally endoscopic LND, and endoscope-assisted LND are separately discussed.

Conclusions: Endoscopic LND is a feasible and safe technique in terms of complete resection of the selected neck levels, complications, and cosmetic outcomes. However, it is recommended to strictly select criteria when expanding the population of eligible patients. A formal indication for endoscopic LND has not yet been established. Thus, a well-designed, multicenter study with a large cohort is necessary to confirm the feasibility, long-term outcomes, oncological safety, and influence of endoscopic LND on patient quality of life (QoL).

Keywords: endoscopic thyroidectomy, robotic thyroidectomy, lateral neck dissection, quality of life, cosmetic outcome

1 BACKGROUND

In the past 10 years, the incidence of thyroid cancer (TC) has risen significantly among many districts and countries (1). Among the various subtypes, differentiated TC (DTC) accounts for approximately 95% of all TCs, and surgery is widely accepted as the most effective treatment for most DTC patients (2, 3). To date, conventional open thyroidectomy through a collar incision is the standard approach to thyroidectomy (4). While the majority of patients accept a thyroidectomy scar, a certain percentage of patients are not satisfied with a visible scar on the neck. Some of them with cosmetic needs may even seek out further plastic surgery to improve the appearance of the scar (5, 6). With the growing appreciation of cosmetic needs, as well as the progression of endoscopic technologies, many thyroidectomy approaches have undergone significant development and modification to minimize potential scars, including minimally invasive cervical approaches and remote-access approaches (7).

Neck appearance has an important influence on the quality of life (QoL) of TC patients. Endoscopic thyroidectomy and robotic thyroidectomy have been shown to be effective and safe surgical options for thyroid surgery while providing excellent cosmetic results (8, 9). For patients who need lateral neck dissection (LND) due to metastatic lateral neck lymph nodes (LNs), a conspicuous scar (L-shaped, U-shaped, or extended collar) is often created, causing unsatisfactory experiences after the surgery. In fact, much effort has been made to alleviate cervical disfigurement derived from long incisions (10). Endoscopic LND has limited acceptance for TCs with local metastasis, and only strictly selected patients are eligible for the technique. Technologic innovations have enabled LND without extending the cervical incision and allowing access to remote sites, including axillary, chest–breast, face-lift, transoral, and hybrid approaches. These techniques can also be divided into robotic approaches and endoscopic approaches, depending on the types of instruments used. The endoscopic approaches can be subdivided into total endoscopic and endoscope-assisted approaches by the way the devices are used.

In this review, we discussed the current knowledge regarding endoscopic LND. We specifically addressed the following points: 1) the surgical procedure, 2) the indications and contraindications, 3) the complications and surgical outcomes, and 4) the technical advantages and limitations. LND achieved through a robotic surgery system is recognized as robotic LND. Although there is an ambiguous border between total endoscopic LND and endoscope-assisted LND, we attempted to distinguish them in this review. Total endoscopic LND is performed with trocars in an enclosed area with or without CO_2 insufflation, while endoscope-assisted LND is performed in a semiopen area without a trocar or CO_2 insufflation.

2 ROBOTIC LATERAL NECK DISSECTION

2.1 Surgical Procedures

2.1.1 Gasless, Transaxillary Approach

The robotic transaxillary approach is the most commonly reported robotic LND technique in the literature. A transaxillary approach was attempted *via* a 7- to 8-cm vertical incision located in the anterior axillary fold, and then a flap was created above the anterior surface of the pectoralis major muscle from the axilla to the clavicle (**Figure 1A**). The dissection should be continuously made until the submandibular gland and the posterior belly of the digastric muscle are reached. The skin flap is extended at the subplatysmal level in the neck superiorly to the mandible, posteriorly to the anterior border of the trapezius muscle, and anteriorly to the midline of the neck. The omohyoid muscle is interrupted at the thyroid cartilage, with the identification and dissociation of the internal jugular vein (IJV). A long and wide retractor blade is placed through the tunnel, and the flap and sternocleidomastoid muscle (SCM) are lifted to create a space for the operation. All four robotic arms are inserted through the same tunnel, and thyroidectomy and central neck dissection (CND) are performed as in conventional procedures. After the IJV is skeletonized and level III, IV, and VB dissections are performed, re-docking may be necessary for additional level II dissections. In addition, LNs located in levels IIB and VA, which are not routinely included in lymphadenectomy, can also be exposed and dissected (11–21).

2.1.2 Bilateral Axillary Breast Approach

This approach requires four incisions, including a circumareolar incision in each breast and a vertical incision in each axilla. Compared with a simple thyroidectomy, a larger flap, up to the inferior border of the submandibular gland, superiorly to the angle of the mandible and posteriorly to the anterior edge of the trapezius, is needed for LND (**Figure 1B**). Two suture lines are used to pull the SCM laterally to expose the lateral cervical compartment, which can also be achieved by separating the SCM and the strap muscles. Similar to TA, the camera may need to be moved for better level II dissection. It is very important to preserve the brachial plexus and spinal accessory nerve (SAN) while dissecting level V LNs. Clipped level V LNs are moved to level IV through the bottom of the SCM. Additionally, to preserve the SAN, the posterior belly of the digastric muscle should be exposed while dissecting (22–25).

2.1.3 Unilateral Retroauricular Approach

The retroauricular approach (RA) needs an L-shaped incision behind the auricle, and a flap is created above the SCM, proceeding anteriorly to the midline of the neck and extending superiorly to the submandibular gland and inferiorly to the level of the clavicle and sternal notch (**Figure 1C**). The flap is subsequently retracted and maintained by self-retaining retractors, and three arms of the da Vinci Surgical System are usually used in this approach. Specifically, the dissections are usually performed with the assistance of the robotic arms, while the exposure and dissection of the accessory nerve and LNs of levels II and III can be achieved under direct vision with regular surgical instruments (26, 27).

Kim and Byeon et al. reported a modified transaxillary and retroauricular (TARA) robot-assisted neck dissection. SAN can be identified through the RA incision. LNs of level II, VA, and upper level III can be recognized and dissected under direct vision, while the LNs of levels III, VB, and IV can be recognized and dissected with the assistance of robotic arms through the transaxillary approach. Thyroidectomy and CND can also be accomplished *via* TA (28, 29).

2.1.4 Transoral Approach

Few studies have applied TO during robotic dissection. Tae et al. reported one case of dissecting LNs of levels III and IV.

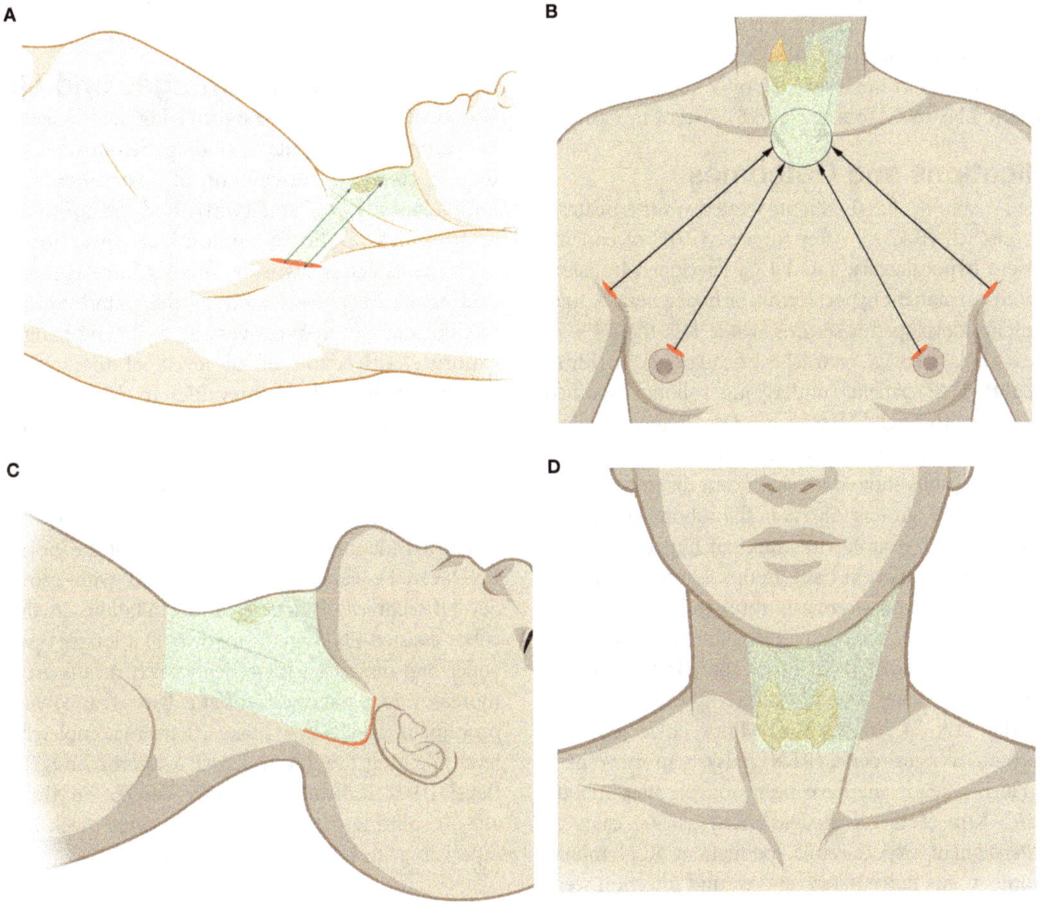

FIGURE 1 | Robotic lateral neck dissection (LND) approaches. **(A)** Transaxillary approach. **(B)** Bilateral axillary breast approach (BABA). **(C)** Unilateral retroauricular approach (RA). **(D)** Transoral approach (TO); incision sites were the same in totally endoscopic TO approach. The area of raised skin flap was marked with green wireframes.

One central incision and two lateral incisions were made on the base of the lower lip frenulum and the oral commissure. A flap is required inferiorly to the sternal and clavicle notch and laterally to the SCM. Another incision is required in the right axillary region for a third robotic instrument (**Figure 1D**). Total thyroidectomy and bilateral CND are similar to those of the endoscopic transoral approach. The SCM can be retracted to obtain a better view of the operation. With good exposure and protection of the IJV, the LNs of levels III and IV can be subsequently dissected (30).

2.2 Indications and Contraindications

2.2.1 Gasless, Transaxillary Approach

Based on the experience of centers that have performed this procedure thus far, the inclusion criteria are as follows: 1) unilateral DTC with cervical LN metastasis and 2) without previous surgical treatments of TC. The exclusion criteria are usually as follows: 1) unrelated pathologic conditions of the neck or shoulder; 2) extensive extrathyroidal spread; 3) metastatic LNs are fused or fixed; 4) metastatic LNs on the substernal or the infraclavicular area; 5) recurrent disease; and 6) distant metastasis.

2.2.2 Bilateral Axillary Breast Approach

The inclusion criteria are as follows: 1) primary tumor size <3 cm without local invasion; 2) LN metastasis derived from DTC; 3) largest LN diameter <2 cm; and 4) an advanced cosmetic need. The exclusion criteria are usually as follows: 1) previous neck or chest surgery; 2) body mass index (BMI) >30 or short neck; 3) extensive extrathyroidal spread; 4) metastatic LNs in the level V regions or below the sternoclavicular joint; 5) metastatic LNs fused or fixed; and 6) distant metastasis.

2.2.3 Unilateral Retroauricular Approach

The inclusion criteria for RA are as follows: 1) unilateral tumor and 2) with no previous history of treatment for thyroid carcinoma. The exclusion criteria are as follows: 1) recurrent disease; 2) unrelated pathologic conditions of the retroauricular area; 3) extensive extrathyroidal spread; 4) metastatic LNs fused or fixed; and 5) distant metastasis.

2.2.4 Transoral Approach

The inclusion criteria for the transoral approach are as follows: 1) primary tumor size <2 cm in the unilateral lobe; 2) without capsular invasion; 3) suspected level III/IV LN metastases; 4) an advanced cosmetic need; and 5) no evidence of thyroiditis. The exclusion criteria are as follows: 1) previous neck or chest surgery; 2) BMI > 30 or short neck; 3) extensive extrathyroidal spread; 4) metastatic LNs in the level I, II, or V regions; 5) level III or IV metastatic LNs fused or fixed; and 6) distant metastasis.

2.3 Complications and Outcomes

He et al. reported a cohort of 260 patients treated *via* the bilateral axillary breast approach (BABA). After surgery, 19.6% of patients developed transient hypocalcemia, and 1.15% developed transient hoarseness without permanent hypocalcemia or hoarseness. A total of 1.15% of patients developed a seroma, while less than 1% of patients have less chylar leakage or tracheal fistula (24). In Kim's cohort, they reported 42 patients undergoing robotic modified radical neck dissection through TA with a 5-year follow-up time, and a 1:3 matching analysis with the conventional open procedure was conducted. Their results showed no significant difference in the complication rate between groups (58.5% in the robotic group and 62.7% in the conventional group), with transient hypocalcemia as the most common complication in both groups. Lymphatic fistula in one case and transient hypocalcemia in three (6.2%) cases were reported in Lira's cohort with an RA. No other surgical complications were described (26). In other comparative studies, the reported complication rates were not different between robotic and open surgeries (12, 14, 20, 23, 26). Minor chyle leakages, temporary recurrent laryngeal nerve (RLN) palsy, arm movement disorders, and Horner syndrome have been noticed after robotic surgeries (12, 20). Kim et al. reported as many as 500 cases of robotic LND. Permanent hypocalcemia, permanent RLN injury, Horner's syndrome, vagus nerve injury, and wound infection were noticed with extremely low rates (21). The general characteristics, technical safety (complications), and oncological outcomes of robotic surgeries are listed in **Table 1**.

In He's cohort of BABA procedures, all 260 patients experienced varying degrees of paraesthesia in the neck and chest; however, they mainly recovered within 4–12 months. All of the patients were extremely satisfied or satisfied with the cosmetic results. Only one case was identified with a tumor recurrence in the short-term follow-up period (1–48 months) (24). Lee's comparative study concerning TA and conventional thyroidectomy investigated pain scores, paraesthesia, and cosmetic satisfaction. While no significant difference was detected in pain scores, paraesthesia of the neck was found more frequently after conventional thyroidectomy; however, paraesthesia of the chest was more frequent in the robotic group. Moreover, the robotic group had better cosmetic satisfaction than the conventional group, and the neck and shoulder function scores were not different between the two groups (14). The cosmetic effects and other QoL results are listed in **Table 2**.

Meanwhile, robotic surgeries are as effective in harvesting LNs as conventional surgery (20). Serum triglyceride (TG) levels (thyroid-stimulating hormone (TSH) suppressed), neck ultrasound, ultrasound-guided fine-needle aspiration (FNA), CT, and PET-CT were used to evaluate disease recurrence. Multiple studies have revealed that the recurrence and mortality rates are not different between robotic and open surgeries (13, 16, 20, 23, 24). In Kim's two cohorts investigating cancer recurrence, recurrence rates over 5 years (the longest follow-up period as reported) did not differ between the robotic and open groups (2.4 vs. 2.9%), showing a consistent oncological effect (12, 21).

2.4 Technical Advantages and Limitations

Robotic instruments have shown additional superiorities, over other endoscopic instruments, including tremor-free, stabilized, and 7-degree freedom movement of instruments; 3-dimensional endoscopic view; self-controlled traction; and optimized ergonomics. Delicate anatomical operation with versatile instruments can assist with complex intraoperative situations and lead to easier preservation of the parathyroid gland and the identification of nerves, vessels, and lymphangion. With good exposure, dissection of all levels of the neck compartments can be theoretically achievable. In Kim's experience, setting contraindications of robotic LND according to the TNM staging system is unnecessary. They believe that experienced surgeons can determine whether they can complete robotic LND even though a patient may have metastatic nodes in level VII or primary cancer can be a T4 lesion (21). This suggests that the indication for robotic LND can be easily further expanded with growing experience. Several technical difficulties and limitations in the application of robot-assisted LND are as follows: 1) a longer operative time; 2) a wider flap dissection is needed, which means greater trauma and more severe paraesthesia of the flap area; 3) higher costs; 4) a prominent clavicle may make it hard to completely remove LNs of level IV using the TA and BABA approaches; 5) the upper neck (level II) is difficult to remove (except in the RA approach); and 6) splitting the SCM may exaggerate neck pain and stiffness, especially with bilateral procedures.

3 TOTALLY ENDOSCOPIC LATERAL NECK DISSECTION

3.1 Surgical Procedures

3.1.1 Chest–Breast Approach

The chest–breast approach is characterized by CO_2 gas usage and the presence of all of the incisions and working space confined to the anterior chest wall, including the breast. Various total endoscopic approaches have been described, such as approaches *via* the parasternum and bilateral mammary areolas (chest–breast, **Figure 2A**) (37) and total mammary areolas (breast, **Figure 2B**) (38, 39). Epinephrine solution or liquid–gas mix tumescent is used to control bleeding while creating the flap. One 10-mm incision at the margin of the breast (parasternum) or at the right areola for the laparoscope and two 5-mm incisions at the bilateral areola for operating the instruments are made for the trocar location. The working space is filled with CO_2, maintaining a pressure of approximately 7 mmHg. Devices have been introduced in this kind of approach, such as U-shaped retractors, suspension sutures, ultrasonic coagulators, and minilap (31, 37–43).

After thyroidectomy and CND, the working space should be expanded superiorly to the lower edge of the submandibular gland and laterally to the lateral edge of the SCM. The steps of LND are

TABLE 1 | General characteristics, technical safety, and oncological outcomes of robotic studies.

Surgeons	Instruments/ approaches	No. of cases	Study type	Dissected neck levels	Complications (n)	Difference in retrieved nodes*	Follow-up time (months) and recurrence (n)	Ref
Kim et al.	Robotic transaxillary#	42	Retrospective/ comparative	IIA, IIB, III, IV, and Vb	Seroma, 4 Chyle leakage, 4 Temporary vocal cord paresis, 3 Transient hypocalcemia, 18 Arm movement disorder, 1	No difference	5 years 1	(12)
Lira et al.	Robotic retroauricular	12	Retrospective/ case series	II–V	Reoperation, 1 Transient hypocalcemia, 2 Vocal cord paresis, 3 Surgical site infection, 1	NA	17.4 (mean) 0	(26)
Tae et al.	Robotic transoral	1	Case report	III, IV	None	NA	NA NA	(30)
Yu et al.	Robotic BABA	15	Retrospective/ case series	II–V	Transient hypocalcemia, 7 Temporary vocal cord paresis, 1 Horner's syndrome, 1	NA	18.7 (mean) 0	(22)
Byeon et al.	Robotic retroauricular	4	Retrospective/ case series	II–V	Seroma, 1 Transient hypocalcemia, 2 Chyle leakage, 1	NA	NA NA	(27)
Kim et al.	Robotic BABA	13	Retrospective/ comparative	II, III, IV, and Vb	Chyle leakage, 1	No difference	15.9 (mean) 0	(23)
He et al.	Robotic BABA	260	Retrospective/ case series	II, III, IV, and Vb**	Transient hypocalcemia, 51 Temporary vocal cord paresis, 3 Seroma, 3 Surgical site infection, 1 Tracheal fistula, 1	Presenting as number of retrieved nodes	28.6 (mean) 0	(24)
Byeon et al.	Robotic TARA	1	Case report	III, IV	None	Presenting as number of retrieved nodes	NA NA	(29)
Kim et al.	Robotic TARA	22	Retrospective/ comparative	II–V	Seroma/hematoma, 3 Transient hypocalcemia, 6 Chyle leakage, 1 Earlobe numbness, 6 Temporary vocal cord paresis, 2	No difference	15.9 (mean) 0	(28)
Song et al.	Robotic BABA	4	Retrospective/ case series	Bilateral MRND***	Pleural effusion (not chylous)	Presenting as number of retrieved nodes	17-36 (range) 0	(25)
Kang et al.	Robotic transaxillary	56	Retrospective/ comparative	IIA, III, IV, and Vb	Seroma/hematoma, 5 Transient hypocalcemia, 27 Chyle leakage, 5 Temporary vocal cord paresis, 2 Reoperation, 1	No difference	One year (fixed time point) 0	(20)
Lee et al.	Robotic transaxillary	62	Retrospective/ comparative	IIA, III, IV, and Vb	Seroma/hematoma, 2 Transient hypocalcemia, 24	No difference	8.4 (mean) 0	(14)

(Continued)

TABLE 1 | Continued

Surgeons	Instruments/ approaches	No. of cases	Study type	Dissected neck levels	Complications (n)	Difference in retrieved nodes*	Follow-up time (months) and recurrence (n)	Ref
					Chyle leakage, 1 Temporary vocal cord paresis, 2			
Kim et al.	Robotic transaxillary	500	Retrospective/ case series	II–V	Transient hypocalcemia, 151 Permanent hypocalcemia, 20 Temporary vocal cord paresis, 20 Permanent vocal cord paresis, 5 Seroma/hematoma, 19 Chyle leakage, 26 Horner's syndrome, 2 Vagus nerve injury, 1 Wound infection, 1	Presenting as number of retrieved nodes	NA 5	(21)

NA, not available; MRND, modified radical neck dissection; LND, lateral neck dissection.
#Only studies regarding robotic transaxillary approaches with case number >40 have been included.
**Compared with those retrieved in conventional open surgery.*
***Unilateral LND was performed in 239 cases and bilateral LND in 21 cases.*
****Dissected levels were not described.*

basically identical to those of conventional thyroidectomy after the SCM is split longitudinally to expose the lateral cervical compartment. Particularly, the posterior border of the IJV and the SAN should be carefully anatomized when removing the LNs of levels 2A and 2B. The transverse cervical artery, phrenic nerve, vagus nerve, brachial plexus, and cervical plexus are exposed and protected (31, 37–43).

3.1.2 Transoral Approach

Tan et al. reported selective LND *via* a transoral endoscopic approach in 20 PTC cases. Ngo et al. also reported a case of LND *via* a transoral endoscopic approach. Three vestibular incisions were made in the mouth vestibular (**Figure 1D**). The working space is described as between the sternohyoid muscles and the platysma muscle. Upon completing the thyroid lobectomy and

TABLE 2 | Cosmetic results and other quality of life (QoL) results in retrieved references.

Surgeons	Cosmetic evaluation methods	Cosmetic results	Other QoL evaluation	Other results	Ref
He et al.	Five-point scale	4.68 ± 0.35 (score)*	None	None	(24)
Kim et al.	Five-point scale	3.9 ± 1.0, better than open group	None	None	(28)
Lee et al.	Five-point scale	Better than open group**	Pain score, voice handicap index, etc.#	No difference	(14)
Song et al.	Five-point scale	1.64 ± 0.61 (one month), better than open group	Pain and paresthesia scores of the neck and anterior chest area	No difference or higher in robotic group***	(13)
Guo et al.	NA	8.3 ± 0.7, better than open group	Pain scores	No difference	(31)
Lin et al.	Visual analog scale (VAS)	9 (mean, range 5–10)*	Pain score, voice handicap index, etc.#	Presenting as scores	(32)
Zhang et al.	Verbal response scale and numeric rating scale	2.8 ± 0.5 and 7.0 ± 0.9, better than open group	Pain score (VAS)	Better in endoscopic assisted group	(33)
Zhang et al.	Verbal response scale and numeric rating scale	7.0 ± 1.2 and 2.7 ± 0.6, Better than open group	None	None	(34)
Lin et al.	Verbal response scale	9 (mean, range 9–10), better than open group	Pain score, voice handicap index, etc.#	No difference	(35)
Zhang et al.	Five-point scale	1.4 ± 0.6 (3 months), better than open group	Pain and paresthesia scores of the neck	Better in endoscopic assisted group	(36)

NA, not available.
**Case series studies.*
***Presenting as numbers of satisfied or dissatisfied patients.*
****Pain and paresthesia scores of the neck were similar as those in open surgery, while pain and paresthesia scores of the anterior chest area were higher.*
#Other QoL evaluation included swallowing impairment score (SIS-6), neck dissection impairment index (NDII), and arm abduction test (AAT) in these studies.

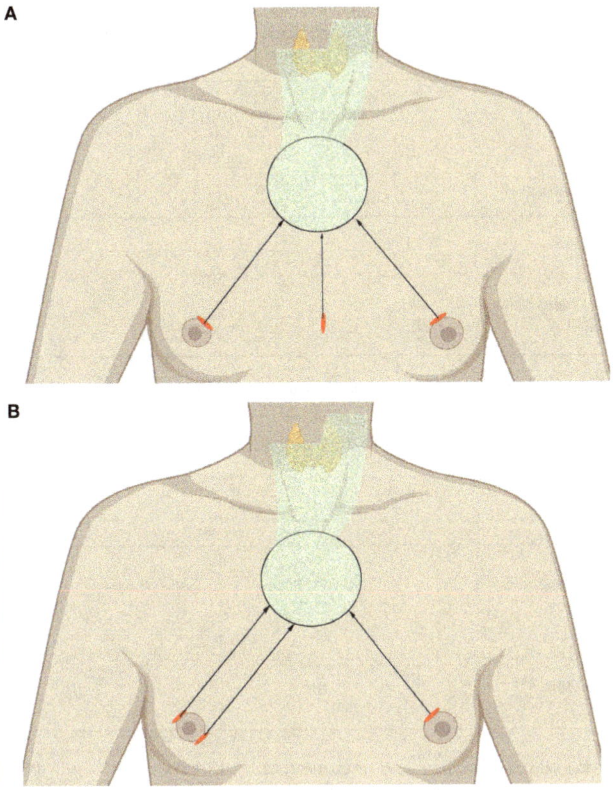

FIGURE 2 | Totally endoscopic lateral neck dissection (LND) approaches. **(A)** Chest-breast approach. **(B)** Total mammary areolas approach. The area of raised skin flap was marked with green wireframes.

CND, selective LND is performed through the two heads of the SCM. After removal of the omohyoid muscle to create a larger space, the IJV should be anatomized and well protected. The LNs of levels III and IV can be subsequently resected starting from the level of the carotid bifurcation to the clavicle (44, 45).

3.2 Indications and Contraindications

3.2.1 Chest-Breast Approach

Based on the experience of centers that have performed this procedure thus far, the inclusion criteria for chest-breast approach are as follows: 1) primary tumor size <3 cm without local invasion; 2) LN metastasis derived from DTC; 3) largest LN diameter <2 cm; and 4) an advanced cosmetic need. The exclusion criteria are usually as follows: 1) previous neck or chest surgery; 2) BMI >30 or short neck; 3) extensive extrathyroidal spread; 4) metastatic LNs in the level V regions or below the sternoclavicular joint; 5) metastatic LNs fused or fixed; and 6) distant metastasis (39, 40, 42).

3.2.2 Transoral Approach

The inclusion criteria for the transoral approach are as follows: 1) primary tumor size <2 cm in the unilateral lobe; 2) without capsular invasion; 3) suspected level III/IV LN metastases; 4) an advanced cosmetic need; and 5) no evidence of thyroiditis. The exclusion criteria are as follows: 1) previous neck or chest surgery; 2) BMI > 30 or short neck; 3) extensive extrathyroidal spread; 4) metastatic LNs in the level I, II, or V regions; 5) level III or IV metastatic LNs fused or fixed; and 6) distant metastasis (44).

3.3 Complications and Outcomes

Several centers have reported the perioperative complications of totally endoscopic LND. Common complications of thyroidectomy and lymphadenectomy may also occur during endoscopic surgery. Yan et al. performed and reported their rich experience with endoscopic thyroidectomy *via* a breast approach with levels II, III, and IV LND. They retrospectively compared the endoscopic LND group with 155 patients and the conventional open LND group with 102 patients. Operation-related complications, such as transit hoarseness, hematoma, IJV rupture, and limb lift restriction occurred in both the endoscopic LND group and the open group. No significant difference was found for the complication incidences between the groups. However, the mean operating duration was longer in the endoscopic LND group than in the open group (40). Guo et al. also confirmed the prolonged LND time of endoscopic thyroidectomy. Consistently, no significant difference was found in transient voice change, transient hypoparathyroidism, postoperative lymphatic leakage, or intraoperative large blood vessel injury, while no severe complications, such as hematoma, permanent hypoparathyroidism, and permanent nerve injury were found to occur (31). Wang et al. reported one case of conversion to open surgery due to right RLN invasion. Injury to the SAN was found in 2 patients, who subsequently developed light SCM dystrophy (41). Cervical plexus and hypoglossal nerve injury have been reported in Chen's study (46). The general characteristics, technical safety (complications), and oncological outcomes of totally endoscopic surgeries are listed in **Table 3**.

In contrasting analyses, no difference was found in the number of dissected lateral LNs between the endoscopic LND group and the conventional open LND group (31). Yan et al. calculated the number of dissected LNs in levels II, III, and IV. The numbers at each level were statistically identical in the endoscopic group and open group (40). Cosmetic satisfaction scores were mentioned in only one study, and the endoscopic group had a higher score than the open group (**Table 2**) (31). The median follow-up period in Wang's cohort was 24 months, ranging from 4 to 59 months. Postoperative thyroglobulin (Tg) levels were used to evaluate tumor recurrence, and Tg < 1 ng/ml was achieved in 80% of individuals 1 year after surgery, with only one recurrence at the LNs of level VII. All 37 patients were satisfied with the cosmetic results (41). The study by Yan et al. reported local recurrence in four patients (2 in the endoscopic group and 2 in the open group) during follow-up, while no patients developed distant metastases or tumor-related death (40).

3.4 Technical Advantages and Limitations

Although the endoscopic device is not as versatile as the robotic device, it is easy and economical to apply in most hospitals. The effectiveness and safety of endoscopic surgery have been widely proven to be the same as those of robotic surgery in the treatment

TABLE 3 | General characteristics, technical safety, and oncological outcomes of totally endoscopic and endoscope-assisted studies.

Surgeons	Instruments/ approaches	No. of cases	Study type	Dissected neck levels	Complications (n)	Difference in retrieved nodes*	Follow-up time (months) and Recurrence (n)	Ref
Guo et al.	Totally endoscopic/ chest–breast#	24	Retrospective/ case series and comparative	II, III, IV	Blood vessels injury, 2 Transient hypocalcemia, 4 Chyle leakage, 2 Temporary vocal cord paresis, 1	No difference	NA 0	(31, 47)**
Huo et al.	Totally endoscopic/ chest–breast	20	Retrospective/ case series	II, III, IV	Blood vessels injury, 2 Chyle leakage, 1 Temporary vocal cord paresis, 1 Transient hypocalcemia, 4	NA	NA NA	(43)
Wang et al.	Totally endoscopic/ chest–breast	37	Retrospective/ case series	II– V	Temporary vocal cord paresis, 3 Transient hypocalcemia, 12 Permanent hypocalcemia, 1 Spinal accessory nerve injury, 2 Chyle leakage, 1 Chest wall ecchymosis, 1	Presenting as number of retrieved nodes	24 (mean) 1	(41)
Wang et al.	Totally endoscopic/ chest–breast	155	Retrospective/ comparative	II, III, IV	Temporary vocal cord paresis, 8 Seroma, 3 Chyle leakage, 4 Infection, 2 Internal jugular vein rupture, 19 Limb lift restriction, 6	No difference	10 years (max) 2	(37, 40, 42)**
Chen et al	Totally endoscopic/ chest–breast	35	Retrospective/ case series	IIA, III, IV	Chyle leakage, 1 cervical plexus injury, 7 hypoglossal nerve injury, 1 accessory nerve injury, 3 internal jugular vein injuries, 2	Presenting as number of retrieved nodes	18.1 (mean) None	(46)
Huo et al.	Totally endoscopic/ chest–breast	12	Retrospective/ comparative	II, III, IV, VB	Chyle leakage, 1 Temporary vocal cord paresis, 2	No difference	NA None	(48)
Kitagawa et al.	Endoscope assisted/ anterior chest	3	Retrospective/ case series	Lateral zone***	None	NA	NA NA	(49)
Wu et al.	Endoscope assisted	26	Retrospective/ case series	IIA, III, IV	Temporary vocal cord paresis, 2 Transient hypocalcemia, 4	Presenting as number of retrieved nodes	19 (mean) None	(10)
Zhang et al.	Endoscope assisted	26	Retrospective/ case series	II– V	Spinal accessory nerve injury, 1	Presenting as number of retrieved nodes	NA NA	(50, 51)**
Zhang et al	Endoscope assisted	130	Retrospective/ case series	II– IV or II–V	Transient hypocalcemia, 19 Temporary vocal cord paresis, 7 Permanent vocal cord paresis, 3 Spinal accessory nerve injury, 2 Chyle leakage, 4 Seroma, 1	Presenting as number of retrieved nodes	19 (mean) None	(34, 52)**
Lin et al.	Endoscope assisted	18	Retrospective/ case series	II– IV	Transient hypocalcemia, 1	NA	54.5 (mean) None	(32)
Zhang et al.	Endoscope assisted	32	Prospective/ comparative	II– IV, VB	Temporary vocal cord paresis, 1 transient hypocalcemia, 4 Seroma, 1 Horner's syndrome, 1 Chyle leakage, 1	No difference	NA None	(33)

(Continued)

TABLE 3 | Continued

Surgeons	Instruments/ approaches	No. of cases	Study type	Dissected neck levels	Complications (n)	Difference in retrieved nodes*	Follow-up time (months) and Recurrence (n)	Ref
Lin et al.	Endoscope assisted/ anterior chest	31	Retrospective/ comparative	II– IV	Transient hypocalcemia, 2	No difference	NA None	(35)
Zhang et al	Endoscope assisted	18	Prospective/ comparative	II– V	Temporary vocal cord paresis, 6 Transient hypocalcemia, 3	No difference	NA NA	(36)

NA, not available.
#Only studies regarding total totally endoscopic/chest-breast and endoscope assisted (collar incision) with case number >10 have been included.
**Compared with those retrieved in conventional open surgery.*
***These studies may include repeatedly reported cases.*
****Dissected levels were not described.*

of TC. However, it is slightly inferior to robotic surgery in terms of the diversity of surgical approaches and the range of indications. Several technical difficulties and limitations in the application of endoscopic thyroidectomy and LND are as follows: 1) unexpected complications in endoscopic instrument usage, such as CO_2 embolism, tumor or metastatic LN rupture, and chest wall ecchymosis. 2) Poor surgical techniques, working space building, and lateral compartment exposure lead to a longer surgical time, which means a longer anesthesia time, increased cost, and a higher incidence of possible complications. 3) At present, the cosmetic evaluations are only descriptive. A quantitative, reproducible scoring system is needed. 4) In the breast approaches, level IV and VI lymph dissections are restricted by claviculation, while level V lymph dissections are restricted by the lateral border of the SCM. Due to endoscopic magnification and less space restriction, it will be easier to perform level IIB LND with endoscopic techniques than with open surgery. 5) Difficulty in level II and V lymph dissection with oral approaches: it will be difficult to expose level II LNs during surgical manipulation from the superior to inferior direction. Level V LNs are also restricted by the lateral border of the SCM. 6) SCM stiffness: in all of the studies, the SCM was split longitudinally to expose the lateral cervical compartment. However, the consequences of SCM splitting, such as stiffness, numbness, pain, and constriction, have not been evaluated.

4 ENDOSCOPE-ASSISTED LATERAL NECK DISSECTION

4.1 Surgical Procedure

Endoscope-assisted LND is characterized by the endoscopic removal of lateral LNs through an incision of approximately 2-4 cm without a trocar. Unlike total endoscopic LND, the working space of endoscope-assisted LND is not fully enclosed and is often remedied by a gasless traction system. Special instruments are introduced to lift the anterior neck skin without CO_2 gas as originally described by Miccoli and Lombardi (53, 54). Zhang et al. invented a working space creator and reported a cohort with the largest number of cases by using this instrument (34, 52). The working space is created from the posterior belly of the digastric muscle to the posterior border of the SCM (**Figure 3A**). The SCM and IJV are dissected and retracted reversely to expose the lateral lymph. The vagus nerve is carefully anatomized, followed by the removal of the LNs and surrounding fibroadipose tissue. Level II, III, and IV LNs can be dissected in the caudad to cephalad direction, while level III and IV LNs can also be dissected in the cephalad to caudad direction due to freedom from restriction. The SAN, cervical plexus, phrenic nerve, brachial plexus, and transverse cervical should be carefully protected (10, 32–34, 50–53).

Kitagawa and Lin et al. reported a totally gasless anterior chest approach. A 3.5-cm incision and another 0.5-cm incision were made on the tumor side of the chest wall and the lateral neck with a widely created working space (**Figure 3B**). The incision on the lateral neck should be widened to 2 cm when LND is required. The working space is subsequently widened to the

A

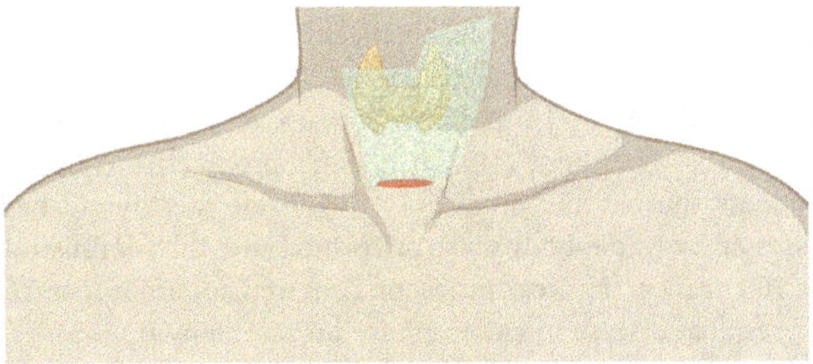

B

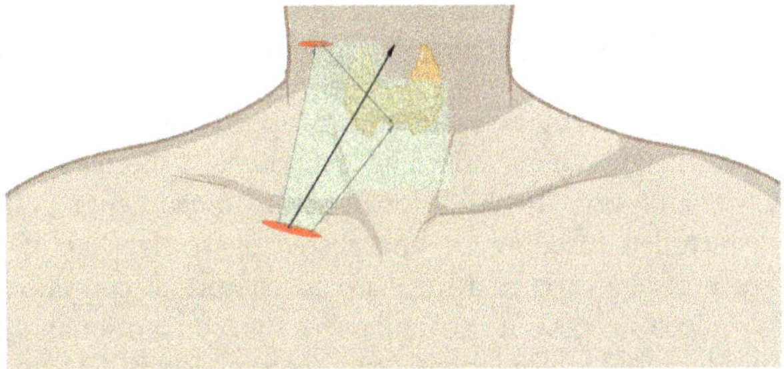

FIGURE 3 | Endoscope-assisted LND approaches. **(A)** Approach through the collar incision. **(B)** Approach through chest wall incision (infraclavicular incision). The area of raised skin flap was marked with green wireframes.

level of the lobulus auriculae, the posterior belly of the digastric muscle, the posterior border of the SCM, and the space beneath the SCM (35, 49).

4.2 Indications and Contraindication

The eligibility criteria were usually as follows: 1) unilateral tumor and 2) largest diameter <4 cm. The exclusion criteria were usually as follows: 1) extrathyroidal extension; 2) distant metastases; 3) LN metastases in level I or VA; and 4) history of previous neck surgery or radiation therapy (33, 34, 49).

4.3 Complications and Outcomes

Thyroidectomy and CND are performed as conventional open procedures. Transient RLN palsy and hypoparathyroidism rates are similar to those of the conventional open procedure. Wu et al. reported no conversion to open surgery, no significant blood loss, and only mild postoperative pain in their 26 cases (10). Zhang et al. reported an injury of the trapezius branch of the accessory nerve, causing weakness that recovered within 2 years (50). Kitagawa reported lateral LN clearance in three patients through a totally gasless anterior neck skin lifting method without any severe complications (49). Zhang et al. designed a prospective randomized study to compare video-assisted and open LND. One transient sympathetic nerve injury and one minor chyle leak were observed in the video-assisted group (33).

Cosmetic outcomes were generally better in endoscope-assisted surgery than in open surgery (32, 34, 36, 52). In Zhang's cohort, postoperative pain was significantly less severe in the endoscope-assisted group at 24 and 48 h after surgery (33). The incidence of voice change, swallowing, neck impairment, and arm abduction was not significantly different in Lin's cohort (the details can be found in **Table 2**) (35). In Wu's cohort, the postoperative Tg level was dramatically decreased to zero in most patients. Eleven patients received ^{131}I diagnostic whole-body scans at the 6- to 12-month follow-up, and no recurrence or metastasis was found (10). In Zhang's prospective cohorts, no patients showed any uptake of ^{131}I outside the thyroid bed as assessed by whole-body scans performed after the administration of 100 mCi of ^{131}I. Neck ultrasound showed no tumor recurrence or residual disease in either group during follow-up (33).

4.4 Technical Advantages and Limitations

Unlike other remote extracervical approaches, endoscope-assisted LND is characterized by less trauma, a shorter learning curve, and less demand for specific instruments. When uncontrolled bleeding or unexpected aggressiveness of the disease occurs, it is also not hard to convert to conventional thyroidectomy. As it is similar to the conventional open procedure, the indications for endoscope-assisted LND can be easily extended with growing experience. The extension of lateral neck clearance has been reported to include levels IIA, IIB, III, IV, and partly V (33). Zhang et al. have made some efforts to extend the indications, showing the feasibility of endoscopic upper mediastinal LN dissection in the treatment of papillary thyroid carcinoma with promising results (55).

Several technical difficulties and limitations in the application of endoscope-assisted LND still exist: 1) it leaves an obvious scar on the neck, although it is better than the scar from conventional thyroidectomy. 2) LNs of level I and VA are hard to reach and remove. 3) It has a longer operative time (which will decline rapidly with greater experience).

CONCLUSIONS AND FUTURE PERSPECTIVES

Endoscopic LND allows comprehensive en bloc removal of all lateral neck levels through a remote extracervical incision or an unextended collar incision. They are feasible and safe techniques in terms of the complete resection of selected neck levels, complications, and cosmetic outcomes. As the most commonly reported approach, robotic LND has more selective remote sites for robotic system docking. Device intelligence makes the theoretical indications less limited, but the obvious disadvantage is the high cost. In general, endoscopic LND is easy to carry out. The completeness of the surgical resection in selected compartments is satisfactory; however, some neck levels are difficult to achieve. Endoscope-assisted LND (cervical approach) is characterized by less trauma, close to open vision, and not limited by local tumor progression, and it can even be feasible for mediastinal LN dissection. Nevertheless, an obvious scar is still left on the neck. There is still controversy concerning the technical challenges, the introduction of new complications, and the operative trauma of endoscopic LND. Technical difficulties and limitations affect the different approaches. It is also challenging for all of the techniques to dissect all of the metastatic LNs in hard-to-reach areas or invaded areas. Moreover, unlike other procedures, additional trauma following the creation of the working space is inevitable due to the lack of free space in the neck. Theoretically, endoscopic approaches can provide meticulous dissection in the lateral neck. Complete surgical resection, a reduction in the time required, and less trauma will be achieved with the growing experience of surgeons. Regardless, it is recommended to strictly apply selection criteria when expanding the population of eligible patients in centers with a high volume of thyroid surgery. A formal indication for endoscopic LND has not yet been established. Thus, a well-designed, multicenter study with a large cohort is necessary to confirm the feasibility, long-term outcomes, oncological safety, and influence of endoscopic LND on patient QoL.

AUTHOR CONTRIBUTIONS

All authors contributed to drafting or revising the article, gave final approval of the version to be published, agreed to the submitted journal, and agree to be accountable for all aspects of the work.

REFERENCES

1. Kitahara CM, Sosa JA. The Changing Incidence of Thyroid Cancer. *Nat Rev Endocrinol* (2016) 12:646–53. doi: 10.1038/nrendo.2016.110
2. Cabanillas ME, McFadden DG, Durante C. Thyroid Cancer. *Lancet* (2016) 388:2783–95. doi: 10.1016/S0140-6736(16)30172-6
3. Van Den Heede K, Tolley NS, Di Marco AN, Palazzo FF. Differentiated Thyroid Cancer: A Health Economic Review. *Cancers (Basel)* (2021) 13:2253. doi: 10.3390/cancers13092253
4. Duek I, Duek OS, Fliss DM. Minimally Invasive Approaches for Thyroid Surgery-Pitfalls and Promises. *Curr Oncol Rep* (2020) 22:77. doi: 10.1007/s11912-020-00939-2
5. Best AR, Shipchandler TZ, Cordes SR. Midcervical Scar Satisfaction in Thyroidectomy Patients. *Laryngoscope* (2017) 127:1247–52. doi: 10.1002/lary.26177
6. Russell JO, Sahli ZT, Shaear M, Razavi C, Ali K, Tufano RP. Transoral Thyroid and Parathyroid Surgery via the Vestibular Approach-A 2020 Update. *Gland Surg* (2020) 9:409–16. doi: 10.21037/gs.2020.03.05
7. Rossi L, Materazzi G, Bakkar S, Miccoli P. Recent Trends in Surgical Approach to Thyroid Cancer. *Front Endocrinol (Lausanne)* (2021) 12:699805. doi: 10.3389/fendo.2021.699805
8. Song CM, Bang HS, Kim HG, Park HJ, Tae K. Health-Related Quality of Life After Transoral Robotic Thyroidectomy in Papillary Thyroid Carcinoma. *Surgery* (2021) 170(1):99–105. doi: 10.1016/j.surg.2021.02.042
9. Nguyen HX, Nguyen LT, Nguyen HV, Nguyen HX, Trinh HL, Nguyen TX, et al. Comparison of Transoral Thyroidectomy Vestibular Approach and Unilateral Axillobreast Approach for Endoscopic Thyroidectomy: A Prospective Cohort Study. *J Laparoendosc Adv Surg Tech A* (2021) 31:11–7. doi: 10.1089/lap.2020.0272
10. Wu B, Ding Z, Fan Y, Deng X, Guo B, Kang J, et al. Video-Assisted Selective Lateral Neck Dissection for Papillary Thyroid Carcinoma. *Langenbecks Arch Surg* (2013) 398:395–401. doi: 10.1007/s00423-012-1045-2
11. Kang SW, Kim MJ, Chung WY. Gasless, Transaxillary Robotic Neck Dissection: The Technique and Evidence. *Gland Surg* (2018) 7:466–72. doi: 10.21037/gs.2017.09.09
12. Kim MJ, Lee J, Lee SG, Choi JB, Kim TH, Ban EJ, et al. Transaxillary Robotic Modified Radical Neck Dissection: A 5-Year Assessment of Operative and Oncologic Outcomes. *Surg Endosc* (2017) 31:1599–606. doi: 10.1007/s00464-016-5146-9
13. Song CM, Ji YB, Sung ES, Kim DS, Koo HR, Tae K. Comparison of Robotic Versus Conventional Selective Neck Dissection and Total Thyroidectomy for Papillary Thyroid Carcinoma. *Otolaryngol Head Neck Surg* (2016) 154:1005–13. doi: 10.1177/0194599816638084
14. Lee J, Kwon IS, Bae EH, Chung WY. Comparative Analysis of Oncological Outcomes and Quality of Life After Robotic Versus Conventional Open Thyroidectomy With Modified Radical Neck Dissection in Patients With Papillary Thyroid Carcinoma and Lateral Neck Node Metastases. *J Clin Endocrinol Metab* (2013) 98:2701–8. doi: 10.1210/jc.2013-1583
15. Tae K, Ji YB, Song CM, Min HJ, Lee SH, Kim DS. Robotic Lateral Neck Dissection by a Gasless Unilateral Axillobreast Approach for Differentiated Thyroid Carcinoma: Our Early Experience. *Surg Laparosc Endosc Percutan Tech* (2014) 24:e128–132. doi: 10.1097/SLE.0b013e3182a4bfa1
16. Kang SW, Park JH, Jeong JS, Lee CR, Park S, Lee SH, et al. Prospects of Robotic Thyroidectomy Using a Gasless, Transaxillary Approach for the Management of Thyroid Carcinoma. *Surg Laparosc Endosc Percutan Tech* (2011) 21:223–9. doi: 10.1097/SLE.0b013e3182266f31
17. Kang SW, Lee SH, Ryu HR, Lee KY, Jeong JJ, Nam KH, et al. Initial Experience With Robot-Assisted Modified Radical Neck Dissection for the Management of Thyroid Carcinoma With Lateral Neck Node Metastasis. *Surgery* (2010) 148:1214–21. doi: 10.1016/j.surg.2010.09.016
18. Kiriakopoulos A, Linos D. Gasless Transaxillary Robotic Versus Endoscopic Thyroidectomy: Exploring the Frontiers of Scarless Thyroidectomy Through a Preliminary Comparison Study. *Surg Endosc* (2012) 26:2797–801. doi: 10.1007/s00464-012-2281-9
19. Song CM, Park JS, Park W, Ji YB, Cho SH, Tae K. Feasibility of Charcoal Tattooing for Localization of Metastatic Lymph Nodes in Robotic Selective Neck Dissection for Papillary Thyroid Carcinoma. *Ann Surg Oncol* (2015) 22 Suppl 3:S669–675. doi: 10.1245/s10434-015-4860-1
20. Kang SW, Lee SH, Park JH, Jeong JS, Park S, Lee CR, et al. A Comparative Study of the Surgical Outcomes of Robotic and Conventional Open Modified Radical Neck Dissection for Papillary Thyroid Carcinoma With Lateral Neck Node Metastasis. *Surg Endosc* (2012) 26:3251–7. doi: 10.1007/s00464-012-2333-1
21. Kim JK, Lee CR, Kang SW, Jeong JJ, Nam KH, Chung WY. Robotic Transaxillary Lateral Neck Dissection for Thyroid Cancer: Learning Experience From 500 Cases. *Surg Endosc* (2021). doi: 10.1007/s00464-021-08526-7
22. Yu HW, Chai YJ, Kim SJ, Choi JY, Lee KE. Robotic-Assisted Modified Radical Neck Dissection Using a Bilateral Axillo-Breast Approach (Robotic BABA MRND) for Papillary Thyroid Carcinoma With Lateral Lymph Node Metastasis. *Surg Endosc* (2018) 32:2322–7. doi: 10.1007/s00464-017-5927-9
23. Seup Kim B, Kang KH, Park SJ. Robotic Modified Radical Neck Dissection by Bilateral Axillary Breast Approach for Papillary Thyroid Carcinoma With Lateral Neck Metastasis. *Head Neck* (2015) 37:37–45. doi: 10.1002/hed.23545
24. He Q, Zhu J, Zhuang D, Fan Z, Zheng L, Zhou P, et al. Robotic Lateral Cervical Lymph Node Dissection *via* Bilateral Axillo-Breast Approach for Papillary Thyroid Carcinoma: A Single-Center Experience of 260 Cases. *J Robot Surg* (2020) 14:317–23. doi: 10.1007/s11701-019-00986-3
25. Song RY, Sohn HJ, Paek SH, Kang KH. The First Report of Robotic Bilateral Modified Radical Neck Dissection Through the Bilateral Axillo-Breast Approach for Papillary Thyroid Carcinoma With Bilateral Lateral Neck Metastasis. *Surg Laparosc Endosc Percutan Tech* (2020) 30:e18–22. doi: 10.1097/SLE.0000000000000590
26. Lira RB, Chulam TC, Kowalski LP. Variations and Results of Retroauricular Robotic Thyroid Surgery Associated or Not With Neck Dissection. *Gland Surg* (2018) 7:S42–s52. doi: 10.21037/gs.2018.03.04
27. Byeon HK, Holsinger FC, Tufano RP, Chung HJ, Kim WS, Koh YW, et al. Robotic Total Thyroidectomy With Modified Radical Neck Dissection *via* Unilateral Retroauricular Approach. *Ann Surg Oncol* (2014) 21:3872–5. doi: 10.1245/s10434-014-3896-y
28. Kim WS, Koh YW, Byeon HK, Park YM, Chung HJ, Kim ES, et al. Robot-Assisted Neck Dissection *via* a Transaxillary and Retroauricular Approach Versus a Conventional Transcervical Approach in Papillary Thyroid Cancer With Cervical Lymph Node Metastases. *J Laparoendosc Adv Surg Tech A* (2014) 24:367–72. doi: 10.1089/lap.2013.0296
29. Byeon HK, Ban MJ, Lee JM, Ha JG, Kim ES, Koh YW, et al. Robot-Assisted Sistrunk's Operation, Total Thyroidectomy, and Neck Dissection *via* a Transaxillary and Retroauricular (TARA) Approach in Papillary Carcinoma Arising in Thyroglossal Duct Cyst and Thyroid Gland. *Ann Surg Oncol* (2012) 19:4259–61. doi: 10.1245/s10434-012-2674-y
30. Tae K, Kim KH. Transoral Robotic Selective Neck Dissection for Papillary Thyroid Carcinoma: Dissection of Levels III and IV. *Head Neck* (2020) 42 (10):3084–8. doi: 10.1002/hed.26379
31. Guo Y, Qu R, Huo J, Wang C, Hu X, Chen C, et al. Technique for Endoscopic Thyroidectomy With Selective Lateral Neck Dissection *via* a Chest-Breast Approach. *Surg Endosc* (2019) 33:1334–41. doi: 10.1007/s00464-018-06608-7
32. Lin PL, Liang FY, Han P, Chen RH, Yu ST, Cai Q, et al. Gasless Endoscopic Selective Lateral Neck Dissection *via* an Anterior Chest Approach for Papillary Thyroid Carcinomas. *Zhonghua Er Bi Yan Hou Tou Jing Wai Ke Za Zhi* (2017) 52:915–20. doi: 10.3760/cma.j.issn.1673-0860.2017.12.008
33. Zhang D, Gao L, Xie L, He G, Chen J, Fang L, et al. Comparison Between Video-Assisted and Open Lateral Neck Dissection for Papillary Thyroid Carcinoma With Lateral Neck Lymph Node Metastasis: A Prospective Randomized Study. *J Laparoendosc Adv Surg Tech A* (2017) 27:1151–7. doi: 10.1089/lap.2016.0650
34. Zhang D, Xie L, He G, Fang L, Miao Y, Wang Z, et al. A Comparative Study of the Surgical Outcomes Between Video-Assisted and Open Lateral Neck Dissection for Papillary Thyroid Carcinoma With Lateral Neck Lymph Node Metastases. *Am J Otolaryngol* (2017) 38:115–20. doi: 10.1016/j.amjoto.2016.07.005
35. Lin P, Liang F, Cai Q, Han P, Chen R, Xiao Z, et al. Comparative Study of Gasless Endoscopic Selective Lateral Neck Dissection via the Anterior Chest Approach Versus Conventional Open Surgery for Papillary Thyroid Carcinoma. *Surg Endosc* (2020) 35(2):693–701. doi: 10.1007/s00464-020-07434-6

36. Zhang Z, Zhao X. A Comparative Study of Endoscopic Assisted Lateral Neck Dissection and Open Lateral Neck Dissection in the Treatment of Cervical Lymph Node Metastasis of Papillary Thyroid Carcinoma. *Lin Chung Er Bi Yan Hou Tou Jing Wai Ke Za Zhi* (2020) 34:836–9; 843. doi: 10.13201/j.issn.2096-7993.2020.09.015
37. Li Z, Wang P, Wang Y, Xu S, Cao L, Que R, et al. Endoscopic Lateral Neck Dissection *via* Breast Approach for Papillary Thyroid Carcinoma: A Preliminary Report. *Surg Endosc* (2011) 25:890–6. doi: 10.1007/s00464-010-1292-7
38. Zhao W, Wang B, Yan S, Zhang L. Minilaparoscopy-Assisted Modified Neck Dissection Through Bilateral Breast Approach. *VideoEndocrinology* (2016) 3: ve.2015.0038. doi: 10.1089/ve.2015.0038
39. Xiang D, Xie L, Li Z, Wang P, Ye M, Zhu M. Endoscopic Thyroidectomy Along With Bilateral Central Neck Dissection (ETBC) Increases the Risk of Transient Hypoparathyroidism for Patients With Thyroid Carcinoma. *Endocrine* (2016) 53:747–53. doi: 10.1007/s12020-016-0884-y
40. Yan HC, Xiang C, Wang Y, Wang P. Scarless Endoscopic Thyroidectomy (SET) Lateral Neck Dissection for Papillary Thyroid Carcinoma Through Breast Approach: 10 Years of Experience. *Surg Endosc* (2020) 35(7):3540–6. doi: 10.1007/s00464-020-07814-y
41. Wang B, Weng YJ, Wang SS, Zhao WX, Yan SY, Zhang LY, et al. Feasibility and Safety of Needle-Assisted Endoscopic Thyroidectomy With Lateral Neck Dissection for Papillary Thyroid Carcinoma: A Preliminary Experience. *Head Neck* (2019) 41:2367–75. doi: 10.1002/hed.25705
42. Yan H, Wang Y, Wang P, Xie Q, Zhao Q. "Scarless" (in the Neck) Endoscopic Thyroidectomy (SET) With Ipsilateral Levels II, III, and IV Dissection *via* Breast Approach for Papillary Thyroid Carcinoma: A Preliminary Report. *Surg Endosc* (2015) 29:2158–63. doi: 10.1007/s00464-014-3911-1
43. Huo JL, Qu R, Guo YM, Chen C. Endoscopic Selective Lateral Neck Dissection *via* a Chest-Breast Approach for Papillary Thyroid Carcinoma: Preliminary Experience in 20 Cases. *Lin Chung Er Bi Yan Hou Tou Jing Wai Ke Za Zhi* (2019) 33:346–50. doi: 10.13201/j.issn.1001-1781.2019.04.014
44. Tan Y, Guo B, Deng X, Ding Z, Wu B, Niu Y, et al. Transoral Endoscopic Selective Lateral Neck Dissection for Papillary Thyroid Carcinoma: A Pilot Study. *Surg Endosc* (2019) 34(12):5274–82. doi: 10.1007/s00464-019-07314-8
45. Ngo DQ, Tran TD, Le DT, Ngo QX, Van Le Q. Transoral Endoscopic Modified Radical Neck Dissection for Papillary Thyroid Carcinoma. *Ann Surg Oncol* (2021) 28(5):2766. doi: 10.1245/s10434-020-09466-7
46. Chen ZX, Song YM, Chen JB, Zhang XB, Lin ZH, Cai BY, et al. Qin's Seven Steps for Endoscopic Selective Lateral Neck Dissection via the Chest Approach in Patients With Papillary Thyroid Cancer: Experience of 35 Cases. *Surg Endosc* (2021). doi: 10.1007/s00464-021-08540-9
47. Qu R, Hu X, Guo Y, Zhou X, Huo J, Chen Y, et al. Endoscopic Lateral Neck Dissection (IIA, IIB, III, and IV) Using a Breast Approach: Outcomes From a Series of the First 24 Cases. *Surg Laparosc Endosc Percutan Tech* (2020) 31:66–70. doi: 10.1097/SLE.0000000000000849
48. Huo J, Guo Y, Hu X, Chen X, Liu W, Luo L, et al. Endoscopic Thyroidectomy With Level Vb Dissection *Via* a Chest-breast Approach: Technical Updates for Selective Lateral Neck Dissection. *Surg Laparosc Endosc Percutan Tech* (2021) 31:342–5. doi: 10.1097/SLE.0000000000000887
49. Kitagawa W, Shimizu K, Akasu H, Tanaka S. Endoscopic Neck Surgery With Lymph Node Dissection for Papillary Carcinoma of the Thyroid Using a Totally Gasless Anterior Neck Skin Lifting Method. *J Am Coll Surg* (2003) 196:990–4. doi: 10.1016/S1072-7515(03)00130-3
50. Zhang Z, Xu Z, Li Z, An C, Liu J, Zhu Y, et al. Minimally-Invasive Endoscopically-Assisted Neck Dissection for Lateral Cervical Metastases of Thyroid Papillary Carcinoma. *Br J Oral Maxillofac Surg* (2014) 52:793–7. doi: 10.1016/j.bjoms.2014.05.009
51. Zhang ZM, Xu ZG, Li ZJ, An CM, Liu J, Zhu YM, et al. Minimally Invasive Endoscopy-Assisted Neck Dissection to Treat Lateral Cervical Metastasis of Thyroid Papillary Carcinoma. *Zhonghua Er Bi Yan Hou Tou Jing Wai Ke Za Zhi* (2013) 48:712–5.
52. Zhang DG, Gao L, Xie L, He GF, Fang L, Chen J, et al. Modified Minimally Invasive Video-Assisted Lateral Neck Dissection for Papillary Thyroid Carcinoma: A Series of 130 Cases. *Zhonghua Wai Ke Za Zhi* (2016) 54:864–9. doi: 10.3760/cma.j.issn.0529-5815.2016.11.015
53. Lombardi CP, Raffaelli M, Princi P, De Crea C, Bellantone R. Minimally Invasive Video-Assisted Functional Lateral Neck Dissection for Metastatic Papillary Thyroid Carcinoma. *Am J Surg* (2007) 193:114–8. doi: 10.1016/j.amjsurg.2006.02.024
54. Miccoli P, Materazzi G, Berti P. Minimally Invasive Video-Assisted Lateral Lymphadenectomy: A Proposal. *Surg Endosc* (2008) 22:1131–4. doi: 10.1007/s00464-007-9564-6
55. Zhang D, Chen J, He G, Gao L, Fang L, Chen Z. Application of Endoscopic Upper Mediastinal Lymph Node Dissection in Treatment of Papillary Thyroid Carcinoma. *Chin J Gen Surg* (2018) 27:1583–8.

8

Necessity of Routinely Testing the Proximal and Distal Ends of Exposed Recurrent Laryngeal Nerve During Monitored Thyroidectomy

Hsiao-Yu Huang[1], Ching-Feng Lien[1,2], Chih-Chun Wang[1,2], Chien-Chung Wang[1], Tzer-Zen Hwang[1,2], Yu-Chen Shih[3], Che-Wei Wu[4], Gianlorenzo Dionigi[5,6], Tzu-Yen Huang[4] and Feng-Yu Chiang[1,2*]*

[1] *Department of Otolaryngology-Head and Neck Surgery, E-Da Hospital, Kaohsiung, Taiwan,* [2] *School of Medicine, College of Medicine, I-Shou University, Kaohsiung, Taiwan,* [3] *Department of Otolaryngology, E-Da Cancer Hospital, Kaohsiung, Taiwan,* [4] *Department of Otorhinolaryngology-Head and Neck Surgery, International Thyroid Surgery Center, Kaohsiung Medical University Hospital, Faculty of Medicine, College of Medicine, Kaohsiung Medical University, Kaohsiung, Taiwan,* [5] *Division of General Surgery, Endocrine Surgery Section, Istituto Auxologico Italiano Istituto di Ricovero e Cura a Carattere Scientifico (IRCSS), Milan, Italy,* [6] *Department of Pathophysiology and Transplantation, University of Milan, Milan, Italy*

***Correspondence:**
Tzu-Yen Huang
tyhuang.ent@gmail.com
Feng-Yu Chiang
fychiang@kmu.edu.tw

Objectives: Intraoperative neuromonitoring (IONM) is a useful tool to evaluate the function of recurrent laryngeal nerve (RLN) in thyroid surgery. This study aimed to determine the necessity and value of routinely testing the proximal and distal ends of RLN.

Methods: In total, 796 patients undergoing monitored thyroidectomies with standardized procedures were enrolled. All 1346 RLNs with visual integrity of anatomical continuity were routinely stimulated at the most proximal (R2p signal) and distal (R2d signal) ends after complete RLN dissection. The EMG amplitudes between R2p and R2d signals were compared. If the amplitude of R2p/R2d ratio reduction (RPDR) was over 10% or loss of signal (LOS) occurred, the exposed RLN was mapped to identify the injured point. Pre- and post-operative vocal cord (VC) mobility was routinely examined with video-laryngofiberscope.

Results: Nerve injuries were detected in 108 (8%) RLNs, including 94 nerves with incomplete LOS (RPDR between 13%-93%) and 14 nerves with complete LOS. The nerve injuries were caused by traction in 80 nerves, dissecting trauma in 23 nerves and lateral heat spread of energy-based devices in 5 nerves. Symmetric VC mobility was found in 72 nerves with RPDR ≤50%. The occurrence of abnormal VC mobility (weak or fixed) was 14%, 67%, 100%, and 100% among the different RPDR stratifications of 51%-60%, 61%-70%, 71%-80%, and 81-93%, respectively. Of the 14 nerves with complete LOS, all showed fixed VC mobility. Permanent VC palsy occurred in 2 nerves with thermal injury.

Conclusion: Routinely testing the proximal and distal ends of exposed RLN helps detect unrecognized partial nerve injury, elucidate the injury mechanism and determine injury severity. The procedure provides accurate information for evaluating RLN function after nerve dissection and should be included in the standard IONM procedure.

Keywords: recurrent laryngeal nerve (RLN), intraoperative neuromonitoring (IONM), thyroid surgery, electromyography (EMG), vocal cord (VC) mobility

INTRODUCTION

Intraoperative neuromonitoring (IONM) has been commonly applied in thyroid surgery to facilitate the identification of recurrent laryngeal nerve (RLN), evaluate nerve function after dissection, detect nerve injury and elucidate its mechanism, predict the outcome of vocal cord (VC) function and make the decision to perform staged thyroidectomy (1–6).

From the literature review, the era in the absence of standard IONM procedures revealed a high negative predictive value of 92%-100%, but a low and highly variable positive predictive value, ranging from 10% to 90% (7–13). The results suggested that patients with positive EMG signals after thyroid resection generally do not have VC palsy. Conversely, patients with loss of signal (LOS) have unpredictable VC functional outcomes, leading to unnecessary staged operation.

In recent years, through following the standard 4-step IONM procedures (V_1-R_1-R_2-V_2) and troubleshooting algorithms, the positive predictive value has greatly improved. When LOS occurs after RLN dissection, it always indicates nerve injury and the development of postoperative VC palsy (5, 6, 14–16). However, a positive EMG signal at the proximal end of RLN does not guarantee normal nerve function and normal postoperative VC function. In the absence of complete LOS, a partial nerve injury could be unrecognized and an unexpected VC palsy may occur (17, 18). In this study, we hypothesize that routinely testing the proximal and distal ends of exposed RLN may help detect unrecognized nerve injury, elucidating the injury mechanism, and determining injury severity.

MATERIALS AND METHODS

Patients

From January 2015 to October 2019, 796 patients (152 men and 644 women; ages ranging from 12 to 81 years; mean age, 50.4 years) underwent operations for various thyroid diseases by the same surgeon (F.-Y. C) were collected. There were 232 thyroid lobectomies and 564 total thyroidectomies (467 benign and 329 malignant thyroid diseases). Fourteen nerves were excluded from this study due to preoperative cord palsy (10 nerves) and intentional sacrifice due to cancer encasement (4 nerves). Thus, 1346 nerves at risk were enrolled in this study. The study was approved by the Institutional Review Board (IRB) of Kaohsiung Medical University Hospital, Taiwan: KMUHIRB-E (II)-20200348.

IONM Setup and Procedures

The standard procedures for equipment setup and anesthesia were performed by the IONM team of Kaohsiung Medical University Hospital. All patients were intubated with a regular oral endotracheal tube. After dissection of the thyroid pyramidal lobe, two paired subdermal needle electrodes (length 12.0 mm, Medtronic Xomed, Jacksonville, FL, USA) were obliquely inserted into the sub-perichondrium of the lateral thyroid cartilage on each side for EMG signal recording (19, 20).

During the operation, standardized IONM procedures were strictly followed. The VN (without dissecting the carotid sheath to expose the VN) was stimulated with a 5-10 mA stimulus current before and after RLN dissection, and V_1 and V_2 signals were obtained. The RLN was stimulated with 3-5 mA at the first identification, and the R_1 signal was obtained. After complete RLN dissection, the exposed RLN was stimulated at the most proximal end, and distal end near the laryngeal entry point, and R_{2p} and R_{2d} signals were obtained, respectively. The largest amplitudes of these five EMG signals (V_1-R_1-R_{2p}-R_{2d}-V_2) were registered in all cases. The amplitudes of the R_{2p} and R_{2d} signals were compared. If the amplitude of R_{2p}/R_{2d} ratio reduction (RPDR) was over 10% after repeated testing or LOS occurred, the whole exposed RLN was mapped to identify the weak or disrupted point of nerve conduction with 1 mA. The standardized IONM techniques in this study started with a preoperative examination of VC function (L_1), and an intraoperative 5-step procedure (V_1-R_1-R_{2p}-R_{2d}-V_2), and ended with a postoperative examination of VC function (L_2) for all patients (**Table 1**).

For the severity of nerve injury, complete LOS was defined as an absence of EMG signals (R_{2p} amplitude less than 100 μV) after nerve stimulation. Incomplete LOS was defined as when the R_{2p} amplitude was detectable (more than 100 μV), the RDPR was more than 10% and less than 100%. When nerve injury occurred, the mechanism of nerve injury (traction injury, dissecting trauma and thermal injury) and injury site (upper third, middle third and lower third portion of the exposed RLN) were registered. For the type of nerve injury, type 1 LOS was defined as a detectable injury site on the exposed RLN, and type 2 LOS was defined as no detectable injury site on the whole exposed RLN. For VC mobility, normal (symmetric) VC function was correlated with symmetric VC mobility during phonation, weak VC function was correlated with weak VC mobility (asymmetric and sluggish VC movement at the injury side), and VC palsy was correlated with fixed VC mobility. When VC palsy persisted for more than 6 months, it was regarded as permanent palsy.

The percentage and mean value were calculated using Microsoft Excel 2016 (Microsoft Corp., Redmond, WA, USA).

TABLE 1 | Standardized IONM procedures.

Procedures
L_1 Pre-operative examination of VC function with laryngofiberscope
V_1 Vagus nerve stimulation with 5-10 mA before thyroid dissection
R_1 RLN stimulation with 3-5 mA at first RLN identification
(R_{2p})* RLN stimulation with 3-5 mA at the most proximal end after RLN dissection
(R_{2d})* RLN stimulation with 3-5 mA at the distal end near the laryngeal entry point
V_2 Vagus nerve stimulation with 5-10 mA after resection of thyroid lobe
L_2 Post-operative examination of VC function with laryngofiberscope

**RLN mapping with 1 mA if the amplitude reduction of R_{2p}/R_{2d} signals over 10% or LOS*

IONM, intraoperative neuromonitoring; RLN, recurrent laryngeal nerve; VC, vocal cord.

RESULTS

Among 1346 RLNs with anatomical integrity in continuity after nerve dissection, nerve injury was detected in 108 (8%) nerves, including 94 nerves with incomplete LOS (RPDR ranging from 13% to 93%) and 14 nerves with complete LOS.

Of the 94 RLNs with incomplete LOS, the nerve injury site was detectable in all nerves. Seventy-three nerve injuries were caused by traction injury, 19 nerve injuries were caused by dissecting trauma, and 2 nerve injuries were caused by thermal injury. For injured nerves with RPDR ≤50%, the 72 corresponding patients had postoperative symmetric VC mobility; for injured nerves with RPDR between 51%-60%, weak VC mobility was found in 1 (14%) of 7 corresponding patients; for injured nerves with RPDR between 61%-70%, abnormal (2 weak and 2 fixed) VC mobility was found in 4 (67%) of 6 corresponding patients; for injured nerves with RPDR between 71%-80%, abnormal (1 weak and 2 fixed) VC mobility was found in 3 (100%) of 3 corresponding patients; for injured nerves with RPDR between 81%-93%, abnormal VC mobility was found in 6 (100%) of 6 corresponding patients, and all patients had fixed VC mobility (**Tables 2, 3**).

Of the 14 RLNs with complete LOS, the nerve injury site was detectable on the exposed RLN in 11 nerves (type 1 LOS) and was not detectable on the exposed RLN in 3 nerves (type 2 LOS). Seven nerve injuries were caused by traction injury, 4 nerve injuries were caused by dissecting trauma, and 3 nerve injuries were caused by thermal injury. All 14 cases showed fixed VC mobility postoperatively. Temporary VC palsy occurred in 12 nerves, and permanent VC palsy occurred in 2 nerves with thermal injury (**Tables 2, 4**).

Among 105 nerves with a detectable injury site, the weak or disrupted point of nerve conduction was localized at the region of Berry's ligament (within the upper portion of the exposed RLN) in 83 (79%) nerves (77 traction injuries, 3 dissecting traumas, and 3 thermal injuries), on the middle portion of the exposed RLN in 9 (9%) nerves (8 dissecting traumas and 1 thermal injury), and on the lower portion of the exposed RLN in 13 (12%) nerves (12 dissecting traumas and 1 thermal injury).

DISCUSSION

When applying IONM in thyroid surgery, the measurement of EMG amplitude from RLN stimulation may correlate with the number of motor units that contribute to polarization and reflect the neurophysiologic function of the nerve (21, 22). Theoretically, unchanged EMG amplitude after RLN dissection indicates normal nerve and VC functions postoperatively. Conversely, decreased EMG amplitude after nerve dissection indicates a nerve function deficit or a decreased number of motor units participating in polarization. Complete LOS after RLN dissection may indicate complete loss of nerve conduction and postoperative VC palsy. However, the correlation between the residual ratio of EMG amplitude after partial RLN injury and the sufficient muscle strength required for normal VC mobility is still unknown.

The intraoperative 4-step procedure (V_1-R_1-R_2-V_2) has been accepted as a standard IONM procedure by many studies (5, 6, 14–17). It was useful to evaluate nerve function by comparing the EMG signals between pre- and post-dissection of RLN. Unchanged or increased post-dissection EMG amplitudes (comparing R_2 and V_2 signals with R_1 and V_1 signals, respectively) indicated functional integrity of the RLN. Conversely, decreased R_2 and V_2 signals indicated RLN injury and the risk of postoperative VC palsy. However, when using an EMG endotracheal tube for signal recording, unstable EMG amplitudes often occur intraoperatively due to the change in contact quality between the EMG tube and vocal cords. Poor

TABLE 2 | The mechanism and severity of RLN injury and the outcome of VC mobility in 108 RLNs detected with injury.

Severity of nerve injury	Case number	Mechanism of nerve injury and injury site			VC mobility		
		Traction injury (U/M/L)	Dissecting trauma (U/M/L)	Thermal injury (U/M/L)	Sym	Weak	Fixed
Incomplete LOS (RPDR >10%, <100%)	94	73(73/0/0)	19(2/6/11)	2(0/1/1)	80	4	10
11%-20%	35	32	3	0	35	0	0
21%-30%	16	12	3	1	16	0	0
31%-40%	10	6	4	0	10	0	0
41%-50%	11	7	4	0	11	0	0
51%-60%	7	7	0	0	6	1	0
61%-70%	6	5	1	0	2	2	2
71%-80%	3	1	2	0	0	1	2
81%-90%	3	1	1	1	0	0	3
91%-93%	3	2	1	0	0	0	3
Complete LOS	14	7(4/0/0)+	4(1/2/1)	3(3/0/0)	0	0	14*
Total	108	80	23	5	80	4	24

+type 1 complete LOS in 4 nerves with detectable injured point, type 2 complete LOS in 3 nerves without detectable injured point.
*temporary palsy in 12 nerves, permanent palsy in 2 nerve with thermal injury.
U/M/L, upper/middle/lower portion of the exposed RLN.
RLN, recurrent laryngeal nerve; VC, vocal cord; RPDR, R_{2p}/R_{2d} ratio reduction; LOS, loss of signal; sym, symmetric.

TABLE 3 | Intraoperative EMG signals and mechanism of nerve injury in the RLNs without complete LOS (detectable injury site and R_{2p}/R_{2d} reduction >50%).

No.	V_1 (μV)	R_1 (μV)	R_{2p} (μV)	R_{2d} (μV)	V_2 (μV)	R_{2p}/R_{2d} reduction	Injury site	Injury mechanism	VC mobility
1	949	1017	708	1431	655	51%	U(BL)	traction	sym
2	2051	2215	1188	2491	1037	52%	U(BL)	traction	sym
3	3598	3752	1337	2806	1068	52%	U(BL)	traction	sym
4	2728	2899	1393	3110	979	55%	U(BL)	traction	sym
5	1261	1358	512	1214	358	58%	U(BL)	traction	weak
6	1570	2237	989	2441	606	59%	U(BL)	traction	sym
7	1957	2354	954	2325	801	59%	U(BL)	traction	sym
8	2235	3695	1480	3855	1072	62%	U(BL)	traction	weak
9	1153	1278	364	1480	244	66%	U(BL)	traction	sym
10	921	843	396	1230	272	68%	U(BL)	traction	fixed^t
11	752	780	229	724	167	68%	L	trauma	fixed^t
12	2707	4570	1647	5254	903	69%	U(BL)	traction	sym
13	1175	1363	688	2264	462	70%	U(BL)	traction	weak
14	1728	3494	880	3422	543	74%	U(BL)	traction	weak
15	1889	2206	509	2144	577	76%	L	trauma	weak
16	1287	1658	346	1712	247	80%	M	trauma	fixed^t
17	1152	1289	145	755	138	81%	U(BL)	traction	fixed^t
18	1564	1735	351	1837	287	81%	L	thermal	fixed^t
19	1308	1521	188	1810	122	90%	L	trauma	fixed^t
20	2896	3015	250	3109	235	92%	U(BL)	traction	fixed^t
21	2779	3410	323	3822	190	92%	U(BL)	traction	fixed^t
22	2935	3773	232	3351	217	93%	U(BL)	trauma	fixed^t

EMG, electromyography; RLN, recurrent laryngeal nerve; LOS, complete loss of signal; VC, vocal cord; U(BL), upper portion of the exposed RLN (at the region of Berry's ligament); M, middle portion of the exposed RLN; L, lower portion of the exposed RLN; sym, symmetric; fixed ^{t}, temporary palsy.

contact quality caused by EMG tube displacement during the surgical maneuver on the trachea will lead to a significant decrease in EMG amplitudes or false LOS. Therefore, a decrease or loss of the post-dissection EMG amplitude would not necessarily be a nerve injury. Genther et al. reported that the risk of immediate postoperative VC palsy is approximately 72% when post-dissection EMG amplitudes are less than 200 μV (23). Pavier et al. reported that the risk of VC palsy is approximately 50% when post-dissection EMG amplitudes were under the value of 280 μV and suggested a staged thyroidectomy (24). The data of these 2 studies showed that the false-positive rate ranged from 28% to 50% and indicated that many patients might receive unnecessary second operations. Calò et al. reported that staged thyroidectomy was performed in 37 patients due to LOS, but 8 (22%) patients had normal VC function after their first operations (25). Melin et al. reported that the second operation was performed in 18 patients with LOS, but 8 (44%) patients were confirmed to have primarily intact vocal cord function (26).

In this study, we used the trans-thyroid cartilage EMG signal recording method (19, 27–29). The EMG amplitude will not be influenced by EMG tube displacement and the elicited signals remain high and stable during the entire course of operation that is important to monitor the actual status of RLN function. Furthermore, we routinely test the proximal and distal ends of the exposed RLN after complete nerve dissection. The procedure helps detect unrecognized partial nerve injury and determine its severity by comparing R_{2p} with R_{2d} signals. This series found that the outcomes of VC function were highly correlated with the severity of

TABLE 4 | Intraoperative EMG signals and mechanism of nerve injury in the RLNs with complete LOS.

No.	V_1 (μV)	R_1 (μV)	R_{2p} (μV)	R_{2d} (μV)	V_2 (μV)	R_{2p}/R_{2d} reduction	Injury site	Injurymechanism	VC mobility
1	2862	2993	LOS	3279	LOS	=100%	U(BL)	traction	fixed^t
2	1391	1581	LOS	1242	LOS	=100%	U(BL)	traction	fixed^t
3	2430	2882	LOS	2976	LOS	=100%	U(BL)	traction	fixed^t
4	3616	4600	LOS	5019	LOS	=100%	U(BL)	traction	fixed^t
5	1716	2585	LOS	LOS	LOS	=0%	nil	traction	fixed^t
6	2145	2521	LOS	LOS	LOS	=0%	nil	traction	fixed^t
7	1053	1384	LOS	LOS	LOS	=0%	nil	traction	fixed^t
8	2816	2756	LOS	3149	LOS	=100%	U(BL)	trauma	fixed^t
9	1532	3750	LOS	3818	LOS	=100%	L	trauma	fixed^t
10	729	1395	LOS	1289	LOS	=100%	M	trauma	fixed^t
11	1748	1784	1998	LOS	LOS	=100%	M	trauma	fixed^t
12	2154	3823	LOS	3750	LOS	=100%	U(BL)	thermal	fixed^t
13	1421	1600	LOS	1744	LOS	=100%	M	thermal	fixed^p
14	2860	3637	LOS	3171	LOS	=100%	U(BL)	thermal	fixed^p

EMG, electromyography; RLN, recurrent laryngeal nerve; LOS, complete loss of signal; VC, vocal cord; U(BL), upper portion of the exposed RLN (at the region of Berry's ligament); M, middle portion of the exposed RLN; L, lower portion of the exposed RLN; fixed ^{t}, temporary palsy; fixed ^{P}, permanent palsy.

nerve injury. In 14 nerves with post-dissection complete LOS, all cases showed fixed VC mobility postoperatively. In 94 nerves with RPDR over 10% (ranging from 13% to 93%), 72 nerves showed symmetric VC mobility where the RPDR was ≤50%. Abnormal VC mobility (weak or fixed VC movement) was only found in the nerves with RPDR >50%. The possibility of postoperative abnormal VC mobility was approximately 14%, 67%, 100%, and 100% among the different RPDR stratifications of 51%-60%, 61%-70%, 71%-80%, and 81-93%, respectively.

A weak or disrupted point of nerve conduction is important neurophysiological evidence of nerve injury. By mapping the exposed RLN, we can localize the injured point and clarify the possible mechanism of nerve injury. In this study, we found that the region of Berry's ligament is the most common site of nerve injury. Among 105 nerves with an injured point detected, 83 (79%) nerves were injured at this site, including 77 traction injuries, 3 dissecting traumas, and 3 thermal injuries. The injured point was localized at the middle portion of the exposed RLN in 10 (10%) nerves (9 dissecting trauma and 1 thermal injury) and at the lower portion in 12 (11%) nerves (11 dissecting trauma and 1 thermal injury).

This study also found that traction injury was the most common cause of RLN injury, of approximately 74% (80/108). The RLN can be injured at the region of Berry's ligament by stretching dense fibrous tissue or surrounding blood vessels during medial thyroid retraction. Of the 80 nerves with traction injuries, the injury points were located at Berry's ligament region in 73 nerves without LOS (**Figure 1**). In the other 7 nerves with LOS, 4 injury points were located at Berry's ligament region (type 1 LOS) (**Figures 2A, B**), and 3 injury points were not found (type 2 LOS), and the injury point may be located higher above the laryngeal entry point (**Figures 3A, B**). Dissecting trauma was the second most common cause of RLN injury, with a rate of approximately 21% (23/108). Of the 23 nerves injured by dissecting trauma, 3 nerve injuries occurred during dissection of the RLN from Berry's ligament, 8 nerve injuries occurred during dissection of the RLN from malignant tumors or recurrent benign tumors (**Figures 4A, B**), and 12 nerve injuries occurred during paratracheal node dissection. Thermal injury accounted for approximately 5% (5/108), and all 5 nerve injuries were caused by lateral heat spread of the energy-

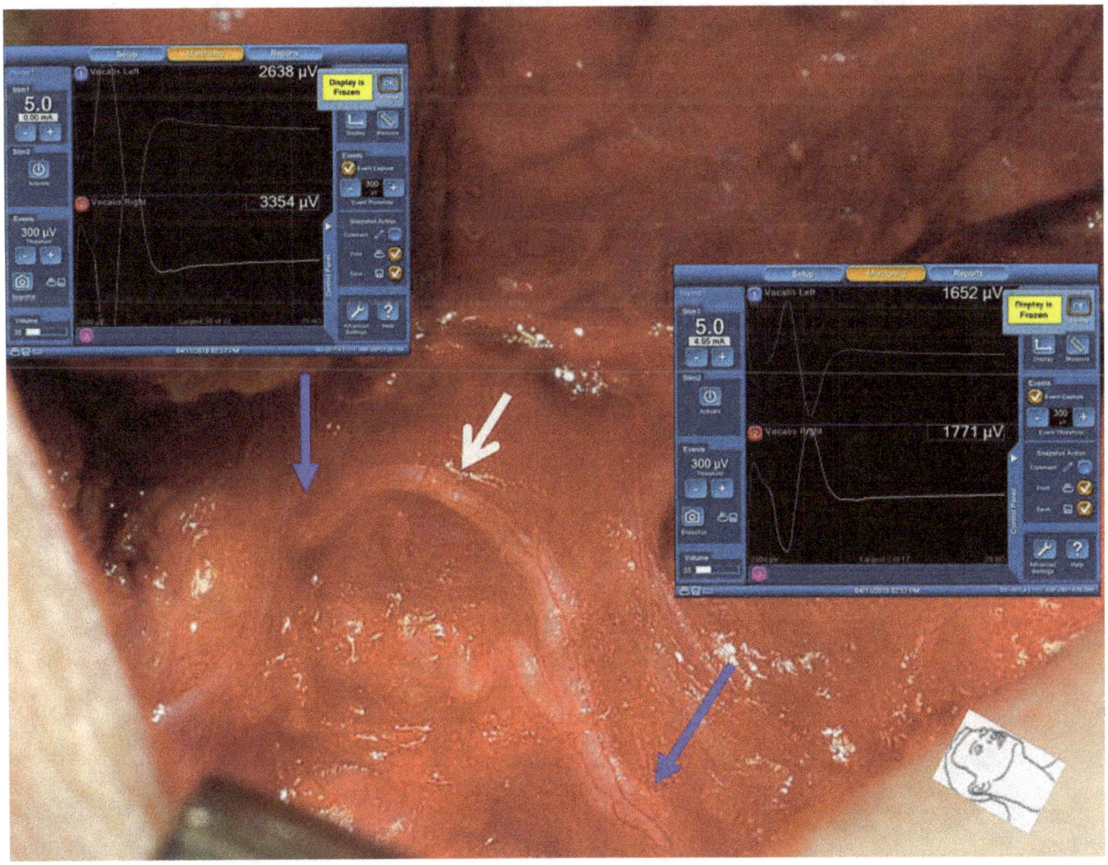

FIGURE 1 | A case of type 1 incomplete LOS. The anterior motor branch of the RLN was stretched upward during medial thyroid traction. After complete RLN dissection and comparing R_{2p} signal (1771 μV) with R_{2d} signal (3354 μV), it showed an amplitude reduction of approximately 47%, and a weak point of nerve conduction was mapped (white arrow).

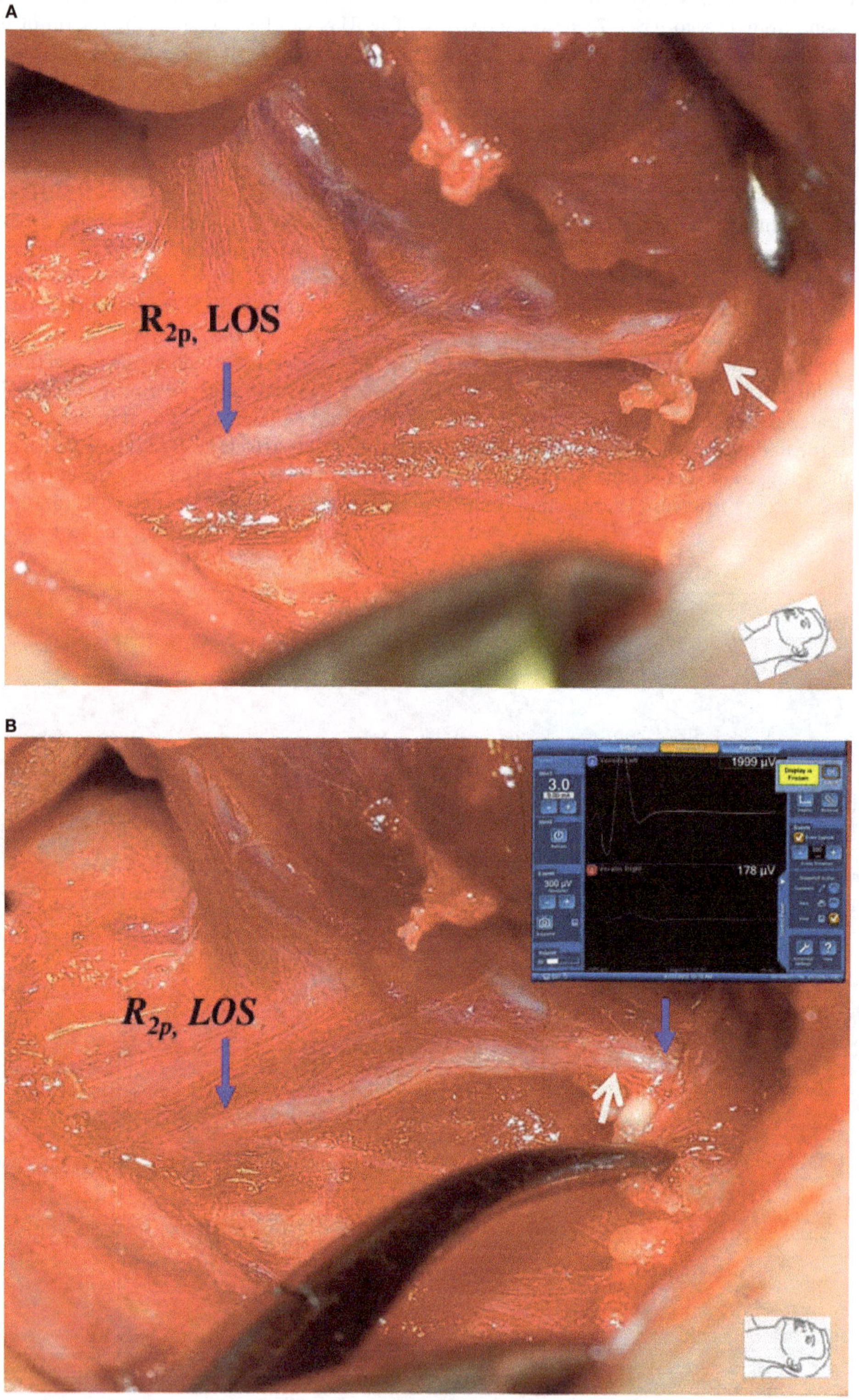

FIGURE 2 | A case of type 1 complete LOS. **(A)** The R_{2p} signal was lost, and a small artery (white arrow) was found to be intertwined with the RLN at the region of Berry's ligament. **(B)** After dissecting the intertwined vessel from the RLN, R_{2d} signal showed 1999 µV and R_{2p} signal showed complete LOS, a disrupted point of nerve conduction (white arrow) was detected. This was a type 1 LOS and the patient had temporary vocal cord palsy.

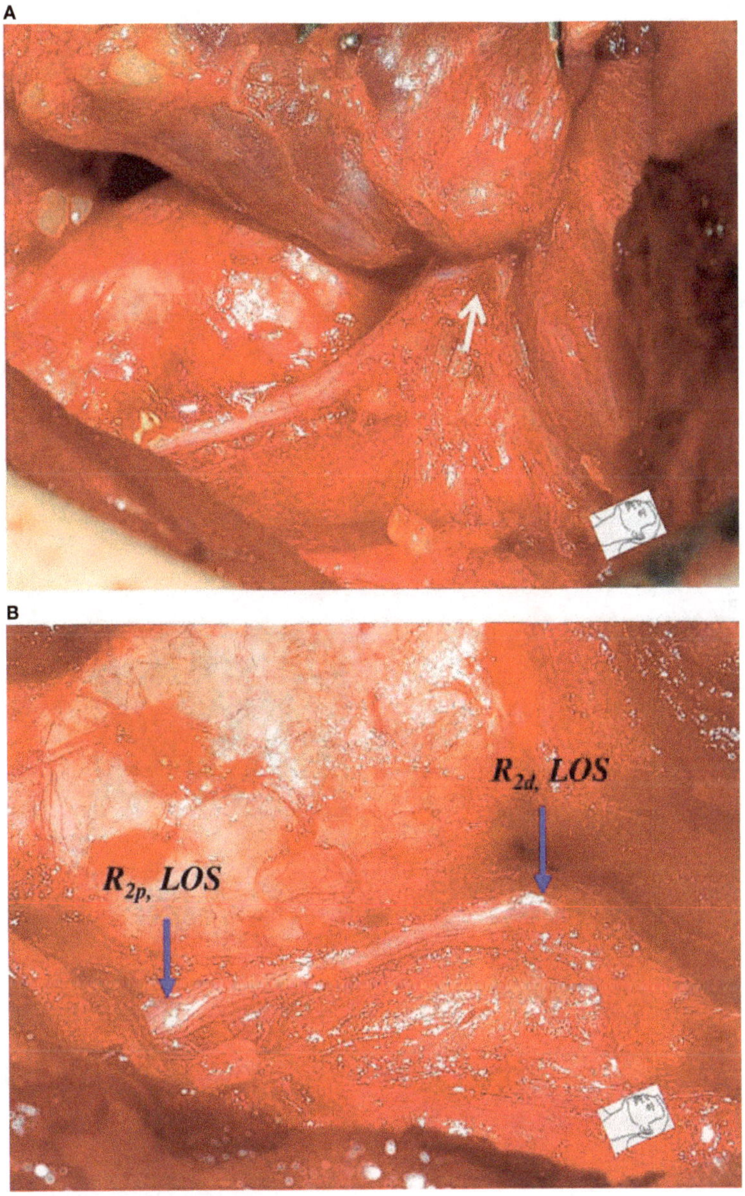

FIGURE 3 | A case of type 2 complete LOS. **(A)** The RLN was stretched upward (white arrow) at the region of Berry's ligament during medial thyroid traction. **(B)** After complete RLN dissection, both R_{2p} and R_{2d} signals showed complete LOS and no injured point was found on the exposed RLN. This was a type 2 LOS and it developed temporary vocal cord palsy.

based device (EBD) or electrocauterization (**Figures 5, 6**). In 3 nerves with LOS, 2 nerves developed permanent VC palsy, and 1 developed temporary VC palsy. Another nerve with RPDR of 81% developed temporary VC palsy. The other nerve with RPDR of less than 50% showed symmetrical VC mobility after surgery.

From the results of this study, it can be found that permanent VC palsy rarely occurred in nerve injuries caused by traction or dissecting trauma, but there was a high rate of permanent VC palsy (40%, 2/5) in thermal injuries. The voice outcome and VC mobility prognosis are worse in patients with thermal RLN injuries than in those with mechanical RLN injuries (30, 31). Therefore, the use of EBDs or electrocauterization near the RLN should pay special attention to the safety distance. Several studies on animals have shown that activations of various EBDs at 2 mm are safe under electrophysiological evidence (32–34), but translating the data to clinical practice must be very careful. When EBD is activated, tissue contraction can reduce the safety distance and increase the risk of thermal injury. Additionally, hot tissue fluid contact with the RLN may also

A

B

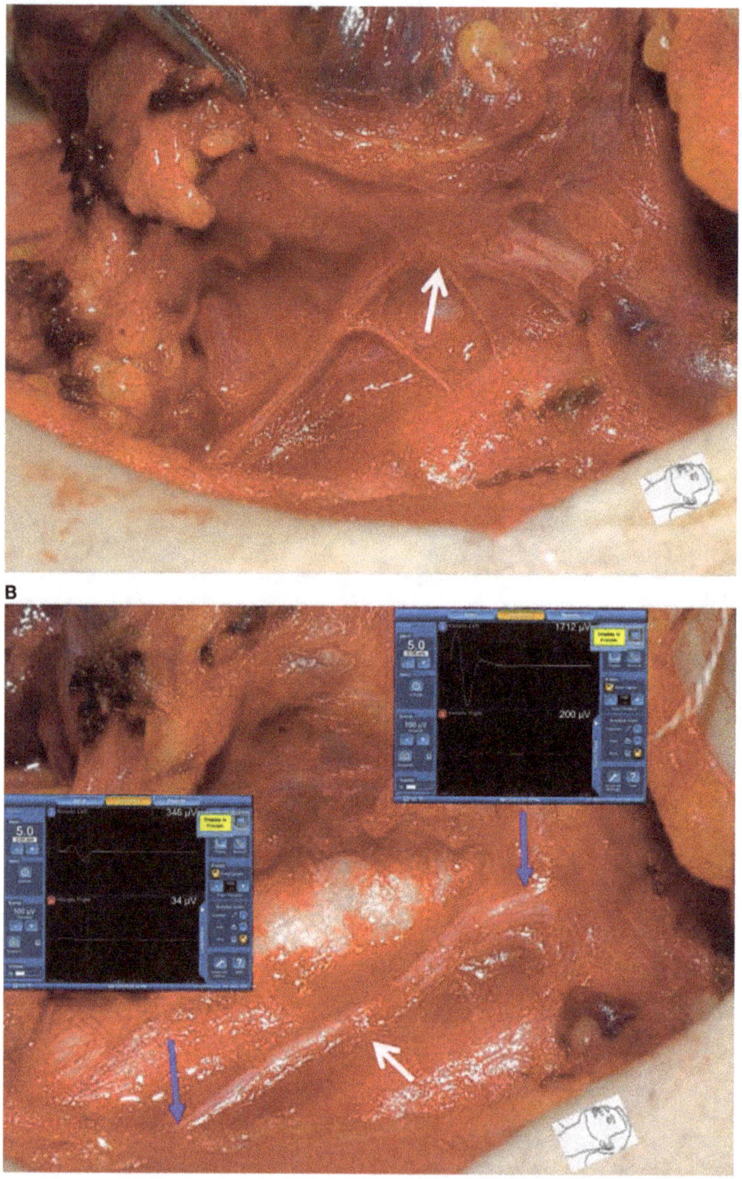

FIGURE 4 | Dissecting trauma of the RLN. **(A)** The RLN was adherent to thyroid cancer. **(B)** After complete RLN dissection and comparing R_{2p} signal (346 μV) with R_{2d} signal (1712 μV), it showed an approximately 80% amplitude reduction and an injured point caused by dissecting trauma was mapped (white arrow). The patient had temporary vocal cord palsy.

cause thermal injury (35). Lin et al. confirmed that complete LOS occurred when the RLN was in contact with hot water at 60°C (36). Therefore, we recommend that the RLN should be clearly visualized and that the safety distance from the nerve is best to have 5 mm (37). If the safe distance is less than 5 mm, particularly at the region of Berry's ligament, a small piece of wet gauze or forceps should be placed between the nerve and the EBD to prevent thermal injury caused by lateral heat spread or by hot tissue fluid. Based on the above, elucidating the mechanism (traction injury, dissecting trauma, and thermal injury) and type (detectable or undetectable injury site) of nerve injury while performing R_{2p} and R_{2d} steps enables thyroid surgeons to continuously improve surgical techniques and reduce surgical complications.

Several limitations should be mentioned in this study. First, this was an observational study without a control group. Second, the number of patients with complete LOS was relatively small; however, the characteristics of severe incomplete LOS and complete LOS can be clearly shown in this study. Last, the functional outcomes and prognosis of type 1 and type 2 LOS

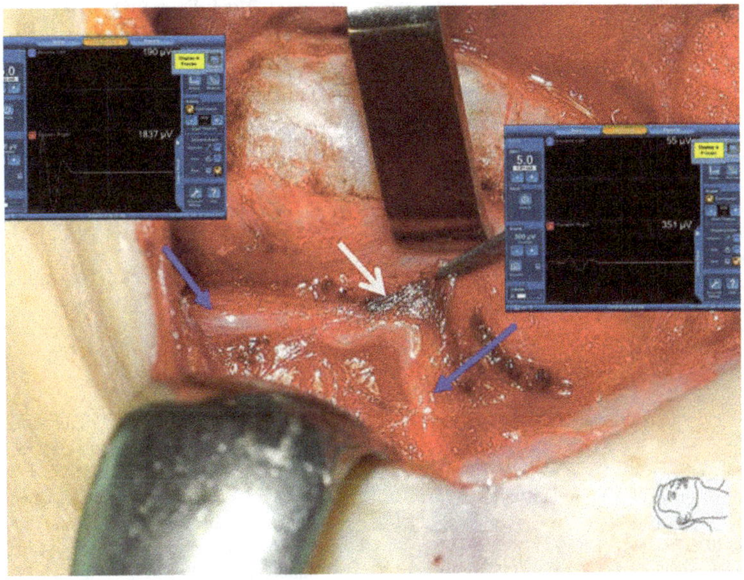

FIGURE 5 | Thermal injury of the RLN with incomplete LOS. The RLN was injured by lateral thermal spread of electrocauterization (white arrow). Comparing R_{2p} signal (351 μV) with R_{2d} signal (1837 μV) showed an approximately 81% amplitude reduction and the development of temporary vocal cord palsy.

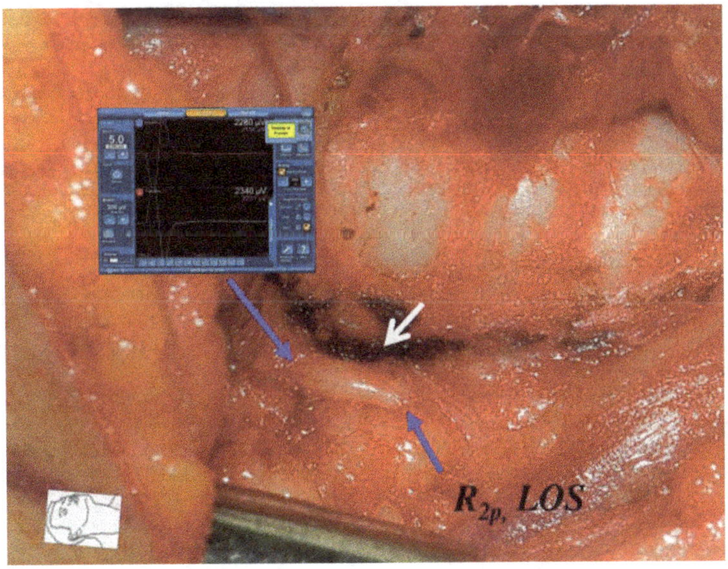

FIGURE 6 | Thermal injury of the RLN with complete LOS. The RLN was injured by lateral thermal spread of energy-based device (white arrow) at the region of Berry's ligament. Complete LOS occurred in R_{2p} signal, and the R_{2d} signal was 2340 μV. The patient had temporary vocal cord palsy.

warrant further study, and a well-designed study would help to highlight the advantages of R_{2p} and R_{2d} steps.

CONCLUSION

Routinely testing the proximal and distal ends of the exposed RLN is a simple and useful procedure to accurately evaluate RLN function after complete dissection. It helps detect unrecognized nerve injury and clarifies where and how the nerve was injured and determines the severity of nerve injury. The provided information will be useful to improve surgeons' surgical techniques and help make decisions regarding staged thyroidectomy. The additional step of testing the distal end of the exposed RLN should be included in the standard IONM procedure.

ETHICS STATEMENT

The studies involving human participants were reviewed and approved by Institutional Review Board (IRB) of Kaohsiung Medical University Hospital, Taiwan: KMUHIRB-E(II)-20200348. Written informed consent for participation was not required for this study in accordance with the national legislation and the institutional requirements.

AUTHOR CONTRIBUTIONS

Supervision - T-ZH, C-WW, GD, and F-YC; Materials - C-FL, T-ZH, Y-CS, T-YH, and F-YC; Data Collection and Processing - H-YH, Chih-CW, Chien-CW, Y-CS; Analysis and Interpretation - H-YH, C-FL, T-YH, and F-YC; Literature Search - H-YH, Chih-CW, Chien-CW, T-YH, and F-YC; Writing Manuscript - All authors. All authors have read and agreed to the published version of the manuscript.

ACKNOWLEDGMENTS

The authors would like to thank all the patients included in this study.

REFERENCES

1. Wu C-W, Randolph G, Barczynski M, Schneider R, Chiang F-Y, Huang T-Y, et al. Training Courses in Laryngeal Nerve Monitoring in Thyroid and Parathyroid Surgery-The INMSG Consensus Statement. *Front Endocrinol* (2021) 12:708. doi: 10.3389/fendo.2021.795281
2. Liu N, Chen B, Li L, Zeng Q, Sheng L, Zhang B, et al. Mechanisms of Recurrent Laryngeal Nerve Injury Near the Nerve Entry Point During Thyroid Surgery: A Retrospective Cohort Study. *Int J Surg* (2020) 83:125–30. doi: 10.1016/j.ijsu.2020.08.058
3. Zhang D, Sun H, Tufano R, Caruso E, Dionigi G, Kim HY. Recurrent Laryngeal Nerve Management in Transoral Endoscopic Thyroidectomy. *Oral Oncol* (2020) 108:104755. doi: 10.1016/j.oraloncology.2020.104755
4. Hayward NJ, Grodski S, Yeung M, Johnson WR, Serpell J. Recurrent Laryngeal Nerve Injury in Thyroid Surgery: A Review. *ANZ J Surg* (2013) 83(1-2):15–21. doi: 10.1111/j.1445-2197.2012.06247.x
5. Chiang F-Y, Lu I-C, Kuo W-R, Lee K-W, Chang N-C, Wu C-W. The Mechanism of Recurrent Laryngeal Nerve Injury During Thyroid Surgery—the Application of Intraoperative Neuromonitoring. *Surgery* (2008) 143 (6):743–9. doi: 10.1016/j.surg.2008.02.006
6. Chiang F-Y, Lee K-W, Chen H-C, Chen H-Y, Lu I-C, Kuo W-R, et al. Standardization of Intraoperative Neuromonitoring of Recurrent Laryngeal Nerve in Thyroid Operation. *World J Surg* (2010) 34(2):223–9. doi: 10.1007/s00268-009-0316-8
7. Dralle H, Sekulla C, Lorenz K, Brauckhoff M, Machens A. Intraoperative Monitoring of the Recurrent Laryngeal Nerve in Thyroid Surgery. *World J Surg* (2008) 32(7):1358–66. doi: 10.1007/s00268-008-9483-2
8. Tomoda C, Hirokawa Y, Uruno T, Takamura Y, Ito Y, Miya A, et al. Sensitivity and Specificity of Intraoperative Recurrent Laryngeal Nerve Stimulation Test for Predicting Vocal Cord Palsy After Thyroid Surgery. *World J Surg* (2006) 30(7):1230–3. doi: 10.1007/s00268-005-0351-z
9. Hamelmann W, Meyer T, Timm S, Timmermann W. Kritische Beurteilung Und Fehlermöglichkeiten Des Intraoperativen Neuromonitoring (IONM) Bei Operationen an Der Schilddrüse. *Zentralbl Für Chirurgie* (2002) 127(05):409–13. doi: 10.1055/s-2002-31982
10. Hermann M, Hellebart C, Freissmuth M. Neuromonitoring in Thyroid Surgery: Prospective Evaluation of Intraoperative Electrophysiological Responses for the Prediction of Recurrent Laryngeal Nerve Injury. *Ann Surg* (2004) 240(1):9. doi: 10.1097/01.sla.0000132260.34503.02
11. Thomusch O, Sekulla C, Machens A, Neumann H-J, Timmermann W, Dralle H. Validity of Intra-Operative Neuromonitoring Signals in Thyroid Surgery. *Langenbeck's Arch Surg* (2004) 389(6):499–503. doi: 10.1007/s00423-003-0444-9
12. Beldi G, Kinsbergen T, Schlumpf R. Evaluation of Intraoperative Recurrent Nerve Monitoring in Thyroid Surgery. *World J Surg* (2004) 28(6):589–91. doi: 10.1007/s00268-004-7226-6
13. Chan W-F, Lo C-Y. Pitfalls of Intraoperative Neuromonitoring for Predicting Postoperative Recurrent Laryngeal Nerve Function During Thyroidectomy. *World J Surg* (2006) 30(5):806–12. doi: 10.1007/s00268-005-0355-8
14. Schneider R, Randolph GW, Dionigi G, Wu CW, Barczynski M, Chiang FY, et al. International Neural Monitoring Study Group Guideline 2018 Part I: Staging Bilateral Thyroid Surgery With Monitoring Loss of Signal. *Laryngoscope* (2018) 128:S1–S17. doi: 10.1002/lary.27359
15. Wu C-W, Wang M-H, Chen C-C, Chen H-C, Chen H-Y, Yu J-Y, et al. Loss of Signal in Recurrent Nerve Neuromonitoring: Causes and Management. *Gland Surg* (2015) 4(1):19. doi: 10.3978/j.issn.2227-684X.2014.12.03
16. Randolph GW, Dralle H, Group IIMS, Abdullah H, Barczynski M, Bellantone R, et al. Electrophysiologic Recurrent Laryngeal Nerve Monitoring During Thyroid and Parathyroid Surgery: International Standards Guideline Statement. *Laryngoscope* (2011) 121(S1):S1–S16. doi: 10.1002/lary.21119
17. Wu C-W, Hao M, Tian M, Dionigi G, Tufano RP, Kim HY, et al. Recurrent Laryngeal Nerve Injury With Incomplete Loss of Electromyography Signal During Monitored Thyroidectomy—Evaluation and Outcome. *Langenbeck's Arch Surg* (2017) 402(4):691–9. doi: 10.1007/s00423-016-1381-8
18. Wojtczak B, Sutkowski K, Kaliszewski K, Głód M, Barczyński M. Experience With Intraoperative Neuromonitoring of the Recurrent Laryngeal Nerve Improves Surgical Skills and Outcomes of non-Monitored Thyroidectomy. *Langenbeck's Arch Surg* (2017) 402(4):709–17. doi: 10.1007/s00423-016-1449-5
19. Chiang FY, Lu IC, Chang PY, Dionigi G, Randolph GW, Sun H, et al. Comparison of EMG Signals Recorded by Surface Electrodes on Endotracheal Tube and Thyroid Cartilage During Monitored Thyroidectomy. *Kaohsiung J Med Sci* (2017) 33(10):503–9. doi: 10.1016/j.kjms.2017.06.014
20. Chiang F-Y, Wu C-W, Chang P-Y, Wu S-H, Chen H-Y, Lin Y-C, et al. Trans-Thyroid Cartilage Recording for Neural Monitoring of the Recurrent Laryngeal Nerve in Thyroid Surgery. *Laryngoscope* (2020) 130(4):E280–E3. doi: 10.1002/lary.28049
21. Behm D, Whittle J, Button D, Power K. Intermuscle Differences in Activation. *Muscle Nerve* (2002) 25(2):236–43. doi: 10.1002/mus.10008
22. Roberts TJ, Gabaldón AM. Interpreting Muscle Function From EMG: Lessons Learned From Direct Measurements of Muscle Force. *Integr Comp Biol* (2008) 48(2):312–20. doi: 10.1093/icb/icn056
23. Genther DJ, Kandil EH, Noureldine SI, Tufano RP. Correlation of Final Evoked Potential Amplitudes on Intraoperative Electromyography of the Recurrent Laryngeal Nerve With Immediate Postoperative Vocal Fold Function After Thyroid and Parathyroid Surgery. *JAMA Otolaryngol Head Neck Surg* (2014) 140(2):124–8. doi: 10.1001/jamaoto.2013.6139
24. Pavier Y, Saroul N, Pereira B, Tauveron I, Gilain L, Mom T. Acute Prediction of Laryngeal Outcome During Thyroid Surgery by Electromyographic Laryngeal Monitoring. *Head Neck* (2015) 37(6):835–9. doi: 10.1002/hed.23676
25. Calò PG, Medas F, Conzo G, Podda F, Canu GL, Gambardella C, et al. Intraoperative Neuromonitoring in Thyroid Surgery: Is the Two-Staged Thyroidectomy Justified? *Int J Surg* (2017) 41:S13–20. doi: 10.1016/j.ijsu.2017.02.001
26. Melin M, Schwarz K, Lammers BJ, Goretzki PE. IONM-Guided Goiter Surgery Leading to Two-Stage Thyroidectomy—Indication and Results. *Langenbeck's Arch Surg* (2013) 398(3):411–8. doi: 10.1007/s00423-012-1032-7
27. Liu C-H, Huang T-Y, Wu C-W, Wang JJ, Wang L-F, Chan L-P, et al. New Developments in Anterior Laryngeal Recording Technique During Neuromonitored Thyroid and Parathyroid Surgery. *Front Endocrinol* (2021) 12. doi: 10.3389/fendo.2021.763170

28. Türk Y, Kıvratma G, Özdemir M, İçöz G, Makay Ö. The Use of Thyroid Cartilage Needle Electrodes in Intraoperative Neuromonitoring During Thyroidectomy: C Ase–Control Study. *Head Neck* (2021) 43(11):3287–93. doi: 10.1002/hed.26810
29. Wu C-W, Chiang F-Y, Randolph GW, Dionigi G, Kim HY, Lin Y-C, et al. Feasibility of Intraoperative Neuromonitoring During Thyroid Surgery Using Transcartilage Surface Recording Electrodes. *Thyroid* (2018) 28(11):1508–16. doi: 10.1089/thy.2017.0680
30. Huang T-Y, Yu W-HV, Chiang F-Y, Wu C-W, Fu S-C, Tai A-S, et al. How the Severity and Mechanism of Recurrent Laryngeal Nerve Dysfunction During Monitored Thyroidectomy Impact on Postoperative Voice. *Cancers* (2021) 13 (21):5379. doi: 10.3390/cancers13215379
31. Huang T-Y, Yu W-HV, Chiang F-Y, Wu C-W, Fu S-C, Tai A-S, et al. Prognostic Indicators of Non-Transection Nerve Injury and Vocal Fold Motion Impairment After Thyroid Surgery–Correlation Between Intraoperative Neuromonitoring Findings and Perioperative Voice Parameters. *Front Endocrinol* (2021) 12. doi: 10.3389/fendo.2021.755231
32. Wu CW, Chai YJ, Dionigi G, Chiang FY, Liu X, Sun H, et al. Recurrent Laryngeal Nerve Safety Parameters of the H Armonic F Ocus During Thyroid Surgery: Porcine Model Using Continuous Monitoring. *Laryngoscope* (2015) 125(12):2838–45. doi: 10.1002/lary.25412
33. Huang TY, Lin YC, Tseng HY, Dionigi G, Kim HY, Chai YJ, et al. Safety Parameters of Ferromagnetic Device During Thyroid Surgery: Porcine Model Using Continuous Neuromonitoring. *Head Neck* (2020) 42(10):2931–40. doi: 10.1002/hed.26334
34. Huang T-Y, Lin Y-C, Tseng H-Y, Dionigi G, Kim H-Y, Lu I-C, et al. Safety of Ligasure Exact Dissector in Thyroidectomy With Continuous Neuromonitoring: A Porcine Model. *Gland Surg* (2020) 9(3):702. doi: 10.21037/gs.2020.03.17
35. Yu X, Liu C, Yan M, Gong W, Wang Y. Hyperthermal Liquid, Spray, and Smog may be Potential Risk Factors for Recurrent Laryngeal Nerve Thermal Injury During Thyroid Surgeries. *Endocrine* (2021) 72(1):198–207. doi: 10.1007/s12020-020-02451-w
36. Lin YC, Dionigi G, Randolph GW, Lu IC, Chang PY, Tsai SY, et al. Electrophysiologic Monitoring Correlates of Recurrent Laryngeal Nerve Heat Thermal Injury in a Porcine Model. *Laryngoscope* (2015) 125(8): E283–E90. doi: 10.1002/lary.25362
37. Seehofer D, Mogl M, Boas-Knoop S, Unger J, Schirmeier A, Chopra S, et al. Safety and Efficacy of New Integrated Bipolar and Ultrasonic Scissors Compared to Conventional Laparoscopic 5-Mm Sealing and Cutting Instruments. *Surg Endosc* (2012) 26(9):2541–9. doi: 10.1007/s00464-012-2229-0

9

Clinical Characteristics-Assisted Risk Stratification for Extent of Thyroidectomy in Patients with 1–4 cm Solitary Intrathyroidal Differentiated Thyroid Cancer

Fang Dong[1†], *Lin Zhou*[1†], *Shuntao Wang*[1], *Jinqian Mao*[2], *Chunping Liu*[1*] and *Wei Shi*[1*]

[1] *Department of Breast and Thyroid Surgery, Union Hospital, Tongji Medical College, Huazhong University of Science and Technology, Wuhan, China,* [2] *Department of Vascular Surgery, Union Hospital of Tongji Medical College, Huazhong University of Science and Technology, Wuhan, China*

Correspondence:
Chunping Liu
liucpwhxh@hust.edu.cn
Wei Shi
shiweihust@163.com

†These authors have contributed equally to this work

Background: Differentiated thyroid cancer (DTC) is the most common type of thyroid cancer. The 2015 American Thyroid Association (ATA) guidelines recommend that lobectomy is suitable for solitary intrathyroidal DTC (SI-DTC) of 1–4 cm. However, some SI-DTC patients with other high-risk characteristics still have poor prognosis and require more aggressive surgical methods. This study aimed to explore the clinical characteristics that are important for the identification and treatment of high-risk patients with SI-DTC of 1–4 cm.

Methods: The study cohort was obtained from the SEER database, consisting of data between 2004 and 2013. The outcome measures were thyroid carcinoma-specific mortality (CSM) and all-cause mortality (ACM). Patient survival curves were examined using Kaplan–Meier analyses with log-rank tests and Cox proportional hazards regression analyses. Hazard ratios (HRs) were used to show the magnitude of the effect of disease stage on DTC-specific patient mortality.

Results: The study included 55,947 patients with SI-DTC of 1–4 cm and 4,765 patients with DTC >4 cm. Tumor size, surgical approach, age, sex, race, and radiation exposure were independent risk factors for CSM and ACM. SI-DTC patients with female, age ≤45, and 1 cm< tumor size ≤2 cm were at low risk of CSM [HR = 0.014 (0.002–0.115)] and ACM [HR = 0.115 (0.077–0.171)] when stratified by age, sex, and tumor size. Compared to T3 patients, CSM was not significantly different in male patients, age >45, 2 cm< tumor size ≤3 cm [HR = 0.839 (0.414–1.700)] and male patients, age >45, 1 cm< tumor size ≤2 cm [HR = 0.751 (0.410–1.377)]. Furthermore, compared to T3 patients without extrathyroidal extension (ETE) and lymph node metastasis (LNM), more subgroups of SI-DTC of 1–4 cm had a similar prognosis. In addition, patients with SI-DTC of 1–4 cm showed similar rates of CSM and ACM to T3 patients without ETE, LNM, and distant metastasis (DM). Similar results were obtained when we set the age cut-off value as 55 years, according to the 8th edition of AJCC TNM system.

Conclusions: Our study demonstrated that sex, age, and tumor size clearly differentiate SI-DTC of 1–4 cm into low-and high-risk categories. Survival rates were significantly lower in subgroups containing old males with larger tumors compared to younger females with small tumors. Total thyroidectomy may be favored in these high-risk subgroup patients.

Keywords: differentiated thyroid cancer, SEER, surgery approaches, tumor size, thyroidectomy

INTRODUCTION

Thyroid cancer is a frequently encountered endocrine malignancy, and differentiated thyroid cancer (DTC), namely, papillary thyroid cancer (PTC) and follicular thyroid cancer (FTC), are the most common types of thyroid cancer, accounting for about 90% of all thyroid malignancies (1–3). DTC is curable and inert with low mortality, but some patients have an aggressive disease course, such as recurrence (4, 5).

Effective risk stratification based on the evaluation of clinicopathological risk features is important for appropriate treatment of DTC patients to balance treatment, such as surgical benefits and complications (6, 7). This can be referenced in the American Thyroid Association's guidelines (6th, 7th, and 8th versions) on the management of DTC (5, 8, 9). The 8th version (2015 American Thyroid Association (ATA) guideline) recommended that lobectomy is suitable for solitary intrathyroidal DTC (SI-DTC: without extrathyroidal invasion, lymph node metastasis, and distant metastasis) of tumor size between 1 and 4 cm and is accepted by most clinicians for the treatment of thyroid cancer.

However, the worldwide impact of this recommendation on the treatment of thyroid cancer remains controversial (10–12). Because other high-risk characteristics in patients with SI-DTC may also affect survival, this subgroup may not be suitable for union surgical strategy. Therefore, in this study, we tried to investigate the high-risk patients among the ST-DTC of 1-4 cm and attempted to provide clues for precision treatment of SI-DTC of 1-4 cm.

MATERIALS AND METHODS

Patient Population

The DTC study cohort was obtained from the Surveillance, Epidemiology, and End Results (SEER) from 18 regions in the United States, consisting of data between 2004 and 2013. The SEER project is a United States population-based cancer registry that began in 1973 and is supported by the National Cancer Institute and the Centers for Disease Control and Prevention. It covers approximately 30% of the population of the United States and contains data across multiple geographic regions on incidence, prevalence, mortality, population-based variables, primary characteristics of the tumor, and other attributes.

Data Collection

Study participants included patients with a diagnosis of DTC, defined by a combination of International Classification of Diseases for Oncology (ICD-O) site code C73.9 (i.e., thyroid) and diagnostic codes of papillary and/or follicular histology. The diagnostic codes used in the study included "papillary carcinoma", "papillary adenocarcinoma", "follicular adenocarcinoma", and "papillary & follicular adenocarcinoma". Patients without follow-up information were excluded from the study.

Statistical Analyses

Patients were followed up until December 2013. The outcome measures were thyroid carcinoma-specific mortality and all-cause mortality. Patient survival curves were examined using Kaplan–Meier analyses with log-rank tests and Cox proportional hazards regression analyses. Hazard ratios (HRs) were used to show the magnitude of the effect of disease stage on DTC-specific patient mortality, and 95% confidence intervals (CIs) were used to indicate the significance of the risk. All *P*-values were 2-sided, and $P < 0.05$ was considered significant. Analyses were performed using SPSS version 19.0, Stata/SE version 12 (Stata Corp), and GraphPad Prism version 6 (GraphPad Software Inc.).

RESULTS

Characteristics for Patients With SI-DTC of 0–4 cm

This study assessed the prognosis of 55,947 patients with SI-DTC with tumor size 1–4 cm and 4,765 patients with DTC with tumor size >4 cm. The mean age and follow-up duration according to the different histological subtypes are shown in **Table 1**. The clinicopathological features of patients with SI-DTC of 0–4 cm were analyzed according to tumor size (**Table 1**). Age at diagnosis, sex, race, radiation, multifocality, and surgical approaches all showed significant differences among the different tumor size groups.

Risk Factors for Cancer-Specific and All-Cause Mortality

The results of the univariate Cox regression analyses demonstrated that cancer-specific mortality was associated with age, sex, race, tumor size, and treatment approaches (radiation and surgery). Furthermore, all-cause mortality was also found to be associated with age, sex, race, radiation, and surgery. Meanwhile, the multivariate Cox regression model showed that tumor size, surgical approach, age, sex, race, and radiation were independent risk factors for cancer-specific mortality and all-cause mortality (**Table 2**).

TABLE 1 | Charectaristic for patients with EXE (−), N0, M0, tumor size 0–4 cm.

Covariate	Level	0–1 cm	1–2 cm	2–3 cm	3–4 cm	p-value
Age*		51.44 ± 13.75	48.81 ± 14.54	47.74 ± 15.43	47.77 ± 15.99	<0.001
sex	female	24,000 (83.1%)	12,643 (80.9%)	5,893 (77.7%)	2,823 (73.1%)	<0.001
	male	4,879 (16.9%)	2,979 (19.1%)	1,691 (22.3%)	1,039 (26.9%)	
race	white	24,306 (84.2%)	13,106 (83.9%)	6,219 (82.0%)	3,109 (80.5%)	<0.001
	black	2,023 (7.0%)	941 (6.0%)	588 (7.8%)	380 (9.8%)	
	other	2,550 (8.8%)	1,575 (10.1%)	777 (10.2%)	373 (9.7%)	
radiation	none of refused	22,509 (77.9%)	6,948 (44.5%)	2,820 (37.2%)	1,381 (35.8%)	<0.001
	radiation	6,370 (22.1%)	8,674 (55.5%)	4,764 (62.8%)	2,481 (64.2%)	
multifocality	no	19,763 (68.4%)	9,218 (59.0%)	4,774 (62.9%)	2,556 (66.2%)	<0.001
	yes	9,116 (31.6%)	6,404 (41.0%)	2,810 (37.1%)	1,306 (33.8%)	
surgery	lobectomy	7,306 (25.3%)	1,638(10.5%)	991 (13.1%)	579 (15.0%)	<0.001
	subtotal or near total	1,349 (4.7%)	548 (3.5%)	300 (4.0%)	169 (4.4%)	
	total	20,224 (70.0%)	13,436 (86.0%)	6,293 (83.0%)	3,114 (80.6%)	
survival months		48.71 ± 33.22	51.11 ± 33.83	52.40 ± 34.29	52.53 ± 34.29	<0.001

Age at diagnosis.

TABLE 2 | Risk factors for survival: Outcome of thyroid cancer specific mortality and all-cause mortality.

Covariate	Level	Thyroid cancer specific mortality				All-cause mortality			
		Univariate cox regression		Multivariate Cox regression		Univariate Cox regression		Multivariate Cox regression	
		Hazard Ratio (95%CI)	p-value	Hazard Ratio (95%CI)	p-value	Hazard Ratio (95%CI)	p-value	Hazard Ratio (95%CI)	p-value
age at diagnosis		1.096 (1.079–1.114)	<0.001	1.099 (1.081–1.116)	<0.001	1.083 (1.079–1.087)	<0.001	1.081 (1.077–1.085)	<0.001
sex	female	ref		ref		ref		ref	
	male	2.770 (1.845–4.159)	<0.001	1.900 (1.261–2.862)	0.002	2.200 (1.994–2.427)	<0.001	1.680 (1.521–1.856)	<0.001
race	white	ref		ref		ref		Ref	
	black	0.447 (0.150–1.509)	0.208	0.570 (0.180–1.810)	0.341	1.304 (1.106–1.538)	0.002	1.467 (1.243–1.731)	<0.001
	other	1.876 (1.096–3.211)	0.022	2.130 (1.242–3.651)	0.006	0.722 (0.598–0.872)	<0.001	0.871 (0.721–1.051)	0.149
tumor size	0–1 cm	ref		ref		ref		ref	
	1–2 cm	1.476 (0.876–2.486)	0.143	1.170 (0.680–2.014)	0.571	0.897 (0.802–1.002)	0.055	1.085 (0.965–1.219)	0.172
	2–3 cm	2.966 (1.761–4.996)	<0.001	2.217 (1.279–3.843)	0.005	0.993 (0.865–1.140)	0.921	1.195 (1.035–1.380)	0.015
	3–4 cm	3.352 (1.809–6.210)	<0.001	2.171 (1.137–4.148)	0.019	1.074 (0.901–1.281)	0.426	1.160 (0.967–1.392)	0.109
multifocality	No	ref		ref		ref		ref	
	yes	1.200 (0.795–1.810)	0.386	0.886 (0.584–1.345)	0.569	0.938 (0.850–1.035)	0.205	0.982 (0.888–1.087)	0.732
radiation	none of refused	ref		ref		ref		ref	
	radiation	2.371 (1.568–3.586)	<0.001	2.185 (1.377–3.466)	<0.001	0.683 (0.620–0.753)	<0.001	0.827 (0.741–0.923)	0.001
surgery	lobectomy	ref		ref		ref		ref	
	subtotal or near total	2.118 (0.710–6.321)	0.179	1.976 (0.657–5.947)	0.226	0.904 (0.727–1.125)	0.366	1.023 (0.821–1.274)	0.838
	total	2.381 (1.197–4.735)	0.013	1.983 (0.969–4.056)	0.061	0.788 (0.705–0.880)	<0.001	0.987 (0.877–1.109)	0.822

Subgroups Analysis With High-Risk Mortality

When three common clinical factors, age, sex, and tumor size, were included to select the high-risk mortality of SI-DTC, we found that compared to patients with male sex, age >45 years, and 3 cm< tumor size ≤4 cm, female patients with 1 cm <tumor size ≤3 cm aged ≤45 years, female patients with 0< tumor size ≤3 cm aged >45 years, and male patients with 0< tumor size ≤2 cm aged >45 years were at a lower risk of cancer-specific mortality (**Table 3**).

Moreover, age ≤45 years was a low-risk factor for all-cause mortality in all patients regardless of sex or tumor size when compared to male patients with age >45 years old and 3 cm< tumor size ≤4 cm. For patients aged >45 years, female sex and 0< tumor size ≤3 cm were low-risk factors for all-cause mortality (**Table 3**).

Comparison Between SI-DTC With T3 Patients

When T3 patients were included for comparison, we found that the cancer-specific mortality showed no significant difference between T3 patients, SI-DTC patients with male sex, age >45 years, and 2 cm< tumor size ≤3 cm (HR: 0.839, 95%CI: 0.414–1.700), and SI-DTC patients with male sex, age >45 years, and 1 cm< tumor size ≤2 cm (HR: 0.751, 95%CI: 0.410–1.377). Similar results were obtained for all-cause mortality (**Table 4** and **Figure 1**).

Furthermore, when we selected T3 patients with tumor size >4 cm and excluded T3 patients without ETE and LNM for reference, we found that more subgroups of SI-DTC with a tumor size of 1–4 cm had a similar prognosis (cancer-specific mortality) with T3 patients having a tumor size >4 cm. Similar results were obtained for all-cause mortality (**Table 5** and **Figure 2**).

TABLE 3 | Age, sex, tumor size factors for survival: outcome of thyroid cancer specific mortality and all-cause mortality.

Covariate	Level	Thyroid cancer specific mortality		All-cause mortality	
		Univariate Cox regression		Univariate Cox regression	
		Hazard Ratio (95%CI)	p-value	Hazard Ratio (95%CI)	p-value
0		ref		ref	
1		0.014 (0.002–0.115)	<0.001	0.115 (0.077–0.171)	<0.001
2		0.084 (0.022–0.318)	<0.001	0.098 (0.059–0.164)	<0.001
3			0.971	0.068 (0.031–0.150)	<0.001
4			0.975	0.159 (0.084–0.299)	<0.001
5			0.976	0.173 (0.092–0.326)	<0.001
6			0.981	0.217 (0.110–0.429)	<0.001
7			0.985	0.289 (0.137–0.611)	0.001
8		0.120 (0.053–0.272)	<0.001	0.593 (0.442–0.796)	0.001
9		0.217 (0.094–0.502)	<0.001	0.559 (0.411–0.760)	<0.001
10		0.342 (0.140–0.838)	0.019	0.640 (0.460–0.890)	0.008
11		0.427 (0.155–1.177)	0.1	0.817 (0.571–1.169)	0.269
12		0.275 (0.111–0.684)	0.005	1.116 (0.821–1.518)	0.484
13		0.363 (0.136–0.967)	0.043	1.137 (0.821–1.574)	0.441
14		0.910 (0.366–2.264)	0.84	1.310 (0.925–1.855)	0.128
15			0.93	0.086 (0.058–0.128)	<0.001

Ref: age >45 years old, Male, 3< tumor size ≤4 cm.
1: age ≤45 years old, Female, 1< tumor size ≤2 cm.
2: age ≤45 years old, Female, 2< tumor size ≤3 cm.
3: age ≤45 years old, Female, 3< tumor size ≤4 cm.
4: age ≤45 years old, Male, 0< tumor size ≤1 cm.
5: age ≤45 years old, Male, 1< tumor size ≤2 cm.
6: age ≤45 years old, Male, 2< tumor size ≤3 cm.
7: age ≤45 years old, Male, 3< tumor size ≤4 cm.
8: age >45 years old, Female, 0< tumor size ≤1 cm.
9: age >45 years old, Female, 1< tumor size ≤2 cm.
10: age >45 years old, Female, 2< tumor size ≤3 cm.
11: age >45 years old, Female, 3< tumor size ≤4 cm.
12: age >45 years old, Male, 0< tumor size ≤1 cm.
13: age >45 years old, Male, 1< tumor size ≤2 cm.
14: age >45 years old, Male, 2< tumor size ≤3 cm.
15: age ≤45 years old, Female, 0< tumor size ≤1 cm.

In addition, when we selected T3 patients without ETE, LNM, and DM as references, we found that more subgroups and patients with SI-DTC with a tumor size of 1–4 cm showed similar rates of cancer-specific mortality and all-cause mortality (**Table 6** and **Figure 3**). Similar results were obtained when we set the age cut-off value as 55 years according to the 8th edition of the American Joint Committee on Cancer (AJCC) Tumor, Node, Metastasis (TNM) system (13) (**Tables S1–S3** and **Figures S1–S3**).

DISCUSSION

The current trend in the management of DTC has become more conservative. Unilateral lobectomy is now suggested as a viable alternative to total thyroidectomy for patients with SI-DTC 1–4 cm in size based on the ATA 2015 guidelines (4). Although overall prognosis seems to be excellent after lobectomy, some patients that appear to be at low risk, in fact, have high intrinsic risk for poor prognosis and should benefit from an aggressive treatment. Even in papillary thyroid microcarcinoma, cases evaluated as having a low risk of recurrence preoperatively showed intermediate to high-risk disease post-surgery, leading to a higher rate of radioiodine therapy (14).

Lobectomy for low-risk SI-DTC can be beneficial for thyroid function preservation and decreased risk of surgical complications, such as postoperative hypoparathyroidism and recurrent laryngeal nerve injury, according to many reports (15, 16). Despite these advantages, total thyroidectomy is generally accepted for SI-DTC because total thyroidectomy can provide convenience for the use of radioactive iodine in surveillance and postoperative treatment (4). It is easier to detect recurrence early *via* follow-up and dynamically monitoring serum thyroglobulin levels. In addition, Benjamin et al. reported that nearly half of low-risk DTC patients were found to have tumors in the contralateral lobe and may be more adequate for total thyroidectomy (17).

This study suggested that there were still some patients with high-risk prognosis among the SI-DTC with 1–4 cm, and selecting low-risk patients based on ETE, LNM, and DM was not precise. Our results provided some estimate for this possible need for completion of a total thyroidectomy after an initial lobectomy for these otherwise low-risk patients and can provide a future guide for the precision treatment for patients with SI-DTC of 1–4 cm.

In addition, some patients who underwent lobectomy may be reclassified as intermediate or high risk after surgery based on the

TABLE 4 | Analysis of si-DTC patients and patients with total T3 (ETE+, N1, M1).

Covariate	Level	Thyroid cancer specific mortality		All-cause mortality	
		Univariate Cox regression		Univariate Cox regression	
		Hazard Ratio (95%CI)	**p-value**	**Hazard Ratio (95%CI)**	**p-value**
0		ref		ref	
1		0.012 (0.002–0.086)	<0.001	0.150 (0.112–0.200)	<0.001
2		0.071 (0.023–0.221)	<0.001	0.128 (0.083–0.197)	<0.001
3		0		0.088 (0.042–0.186)	<0.001
4		0		0.206 (0.117–0.365)	<0.001
5		0		0.226 (0.128–0.399)	<0.001
6		0		0.284 (0.152–0.529)	<0.001
7		0		0.377 (0.188–0.756)	0.006
8		0.099 (0.063–0.157)	<0.001	0.770 (0.692–0.856)	<0.001
9		0.180 (0.110–0.295)	<0.001	0.726 (0.631–0.834)	<0.001
10		0.285 (0.160–0.510)	<0.001	0.832 (0.693–0.999)	0.049
11		0.355 (0.167–0.754)	0.007	1.063 (0.844–1.337)	0.604
12		0.228 (0.124–0.418)	<0.001	1.448 (1.260–1.664)	<0.001
13		0.301 (0.148–0.609)	0.001	1.475 (1.238–1.757)	<0.001
14		0.751 (0.410–1.377)	0.354	1.699 (1.372–2.103)	<0.001
15		0.839 (0.414–1.700)	0.627	1.311 (0.980–1.755)	0.068
16		0		0.112 (0.084–0.149)	<0.001

Ref: total T3 (includes M1, N1, ETE+).
1: age ≤45 years old, Female, 0< tumor size ≤1 cm.
2: age ≤45 years old, Female, 1< tumor size ≤2 cm.
3: age ≤45 years old, Female, 2< tumor size ≤3 cm.
4: age ≤45 years old, Female, 3< tumor size ≤4 cm.
5: age ≤45 years old, Male, 0< tumor size ≤1 cm.
6: age ≤45 years old, Male, 1< tumor size ≤2 cm.
7: age ≤45 years old, Male, 2< tumor size ≤3 cm.
8: age ≤45 years old, Male, 3< tumor size ≤4 cm.
9: age >45 years old, Female, 0< tumor size ≤1 cm.
10: age >45 years old, Female, 1 <tumor size ≤2 cm.
11: age >45 years old, Female, 2< tumor size ≤3 cm.
12: age >45 years old, Female, 3< tumor size ≤4 cm.
13: age >45 years old, Male, 0< tumor size ≤1 cm.
14: age >45 years old, Male, 1< tumor size ≤2 cm.
15: age >45 years old, Male, 2< tumor size ≤3 cm.
16: age >45 years old, Male, 3< tumor size ≤4 cm.

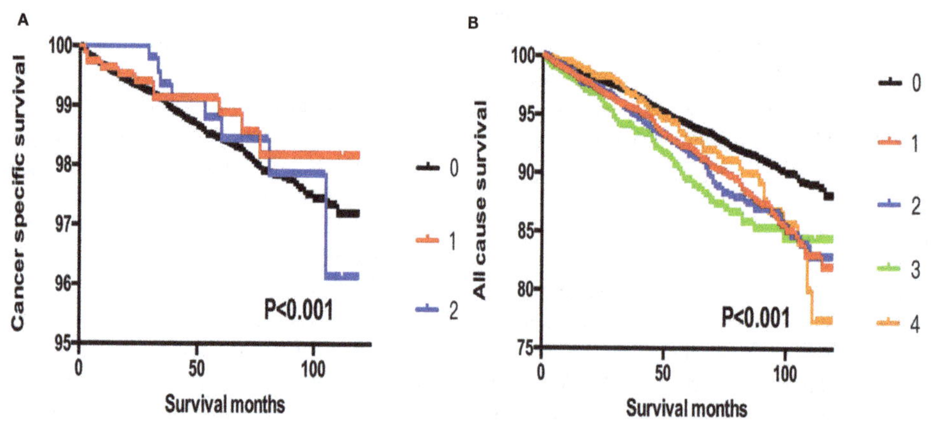

FIGURE 1 | **(A)** Kaplan-Meier curves among patients stratified by tumor size for cancer-specific mortality (Log rank test, p < 0.001). 0 For patients with thyroid cancer > 4 cm in size, gross extrathyroidal extension (clinical T3), or clinically apparent metastatic disease to nodes (clinical N1) or distant sites (clinical M1). 1 Male, > 45 years old, tumor size 2-3 cm. 2 Male, > 45 years old, tumor size 3-4 cm. **(B)** Kaplan-Meier curves among patients stratified by tumor size for all-cause mortality (Log rank test, p < 0.001). 0 For patients with thyroid cancer> 4 cm, gross extrathyroidal extension (clinical T3), or clinically apparent metastatic disease to nodes (clinical N1) or distant sites (clinical M1). 1 Male, > 45 years old, tumor size 0-1 cm. 2 Male, > 45 years old, tumor size 1-2 cm. 3 Male, > 45 years old, tumor size 2-3 cm. 4 Male, > 45 years old, tumor size 3-4 cm.

TABLE 5 | Age, T3 and sex, tumor size factors for survival: outcome of thyroid cancer specific mortality and all-cause mortality.

Covariate	Level	Thyroid cancer specific mortality			All-cause mortality		
		Univariate Cox regression			Univariate Cox regression		
		Hazard Ratio (95%CI)	p-value	Mortality (%)	Hazard Ratio (95%CI)	p-value	Mortality (%)
0		ref			ref		
1		0.019 (0.003–0.136)	<0.001	0.02	0.135 (0.099–0.184)	<0.001	0.85
2		0.110 (0.034–0.354)	<0.001	0.1	0.115 (0.074–0.180)	<0.001	0.72
3			0.967		0.080 (0.038–0.169)	<0.001	0.5
4			0.971		0.187 (0.105–0.333)	<0.001	1.05
5			0.973		0.204 (0.114–0.363)	<0.001	1.27
6			0.978		0.256 (0.136–0.481)	<0.001	1.68
7			0.983		0.340 (0.168–0.687)	0.003	2.17
8		0.154 (0.090–0.262)	<0.001	0.13	0.696 (0.603–0.805)	<0.001	3.82
9		0.279 (0.159–0.491)	<0.001	0.24	0.656 (0.553–0.778)	<0.001	3.73
10		0.442 (0.233–0.842)	0.013	0.4	0.752 (0.611–0.925)	0.007	4.5
11		0.551 (0.247–1.228)	0.145	0.5	0.960 (0.748–1.233)	0.752	5.66
12		0.353 (0.181–0.687)	0.002	0.29	1.310 (1.105–1.553)	0.002	7.07
13		0.466 (0.219–0.994)	0.048	0.39	1.334 (1.091–1.631)	0.005	7.29
14		1.166 (0.599–2.269	0.651	1	1.538 (1.216–1.945)	<0.001	8.57
15		1.301 (0.610–2.776)	0.496	1.19	1.185 (0.872–1.611)	0.279	7.15
16			0.92		0.101 (0.075–0.136)	<0.001	0.59

Ref: T3, with EXE(–), N0.
1: age ≤45 years old, Female, 0< tumor size ≤1 cm.
2: age ≤45 years old, Female, 1< tumor size ≤2 cm.
3: age ≤45 years old, Female, 2< tumor size ≤3 cm.
4: age ≤45 years old, Female, 3< tumor size ≤4 cm.
5: age ≤45 years old, Male, 0< tumor size ≤1 cm.
6: age ≤45 years old, Male, 1< tumor size ≤2 cm.
7: age ≤45 years old, Male, 2< tumor size ≤3 cm.
8: age ≤45 years old, Male, 3< tumor size ≤4 cm.
9: age >45 years old, Female, 0< tumor size ≤1 cm.
10: age >45 years old, Female, 1< tumor size ≤2 cm.
11: age >45 years old, Female, 2< tumor size ≤3 cm.
12: age >45 years old, Female, 3< tumor size ≤4 cm.
13: age >45 years old, Male, 0< tumor size ≤1 cm.
14: age >45 years old, Male, 1< tumor size ≤2 cm.
15: age >45 years old, Male, 2< tumor size ≤3 cm.
16: age >45 years old, Male, 3< tumor size ≤4 cm.

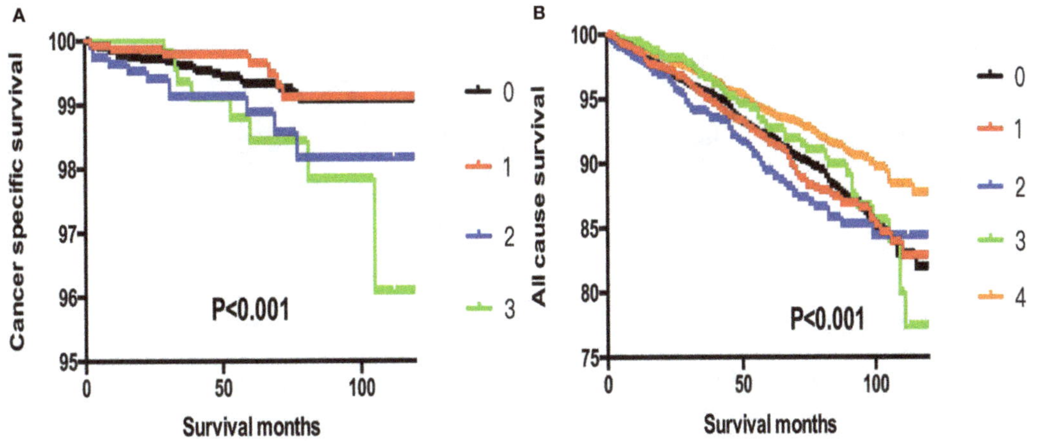

FIGURE 2 | (A) Kaplan-Meier curves among patients stratified by tumor size for cancer-specific mortality (Log rank test, $p < 0.001$). 0 For patients with thyroid cancer>4 cm and without gross extrathyroidal extension (clinical T3) and no clinically apparent metastatic disease to nodes (clinical N0) or distant sites (clinical M0). 1 Male, > 45 years old, tumor size 1-2 cm. 2 Male, > 45 years old, tumor size 2-3 cm. 3 Male, > 45 years old, tumor size 3-4 cm. **(B)** Kaplan-Meier curves among patients stratified by tumor size for all-cause mortality (Log rank test, $p < 0.001$). 0 For patients with thyroid cancer>4 cm and without gross extrathyroidal extension (clinical T3) and no clinically apparent metastatic disease to nodes (clinical N0) or distant sites (clinical M0). 1 Male, > 45 years old, tumor size 0-1 cm. 2 Male, > 45 years old, tumor size 1-2 cm. 3 Male, > 45 years old, tumor size 2-3 cm. 4 Male, > 45 years old, tumor size 3-4 cm.

TABLE 6 | Analysis of SI-DTC and T3 (ETE–, N0, M0) subgroup.

Covariate	Level	Thyroid cancer specific mortality		All-cause mortality	
		Univariate Cox regression		Univariate Cox regression	
		Hazard Ratio (95%CI)	p-value	Hazard Ratio (95%CI)	p-value
0		Ref		ref	
1		0.029 (0.004–0.217)	0.001	0.148 (0.108–0.201)	<0.001
2		0.172 (0.052–0.571)	0.004	0.126 (0.081–0.197)	<0.001
3				0.087 (0.041–0.185)	<0.001
4				0.204 (0.114–0.365)	<0.001
5				0.223 (0.125–0.398)	<0.001
6				0.279 (0.148–0.526)	<0.001
7				0.372 (0.184–0.752)	0.006
8		0.243 (0.135–0.437)	<0.001	0.762 (0.655–0.886)	<0.001
9		0.440 (0.238–0.816)	0.009	0.718 (0.602–0.856)	<0.001
10		0.697 (0.350–1.388)	0.305	0.822 (0.665–1.016)	0.07
11		0.868 (0.376-2.008)	0.741	1.050 (0.815–1.353)	0.705
12		0.558 (0.274–1.134)	0.107	1.433 (1.203–1.709)	<0.001
13		0.736 (0.332–1.633)	0.451	1.460 (1.188–1.793)	<0.001
14		1.844 (0.907–3.747)	0.091	1.682 (1.324–2.136)	<0.001
15		2.051 (0.925–4.548)	0.077	1.296 (0.950–1.767)	0.102
16				0.111 (0.082–0.150)	<0.001

Ref: T3, with EXE(–), N0, M0.
1: age ≤45 years old, Female, 0< tumor size ≤1 cm.
2: age ≤45 years old, Female, 1< tumor size ≤2 cm.
3: age ≤45 years old, Female, 2< tumor size ≤3 cm.
4: age ≤45 years old, Female, 3< tumor size ≤4 cm.
5: age ≤45 years old, Male, 0< tumor size ≤1 cm.
6: age ≤45 years old, Male, 1< tumor size ≤2 cm.
7: age ≤45 years old, Male, 2< tumor size ≤3 cm.
8: age ≤45 years old, Male, 3< tumor size ≤4 cm.
9: age >45 years old, Female, 0< tumor size ≤1 cm.
10: age >45 years old, Female, 1< tumor size ≤2 cm.
11: age >45 years old, Female, 2< tumor size ≤3 cm.
12: age >45 years old, Female, 3< tumor size ≤4 cm.
13: age >45 years old, Male, 0< tumor size ≤1 cm.
14: age >45 years old, Male, 1< tumor size ≤2 cm.
15: age >45 years old, Male, 2< tumor size ≤ 3cm.
16: age >45 years old, Male, 3< tumor size ≤ 4cm.

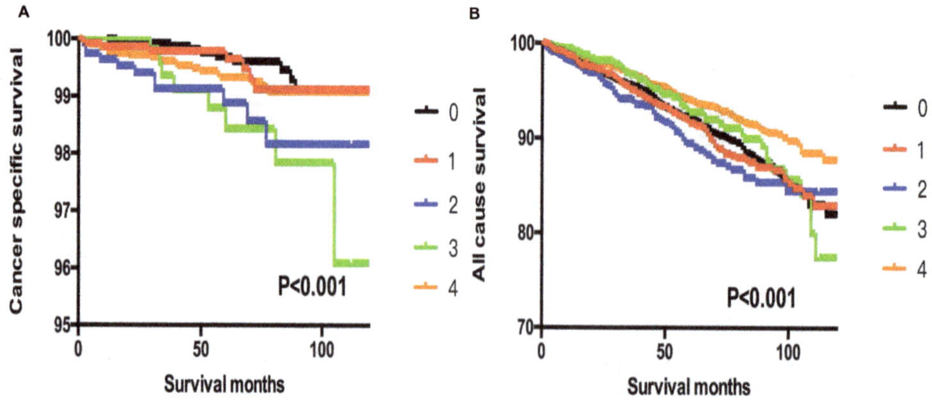

FIGURE 3 | (A) Kaplan-Meier curves among patients stratified by tumor size for cancer-specific mortality (Log rank test, p < 0.001). 0 For patients with thyroid cancer>4 cm and without gross extrathyroidal extension (clinical T3) and no clinically apparent metastatic disease to nodes (clinical N0) and no distant sites (clinical M0). 1 Male, > 45 years old, tumor size 0-1 cm. 2 Male, > 45 years old, tumor size 1-2 cm. 3 Male, > 45 years old, tumor size 2-3 cm. 4 Male, > 45 years old, tumor size 3-4 cm. **(B)** Kaplan-Meier curves among patients stratified by tumor size for all-cause mortality (Log rank test, p < 0.001). 0 For patients with thyroid cancer>4 cm and without gross extrathyroidal extension (clinical T3) and no clinically apparent metastatic disease to nodes (clinical N0) and no distant sites (clinical M0). 1 Male, > 45 years old, tumor size 0-1 cm. 2 Male, > 45 years old, tumor size 1-2 cm. 3 Male, > 45 years old, tumor size 2-3 cm. 4 Male, > 45 years old, tumor size 3-4 cm.

histological findings, and Pedro et al. suggested that total thyroidectomy might be a better option for these patients (13). Previous retrospective studies have estimated that 40–60% of patients with low-risk 1-4 cm PTCs, if initially treated with lobectomy, would require a completion thyroidectomy due to high-risk pathological features in postoperative pathology reports (18, 19). These results underscore the importance of preoperative and intraoperative meticulous assessments by the surgeon during lobectomy for SI-PTCs.

Recently, Huang et al. (20) revealed that in tumors larger than 2.0 to 3.0 cm, recurrences of BRAF V600E mutation-positive SI-PTC were comparable with those of counterpart invasive solitary PTC and need more aggressive treatment. However, these adverse features are only apparent on histopathology and cannot be identified preoperatively. If a lobectomy has been performed, a completion thyroidectomy may be required, which may be associated with certain additional risks. It is essential to know the prevalence of these adverse pathological features to enable surgical planning and patient counseling. A recent study stated that for low-risk PTC patients, identification of intraoperative risk factors such as evidence or suspicion of invasion into local structures (namely, muscle, recurrent laryngeal nerve, esophagus, trachea, or other structures) or positive lymph nodes confirmed on intraoperative frozen section analysis can reduce the need for a later completion thyroidectomy in 21% of cases, but not exclude this need completely. Up to 30% of patients would be deemed intermediate or high risk, requiring a second operation (21). Thus, further studies are needed on preoperative risk stratification.

In this study, we included more clinicopathological factors (age, sex, and tumor size) for analysis to evaluate the reclassification of SI-DTC. Considering that age and sex are easily available preoperatively, including these characteristics for analysis may be more reasonable to select high-risk patients with SI-DTC and reconsider the treatment approaches. We found that survival rates were significantly lower in patients with male sex, age >45 years, and larger tumor size when compared to female patients with age ≤45 years and smaller tumor size, indicating that the former group have a poor prognosis and may require a more radical treatment plan. Our findings are consistent with the role of tumor size in the aggressiveness of PTC. Given that cancer-specific mortality occurred frequently in patients with 3-4 cm in size compared to other subgroups, a close preoperative and intraoperative evaluation of tumor size is important in SI-DTC patients.

A common clinical scenario for SI-DTC with 1–4 cm tumor size is that preoperative ultrasonography does not show suspicious LNM and extrathyroidal extension, as preoperative ultrasonography has a limited sensitivity in detecting central LNM; therefore, many patients with SI-DTC may have occult LNM and ETE, which can synergize with other high-risk characteristics, such as male sex and old age, in promoting DTC mortality. If such patients are treated by lobectomy without neck dissection and radioiodine ablation, the mortality risk could be higher. The present study found that the prognosis of SI-DTC was affected by other clinicopathological characteristics such as sex, age, and tumor size; thus, lobectomy for SI-DTC regardless of the specific clinical status seems to be unreasonable.

Some inherent limitations must be considered when interpreting our results. First, all the risk characteristics included clinicopathological features from the SEER database, but other factors such as ultrasonic data, molecular mutations, vascular invasion, and family history were not obtained nor included in our analysis. Second, data regarding recurrence are not captured in the SEER database, and the designation of cancer-specific death is susceptible to overestimation bias, particularly for diseases such as DTC. Furthermore, given the generally favorable prognosis of PTC, the relatively short study period and follow-up period (2010–2013) is a limitation of our analysis.

Conclusion

Our study demonstrated that sex, age, and tumor size clearly differentiate SI-DTC with a tumor size of 1–4 cm into low and high risk categories. Survival rates were significantly lower in subgroups containing males, older patients, and patients with larger tumor size compared to females, younger patients, and patients with smaller tumor size. Therefore, total thyroidectomy may be favored for these high-risk subgroup patients, and more clinicopathological factors should be included for risk stratification in managing patients with SI-DTC with tumors that are 1–4 cm in size.

AUTHOR CONTRIBUTIONS

SW, LZ, FD, and CL designed the study. FD, LZ, WS, and JM collected and analyzed the data. FD and LZ wrote the manuscript. All authors contributed to the article and approved the submitted version.

ACKNOWLEDGMENTS

All authors are grateful to all subjects who participated in this study.

REFERENCES

1. Chen W, Zheng R, Baade PD, Zhang S, Zeng H, Bray F, et al. Cancer Statistics in China, 2015. *CA Cancer J Clin* (2016) 66(2):115–32. doi: 10.3322/caac.21338
2. Davies L, Hoang JK. Thyroid Cancer in the USA: Current Trends and Outstanding Questions. *Lancet Diabetes Endocrinol* (2021) 9(1):11–2. doi: 10.1016/S2213-8587(20)30372-7
3. Liu C, Chen T, Zeng W, Wang S, Xiong Y, Liu Z, et al. Reevaluating the Prognostic Significance of Male Gender for Papillary Thyroid Carcinoma and Microcarcinoma: A SEER Database Analysis. *Sci Rep* (2017) 7(1):11412. doi: 10.1038/s41598-017-11788-8
4. Liu C, Wang S, Zeng W, Guo Y, Liu Z, Huang T. Total Tumour Diameter is Superior to Unifocal Diameter as a Predictor of Papillary Thyroid Microcarcinoma Prognosis. *Sci Rep* (2017) 7(1):1846. doi: 10.1038/s41598-017-02165-6
5. Haugen BR, Alexander EK, Bible KC, Doherty GM, Mandel SJ, Nikiforov YE, et al. 2015 American Thyroid Association Management Guidelines for Adult

Patients With Thyroid Nodules and Differentiated Thyroid Cancer: The American Thyroid Association Guidelines Task Force on Thyroid Nodules and Differentiated Thyroid Cancer. *Thyroid* (2016) 26(1):1–133. doi: 10.1089/thy.2015.0020

6. Zhang F, Zheng B, Yu X, Wang X, Wang S, Teng W. Risk Factors for Contralateral Occult Carcinoma in Patients With Unilateral Papillary Thyroid Carcinoma: A Retrospective Study and Meta-Analysis. *Front Endocrinol (Lausanne)* (2021) 12:675643. doi: 10.3389/fendo.2021.675643
7. Luo H, Yan F, Lan L, Ma B, Zhao H, He Y, et al. Ultrasonographic Features, Nodule Size, Capsular Invasion, and Lymph Node Metastasis of Solitary Papillary Carcinoma of Thyroid Isthmus. *Front Oncol* (2020) 10:558363. doi: 10.3389/fonc.2020.558363
8. Tran CH, Johnston LE, Chang DC, Bouvet M. A Critical Analysis of the American Joint Committee on Cancer (AJCC) Staging System for Differentiated Thyroid Carcinoma in Young Patients on the Basis of the Surveillance, Epidemiology, and End Results (SEER) Registry. *Surgery* (2012) 152(2):145–51. doi: 10.1016/j.surg.2012.02.015
9. Perrier ND, Brierley JD, Tuttle RM. Differentiated and Anaplastic Thyroid Carcinoma: Major Changes in the American Joint Committee on Cancer Eighth Edition Cancer Staging Manual. *CA Cancer J Clin* (2018) 68(1):55–63. doi: 10.3322/caac.21439
10. Liu W, Yan X, Cheng R. Continuing Controversy Regarding Individualized Surgical Decision-Making for Patients With 1-4 Cm Low-Risk Differentiated Thyroid Carcinoma: A Systematic Review. *Eur J Surg Oncol* (2020) 46 (12):2174–84. doi: 10.1016/j.ejso.2020.08.014
11. Xu Y, Huang K, Huang P, Ke N, Zeng J, Wang L, et al. Benefits and Harms of Hemithyroidectomy, Total or Near-Total Thyroidectomy in 1-4 Cm Differentiated Thyroid Cancer. *Clin Endocrinol (Oxf)* (2021) 95(4):668–76. doi: 10.1111/cen.14495
12. Wang X, Zhang C, Srivastava A, Yu W, Liu C, Wei D, et al. Risk Factors That Influence Surgical Decision-Making for Patients With Low-Risk Differentiated Thyroid Cancer With Tumor Diameters of 1-4 Cm. *Cancer Manag Res* (2020) 12:12423–8. doi: 10.2147/CMAR.S268716
13. Schmid KW, Synoracki S, Dralle H, Wittekind C. Proposal for an Extended pTNM Classification of Thyroid Carcinoma: Commentary on Deficits of the 8th Edition of the TNM Classification. *Pathologe* (2019) 40(Suppl 1):18–24. doi: 10.1007/s00292-018-0418-x
14. Gao R, Jia X, Liang Y, Fan K, Wang X, Wang Y, et al. Papillary Thyroid Micro Carcinoma: The Incidence of High-Risk Features and Its Prognostic Implications. *Front Endocrinol (Lausanne)* (2019) 10:74. doi: 10.3389/fendo.2019.00074
15. Liang J, Li Z, Fang F, Yu T, Li S. Is Prophylactic Central Neck Dissection Necessary for Cn0 Differentiated Thyroid Cancer Patients at Initial Treatment? A Meta-Analysis of the Literature. *Acta Otorhinolaryngol Ital* (2017) 37(1):1–8. doi: 10.14639/0392-100X-1195
16. McMullen C, Rocke D, Freeman J. Complications of Bilateral Neck Dissection in Thyroid Cancer From a Single High-Volume Center. *JAMA Otolaryngol Head Neck Surg* (2017) 143(4):376–81. doi: 10.1001/jamaoto.2016.3670
17. Papachristos AJ, Glover A, Sywak MS, Sidhu SB. Pros and Cons of Hemi-Thyroidectomy for Low-Risk Differentiated Thyroid Cancer. *ANZ J Surg* (2021) 91(9):1704–10. doi: 10.1111/ans.16553
18. Murthy SP, Balasubramanian D, Subramaniam N, Nair G, Babu M, Rathod PV, et al. Prevalence of Adverse Pathological Features in 1 to 4 Cm Low-Risk Differentiated Thyroid Carcinoma. *Head Neck* (2018) 40(6):1214–8. doi: 10.1002/hed.25099
19. DiMarco AN, Wong MS, Jayasekara J, Cole-Clark D, Aniss A, Glover AR, et al. Risk of Needing Completion Thyroidectomy for Low-Risk Papillary Thyroid Cancers Treated by Lobectomy. *BJS Open* (2019) 3(3):299–304. doi: 10.1002/bjs5.50137
20. Huang Y, Qu S, Zhu G, Wang F, Liu R, Shen X, et al. BRAF V600E Mutation-Assisted Risk Stratification of Solitary Intrathyroidal Papillary Thyroid Cancer for Precision Treatment. *J Natl Cancer Inst* (2018) 110(4):362–70. doi: 10.1093/jnci/djx227
21. Craig SJ, Bysice AM, Nakoneshny SC, Pasieka JL, Chandarana SP. The Identification of Intraoperative Risk Factors Can Reduce, But Not Exclude, the Need for Completion Thyroidectomy in Low-Risk Papillary Thyroid Cancer Patients. *Thyroid* (2020) 30(2):222–8. doi: 10.1089/thy.2019.0274

10

A Clinical Predictive Model of Central Lymph Node Metastases in Papillary Thyroid Carcinoma

Zipeng Wang[1†], Qungang Chang[1†], Hanyin Zhang[2], Gongbo Du[1], Shuo Li[1], Yihao Liu[1], Hanlin Sun[1] and Detao Yin[1,3,4]*

[1] Department of Thyroid Surgery, The First Affiliated Hospital of Zhengzhou University, Zhengzhou, China, [2] Department of Dermatology, First Affiliated Hospital of Zhengzhou University, Zhengzhou, China, [3] Engineering Research Center of Multidisciplinary Diagnosis and Treatment of Thyroid Cancer of Henan Province, Zhengzhou, China, [4] Key Medicine Laboratory of Thyroid Cancer of Henan Province, Zhengzhou, China

***Correspondence:**
Detao Yin
detaoyin@zzu.edu.cn

†These authors have contributed equally to this work and share first authorship

Background: Thyroid carcinoma is one of the most common endocrine tumors, and papillary thyroid carcinoma (PTC) is the most common pathological type. Current studies have reported that PTC has a strong propensity for central lymph node metastases (CLNMs). Whether to prophylactically dissect the central lymph nodes in PTC remains controversial. This study aimed to explore the risk factors and develop a predictive model of CLNM in PTC.

Methods: A total of 2,554 patients were enrolled in this study. The basic information, laboratory examination, characteristics of cervical ultrasound, genetic test, and pathological diagnosis were collected. The collected data were analyzed by univariate logistic analysis and multivariate logistic analysis. The risk factors were evaluated, and the predictive model was constructed of CLNM.

Results: The multivariate logistic analysis showed that Age ($p < 0.001$), Gender ($p < 0.001$), Multifocality ($p < 0.001$), *BRAF* ($p = 0.027$), and Tumor size ($p < 0.001$) were associated with CLNM. The receiver operating characteristic curve (ROC curve) showed high efficiency with an area under the ROC (AUC) of 0.781 in the training group. The calibration curve and the calibration of the model were evaluated. The decision curve analysis (DCA) for the nomogram showed that the nomogram can provide benefits in this study.

Conclusion: The predictive model of CLNM constructed and visualized based on the evaluated risk factors was confirmed to be a practical and convenient tool for clinicians to predict the CLNM in PTC.

Keywords: papillary thyroid carcinoma (PTC), predictive model, central lymph node metastasis (CLNM), nomogram, risk factors

INTRODUCTION

Thyroid carcinoma is one of the most popular endocrine tumors, and papillary thyroid carcinoma (PTC) is the most common pathological type (1, 2). The increased incidence of PTC is attributed to both the truly increased prevalence of thyroid diseases and the advances in imaging technology. Current studies have reported that PTC has a strong propensity for CLNM (3), and it is difficult to effectively detect central lymph node metastases (CLNMs) preoperatively (4–6). The most commonly involved central lymph nodes in thyroid carcinoma are the prelaryngeal (Delphian), pretracheal, and the right and left paratracheal nodes; the paratracheal nodes may be anterior as well as posterior to the recurrent laryngeal nerves (3). Whether to prophylactically dissect the central lymph nodes in PTC remains controversial (7). Dissection of the lymph nodes in the central region of the neck is considered necessary. Central lymph node dissection (CLND) is beneficial in eliminating macroscopic or microscopic metastatic sites. When CLNM is found in patients after surgery, a second operation is often necessary. Extra surgery not only is difficult but also increases the risk of complications (8). Prophylactic lymph node dissection of the central cervical facilitates accurate clinical staging (9). However, it has been argued that prophylactic dissection of the central lymph nodes is not necessary. Routine prophylactic CLND is considered uneconomical (10). Routine prophylactic central compartment dissection is particularly associated with temporary and permanent hypoparathyroidism and recurrent laryngeal nerve injury (4, 11, 12). Although numerous retrospective studies determined the benefits of prophylactic CLND by various investigators, the published results have been inconclusive. Due to the indolent nature of PTC, a very large sample size with extended follow-up for a randomized control trial examination is urgently needed. Therefore, preoperative access is of great clinical significance to accurately assess patients for CLNM. In this study, we analyzed the risk factors of CLNM and constructed a predictive model of CLNM to more accurately assess the risk of CLNM preoperatively and provide a practical and convenient tool for clinicians to predict the CLNM in PTC for clinical decision-making.

METHODS

Study Design

We screened all the patients who underwent thyroidectomy for PTC in Thyroid Surgery who were admitted to the First Affiliated Hospital of Zhengzhou University from January 2018 to October 2019. The inclusion criteria were as follows: 1) patients underwent thyroid surgery for the first time; 2) clinically and pathologically diagnosed as PTC. The exclusion criteria included the following: 1) other malignancies combined; 2) preoperative hyperthyroidism or hypothyroidism; 3) other diseases that cause swollen lymph nodes in the neck; 4) two or more thyroidectomies. A total of 2,554 patients including 982 patients with CLNMs (CLNM(+)), and 1,572 patients without CLNMs (CLNM(−)) were enrolled in this study. The enrollment flowchart of the participants is shown in **Figure 1**. The patients with CLNMs (CLNM(+)) and without CLNMs (CLNM(−)) were divided into the training group (n = 1,787) and the validation group (n = 767).

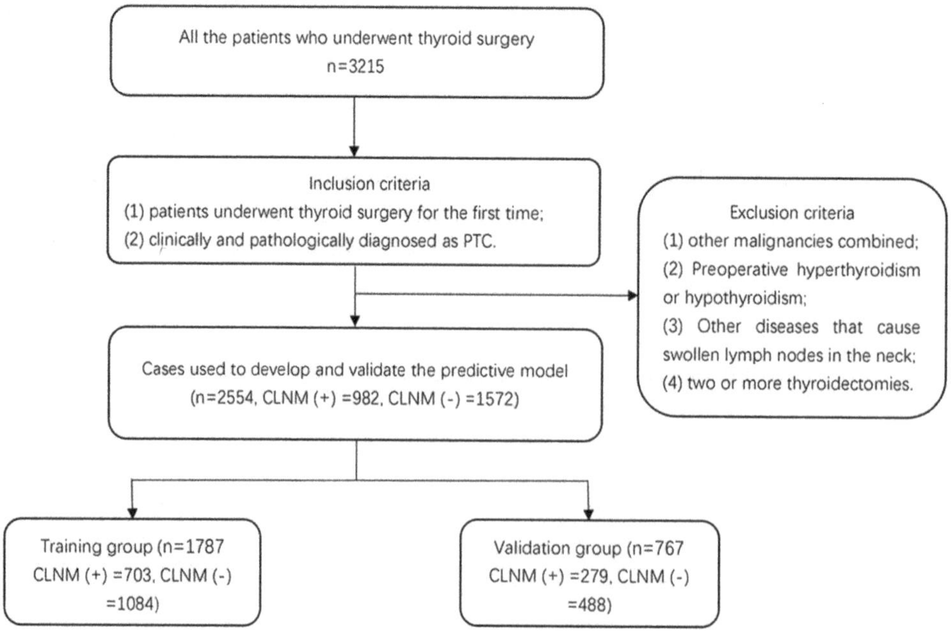

FIGURE 1 | Enrollment flowchart of participants used for model development and validation. PTC, papillary thyroid carcinoma; CLNM, central lymph node metastasis.

Data Collection

The basic information, laboratory examination, cervical ultrasound, genetic test, and pathological diagnosis were collected. The basic information included age and gender. The laboratory indices included free triiodothyronine (FT_3), free tetraiodothyronine (FT_4), thyroid-stimulating hormone (TSH), thyroid peroxidase antibodies (TPOAb), thyroglobulin antibodies (TgAb), and thyroglobulin (Tg). The characteristics of cervical ultrasound include multifocality and tumor size. Multifocality was defined as more than one lesion observed in cervical ultrasound and pathologically confirmed as PTC. Tumor size was the maximum diameter of the suspected nodule under ultrasound that was pathologically confirmed as PTC (8). All patients had a review of the cervical ultrasound with the same sonographer preoperatively. Genetic test results included *BRAF* and *TERT*. Pathological diagnosis included reports of the paraffin section of the primary lesion and central lymph node.

Statistical Analysis

Multivariate multiple imputations with chained equations were used to deal with a few missing data of several variables to decrease the bias (13). All the statistical analysis processes involved were completed by R software, version 4.1.1. p-Value <0.05 was considered statistically significant. The classification data were expressed as percentages, and means ± SD or medians (quartile 1, quartile 3) were described as continuous variables that satisfy or do not satisfy the normal distribution, respectively. The odds ratio (OR) values were calculated by univariate logistic regression of the variables. After the collinearity among variables was calculated and the colinear factors were eliminated, the potential variables with a p-value <0.05 were selected to perform the multivariate logistic regression. A clinical predictive model of CLNM in PTC was built based on the variables with statistical senses.

RESULTS

Baseline Characteristics of the Variables

The baseline characteristics of CLNM(+) and CLNM(−) are shown in **Table 1**. All the enrolled patients were randomly divided into the training group (n = 1,787) and the validation group (n = 767). There was no significant difference in the levels of these variables between the two groups (**Table 2**). Six potential predictors from 12 candidates were considered to have statistical significance ($p < 0.05$).

TABLE 1 | Baseline characteristics of enrolled patients.

Variables	CLNM (−) (n = 1,572)	CLNM (+) (n = 982)	p-Value
Age [years (IQR)]	47.000 (39.000, 54.000)	41.000 (32.000, 50.000)	<0.0001
Gender, n [male (%)]	269 (17.11)	285 (29.02)	<0.0001
FT_3 [pmol/L (IQR)]	4.910 (4.530, 5.320)	5.010 (4.630, 5.420)	<0.0001
FT_4 [pmol/L (IQR)]	11.185 (10.140, 12.322)	11.180 (10.162, 12.190)	0.6288
TSH [μIU/ml (IQR)]	2.530 (1.647, 3.720)	2.504 (1.640, 3.718)	0.3996
TPOAb [(+) (n (%)]	262 (16.67)	170 (17.31)	0.7123
TgAb [(+) (n (%)]	263 (16.73)	190 (19.35)	0.1027
Tg [ng/ml (SD)]	63.154 (404.596)	66.110 (290.648)	0.8422
BRAF [(+) (n (%)]	1,290 (82.06)	841 (85.64)	0.0207
TERT [(+) (n (%)]	4 (0.25)	1 (0.10)	0.6549
Multifocality [n (%)]	308 (19.59)	380 (38.70)	<0.0001
Tumor size (D ≥ 1 cm) (n, %)	382 (24.30)	600 (61.10)	<0.0001

CLNM, central lymph node metastasis; IQR, interquartile range; FT_3, free triiodothyronine; FT_4, free tetraiodothyronine; TSH, thyroid-stimulating hormone; TPOAb, thyroid peroxidase antibodies; TgAb, thyroglobulin antibodies; Tg, thyroglobulin.

TABLE 2 | Baseline characteristics showed there was no statistical difference between the training group and validation group.

Variables	Training group (n = 1,787)	Validation group (n = 767)	p-Value
Age [years (IQR)]	45.000 (36.000, 52.000)	45.000 (36.000, 52.000)	0.6943
Gender, n [male (%)]	392 (21.94)	162 (21.12)	0.685
FT_3 [pmol/L (IQR)]	4.950 (4.570, 5.350)	4.950 (4.580, 5.380)	0.8916
FT_4 [pmol/L (IQR)]	11.160 (10.090, 12.250)	11.260 (10.265, 12.295)	0.2107
TSH [μIU/ml (IQR)]	2.520 (1.660, 3.765)	2.508 (1.630, 3.620)	0.5867
TPOAb [(+) (n (%)]	318 (17.80)	114 (14.86)	0.0794
TgAb [(+) (n (%)]	322 (18.02)	131 (17.08)	0.6078
Tg [(ng/ml, (SD)]	16.100 (7.200, 33.690)	14.700 (6.380, 33.200)	0.2861
BRAF [(+) (n (%)]	1,503 (84.11)	628 (81.88)	0.183
TERT [(+) (n (%)]	4 (0.22)	1 (0.13)	1
Multifocality [n (%)]	482 (26.97)	206 (26.86)	0.991
Tumor size (D ≥ 1 cm) (n, %)	687 (38.44)	295 (38.46)	1

FT_3, free triiodothyronine; FT_4, free tetraiodothyronine; TSH, thyroid-stimulating hormone; TPOAb, thyroid peroxidase antibodies; TgAb, thyroglobulin antibodies; Tg, thyroglobulin.

Risk Factors and Predictive Model of Central Lymph Node Metastasis

Multivariate logistic analysis showed that Age (OR 0.947–0.966), Gender (OR 1.541–2.589), Multifocality (OR 2.348–3.815), *BRAF* (OR 1.044–1.926), and Tumor size (OR 4.127–6.416) were associated with CLNM (**Table 3**). The receiver operating characteristic curve (ROC curve) was drawn to evaluate the diagnostic effectiveness of the model (**Figure 2**). The ROC showed a high efficiency with an area under the ROC (AUC) of 0.781 (specificity 0.778, sensitivity 0.662, **Figure 2A**) in the training group. The effectiveness was verified in the validation group with an AUC of 0.736 (specificity 0.631, sensitivity 0.774), and the result is shown in **Figure 2B**. The model showed a great ability to distinguish the presence or absence of CLNM in the training group with a high value of AUC.

Then the model was evaluated by the calibration curve. The predicted values had good consistency in the training group (mean absolute error = 0.004) and the validation group (mean absolute error = 0.008) with the observed variables. The calibration curve showed that the model had a strong calibration ability (**Figure 3**).

To visualize the model, we plotted the nomogram of our predictive model based on the five variables: Age, Gender, Focal, *BRAF*, and Tumor size. Every variable was scored by drawing a straight line upward the "Points" line. The total points were the sum of the points obtained by the five variables. A straight line down to the axis named "CLNM risk" represents the risk of CLNM (**Figure 4**).

In the training group, we constructed a decision curve analysis (DCA) to identify the net benefit of the nomogram (**Figure 5**). The curve showed that when the threshold probability of patients is between 0.11 and 0.90, the nomogram can provide benefits.

DISCUSSION

PTC metastasis occurs most often in the central lymph nodes, with few distant metastases and low mortality, and the rate of

TABLE 3 | Potential risk factors identified by univariate and multivariate logistic regression analyses.

Variable	Univariable		Multivariable	
	OR (95% CI)	p	OR (95% CI)	p
Age (years)	0.960 (0.952–0.969)	<0.001	0.957 (0.947–0.966)	<0.001
Gender (male, %)	1.948 (1.554–2.445)	<0.001	1.996 (1.541–2.589)	<0.001
FT_3 (pmol/L)	1.364 (1.158–1.607)	<0.001		
FT_4 (pmol/L)	0.989 (0.935–1.045)	0.682		
TSH (µIU/ml)	0.990 (0.948–1.031)	0.633		
TPOAb(+) %	1.064 (0.830–1.361)	0.622		
TgAb(+) %	1.232 (0.964–1.572)	0.0935		
Tg (ng/ml)	1.000 (0.999–1.001)	0.349		
BRAF(+) %	1.327 (1.019–1.737)	0.0377	1.414 (1.044–1.926)	0.027
TERT(+) %	0.513 (0.025–4.018)	0.564		
Multifocality %	2.822 (2.278–3.500)	<0.001	2.989 (2.348–3.815)	<0.001
Tumor size (D ≥ 1 cm) %	5.299 (4.313–6.528)	<0.001	5.138 (4.127–6.416)	<0.001

FT_3, free triiodothyronine; FT_4, free tetraiodothyronine; TSH, thyroid-stimulating hormone; TPOAb, thyroid peroxidase antibodies; TgAb, thyroglobulin antibodies; Tg, thyroglobulin.

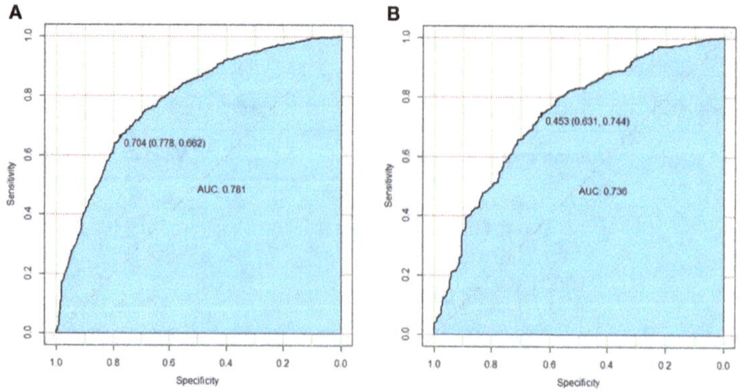

FIGURE 2 | The differential capability of the nomogram. **(A)** ROC curve based on the potential risk factors identified by multivariate logistic regression analysis showed great ability to distinguish the presence or absence of CLNM in the training group with a high value of AUC. **(B)** ROC curve based on the potential risk factors identified by multivariate logistic regression analysis showed great ability to distinguish the presence or absence of CLNM in the validation group. ROC, receiver operating characteristic; CLNM, central lymph node metastasis; AUC, area under the curve.

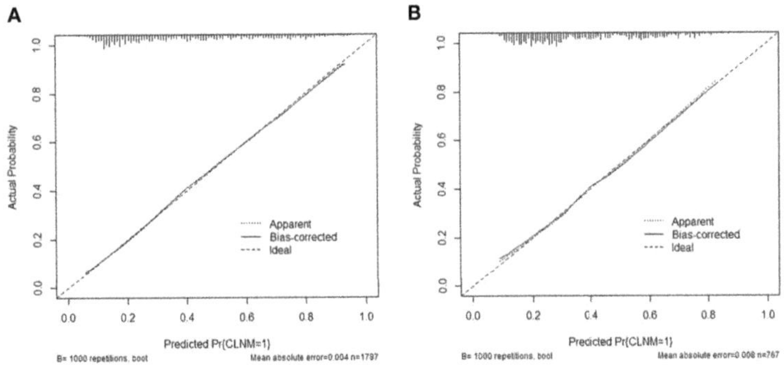

FIGURE 3 | Calibration curve of the predictive nomogram in the **(A)** training group or **(B)** validation group.

cervical lymph node metastasis detection by ultrasound is unsatisfactory, especially for CLNM (5, 14). Information gathered by prospective and randomized clinical studies is the key to determining whether prophylactic dissection of the central lymph nodes in PTC is necessary, but it is probably unavailable currently. Therefore, identification of patients with PTC preoperatively at greater risk of CLNM would be valuable. Prediction models and risk factors analysis based on clinical data have been developed increasingly in a wide variety of diseases in recent years.

To solve these problems, in this study, we collected and analyzed the risk factors and constructed a predictive model of CLNM. The model also showed a high calibration capacity. To the best of our knowledge, it is the first study aiming to construct and visualize a predictive model of CLNM. It is a predictive model that can help clinicians make appropriate treatments and help clinicians assess whether patients need CLND in PTC.

Some studies suggested that CLNM is significantly correlated with age (15, 16), which was similar to our study. Patients with younger age were more likely to be considered at a higher risk of CLNM.

Recent studies have shown that estrogen is a powerful stimulant for benign and malignant thyroid nodules. This explains why thyroid cancer is highly prevalent in women (17). However, in this study, there was a higher rate of CLNM in men. Some scholars confirmed that there were different subtypes of

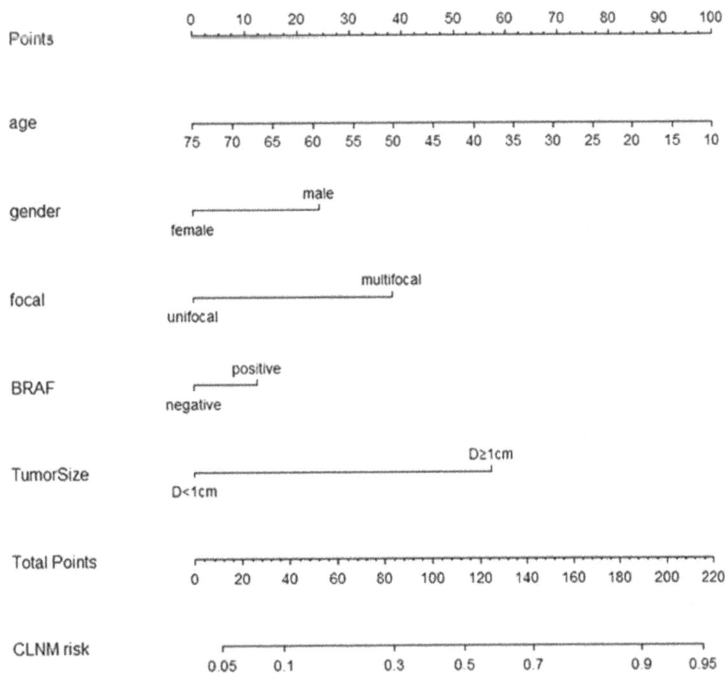

FIGURE 4 | Nomogram based on the five variables including Age, Gender, Focal, BRAF, and Tumor size.

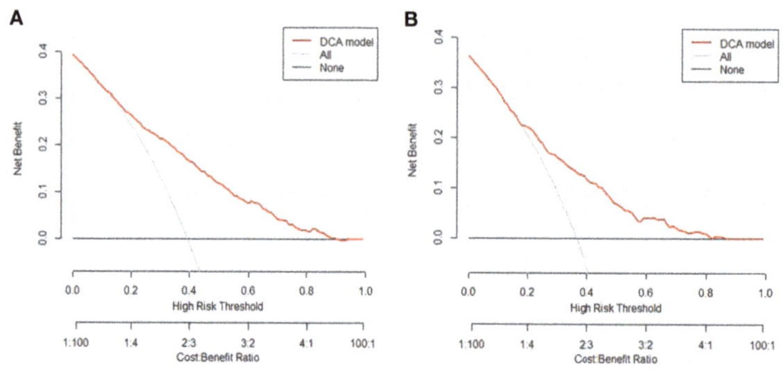

FIGURE 5 | Decision curve for the nomogram predicting CLNM in **(A)** training group or **(B)** validation group. CLNM, central lymph node metastasis.

estrogen receptors (ERs) that were considered a protective factor in PTC (17). This may be a potential cause of a higher rate of CLNM in male patients. The detailed knowledge of this regulation in thyroid cancer is still being debated.

Studies have shown that the risk of CLNM increases with the number of foci (11). The multifocal disease was defined as the presence of 2 or more foci of PTC, and each focus was recorded separately. In this study, CLNM rates were high in multifocal PTC with an OR of 2.989 (95% CI 2.348–3.815). With the application of high-resolution ultrasound, the preoperative diagnostic technology of PTC has made a huge breakthrough (18). Therefore, multifocality should be taken seriously during the preoperative ultrasound. When the cervical ultrasound showed that the suspicious lesions have significant multifocality, lobectomy and prophylactic CLNM should be considered.

BRAF genetic test was valuable for the diagnosis, prognosis, and therapy of PTC (19). In addition, some scholars revealed that *BRAF* mutations were associated with markers of clinical aggressiveness such as larger tumors, lymph node metastases, and poor clinical outcomes (20). In general, *BRAF* genetic test had strong practicability. Genetic testing in preoperative fine-needle aspiration biopsy (FNAB) was helpful to confirm the diagnosis, patients with a positive result for *BRAF* genetic test should be further evaluated, and there were stronger recommendations for prophylactic CLND.

Tumor size is an important risk factor for CLNM in PTC in the present study. This finding was similar to other studies that the risk of CLNM in PTC increases with tumor size (21, 22). In clinical practice, suspicious nodules larger than 10 mm should be managed with caution. Clinicians need to evaluate the patient's cervical lymph nodes to decide whether to perform prophylactic dissection of the lymph nodes. Our research, especially the nomogram, provides a good reference for clinicians.

In the univariate logistic regression model, the titer of FT_3 was statistically significant between the two groups. We searched the relevant literature and found that there is no clear relationship between thyroid hormone and CLNM of PTC. However, one scholar's research results caught our attention; this study showed a high correlation between PTC microcalcification and thyroid hormones (23). Microcalcification of thyroid nodules indicates that it was more likely to be malignant (24). Therefore, the titer of thyroid hormone may be related to the pathology of thyroid nodules, but it cannot be considered a risk factor for CLNM.

Some scholars have reached similar conclusions (25, 26); younger age, male sex, multifocality, and larger tumor size are the risk factors for cervical lymph node metastases in PTC. The predictive model was also constructed and visualized with a nomogram. However, our study aimed at risk factor analysis and predictive model construction for CLNM with a high AUC. In addition, not only the clinical baseline characteristics but also the genetic test result was included in this study. This was more instructive for patients with preoperative FNAB and *BRAF* genetic test.

The decision curve and nomogram in this study show the great utility of our model, and the 5 items in the nomogram are routine clinical variables that can easily be obtained by clinicians, indicating that it may be beneficial for clinicians to assess the need for prophylactic CLND. Our study has a large sample size of 2,554 patients and has excellent diagnostic effectiveness of CLNM with an AUC of 0.781 in the training group. The operation of the model is simple and fast, which can provide a reference for timely prophylactic CLND.

However, there are also several limitations in our study. First, all the enrolled patients came from the same hospital without external validation. Moreover, we still need to expand the sample size to reduce the heterogeneity. In addition, our predictive model is only suitable for PTC; there is still a lack of predictive ability of our model for other types of thyroid carcinoma.

ETHICS STATEMENT

The studies involving human participants were reviewed and approved by The First Affiliated Hospital of Zhengzhou

University Ethics Review Committee. Written informed consent for participation was not required for this study in accordance with the national legislation and the institutional requirements.

AUTHOR CONTRIBUTIONS

DY conceived of the idea and provided guidance. ZW wrote the manuscript and completed the figures. QC and HZ contributed to organizing the database. SL, YL, and HS carefully reviewed the manuscript. GD made critical revisions to the manuscript. All authors contributed to the article and approved the submitted version.

ACKNOWLEDGMENTS

We acknowledge Qungang Chang for the data collection.

REFERENCES

1. Xu S, Huang H, Qian J, Liu Y, Huang Y, Wang X, et al. Prevalence of Hashimoto Thyroiditis in Adults With Papillary Thyroid Cancer and Its Association With Cancer Recurrence and Outcomes. *JAMA Netw Open* (2021) 4(7):e2118526. doi: 10.1001/jamanetworkopen.2021.18526
2. Yasuhiro Ito MK, Takamura Y, Kobayashi K, Miya A, Miyauchi A. Prognosis and Prognostic Factors of Patients With Papillary Thyroid Carcinoma Requiring Resection of Recurrent Laryngeal Nerve Due to Carcinoma Extension. *Endocrine J* (2012) 59(3):247–52. doi: 10.1507/endocrj.ej11-0355
3. Carty SE, Doherty GM, Duh Q-Y, Kloos RT, Mandel SJ, Randolph GW, et al. Consensus Statement on the Terminology and Classification of Central Neck Dissection for Thyroid Cancer. *Thyroid* (2009) 11:2009. doi: 10.1089/thy.2009.0159
4. Sturgeon C, Yang A, Elaraj D. Surgical Management of Lymph Node Compartments in Papillary Thyroid Cancer. *Surg Oncol Clin N Am* (2016) 25(1):17–40. doi: 10.1016/j.soc.2015.08.013
5. Kim KE, Kim EK, Yoon JH, Han KH, Moon HJ, Kwak JY. Preoperative Prediction of Central Lymph Node Metastasis in Thyroid Papillary Microcarcinoma Using Clinicopathologic and Sonographic Features. *World J Surg* (2013) 37(2):385–91. doi: 10.1007/s00268-012-1826-3
6. Mazzaferri ELMD, Doherty GM, Steward DL. The Pros and Cons of Prophylactic Central Compartment Lymph Node Dissection for Papillary Thyroid Carcinoma. *Thyroid* (2009) 19(7) 2009. doi: 10.1089/thy.2009.1578
7. Fritze D, Doherty GM. Surgical Management of Cervical Lymph Nodes in Differentiated Thyroid Cancer. *Otolaryngol Clin North Am* (2010) 43(2):285–300. doi: 10.1016/j.otc.2010.01.005
8. Guang Y, He W, Zhang W, Zhang H, Zhang Y, Wan F. Clinical Study of Ultrasonographic Risk Factors for Central Lymph Node Metastasis of Papillary Thyroid Carcinoma. *Front Endocrinol (Lausanne)* (2021) 12:791970. doi: 10.3389/fendo.2021.791970
9. Hughes DT, White ML, Miller BS, Gauger PG, Burney RE, Doherty GM. Influence of Prophylactic Central Lymph Node Dissection on Postoperative Thyroglobulin Levels and Radioiodine Treatment in Papillary Thyroid Cancer. *Surgery* (2010) 148(6):1100–6; discussion 006-7. doi: 10.1016/j.surg.2010.09.019
10. Garcia A, Palmer BJ, Parks NA, Liu TH. Routine Prophylactic Central Neck Dissection for Low-Risk Papillary Thyroid Cancer Is Not Cost-Effective. *Clin Endocrinol (Oxf)* (2014) 81(5):754–61. doi: 10.1111/cen.12506
11. Al Afif A, Williams BA, Rigby MH, Bullock MJ, Taylor SM, Trites J, et al. Multifocal Papillary Thyroid Cancer Increases the Risk of Central Lymph Node Metastasis. *Thyroid* (2015) 25(9):1008–12. doi: 10.1089/thy.2015.0130
12. Sancho JJ, Lennard TW, Paunovic I, Triponez F, Sitges-Serra A. Prophylactic Central Neck Disection in Papillary Thyroid Cancer: A Consensus Report of the European Society of Endocrine Surgeons (ESES). *Langenbecks Arch Surg* (2014) 399(2):155–63. doi: 10.1007/s00423-013-1152-8
13. Buuren SG-O. Mice: Multivariate Imputation by Chained Equations in R. *J Stat Software* (2011) 45(3):1–67. doi: 10.18637/jss.v045.i03
14. Zhao W, He L, Zhu J, Su A. A Nomogram Model Based on the Preoperative Clinical Characteristics of Papillary Thyroid Carcinoma With Hashimoto's Thyroiditis to Predict Central Lymph Node Metastasis. *Clin Endocrinol (Oxf)* (2021) 94(2):310–21. doi: 10.1111/cen.14302
15. Ito Y, Miyauchi A, Kihara M, Higashiyama T, Kobayashi K, Miya A. Patient Age is Significantly Related to the Progression of Papillary Microcarcinoma of the Thyroid Under Observation. *Thyroid* (2014) 24(1):27–34. doi: 10.1089/thy.2013.0367
16. Zheng X, Peng C, Gao M, Zhi J, Hou X, Zhao J, et al. Risk Factors for Cervical Lymph Node Metastasis in Papillary Thyroid Microcarcinoma: A Study of 1,587 Patients. *Cancer Biol Med* (2019) 16(1):121–30. doi: 10.20892/j.issn.2095-3941.2018.0125
17. Derwahl M, Nicula D. Estrogen and Its Role in Thyroid Cancer. *Endocr Relat Cancer* (2014),21(15) T273–83. doi: 10.1530/ERC-14-0053
18. Khokhar MT, Day KM, Sangal RB, Ahmedli NN, Pisharodi LR, Beland MD, et al. Preoperative High-Resolution Ultrasound for the Assessment of Malignant Central Compartment Lymph Nodes in Papillary Thyroid Cancer. *Thyroid* (2015) 25(12):1351–4. doi: 10.1089/thy.2015.0176
19. Chen H, Song A, Wang Y, He Y, Tong J, Di J, et al. BRAF(V600E) Mutation Test on Fine-Needle Aspiration Specimens of Thyroid Nodules: Clinical Correlations for 4600 Patients. *Cancer Med* (2021) 11(1):40–9. doi: 10.1002/cam4.4419
20. Melo M, Gaspar da Rocha A, Batista R, Vinagre J, Martins MJ, Costa G, et al. TERT, BRAF, and NRAS in Primary Thyroid Cancer and Metastatic Disease. *J Clin Endocrinol Metab* (2017) 102(6):1898–907. doi: 10.1210/jc.2016-2785
21. Machens A, Holzhausen HJ, Dralle H. The Prognostic Value of Primary Tumor Size in Papillary and Follicular Thyroid Carcinoma. *Cancer* (2005) 103 (11):2269–73. doi: 10.1002/cncr.21055
22. Machens A, Hinze R, Thomusch O, Dralle H. Pattern of Nodal Metastasis for Primary and Reoperative Thyroid Cancer. *World J Surg* (2002) 26(1):22–8. doi: 10.1007/s00268-001-0176-3
23. Ha J, Lee J, Jo K, Han JS, Kim MH, Jung CK, et al. Calcification Patterns in Papillary Thyroid Carcinoma Are Associated With Changes in Thyroid Hormones and Coronary Artery Calcification. *J Clin Med* (2018) 7(8):183. doi: 10.3390/jcm7080183
24. Bu Kyung Kim YSC, Kwon HJ, Lee JS, Heo JJ, Han YJ, Park Y-H, et al. Relationship Between Patterns of Calcification in Thyroid Nodules and Histopathologic Findings. *Endocrine J* (2012) 60(2):150–60. doi: 10.1507/endocrj.ej12-0294
25. Feng Y, Min Y, Chen H, Xiang K, Wang X, Yin G. Construction and Validation of a Nomogram for Predicting Cervical Lymph Node Metastasis in Classic Papillary Thyroid Carcinoma. *J Endocrinol Invest* (2021) 44 (10):2203–11. doi: 10.1007/s40618-021-01524-5
26. Tian X, Song Q, Xie F, Ren L, Zhang Y, Tang J, et al. Papillary Thyroid Carcinoma: An Ultrasound-Based Nomogram Improves the Prediction of Lymph Node Metastases in the Central Compartment. *Eur Radiol* (2020) 30 (11):5881–93. doi: 10.1007/s00330-020-06906-6

11

Successful Applications of Food-Assisted and-Simulated Training Model of Thyroid Radiofrequency Ablation

Yan-Rong Li[1,2], *Wei-Yu Chou*[1], *Wai-Kin Chan*[1], *Kai-Lun Cheng*[3,4], *Jui-Hung Sun*[1], *Feng-Hsuan Liu*[1,2], *Szu-Tah Chen*[1,2] *and Miaw-Jene Liou*[1,2*]

[1] *Division of Endocrinology and Metabolism, Department of Internal Medicine, Linkou Chang Gung Memorial Hospital, Taoyuan, Taiwan,* [2] *College of Medicine, Chang Gung University, Taoyuan, Taiwan,* [3] *Department of Medical Imaging, Chung Shan Medical University Hospital, Taichung, Taiwan,* [4] *School of Medical Imaging and Radiological Sciences, Chung Shan Medical University, Taichung, Taiwan*

Correspondence:
Miaw-Jene Liou
lioumj@cgmh.org.tw

Background: Radiofrequency ablation (RFA) for benign thyroid nodules is one kind of scarless treatment for symptomatic or cosmetic benign thyroid nodules. However, how to train RFA-naive physicians to become qualified operators for thyroid RFA is an important issue. Our study aimed to introduce a successful training model of thyroid RFA.

Materials and Methods: We used a food-assisted and -simulated training model of thyroid RFA. Chicken hearts were simulated into thyroid nodules, three-layer pork meats were simulated into peri-thyroid structure, and gel bottles were simulated into trachea, respectively. Successful training ablations were defined as chicken hearts that were fully cooked. After repeating training ablations of chicken hearts at least 100 times with the nearly 100% success rates for three young trainees, they served as the first assistant for the real procedures of thyroid RFA and then were qualified to perform thyroid RFA on real patients under the supervision of one experienced interventional radiologist.

Results: 23 real patients who received RFA and follow-up at least 6 months after treatment were included in Linkou Chang Gung Memorial Hospital from January 1, 2020 to October 1, 2021. Three young endocrinologists performed thyroid RFA independently. The outcomes were volume reduction rate (VRR), major complications and minor complications. The median VRR at 12 months was 82.00%, two major complications were transient hoarseness, and three minor complications were wound pain. All complications were completely recovered within three days.

Conclusions: For young and RFA-native physicians without any basic skills of echo-guided intervention, this food-assisted and -simulated training model of thyroid RFA was useful for medical training and education.

Keywords: thyroid, nodule, radiofrequency ablation, training model, medical education

INTRODUCTION

With the exams by ultrasonography, thyroid nodules are common in general populations, and the prevalence was ever reported 50-60% (1, 2). Among of them, around 7-15% nodules are malignant; therefore, most thyroid nodules are benign (1, 2). For benign thyroid nodules with symptoms and signs of compression or cosmetic problem, treatment should be considered to alleviate the patients' suffering, such as dyspnea, dysphagia, voice change, or the cosmetic reasons of neck. Radiofrequency ablation (RFA) for benign thyroid nodules is one kind of treatment for symptomatic benign thyroid nodules, especially for cosmetic problem because thyroid RFA is a scarless procedure (3).

Thyroid RFA is a minimally invasive procedure using friction heat productions due to tissue ions agitated by alternating electric current of electrodes and performed with generators and 7-cm electrodes which are 18-gauge, and internally cooled with an active tip measuring 5, 7, or 10 mm (4, 5). The reported volume reduction rate (VRR) by thyroid RFA was from 69% to 78% after 1-year follow-up (6, 7). Some guidelines suggested that thyroid RFA can be used for treating benign thyroid nodules for volume reduction to relieve compression or cosmetic problem (8–10). The core skills are trans-isthmic approach method and moving-shot technique (11). Although knowing these two core techniques, young physicians who have never received step-by-step training by experienced operators and lack in practical experience in real patients may be unable to perform thyroid RFA well and still need a longer learning curve. In addition, young physicians with immature basic and core skills may lead to more complications while learning thyroid RFA in real patients.

As a result, the aim of our study was to investigate the feasibility of the food-assisted and -simulated training model of thyroid RFA in three young endocrinologists who had never performed echo-guided aspiration cytology and thyroid RFA in real patients.

MATERIALS AND METHODS

We used a food-assisted and -simulated training model of thyroid RFA for three young endocrinologists who never performed echo-guided aspiration cytology and RFA. Chicken hearts (size around 2 x 1.5 x 1 cm^3) were simulated into thyroid nodules and three-layer pork meats (size around 25-30 x 15-20 x 7-10 cm^3) were simulated into peri-thyroid structure, and gel bottles were simulated into trachea, respectively (**Figure 1**). The generators of RFA were RF Medical Radiofrequency Generator (Mygen M-2004 and M-3004). The electrodes of RFA were RF Electrodes (RFT Series: RFT0707LN). Sequential echo-guided procedures for training the trans-isthmic approach method and the moving shot technique were performed with the food-assisted and -simulated training model of thyroid RFA (**Figure 2**). The successful ablations were defined as the color of chicken hearts from bright red to off-white, indicating that the meat was fully cooked (**Figure 3**).

After repeating ablations of chicken hearts at least 100 times with the nearly 100% success rates for three young endocrinologists and the trainees can performed echo-guided aspirations for cytology of small nodules/lesions on real patients smoothly, they served as the first assistant for the real procedures of thyroid RFA at least five times and then were qualified to perform thyroid RFA on real patients independently under the supervision of one experienced interventional radiologist for patients' safety. This is a retrospective study of thyroid RFA treatment effectiveness and prognosis after our learning model. Therefore, after training by this model and under the supervision of the leader in our hospital, our hospital permitted that we performed RFA in real patients with patients' consent and collected data retrospectively after getting certificate of IRB for a retrospective study. This study was approved by the Institutional Review Board, Chang Gung Memorial Hospital, Taiwan (IRB No.: 202101301B0).

Patients with nodular goiter (2 cm in at least one diameter), and predominantly solid nodules which contributed to compressive symptoms and/or cosmetic problem were

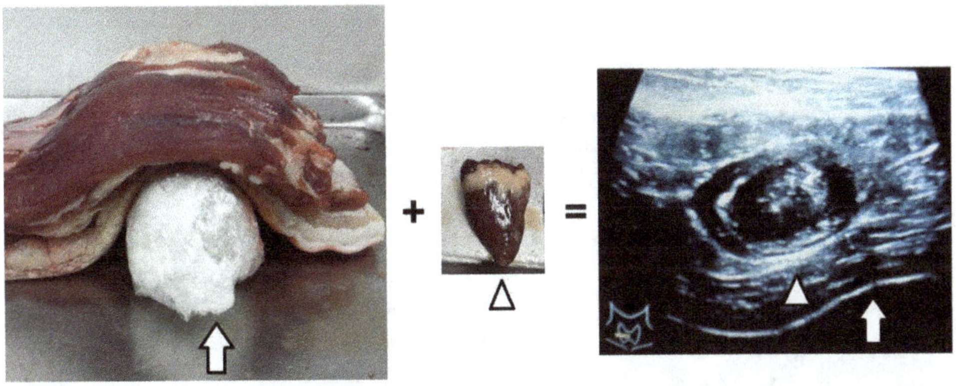

FIGURE 1 | Chicken hearts simulated into thyroid nodules (arrowhead), three-layer pork meats simulated into peri-thyroid skin structure, and gel bottles simulated into trachea (arrow).

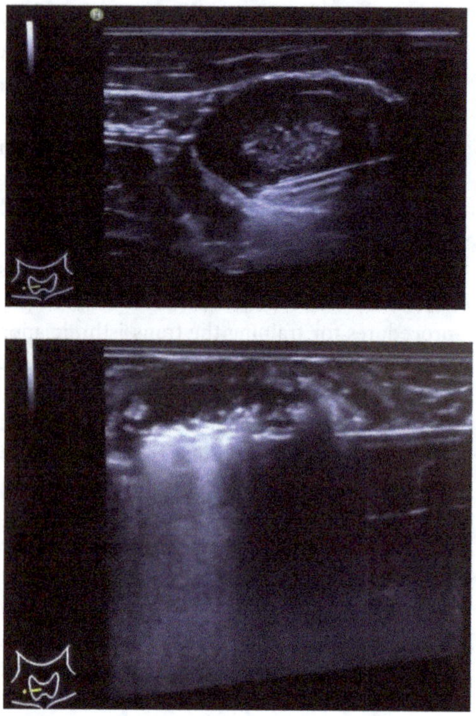

FIGURE 2 | Sequential echo-guided procedures for training the trans-isthmic approach method and the moving shot technique.

arranged to receive echo-guided fine-needle aspiration cytology. If the results of cytology showed benign lesions at least twice and patient refused surgical intervention, there were suggested to receive thyroid RFA for the treatment. If patients had multinodular goiter, the predominant and growing nodule was thought to be responsible for symptoms or cosmetic problems and was selected for the thyroid RFA. Patients with nodules > 5 cm in at least one diameter who may need multiple sessions of thyroid RFA were excluded from this study.

From January 1, 2020 to October 1, 2021, a total of 23 real patients who received thyroid RFA and had follow-up for at least 6 months after treatment in Linkou Chang Gung Memorial Hospital were included in the analysis finally.

OUTCOME MEASUREMENT

The patients were retrospectively reviewed with the medical records to assess the efficacy and the complications of thyroid RFA at the baseline and during the follow-up. The follow-up ultrasonography was performed at 1, 3, 6, and 12 months after thyroid RFA. The volume of nodule and the VRR were calculated

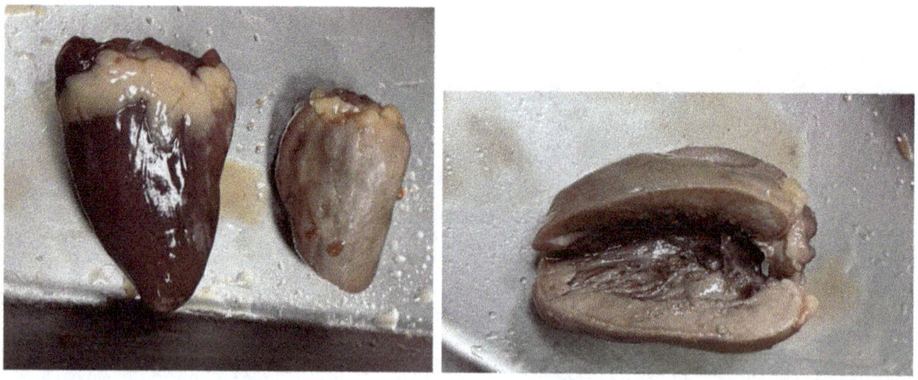

FIGURE 3 | The successful ablations were defined as the color of chicken hearts from bright red to off-white, indicating that the meat was fully cooked.

using the following equations: volume (mL) = length (cm) × width (cm) × depth (cm) × π/6 and VRR = [(initial volume – final volume)/initial volume] × 100%, respectively.

The major outcomes were changes in the volume of nodules, VRR, major complications, and minor complications one year after thyroid RFA. Major complications included voice change, Horner syndrome, brachial plexus injury, and nodule rupture. Minor complications included wound pain, skin burn and hematoma.

STATISTICAL ANALYSIS

Categorical data were determined by frequency and percentage. Kolmogorov-Smirnov test was applied to check the normality of continuous data. Continuous data without normal distributions were expressed as medians with interquartile ranges (IQR). Differences in various continuous parameters during the period of follow-up were examined for statistical significance by using Wilcoxon signed rank test as appropriate because of repeated and non-parametric measurements from a single group. A p value < 0.05 was considered statistically significant. All data analyses were performed using IBM SPSS Statistics for Windows, Version 22.0. (IBM Corp., Armonk, NY, USA).

RESULTS

Baseline Characteristics of Study Patients

23 patients (17 women and 6 men) with 23 benign nodules received thyroid RFA for the treatment. Two trainees performed 8 cases respectively, and the other trainee performed 7 cases. The median age of patients was 51 years (IQR, 43-55 years). The nodules had a median volume of 7.23 mL (IQR, 4.49-13.09 mL) before the thyroid RFA. All nodules were > 50% solidity and 95.65% of nodules were > 90% solidity. All patients had euthyroid status before the treatment of thyroid RFA. The baseline characteristics of study patients are summarized in **Table 1**. No patients had previous surgical intervention, radioactive iodine therapy, thermal/cryo ablation, or radiotherapy which may have an influence on the VRR after thyroid RFA.

TABLE 1 | Baseline characteristics in 23 patients with thyroid radiofrequency ablation.

Clinical characteristics	Value
Main nodule for RFA	23
Age at treatment (year)	51 (43-55)
Female gender	17 (73.91)
Largest diameter (cm)	3.50 (2.80-4.01)
Initial volume	7.23 (4.49-13.09)
Small (< 10 ml)	9 (39.13)
Medium (> 10 to ≤ 20 ml)	5 (21.74)
Large (> 20 to ≤ 30 ml)	6 (26.09)
Very large (> 30 ml)	3 (13.04)
Solidity > 50%	23 (100)
Solidity > 90%	22 (95.65)
Euthyroid status	23 (100)

Data were presented as median (interquartile range) or number (percentage).

Treatment Outcomes and Complications

The sequential changes in the median volume of nodules before and after thyroid RFA were 7.23 mL (IQR, 4.49-13.09 mL) at baseline, 3.49 mL (IQR, 2.36-6.13 mL) at one month, 1.93 mL (IQR, 1.29-4.45 mL) at three months, 1.42 mL (IQR, 0.63-2.30 mL) at six months and 1.30 mL (IQR, 0.22-2.42 mL) at 12 months, respectively (**Table 2** and **Figure 4**). The sequential median VRR after thyroid RFA were 40.89% (IQR, 32.26-56.78%) at one month, 69.62% (IQR, 60.17-79.06%) at three months, 79.89% (61.91-85.44%) at six months and 82.00% (62.17-87.63%) at 12 months, respectively (**Table 2** and **Figure 4**). Each nodule was ablated with single session. One of our real patients was with good response after thyroid RFA and had near 97% VRR at 12 months (**Figures 5A, B**).

Hoarseness could be one kind of major complications after thyroid RFA. There were two patients having transient voice change and both patients recovered totally; one was within five minutes and another was within one day. There were three patients having wound pain and needed non-steroidal anti-inflammatory drugs (NSAIDs) for pain control. Wound pain of these three patients was improved and all patients discontinued NSAIDs within three days. During the follow-up, there was no event of Horner syndrome, brachial plexus injury, nodule rupture, skin burn or hematoma. Due to the small case number of each trainee, the differences of efficacy/complications among these three physicians were not statistically significant.

DISCUSSION

There could be a long learning curve for some physicians to perform thyroid RFA. One recent study showed that there was a measurable learning curve in thyroid RFA until a total of 90 patients for the efficacy of benign thyroid nodules (12). In other words, there could be a minimum number of thyroid RFA for a physician to optimize patients' outcomes. The acceptable VRR after thyroid RFA is at least ≥ 50% at 12 months (13). This concept is like a previous study for evaluation of outcomes in thyroidectomy and the result showed that a surgeon volume threshold (> 25 total thyroidectomies per year) is correlated with improved patients' outcomes (14).

The strength of our study is that it is the first established food-assisted and -simulated training model of thyroid RFA and the result showed successful outcomes (the median VRR at 12 months: 82.00%) for medical training and education. This kind of simulated training model may shorten the learning curve in real patients and could prevent the bad outcomes in the initial 90 patients undergoing thyroid RFA. In other words, by our learning model, trainees can improve their major skills and ability and may be able to prevent excessive trial-and-error learning in the initial 90 real patients.

In Taiwan, thyroid RFA developed later than Korea. In the search of literatures, the first documented case of thyroid RFA in

TABLE 2 | Outcomes of main nodules after thyroid radiofrequency ablation.

	Initial (N = 23)	1 month after RFA (N = 23)	3 month after RFA (N = 23)	6 month after RFA (N = 23)	12 month after RFA (N = 18)
Volume of nodule (mL)	7.23 (4.49-13.09)	3.49 (2.36-6.13)*	1.93 (1.29-4.45)*	1.42 (0.63-2.30)*	1.30 (0.22-2.42)*
VRR (%)	0	40.89 (32.26-56.78)*	69.62 (60.17-79.06)*	79.89 (61.91-85.44)*	82.00 (62.17-87.63)*
Major complications					
Voice change	2	0	0	0	0
Horner syndrome	0	0	0	0	0
Brachial plexus injury	0	0	0	0	0
Nodule rupture	0	0	0	0	0
Minor complications					
Wound pain	3	0	0	0	0
Skin burn	0	0	0	0	0
Hematoma	0	0	0	0	0
Euthyroid status (%)	100	100	100	100	100

RFA, radiofrequency ablation; VRR, volume reduction rate; N, number.
Data were presented as median (interquartile range), number, or percentage.
**p value < 0.05 when compared with the initial nodules.*

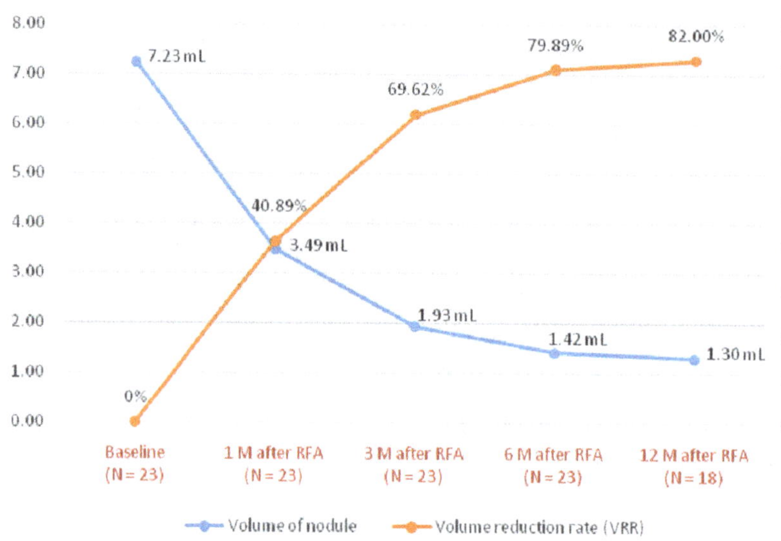

FIGURE 4 | The median changes in the volume of nodules and volume reduction rate during the follow-up.

Taiwan was published in 2016 (15). In Korea, Professor Jung Hwan Baek started thyroid RFA since 2002 (16) and ever published a large population study of thyroid RFA in 2008 (17). Nowadays, many guidelines in different countries have suggested thyroid RFA can be a standard of care to treat benign thyroid nodules for volume reduction to relieve compression or cosmetic problem (3, 8–10). However, in Taiwan, for most clinical physicians who have interests in thyroid RFA, they still have no idea how to learn thyroid RFA efficiently. Traditionally, learning a new invasive procedure requires someone who has a lot of experience to teach the trainee step by step. Two most famous physicians in Taiwan, both Dr. Wei-Che Lin and Dr. Kai-Lun Cheng have performed over one hundred cases of thyroid RFA and mainly contributed to publish a multicenter study of 762 cases after thyroid RFA which established the efficacy and safety of RFA for benign thyroid nodules in Taiwan (18) but they can not teach every trainee by the real patients in Taiwan step by step. Therefore, under the supervision of Dr. Kai-Lun Cheng, one experienced interventional radiologist in Taiwan, we worked together to build this kind of food-assisted and -simulated model for thyroid RFA training. Setting a good training model to learn a new invasive procedure is very important. A good simulated training model consists of hands-on training, deliberate practice, training to proficiency, cognitive teaching, and effective provision of feedback (19). Our training model meets the above points and showed good clinical results after training. The key components of our training model were as the followings: ablations of chicken hearts at least 100 times with the nearly 100% success rates, already performing trans-isthmic approach method with moving-shot technique very well, and understanding the critical structures associated with thyroid RFA, such as danger triangle, middle cervical sympathetic ganglion, and vagal nerve after serving as

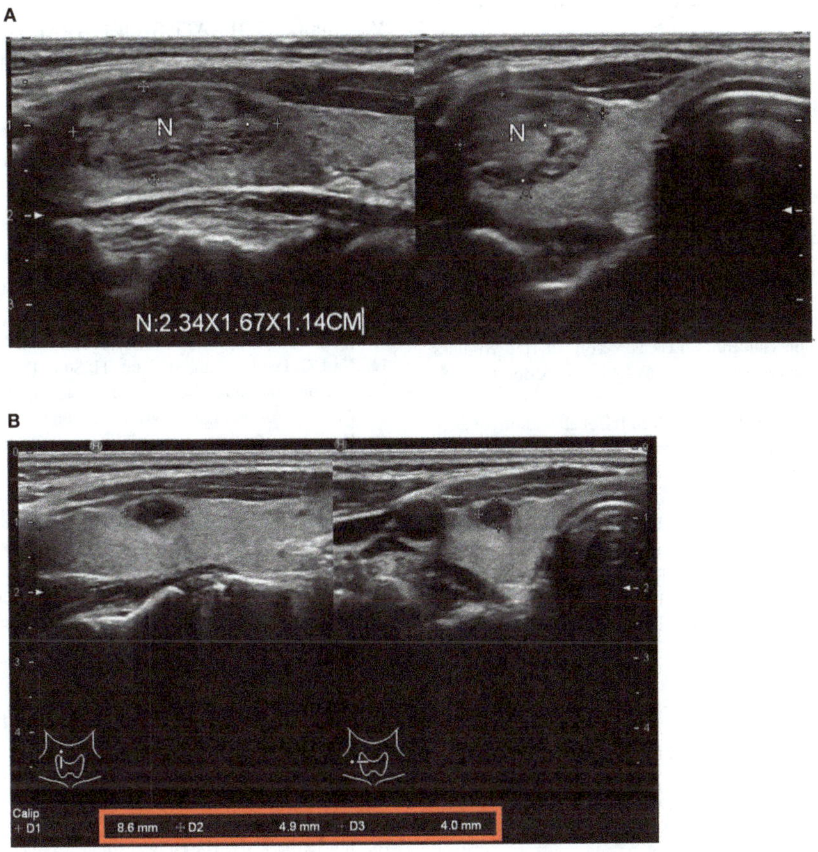

FIGURE 5 | One of our real patients with good response after thyroid radiofrequency ablation (RFA). **(A)** before thyroid RFA **(B)** near 97% volume reduction rate 12 months after thyroid RFA.

the first assistant for the real procedures of thyroid RFA at least five times. Besides, this training model is not expensive, easy to prepare materials and to facilitate the promotion of education. Each round of practice cost around 2500-3500 New Taiwan Dollar and can train multiple trainees at the same time and in the same place. Using this model, we successfully trained and cultivated three physicians simultaneously.

This present study had several major limitations. First, although we tried our best to simulate the peri-thyroid structure but we were unable to simulate the blood vessel, nerves, and esophagus. Therefore, the trainees needed to imagine the locations of the common coratid artery, internal jugular vein, vagal nerve, cervical sympathetic ganglion, danger triangle, and esophagus while practicing the trans-isthmic approach method and moving-shot technique. Second, although the current results of our study showed good applications of our training model with the median VRR 82.00% in real patients, the number of our study subjects is only 23 patients. Third, the longest time of follow-up in our study was 12 months which means we could not confidently evaluate whether the nodular regrowth will occur. Despite these disadvantages, our present study can still provide a valuable training model for those who want to learn how to practice thyroid RFA but do not know where to start.

CONCLUSIONS

For young and RFA-native physicians without any basic skills of echo-guided intervention, this food-assisted and -simulated training model of thyroid RFA was successful for medical training and education.

ETHICS STATEMENT

This study was approved by the Institutional Review Board, Chang Gung Memorial Hospital, Taiwan (IRB No.: 202101301B0). The patients/participants provided their written informed consent to participate in this study.

AUTHOR CONTRIBUTIONS

The conceptualization and design of the study was headed by Y-RL, W-KC, K-LC, and M-JL. The manuscript draft was written by Y-RL and M-JL. While the data analysis and interpretation were done by Y-RL, W-YC, W-KC, K-LC, J-HS, F-HL, S-TC, and M-JL. All authors contributed to the article and approved the submitted version.

ACKNOWLEDGEMENTS

We thank GOLEAD BIOPHARM INC for their assistance of providing the food model, generators, and electrodes of thyroid RFA.

REFERENCES

1. Burman KD, Wartofsky L. Clinical Practice. Thyroid Nodules. *N Engl J Med* (2015) 373(24):2347–56. doi: 10.1056/NEJMcp1415786
2. Haugen BR, Alexander EK, Bible KC, Doherty GM, Mandel SJ, Nikiforov YE, et al. American Thyroid Association Management Guidelines for Adult Patients With Thyroid Nodules and Differentiated Thyroid Cancer: The American Thyroid Association Guidelines Task Force on Thyroid Nodules and Differentiated Thyroid Cancer. *Thyroid* (2016) 26(1):1–133. doi: 10.1089/thy.2015.0020
3. Ha EJ, Baek JH, Che Y, Chou YH, Fukunari N, Kim JH, et al. Radiofrequency Ablation of Benign Thyroid Nodules: Recommendations From the Asian Conference on Tumor Ablation Task Force. *Ultrasonography* (2021) 40 (1):75–82. doi: 10.14366/usg.20112
4. Baek JH, Lee JH, Valcavi R, Pacella CM, Rhim H, Na DG. Thermal Ablation for Benign Thyroid Nodules: Radiofrequency and Laser. *Korean J Radiol* (2011) 12(5):525–40. doi: 10.3348/kjr.2011.12.5.525
5. Park HS, Baek JH, Choi YJ, Lee JH. Innovative Techniques for Image-Guided Ablation of Benign Thyroid Nodules: Combined Ethanol and Radiofrequency Ablation. *Korean J Radiol* (2017) 18(3):461–9. doi: 10.3348/kjr.2017.18.3.461
6. Cesareo R, Pasqualini V, Simeoni C, Sacchi M, Saralli E, Campagna G, et al. Prospective Study of Effectiveness of Ultrasound-Guided Radiofrequency Ablation Versus Control Group in Patients Affected by Benign Thyroid Nodules. *J Clin Endocrinol Metab* (2015) 100(2):460–6. doi: 10.1210/jc.2014-2186
7. Deandrea M, Sung JY, Limone P, Mormile A, Garino F, Ragazzoni F, et al. Efficacy and Safety of Radiofrequency Ablation Versus Observation for Nonfunctioning Benign Thyroid Nodules: A Randomized Controlled International Collaborative Trial. *Thyroid* (2015) 25(8):890–6. doi: 10.1089/thy.2015.0133
8. Dobnig H, Zechmann W, Hermann M, Lehner M, Heute D, Mirzaei S, et al. Radiofrequency Ablation of Thyroid Nodules: "Good Clinical Practice Recommendations" for Austria: An Interdisciplinary Statement From the Following Professional Associations: Austrian Thyroid Association (OSDG), Austrian Society for Nuclear Medicine and Molecular Imaging (OGNMB), Austrian Society for Endocrinology and Metabolism (OGES), Surgical Endocrinology Working Group (ACE) of the Austrian Surgical Society (OEGCH). *Wien Med Wochenschr* (2020) 170:6–14. doi: 10.1007/s10354-019-0682-2
9. Papini E, Pacella CM, Solbiati LA, Achille G, Barbaro D, Bernardi S, et al. Minimally-Invasive Treatments for Benign Thyroid Nodules: A Delphi-Based Consensus Statement From the Italian Minimally-Invasive Treatments of the Thyroid (MITT) Group. *Int J Hyperthermia* (2019) 36:376–82. doi: 10.1080/02656736.2019.1575482
10. Kim JH, Baek JH, Lim HK, Ahn HS, Baek SM, Choi YJ, et al. Thyroid Radiofrequency Ablation Guideline: Korean Society of Thyroid Radiology. *Korean J Radiol* (2018) 19:632–55. doi: 10.3348/kjr.2018.19.4.632
11. Na DG, Lee JH, Jung SL, Kim JH, Sung JY, Shin JH, et al. Korean Society of Thyroid Radiology (KSThR); Korean Society of Radiology. Radiofrequency Ablation of Benign Thyroid Nodules and Recurrent Thyroid Cancers: Consensus Statement and Recommendations. *Korean J Radiol* (2012) 13 (2):117–25. doi: 10.3348/kjr.2012.13.2.117
12. Russ G, Ben Hamou A, Poirée S, Ghander C, Ménégaux F, Leenhardt L, et al. Learning Curve for Radiofrequency Ablation of Benign Thyroid Nodules. *Int J Hyperthermia* (2021) 38(1):55–64. doi: 10.1080/02656736.2021.1871974
13. Negro R, Rucco M, Creanza A, Mormile A, Limone PP, Garberoglio R, et al. Machine Learning Prediction of Radiofrequency Thermal Ablation Efficacy: A New Option to Optimize Thyroid Nodule Selection. *Eur Thyroid J* (2020) 9 (4):205–12. doi: 10.1159/000504882
14. Adam MA, Thomas S, Youngwirth L, Hyslop T, Reed SD, Scheri RP, et al. Is There a Minimum Number of Thyroidectomies a Surgeon Should Perform to Optimize Patient Outcomes? *Ann Surg* (2017) 265(2):402–7. doi: 10.1097/SLA.0000000000001688
15. Lee MT, Wang CY. Case Experience of Radiofrequency Ablation for Benign Thyroid Nodules: From an Ex Vivo Animal Study to an Initial Ablation in Taiwan. *J Med Ultrasound* (2016) 24(1):32–8. doi: 10.1016/j.jmu.2016.03.003
16. Sim JS, Baek JH. Unresolved Clinical Issues in Thermal Ablation of Benign Thyroid Nodules: Regrowth at Long-Term Follow-Up. *Korean J Radiol* (2021) 22(8):1436–40. doi: 10.3348/kjr.2021.0093
17. Jeong WK, Baek JH, Rhim H, Kim YS, Kwak MS, Jeong HJ, et al. Radiofrequency Ablation of Benign Thyroid Nodules: Safety and Imaging Follow-Up in 236 Patients. *Eur Radiol* (2008) 18(6):1244–50. doi: 10.1007/s00330-008-0880-6
18. Lin WC, Wang CK, Wang WH, Kuo CY, Chiang PL, Lin AN, et al. Multicenter Study of Benign Thyroid Nodules With Radiofrequency Ablation: Results of 762 Cases Over 4 Years in Taiwan. *J Pers Med* (2022) 12(1):63. doi: 10.3390/jpm12010063
19. Palter VN. Comprehensive Training Curricula for Minimally Invasive Surgery. *J Grad Med Educ* (2011) 3(3):293–8. doi: 10.4300/JGME-D-11-00091.1

12

Endoscopic-Assisted Transoral Thyroglossal Cyst Resection

_Shanwen Chen, Dong Wang, Jianxin Qiu, Yehai Liu and Yi Zhao_*

Department of Otorhinolaryngology-Head and Neck Surgery, The First Affiliated Hospital of Anhui Medical University, Hefei, China

Sistrunk procedure is the standard method for thyroglossal duct cyst resection. While this procedure is successful and safe, it results in postoperative scars on the front of neck. We propose a total transoral technique without external incision that starts with careful separation of the floor of the mouth and genioglossus muscle followed by the exact localization of the cyst using methylene blue. Simultaneously, the hyoid bone connected to the cyst and tract was removed. Finally, routine hemostasis is conducted, and the operative cavity is closed. All patients who received this operation in our department recovered successfully without experiencing severe intraoperative or postoperative complications.

Keywords: endoscopic surgery, thyroglossal cyst, transoral procedures, outcome, cosmetic (plastic) surgery

***Correspondence:**
Yi Zhao
zhaoyi112659@163.com

INTRODUCTION

Thyroglossal duct cyst (TGDC) is one of the most commonly observed neck masses in clinical medicine. It is characterized by an active, painless mass in the midline or slightly to one side of the neck, usually located below the hyoid bone (about 75% of patients), and can move along with the tongue. This cyst develops embryologically when the thyroid primordium descends from the base of the tongue to its typical location in front of the trachea. If the tract does not degenerate, clinical cysts may develop (1).

Sistrunk procedure is the widely accepted surgical treatment for TGDC and is similar to open thyroid surgery. This procedure entails the removal of the central part of hyoid bone and thyroid remnants. However, the procedure leaves a roughly 5 cm scar in front of the neck.

Kim et al. (2) were the first to report a successful transoral TGDC resection. No other teams have reported the clinical application of this method. Considering different details, our goal is to share our experience with this approach. Informed consent and ethical review were obtained (IRB number: PJ2021-03-22).

METHODS

We describe this procedure using the example of a 24-year-old woman who required it for cosmetic purposes. Therefore, we decided to perform a scarless procedure. **Figure 1** illustrates relevant anatomical diagrams. The proposed technique was conducted under general anesthesia and oral endotracheal intubation. To maintain oral operating space, a unilateral oral distractor was employed. Subsequently, methylene blue was injected into the cyst from the outside (**Figure 2A**).

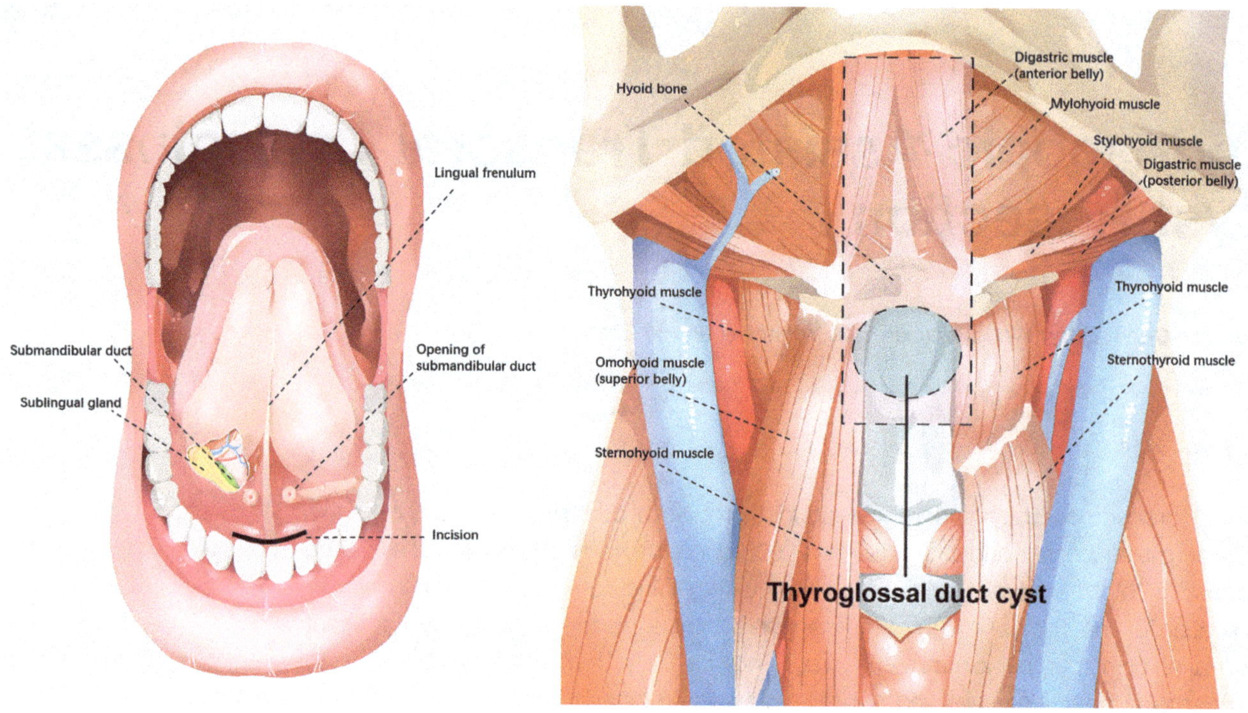

FIGURE 1 | Illustration of anatomy.

At the oral lingual frenulum, a transverse incision of about 2 cm in length was made (**Figure 2B**). The soft tissue of the mouth floor was meticulously dissected, and genioglossus muscles with marked morphological characteristics were identified, separated, and retracted bilaterally (**Figure 2C**). Using a 4 mm rigid nasal endoscope, we longitudinally separated and transected suprahyoid muscles (**Figure 2D**). Then the hyoid bone was located and identified (**Figure 3A**). The hyoid bone's body was then cut using a Kerrison rongeur (**Figure 3B**). Following this step, it was often found that the partially blue-stained cyst remained in the operation cavity. We employed a cryogenic plasma knife to transect the infrahyoid muscles at a distance of 0.5 cm from the hyoid bone. By pulling the hyoid bone upward using forceps, the cyst was completely exposed. Using a plasma knife, the tissue surrounding the cyst was meticulously dissected, and the hyoid bone was pulled out (**Figure 3C**). The hyoid bone and cyst were removed together (**Figure 3D**). After sufficient hemostasis, the operative cavity was flushed with distilled water. A drainage tube was inserted from the mouth floor and fixed under the chin. Finally, the oral mucosa was sutured with a 4-0 suture and bandaged with external neck pressure (**Video 1, Supporting Information**).

The drain was removed when drainage volume was less than 5 mL per 24 h. After operation, no special dietary restrictions were found, and patients were given saline to gargle and maintain their mouth clean. Patients were discharged two days following extubation unless there were special circumstances and were required to comply with regular outpatient follow-up.

RESULTS

Our technique was successful in five patients. The characteristics of patients and operations are listed in **Table 1**. During at least a half-year follow-up, no recurrences or peri/postoperative complications were observed, and all patients achieved excellent cosmetic outcomes with their necks (**Figures 4** and **5**).

DISCUSSION

After diagnosis with a thyroglossal duct cyst, patients tended to seek surgical treatment with an otolaryngologist. A standard Sistrunk procedure is often adopted to resect the lesion. However, growing esthetic concerns motivate patients to seek cosmetic treatment for their unsightly scar in the neck. While the auxiliary use of local drugs and the improvement of surgical hardware can indeed reduce the obvious degree of postoperative scarring, they can also introduce complications such as pruritus and local pain.

Currently, researchers have focused on hidden scars or scarless cosmetic surgery. Cai et al. (3) used endoscope-assisted surgery to successfully resect TGDC *via* a small submental incision, but scarring remains inevitable. One study published by Qu et al. (4) presented a study in which they successfully executed the breast approach on 13 patients, but one had an infection, one developed skin bruising, and another had subcutaneous fluid. Anuwong et al. (5) also completed this

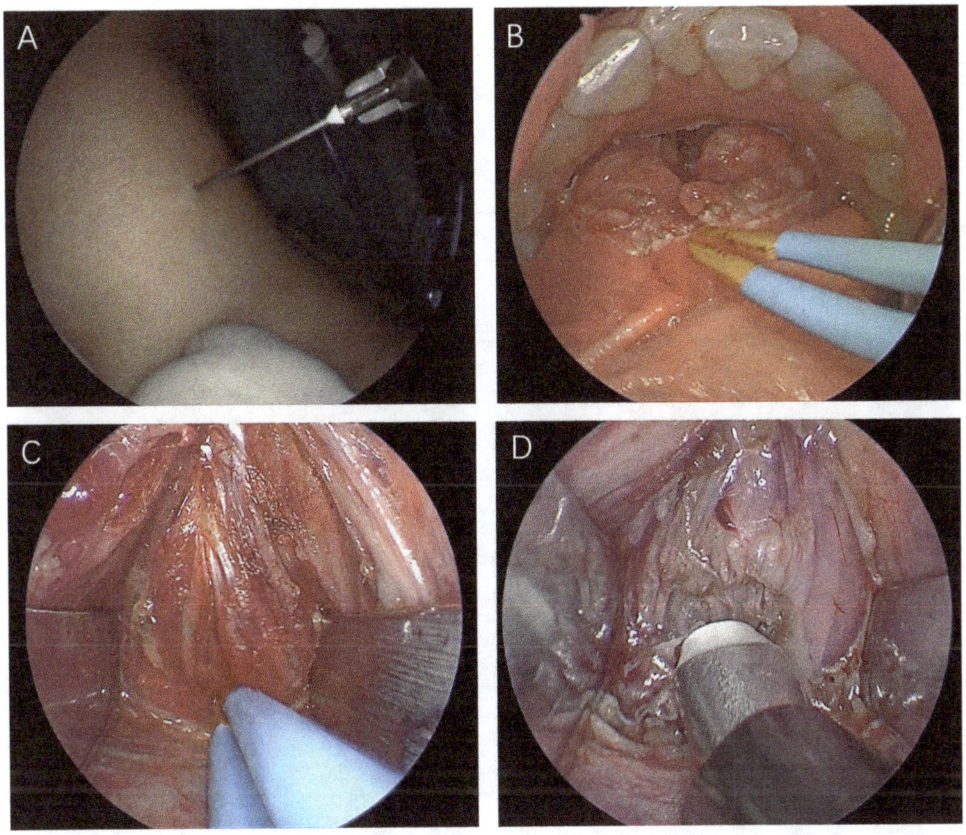

FIGURE 2 | **(A)** Methylene blue injection. **(B)** Transverse frenotomy incision. **(C)** The genioglossus muscles were retracted bilaterally. **(D)** Transection of suprahyoid muscles.

operation with the bilateral areola approach. Considering the author's experience with endoscopic surgery, none of the 11 patients included in their study experienced postoperative complications, and the operation time was shorter. Paek et al. (6) successfully completed TGDC resection for two patients using the bilateral axillo-breast approach. However, this procedure requires more incisions. Kim et al. (7) and Lee et al. (8) selected the retroauricular approach, successfully removed TGDC with robot assistance, and the incision can be hidden, but the costs and hardware constraints obstruct wider accessibility. Han et al. (9) and Banuchi et al. (10) completed the operation by employing the transoral vestibular approach. The former adopts a single incision without insufflation, while the latter adopts the same three incisions with CO_2 insufflation as the vestibular approach for thyroid. Both operations were completed successfully without complications. However, the single incision method of Han et al. (9) does not avoid the problem of narrow operation space. Asians have a relatively flat jaw, which may impede the use of this

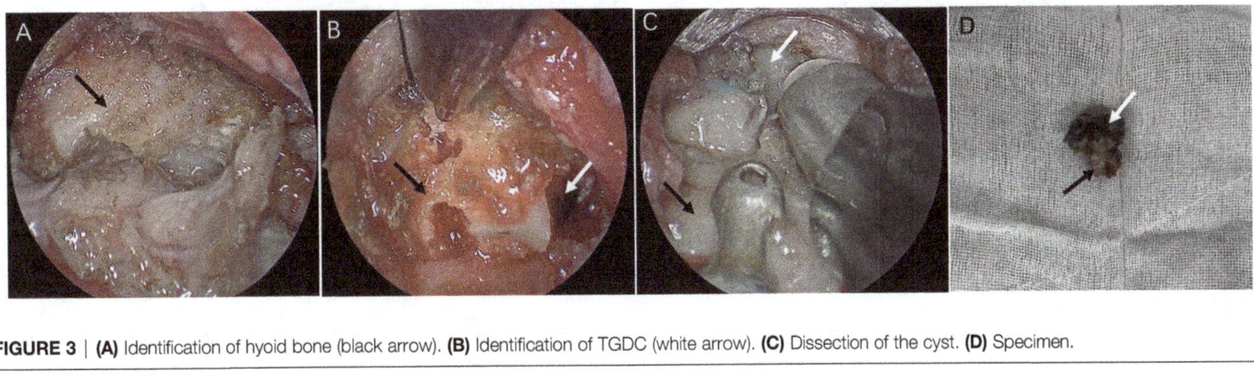

FIGURE 3 | **(A)** Identification of hyoid bone (black arrow). **(B)** Identification of TGDC (white arrow). **(C)** Dissection of the cyst. **(D)** Specimen.

TABLE 1 | Patient demographics and outcomes for undergoing transoral approach for TGDC.

Patient	Age,y	Sex	Lesion size (cm)	Operative time (min)	Bleeding volume (ml)	Drainage volume (ml)	Complication
1	43	Female	1.5×1.2×0.5	180	10	10	None
2	42	Female	2.0×2.0×1.0	190	10	35	None
3	24	Female	1.5×1.0×0.6	210	15	10	None
4	34	Female	2.0×1.0×0.5	165	15	20	None
5	22	Female	2.0×1.4×0.4	130	5	30	None

TGDC, thyroglossal duct cyst.

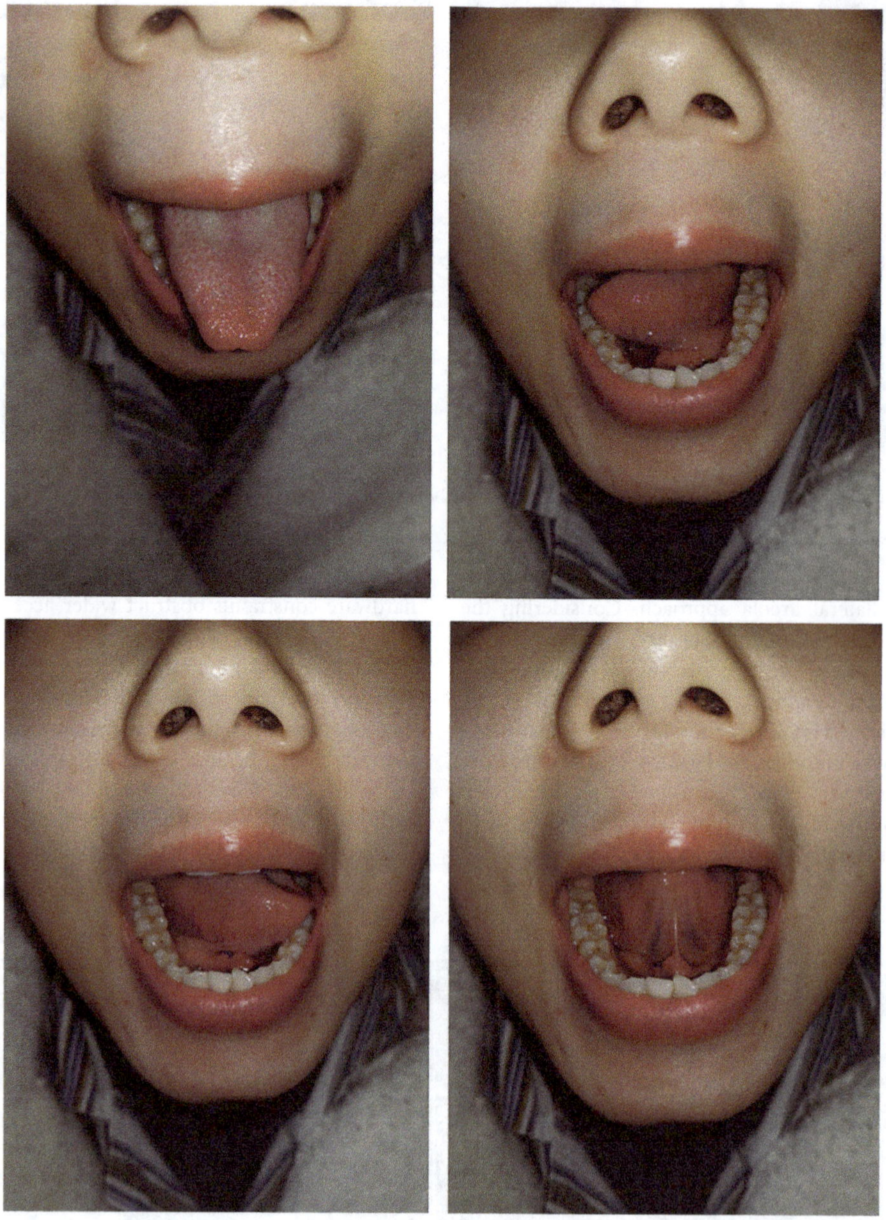

FIGURE 4 | Tongue movement after operation.

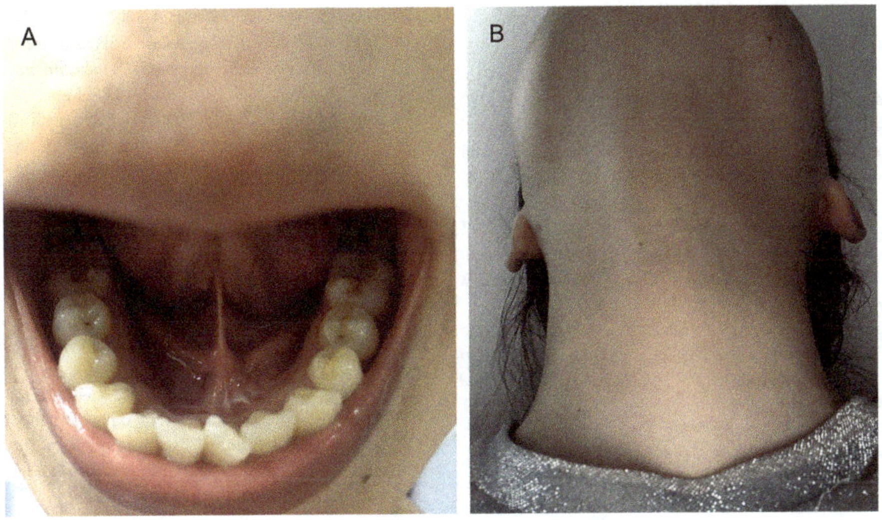

FIGURE 5 | **(A)** Incision at 6-month follow-up. **(B)** Appearance at 6-month follow-up.

technology among other races. Compared with the above approaches, the distance of frenotomy incision is the shortest, and this approach conforms to the law of anatomy. The surgical path is positioned in the midline without important vessels and nerves and does not require extensive tissue dissection and CO_2 insufflation, which avoids possible complications of hypercapnia and numbness in the operation area. However, it should be noted that limitations are still present. The frenotomy incision may bring the risk of incision infection; sublingual edema may cause airway obstruction; narrow operation space significantly increases the difficulty of this procedure, requiring more patience and time. Our operation time was between two and four hours, while the time reported by Woo et al. (11) was about one hour. Similarly, the operation time of Anuwong et al. (5) is also shorter compared with Qu et al. (4) We believe that this technique can be executed more efficiently as experience grows.

The tongue must be retracted upward to expose the mouth floor and the frenum. After recognizing Wharton's duct orifice, we made a frenotomy incision closer to the mandible. Then, blunt separation was used for tissue dissection. In so doing, risk of Wharton's duct injury can be avoided (12). The next issue is the limited operating space, implying why we used 4 mm nasal endoscope. Based on our experience, it is critical to precisely locate the cyst when using the transoral approach. As a result, we used methylene blue for intraoperative localization. The next step requires the surgeon to have extensive experience with endoscopic procedures to avoid cyst rupture because the rupture would lead to blue staining in the operation field, making boundary identification is difficult.

At present, there remain a few reports on endoscopic TGDC surgery, and there are insufficient materials to define indications and contraindications of this operation. In our study, the patients had strong cosmetic intentions and had no history of neck surgery, neck radiotherapy, thyroglossal cyst infection, or thyroglossal fistula. In the above literature, most specimens are 2-3 cm, with the largest specimen of 6 cm in the study of Woo et al. (11) There is no consensus on lesion size limitation. In our method, syringe can be utilized to extract part of the capsule, which may overcome the sample size limitation, but this must be confirmed by follow-up research.

CONCLUSION

TGDC removal using a frenotomy incision is an alternative to conventional procedure with a safe, effective, cosmetic, and well-tolerated outcome. However, because the sample size was relatively small, additional research on indications, complications, and recurrences is still required.

ETHICS STATEMENT

The studies involving human participants were reviewed and approved by Ethics Committee of the First Affiliated Hospital of Anhui Medical University. The patients/participants provided their written informed consent to participate in this study.

AUTHOR CONTRIBUTIONS

Concept and design: All authors. Acquisition, analysis, or interpretation of data: All authors. Drafting of the manuscript: SC. Critical revision of the manuscript for important intellectual content: All authors. Statistical analysis: SC. Administrative, technical, or material support: All authors. Supervision: YZ. All authors contributed to the article and approved the submitted version.

REFERENCES

1. Thompson LD. Thyroglossal Duct Cyst. *Ear Nose Throat J* (2017) 96:54–5. doi: 10.1177/014556131709600204
2. Kim JP, Park JJ, Lee EJ, Woo SH. Intraoral Removal of a Thyroglossal Duct Cyst Using a Frenotomy Incision. *Thyroid* (2011) 21:1381–4. doi: 10.1089/thy.2011.0180
3. Cai Q, Huang X, Liang F, Chen J, Liang M, Pan Y, et al. Endoscope-Assisted Concurrent Resection of Thyroglossal Duct Cysts and Benign Thyroid Nodules *via* a Small Submental Incisions. *Eur Arch Otorhinolaryngol* (2014) 271:1771–5. doi: 10.1007/s00405-013-2688-5
4. Qu R, Wang C, Dong Z, Li J, Liu D. Another Strategy for the Treatment of Thyroglossal Duct Cyst: Totally Endoscopic Surgery by Breast Approach. *Surg Laparosc Endosc Percutan Tech* (2018) 28:118–22. doi: 10.1097/SLE.0000000000000514
5. Anuwong A, Jitpratoom P, Sasanakietkul T. Bilateral Areolar Endoscopic Sistrunk Operation: A Novel Technique for Thyroglossal Duct Cyst Surgery. *Surg Endosc* (2017) 31:1993–8. doi: 10.1007/s00464-016-5137-x
6. Paek SH, Choi JY, Lee K-E, Youn Y-K. Bilateral Axillo-Breast Approach (BABA) Endoscopic Sistrunk Operation in Patients With Thyroglossal Duct Cyst: Technical Report of the Novel Endoscopic Sistrunk Operation. *Surg Laparosc Endosc Percutan Tech* (2014) 24:e95–8. doi: 10.1097/SLE.0b013e31828fa7bf
7. Kim C-H, Byeon HK, Shin YS, Koh YW, Choi EC. Robot-Assisted Sistrunk Operation *via* a Retroauricular Approach for Thyroglossal Duct Cyst. *Head Neck* (2014) 36:456–8. doi: 10.1002/hed.23422
8. Lee DW, Tae K. Robot-Assisted Excision of Thyroglossal Duct Cyst by a Postauricular Facelift Approach. *Wideochir Inne Tech Maloinwazyjne* (2020) 15:245–8. doi: 10.5114/wiitm.2019.88751
9. Han P, Liang F, Cai Q, Chen R, Yu S, Huang X. Endoscope-Assisted Resection of Thyroglossal Duct Cysts *via* a Submaxillary Vestibular Approach. *Head Neck* (2018) 40:377–83. doi: 10.1002/hed.24972
10. Banuchi VE, Long SM, Sachs BY, Kostas JC, Ali KM, Russell JO. Transoral Endoscopic Vestibular Approach Sistrunk Procedure: First Reported Case Series. *Head Neck* (2021) 44:1–5. doi: 10.1002/hed.26889
11. Woo SH, Park JJ, Hong JC, Wang S-G, Park GC, Eun YG, et al. Endoscope-Assisted Transoral Removal of a Thyroglossal Duct Cyst Using a Frenotomy Incision: A Prospective Clinical Trial. *Laryngoscope* (2015) 125:2730–5. doi: 10.1002/lary.25508
12. Wilhelm T, Harlaar JJ, Kerver A, Kleinrensink G-J, Benhidjeb T. Surgical Anatomy of the Floor of the Oral Cavity and the Cervical Spaces as a Rationale for Trans-Oral, Minimal-Invasive Endoscopic Surgical Procedures: Results of Anatomical Studies. *Eur Arch Otorhinolaryngol* (2010) 267:1285–90. doi: 10.1007/s00405-010-1219-x

13

Comparison of Different Mandibular Jawlines Classifications on Transoral Endoscopic Thyroidectomy for Papillary Thyroid Carcinoma

Xing Yu[1], Yuancong Jiang[2], Yujun Li[2], Qionghua He[2], Lei Pan[2], Peifeng Zhu[2], Yong Wang[1] and Ping Wang[1*]*

[1] *Department of Thyroid Surgery, The Second Affiliated Hospital, Zhejiang University School of Medicine, Hangzhou, China,*
[2] *College of Medicine, Zhejiang University, Hangzhou, China*

Correspondence:
Yong Wang
surgwy@zju.edu.cn
Ping Wang
p.wang@zju.edu.cn

Background: The influences of patients' different mandibular jawlines on transoral endoscopic thyroidectomy *via* vestibular approach (TOETVA) have not been described before. The objective of this study was to introduce a new classification to assess different mandibular jawlines, and to evaluate the effects on TOETVA in terms of safety, feasibility, and postoperative feelings in the treatment of papillary thyroid carcinoma (PTC).

Methods: The crossing angle of esthetic plane and mandibular plane was defined as Wang Angle, used to assess patients' different mandibular jawlines. Mandibular classifications of A (angle: 80° ~ 110°), B (angle > 110°), and C (angle < 80°) types were compared to evaluate the surgical outcomes of TOETVA by a retrospective study. 690 patients of PTC who received TOETVA were included in this study, which were divided into three groups according to mandibular classifications.

Results: Clinicopathological characteristics of the patients including age, gender, body mass index, tumor size, Hashimoto thyroiditis were similar in the three groups. Patients' length of jay in group C was significantly longer than group A and group B ($P < 0.01$). The ratios of using suspension system in group C were significantly higher than group A and group B ($P < 0.01$). The scores of postoperative visual analogue scale (VAS) and ratios of mandibular swell in group C were significantly higher than group A and group B ($P < 0.01$). There was no significant difference in the three groups regarding surgical outcomes, including postoperative vocal cord paralysis, hypocalcemia, serum white blood cells and C-reactive protein levels.

Conclusions: The Wang angle and mandibular jawline classifications were firstly introduced in TOETVA. All the patients of class A, B, and C mandibular jawline can achieve safe and effective surgical outcomes in the treatment of PTC with TOETVA. Patients of class C need more assistance of suspension system, would experience higher scores of VAS, and higher ratios of mandibular swell compared with class A and B.

Keywords: mandibular jawlines, length of jay, transoral endoscopic thyroidectomy, papillary thyroid carcinoma, surgical outcomes

INTRODUCTION

Transoral endoscopic thyroidectomy is new that does not cause neck scarring and requires a smaller subcutaneous flap elevation than that of remote access thyroid surgery methods (1). Because of these advantages above, there has been a rapid development of transoral endoscopic thyroidectomy *via* vestibular approach (TOETVA) in the past 10 years (2). However, the influences of patients' different mandibular jawlines on TOETVA have not been described before (3). The angle's classifications of malocclusion were initially used to assess the mesio-distal relationships of the dental arches (4), which was modified by us and used to assess the mandibular jawlines. The objective of this study was to introduce a new classification of mandibular jawlines into transoral endoscopic thyroidectomy, and to evaluate the effects on TOETVA in terms of safety, feasibility, surgical outcomes, and postoperative feelings in the treatment of papillary thyroid carcinoma (PTC).

MATERIALS AND METHODS

Patients' Enrollment

Between January 2015 and June 2020, we retrospectively enrolled 690 patients with PTC who underwent total thyroidectomy or ipsilateral thyroidectomy and lymph node dissection of central compartment in the Second Affiliated Hospital, Zhejiang University School of Medicine. All enrolled patients had cosmetic requirements, and they chose the operation of TOETVA. Patients were divided into three groups according to the different types of mandibular jawlines. The clinicopathological characteristics such as age, gender, body mass index (BMI), tumor size, multiple lesions ratio, and Hashimoto's thyroiditis ratio were compared in the three groups. This study was approved by the ethical committee of the Second Affiliated Hospital of Zhejiang University School of Medicine.

Introduction of Wang Angle and Mandibular Jawlines Classifications

The crossing angle of esthetic plane and mandibular plane was defined as Wang Angle (**Figure 1**). Patients' different mandibular jawlines were classified into three types according to the degree of Wang Angle, including A (angle: 80° ~ 110°), B (angle > 110°), and C (angle < 80°) types. This new classification was firstly introduced in TOETVA. As shown in the **Figure 1**, patients' different mandibular jawlines were exhibited with schematic diagrams and realistic photos. The Wang Angle of each patient was defined as the crossing of esthetic plane and mandibular plane (red line), which was used to assess the different mandibular jawline classifications.

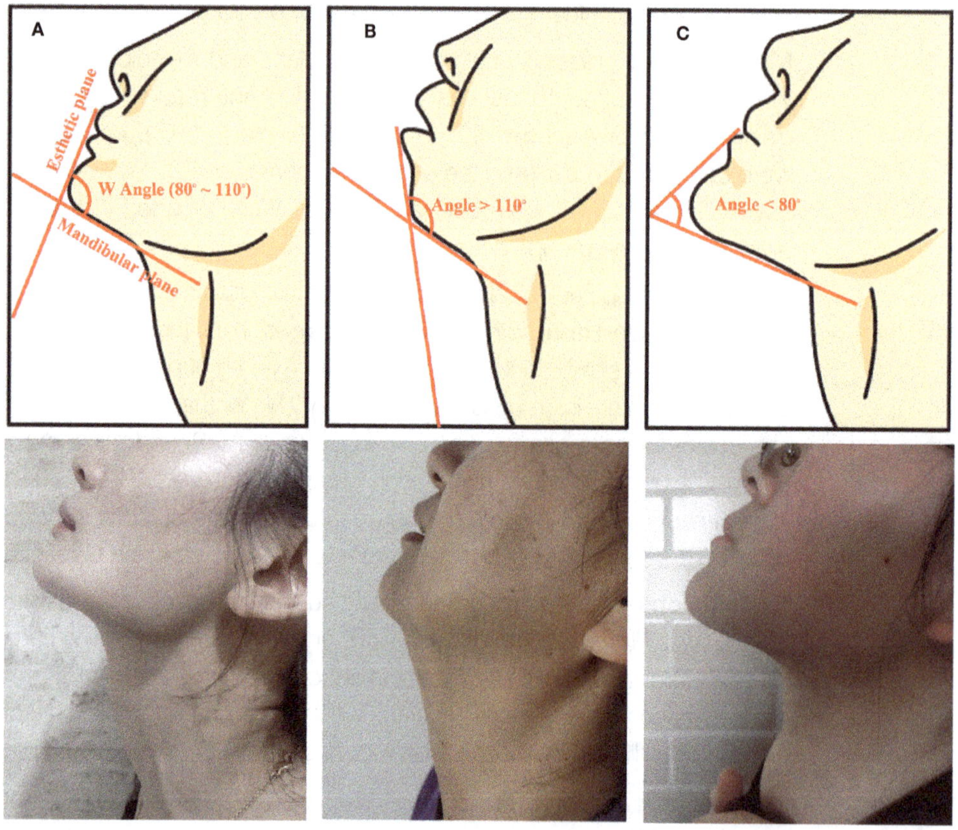

FIGURE 1 | Schematic diagram and realistic photos of the three classifications: **(A)** (angle: 80° ~ 110°), **(B)** (angle > 110°), and **(C)** (angle < 80°) types.

Measure the Length of Jaw

The length of jaw was measured in the A, B, and C types of mandibular jawlines. The length of jaw is a quantitative index, which may be useful to evaluate the level of difficulty to maintain the surgical space in TOETVA. As shown in **Figure 2**, patients were chosen horizontal position, and the length of jaw was defined as the distance from anterior neck plane to the anterior border plane of jaw (red line). The length was measured by a flexible ruler, which was analyzed and compared in the three groups.

Procedures of TOETVA

The procedures of TOETVA were briefly described in the following. A 10-mm incision for the camera port was cautiously made in the middle of the vestibule and frenulum. Another two 5-mm trocars were applied through the mucosa incision at the level of the first premolars for auxiliary use. A 30° angled camera was then advanced through the 10-mm port. Ultrasonic coagulation devices (Harmonic Scalpel, Ethicon Endosurgery, USA) were used to manage thyroid surrounding vessels and the inferior thyroid arteries (5). Thyroid gland was completely resected, and central node dissection (CND) was conducted including the prelaryngeal, pretracheal, and paratracheal areas (6).

Comparison of Surgical Outcomes

Preoperative laryngoscope, thyroid hormones, parathyroid hormone (PTH) and calcium were recorded 3 days before surgery. Postoperative laryngoscope, laboratory tests including PTH, calcium, white blood cell (WBC), and C-reactive protein (CRP) were examined at the day next to the operation. Thyroid hormones, PTH, and calcium were detected at one month postoperatively. Patients receive postoperative review every 3 months after surgery, thyroid function and cervical B ultrasound were included each time.

Statistical Analysis

The results are presented as number (%) and average ± SD appropriate. Data were analyzed by one-way ANOVA, Welch ANOVA, student *t*-test, the $\chi 2$ test, Fisher's exact test, and non-parametric Wilcoxon-Mann-Whitney test appropriately using SPSS 20.0 software (SPSS Inc., Chicago, IL, USA). A p value less than 0.05 was considered to be statistically significant.

RESULTS

Clinicopathologic Characteristics

The clinicopathologic characteristics were summarized in **Table 1**. This study enrolled 690 patients, comprising 342 (Type A), 281 (Type B), and 67 (Type C) patients respectively. Patient's age, sex ratio, and BMI were similar in the groups of type A, B, and C. Tumor characteristics were compared in the three groups, and there was no significant difference in the max tumor size, multiple lesions ratio, and Hashimoto's thyroiditis ratio. Total thyroidectomy ratio was similar between the three groups of type A, B, and C respectively. The length of jaw was compared and has significant difference in the three groups ($P < 0.01$). In the pairwise comparison, the length of jaw in group C was significantly more than group A (7.26 ± 0.23 *vs.* 6.85 ± 0.23, $P < 0.01$), and group B (7.26 ± 0.23 *vs.* 6.17 ± 0.42, $P < 0.01$). And the length of jaw in group A was also more than group B significantly (6.85 ± 0.23 *vs.* 6.17 ± 0.42, $P < 0.01$).

Postoperative Feelings

The ratio of mandibular swell and visual analogue scale (VAS) feeling were compared in the three groups. As shown in **Table 2**, the ratio of mandibular swell was compared and has significant difference in the three groups ($P < 0.01$). In the pairwise comparison, the ratio of mandibular swell in group C was significantly more than group A (10.4% *vs.* 1.2%, $P < 0.01$), and group B (10.4% *vs.* 0.7%, $P < 0.01$). While there was no significant difference in the comparison of mandibular swell between group A and group B (1.2% *vs.* 0.7%, $P = 0.560$). The scores of VAS were compared and has significant difference in the three groups ($P < 0.01$). In the pairwise comparison, the scores of VAS in group C was significantly more than group A (2.1 ± 0.6 *vs.* 1.7 ± 0.5, $P < 0.01$), and group B (2.1 ± 0.6 *vs.* 1.7 ± 0.5, $P < 0.01$). While there was no significant difference in the comparison of VAS scores between group A and group B (1.7 ± 0.5 *vs.* 1.7 ± 0.5, $P = 0.980$).

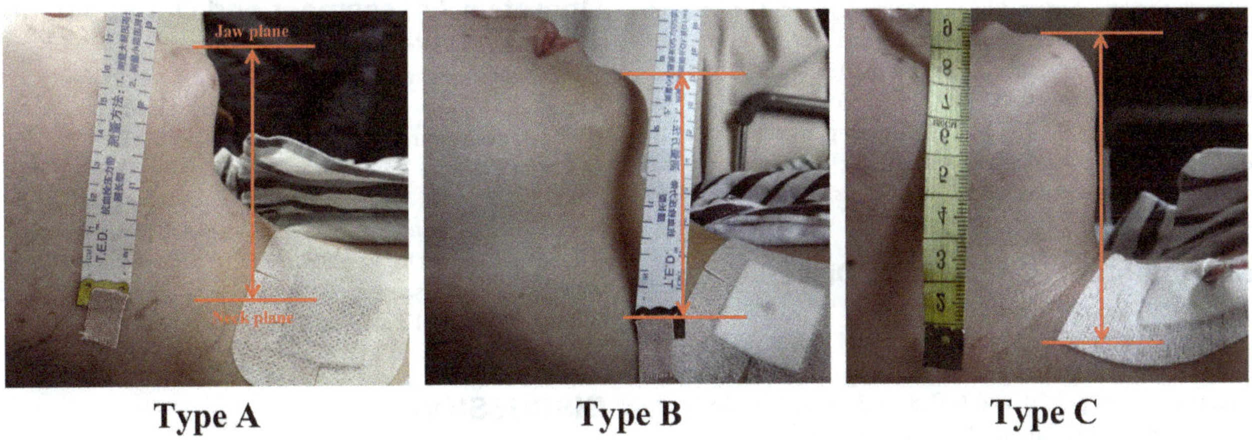

FIGURE 2 | The length of jay was measured from anterior neck plane to the anterior border plane of jaw (red line) in the three groups.

TABLE 1 | Comparation of clinicopathological characteristics in the groups of type A, B, and C.

	Type A (n = 342)	Type B (n = 281)	Type C (n = 67)	*P value*
Age (years)	37.3 ± 9.8	37.6 ± 9.9	35.8 ± 9.2	0.423
Male (%)	90 (26.3%)	74 (26.3%)	25 (37.3%)	0.159
BMI (kg/m^2)	23.7 ± 3.7	23.7 ± 3.7	23.9 ± 3.8	0.825
Max tumor size (cm)	1.23 ± 0.59	1.20 ± 0.61	1.31 ± 0.71	0.175
Multiple lesions (%)	81 (23.7%)	88 (31.3%)	22 (32.8%)	0.065
Hashimoto's thyroiditis (%)	100 (29.2%)	97 (34.5%)	25 (27.3%)	0.238
Total thyroidectomy (%)	111 (32.5%)	98 (34.9%)	25 (37.3%)	0.675
Bilateral CND (%)	108 (31.6%)	96 (34.2%)	19 (28.4%)	0.606
Length of jaw (cm)	6.85 ± 0.23	6.17 ± 0.42	7.26 ± 0.23	<0.01

BMI, body mass index; CND, central node dissection.

TABLE 2 | Effective assessment of surgical results in the groups of type A, B, and C malocclusion.

	Type A (n = 342)	Type B (n = 281)	Type C (n = 67)	*P value*
EMG changes (%)	28 (8.2%)	21 (7.5%)	2 (3.0%)	0.330
Transient vocal cord paralysis (%)	7 (2.0%)	9 (3.2%)	1 (1.5%)	0.563
Postoperative PTH (pg/ml)	34.7 ± 16.5	36.0 ± 18.4	35.7 ± 18.9	0.642
Postoperative calcium	2.09 ± 0.14	2.11 ± 0.13	2.08 ± 0.13	0.360
numbness in limbs (%)	36 (10.5%)	30 (10.7%)	10 (14.9%)	0.559
Total number of CLN	8.83 ± 5.75	9.16 ± 6.14	8.67 ± 4.61	0.715
Number of metastatic CLN	1.70 ± 2.41	1.64 ± 2.37	1.84 ± 2.57	0.827
WBC (×10^9/L)	9.2 ± 2.7	9.5 ± 4.7	9.9 ± 2.9	0.330
Postoperative CRP (mg/L)	8.3 ± 7.0	9.3 ± 8.3	9.4 ± 7.7	0.172
Operative time (min)	116.2 ± 44.3	118.5 ± 46.6	121.7 ± 40.3	0.601
Mandibular swell	4 (1.2%)	2 (0.7%)	7 (10.4%)	<0.01
Visual VAS	1.7 ± 0.5	1.7 ± 0.5	2.1 ± 0.6	<0.01
Hospital stay (days)	3.89 ± 1.09	3.99 ± 1.07	3.88 ± 1.12	0.515
Quality of life	7.89 ± 0.80	7.94 ± 0.71	7.88 ± 0.69	0.609

EMG, electromyography; PTH, parathyroid hormone; CLN, central lymph nodes; WBC, white blood cell; CRP, C-reactive protein; VAS, visual analogue scale.

Surgical Complications

The surgical complications, including postoperative vocal cord paralysis and hypocalcemia were recorded. The electromyography (EMG) changes during the surgery, and the complains of hoarseness and laryngoscope examinations postoperatively were recorded. As shown in **Table 2**, there was no significant difference in the comparison of EMG changes (8.2% *vs.* 7.5% *vs.* 3.0%, $P = 0.330$) and post-operative transient vocal cord paralysis (2.0% *vs.* 3.2% *vs.* 1.5%, $P = 0.563$) in the groups of A, B, and C type. No permanent vocal cord paralysis occurred in all the three groups. The levels of PTH and serum calcium were recorded at the next day postoperatively. It was similar in PTH levels (34.7 ± 16.5 *vs.* 36.0 ± 18.4 *vs.* 35.7 ± 18.9, $P = 0.642$) and serum calcium (2.09 ± 0.14 *vs.* 2.11 ± 0.13 *vs.* 2.08 ± 0.13, $P = 0.360$) in the comparison of type A, B, and C. The incidences of numbness in limbs were also similar in the comparison of type A, B, and C (10.5% *vs.* 10.7% *vs.* 14.9%, $P = 0.559$).

Comparison of Lymph Node Dissection in the Central Compartment

The total number and metastatic central lymph nodes (CLN) were recorded. It was similar in the total number of CLN in the comparison of group A, B, and C (8.83 ± 5.75 *vs.* 9.16 ± 6.14 *vs.* 8.67 ± 4.61, $P = 0.715$). And no difference was found in the number of metastatic CLN in the comparison of group A, B, and C (1.70 ± 2.41 *vs.* 1.64 ± 2.37 *vs.* 1.84 ± 2.57, $P = 0.827$).

Comparison of Postoperative Inflammatory Response

WBC and CRP were recorded to assess the postoperative inflammatory response. There was no difference in the number of WBC in the comparison of group A, B, and C (9.2 ± 2.7 *vs.* 9.5 ± 4.7 *vs.* 9.9 ± 2.9, $P = 0.330$). And it was similar in postoperative CRP level in the comparison of group A, B, and C (8.3 ± 7.0 *vs.* 9.3 ± 8.3 *vs.* 9.4 ± 7.7, $P = 0.172$).

Operative Assessment and Qof Evaluation in the Follow-Up

The operative time and postoperative hospital stay were recorded. And the Quality of life (Qof) was assessed at 3 months postoperatively during the follow-up. The operative time was similar in the three groups of type A, B, and C (116.2 ± 44.3 *vs.* 118.5 ± 46.6 *vs.* 121.7 ± 40.3, $P = 0.601$). And it was similar in the comparation of postoperative hospital stay in the three groups (3.89 ± 1.09 *vs.* 3.99 ± 1.07 *vs.* 3.88 ± 1.12, $P = 0.515$). There was no difference in Qof assessment in the three groups of type A, B, and C (7.89 ± 0.80 *vs.* 7.94 ± 0.71 *vs.* 7.88 ± 0.69, $P = 0.609$).

DISCUSSION

Since a large case series of transoral endoscopic thyroidectomy was reported in 2016, multiple hospital centers worldwide have introduced this technique and reported their initial experience (7). Up to now, transoral endoscopic thyroidectomy *via* vestibular approach (TOETVA) has become one of the most widely used techniques in scarless endoscopic thyroidectomy (8). Our group has reported a large cohort of TOETVA cases, in which we demonstrated that transoral endoscopic thyroidectomy has the same surgical safety compared with total endoscopic thyroidectomy *via* areola approach, and conventional open thyroidectomy (9). Recently, it has been found by us that the surgical outcomes of transoral endoscopic thyroidectomy are safe in the treatment of PTC with a diameter between > 1cm and ≤ 3.5cm (3).

Hence, we compared the different classified types of mandibular jawlines on TOETVA. It was found safe of TOETVA in the treatment of PTC patients with all the three types of mandibular jawlines. No case was needed to transverse conventional open choice in all the 690 cases. No significant difference was found in the comparison of surgical complications in the types of A, B, and C, including postoperative vocal cord paralysis and hypoparathyroidism. Mental nerve injury is a unique complication of TOETVA (10). And the incidence of mental nerve injury is quite diverse (11). In our institute, only 2 cases of mental nerve injury were detected at the initial period after TOETVA performed. There was no mental nerve injury found in this study of 690 PTC cases. These results might provide evidence mental nerve injury rarely occurs with TOETVA in all the patients of class A, B, and C mandibular jawline.

The effect and feasibility were also verified with the largest case series of TOETVA for PTC in the present study. Total and metastatic number of central lymph nodes were similar in the comparison of all the three types, which represents the effect was similar during the implementation of TOETVA in the patients of type A, B, and C. The postoperative inflammatory response, including WBC and CRP, were recorded similar, which represents the feasibility of TOETVA was comparable in type A, B and C.

According to the results of comparative analyses, the length of jaw in the patients of type C was significantly more than type A and B. Due the longer jawline, it had more difficulty in maintaining the surgical space, and the ratios of using suspension assisted system in the patients of type C were also higher than type A and B significantly. Additionally, patients of type C experienced a higher ratio of mandibular swell, and the mandibular swell would be absorbed at 7 ~ 10 days post TOETVA. Patients of type C had higher scores of VAS at the next day post TOETVA, and the pain feelings would be reduced at 3 ~ 5 days post TOETVA according to our experience. Moreover, there was no difference found in the comparison of Qof in the period of follow-up, which represents the longtime postoperative feelings were similar in the comparison of type A, B, and C. Furthermore, several innovative techniques were implemented in TOETVA, which was useful to maintain the surgical space, especially in the patients of type C.

Injecting Epinephrine Solution

Epinephrine solution of diluted adrenaline solution (1:500 000) was injected from the vestibule to the anterior of the neck at the subcutaneous layer (12). The uneven surface of the mandibular would be topped up by the epinephrine solution. Additionally, diluted adrenaline contributed to microvascular constriction, which would be helpful to reduce bleeding during the process of space creating.

Real-Time Observation

We firstly designed a visual separation device, which was used for the separation of skin flap (13). The visual separation bar has a see-through head, could be used for real-time observation during blunt separation. The correct fascia layer is shown white, while a yellow appearance means over superficial or fat layer, and red appearance been over deep or muscle layer. With this help, the tissue separation layer could be adjusted at any time during the process of flap dissection. Additionally, anterior jugular microvascular could also be observed, which would be helpful to avoid bleeding in the procedure of building working space.

Hybrid Space-Maintaining Method

The hybrid space-maintaining system combining constant low pressure gas insufflation with a flap lifting device. We have reported this method before, which was described briefly in the following (14). During the operation, the CO_2 was insufflated and maintained at a low pressure of 6 mm Hg. Additionally, the flap was lifted to expand the space by wires or silk sutures, which retracted by a suspension system. As the critical device of suspension system, a disinfected L-shaped pole was wrapped by a sterile protective cover and then fixed on the side of the head as the suspension frame.

Add Another Vacuum Tube for Working Space Building

The middle curvilinear incision was expanded to 2 cm, which used for observation port and another vacuum tube. Vacuum tube shore up and air inhalation were alternatively used for flap suspension during working space building. Order to reduce the smoke circumstance, the operation space was kept a negative pressure during the whole process. Additional vacuum tube was placed next to the observation port for flap suspension to keep the operation space under negative pressure (**Figure 3**). And the vacuum tube could also be used for air inhalation when much smoke generated in the surgical circumstance.

The Advantages and Disadvantages of TOETVA

TOETVA provides a cranial-caudal perspective that can better expose and more completely central nodes dissection, especially for the lower part including levels VI and VII (15). However, it increases difficulty of handling the thyroid superior pole at the beginning, identifying the superior thyroid artery and superior laryngeal nerve (SLN) (16). Due to the limitations, it is important to evaluate whether different mandibular jawline types would increase the surgical complications in TOETVA. In this study, all tumors were completely removed, and no skin flap disruption or permanent SLN injury occurred. And the different mandibular jawline types, especially for type C, can be overcome with the development of operative proficiency and the improvement of surgical instruments. Additionally, patients chosen TOETVA had

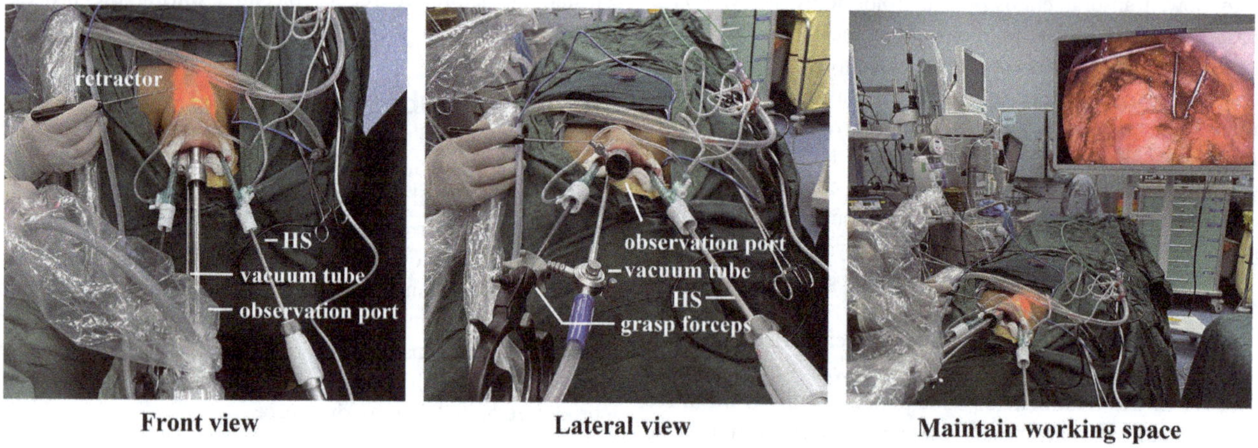

FIGURE 3 | Introduce another vacuum tube for working space building in TOETVA.

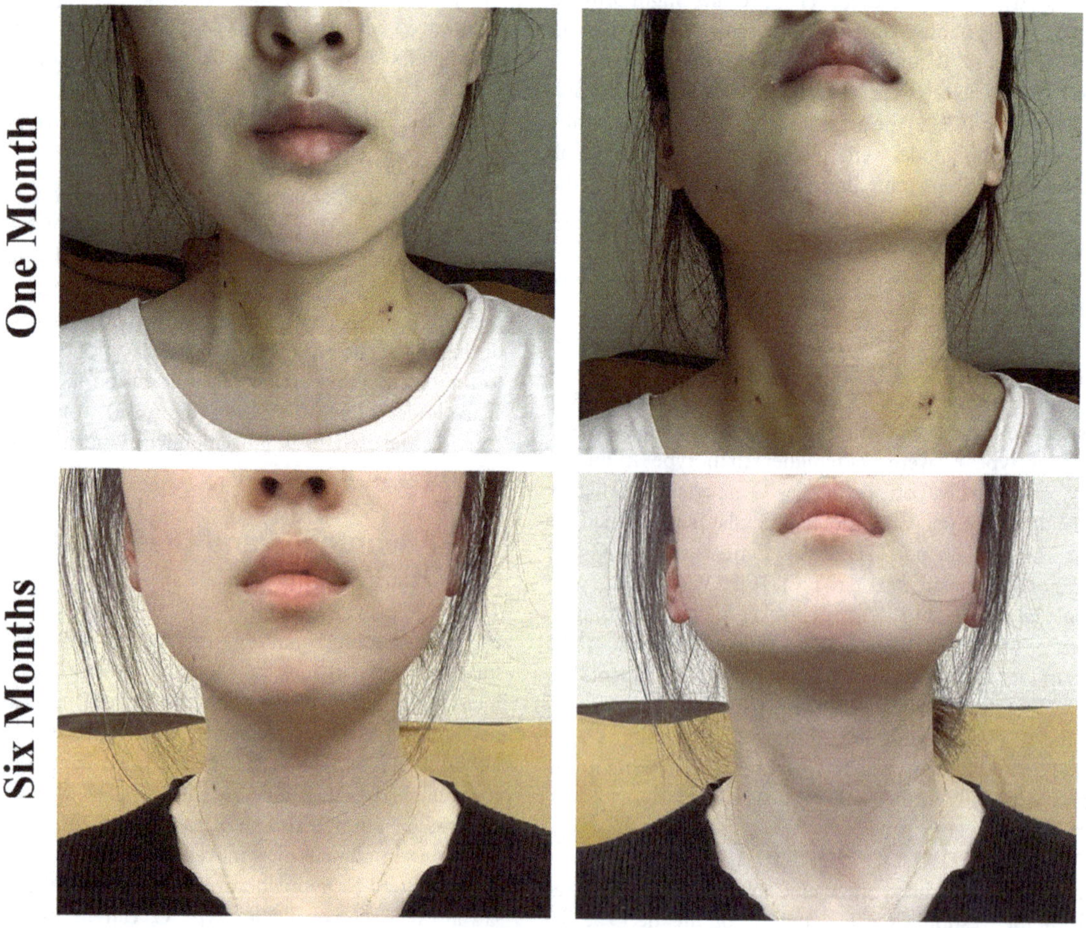

FIGURE 4 | Cosmetic results 1 month and 6 months postoperatively of TOETVA.

much more scores of Qof (17), especially in the aspect of cosmetic result (18), which can hide incisions in the mouth without any scars on the body appearance (**Figure 4**).

Our study has some limitations. Firstly, it was a retrospective study, we only enrolled patients who had a pathological diagnosis of PTC from January 2015 to June 2020 at our single center. Secondly, the operation choices of ipsilateral lobectomy or total thyroidectomy, and central node dissections were according to Chinese guidelines. Additionally, all cases were performed within 18 - 36 months period, and the follow-up time was not long enough to observe tumor recurrence.

CONCLUSION

A new classification was introduced in TOETVA, so as to evaluate the influence of different mandibular jawlines. It has been found that the safety, effect and feasibility were similar in the treatment of PTC with TOETVA in all the mandibular jawlines of type A, B, and C. However, patients of type C would experience a higher ratio of mandibular swell, and higher scores of VAS post TOETVA. New techniques, including real-time observation, hybrid space-maintaining, and adding another vacuum tube may be helpful for working space building of TOETVA, especially in the patients of type C.

ETHICS STATEMENT

Written informed consent was obtained from the individual(s) for the publication of any potentially identifiable images or data included in this article.

AUTHOR CONTRIBUTIONS

XY, YJ, and YW substantial contributed to conception and design. YL, QH, YJ, LP, and PZ contributed to acquisition of data. YL analysis and interpretation of data. YW and XY contributed to draft the article. All authors contributed to the article and approved the submitted version.

REFERENCES

1. Ahn JH, Yi JW. Transoral Endoscopic Thyroidectomy for Thyroid Carcinoma: Outcomes and Surgical Completeness in 150 Single-Surgeon Cases. *Surg Endosc* (2020) 34(2):861–7. doi: 10.1007/s00464-019-06841-8
2. Wang Y, Zhou S, Liu X, Rui S, Li Z, Zhu J, et al. Transoral Endoscopic Thyroidectomy Vestibular Approach vs Conventional Open Thyroidectomy: Meta-Analysis. *Head Neck* (2021) 43(1):345–53. doi: 10.1002/hed.26486
3. Liu Z, Li Y, Wang Y, Xiang C, Yu X, Zhang M, et al. Comparison of the Transoral Endoscopic Thyroidectomy Vestibular Approach and Open Thyroidectomy: A Propensity Score-Matched Analysis of Surgical Outcomes and Safety in the Treatment of Papillary Thyroid Carcinoma. *Surgery* (2021) 170(6):1680–6. doi: 10.1016/j.surg.2021.06.032
4. Masucci C, Oueiss A, Maniere-Ezvan A, Orthlieb JD, Casazza E. What is a Malocclusion? *Orthod Fr* (2020) 91(1-2):57–67. doi: 10.1684/orthodfr.2020.11
5. Yu X, Liu C, Yan M, Gong W, Wang Y. Hyperthermal Liquid, Spray, and Smog may be Potential Risk Factors for Recurrent Laryngeal Nerve Thermal Injury During Thyroid Surgeries. *Endocrine* (2021) 72(1):198–207. doi: 10.1007/s12020-020-02451-w
6. You JY, Kim HY, Park DW, Yang HW, Kim HK, Dionigi G, et al. Transoral Robotic Thyroidectomy Versus Conventional Open Thyroidectomy: Comparative Analysis of Surgical Outcomes Using Propensity Score Matching. *Surg Endosc* (2021) 35(1):124–9. doi: 10.1007/s00464-020-07369-y
7. Anuwong A. Transoral Endoscopic Thyroidectomy Vestibular Approach: A Series of the First 60 Human Cases. *World J Surg* (2016) 40(3):491–7. doi: 10.1007/s00268-015-3320-1
8. Lira RB, De Cicco R, Rangel LG, Bertelli AA, Duque Silva A, de Medeiros Vanderlei JP, et al. Transoral Endoscopic Thyroidectomy Vestibular Approach: Experience From a Multicenter National Group With 412 Patients. *Head Neck* (2021) 43(11):3468–75. doi: 10.1002/hed.26846
9. Sun H, Zheng H, Wang X, Zeng Q, Wang P, Wang Y. Comparison of Transoral Endoscopic Thyroidectomy Vestibular Approach, Total Endoscopic Thyroidectomy *via* Areola Approach, and Conventional Open Thyroidectomy: A Retrospective Analysis of Safety, Trauma, and Feasibility of Central Neck Dissection in the Treatment of Papillary Thyroid Carcinoma. *Surg Endosc* (2020) 34(1):268–74. doi: 10.1007/s00464-019-06762-6
10. You JY, Kim H, Park DW, Yang HW, Dionigi G, Tufano RP. Prevention of Transoral Thyroidectomy Complications: An Analysis of Surgical Outcomes in 423 Consecutive Series. *Surgery* (2021) 170(4):1155–9. doi: 10.1016/j.surg.2021.05.003
11. Tae K. Complications of Transoral Thyroidectomy: Overview and Update. *Clin Exp Otorhinolaryngol* (2021) 14(2):169–78. doi: 10.21053/ceo.2020.02110
12. Yan HC, Xiang C, Wang Y, Wang P. Scarless Endoscopic Thyroidectomy (SET) Lateral Neck Dissection for Papillary Thyroid Carcinoma Through Breast Approach: 10 Years of Experience. *Surg Endosc* (2021) 35(7):3540–6. doi: 10.1007/s00464-020-07814-y
13. Xie QP, Xiang C, Wang Y, Yan HC, Zhao QZ, Yu X, et al. The Patterns and Treatment of Postoperative Hemorrhage and Hematoma in Total Endoscopic Thyroidectomy *via* Breast Approach: Experience of 1932 Cases. *Endocrine* (2019) 63(3):422–9. doi: 10.1007/s12020-018-01837-1
14. Wang Y, Zhang Z, Zhao Q, Xie Q, Yan H, Yu X, et al. Transoral Endoscopic Thyroid Surgery *via* the Tri-Vestibular Approach With a Hybrid Space-Maintaining Method: A Preliminary Report. *Head Neck* (2018) 40(8):1774–9. doi: 10.1002/hed.25157
15. Wang D, Wang Y, Zhou S, Liu X, Wei T, Zhu J, et al. Transoral Thyroidectomy Vestibular Approach Versus non-Transoral Endoscopic Thyroidectomy: A Comprehensive Systematic Review and Meta-Analysis. *Surg Endosc* (2021). doi: 10.1007/s00464-021-08836-w
16. Ji YB, Jeong JH, Wu CW, Chiang FY, Tae K. Neural Monitoring of the External Branch of the Superior Laryngeal Nerve During Transoral Thyroidectomy. *Laryngoscope* (2021) 131(2):E671–6. doi: 10.1002/lary.28883
17. Wongwattana P, Laoveerakul P, Santeerapharp A. A Comparison of Efficacy and Quality of Life Between Transoral Endoscopic Thyroidectomy Vestibular Approach (TOETVA) and Endoscopic Thyroidectomy Axillo-Breast Approach (ETABA) in Thyroid Surgery: non-Randomized Clinical Trial. *Eur Arch Otorhinolaryngol* (2021) 278(10):4043–9. doi: 10.1007/s00405-021-06639-2
18. Lee DW, Bang HS, Jeong JH, Kwak SG, Choi YY, Tae K. Cosmetic Outcomes After Transoral Robotic Thyroidectomy: Comparison With Transaxillary, Postauricular, and Conventional Approaches. *Oral Oncol* (2021) 114:105139. doi: 10.1016/j.oraloncology.2020.105139

14

Post-surgical Thyroid Bed Pyoderma Gangrenosum Mimicking Recurrent Papillary Thyroid Carcinoma

Alessia Dolci[1,2]*, Rita Indirli*[1,2]*, Giovanni Genovese*[3,4]*, Federica Derlino*[5]*, Maura Arosio*[1,2] *and Angelo Valerio Marzano*[3,4*]

[1] *Endocrinology Unit, Fondazione IRCCS Cà Granda Ospedale Maggiore Policlinico, Milan, Italy,* [2] *Department of Clinical Sciences and Community Health, University of Milan, Milan, Italy,* [3] *Dermatology Unit, Fondazione IRCCS Ca' Granda Ospedale Maggiore Policlinico, Milan, Italy,* [4] *Department of Pathophysiology and Transplantation, University of Milan, Milan, Italy,* [5] *Dermatology Unit, Department of Health Sciences, ASST Santi Paolo e Carlo, University of Milan, Milan, Italy*

Correspondence:
Angelo Valerio Marzano
angelo.marzano@unimi.it

Background: Pyoderma gangrenosum (PG) is a rare inflammatory disease presenting with chronic-recurrent cutaneous ulcers histopathologically hallmarked by neutrophilic infiltrates, which may occur more frequently at sites of surgical traumas. The disease is habitually limited to the skin, but it can virtually involve any organ. Nevertheless, no prior cases of PG involving the thyroid bed have ever been reported.

Case Report: A bilateral PG of the breast was diagnosed in a 51-year-old woman and treated with intravenous methylprednisolone pulse-therapy and cyclosporine, with partial improvement. During the hospitalization, cytological examination of two hypoechoic thyroid nodules by fine-needle aspiration (FNA) was consistent with thyroid carcinoma. After total thyroidectomy, histopathology confirmed a papillary thyroid cancer (PTC), and radioactive iodine ablation was performed. At 12-month ultrasonographic follow-up, two hypoechoic avascular areas localized in the empty thyroid bed raised the suspect of PTC recurrence. However, (i) undetectable levels of thyroglobulin without anti-thyroglobulin antibodies, (ii) neutrophilia and increased inflammatory marker levels, and (iii) cytological examination of FNA showing numerous neutrophils induced to suspect thyroid bed PG infiltration. An *ex juvantibus* approach with high-dose methylprednisolone led to dimensional reduction of the hypoechoic areas on ultrasonography, thus confirming the hypothesis of thyroid bed PG.

Conclusion: This case of thyroid bed PG supports the idea that PG reflects a cutaneous phenotype encompassed in the spectrum of systemic neutrophilic diseases. Endocrinologists should be aware that thyroid bed PG involvement is an albeit rare differential diagnosis to consider in patients who had undergone thyroid surgery, especially with a history of PG.

Keywords: pyoderma gangrenosum, differentiated thyroid carcinoma, papillary thyroid carcinoma, pathergy, thyroidectomy

INTRODUCTION

Papillary thyroid carcinoma (PTC), the main variant of differentiated thyroid carcinoma (DTC), is the most common thyroid cancer, accounting for 70–80% of all thyroid carcinomas and occurring predominantly in women, generally with a good prognosis (1). PTC is characterized by a steady and continuous increase in the incidence rate, which has more than doubled within the past three decades all over the world (2).

Pyoderma gangrenosum (PG) is a rare chronic-relapsing inflammatory disease clinically characterized by single or multiple skin ulcers with undermined erythematous-violaceous borders usually developing on the lower extremities (3). It is nowadays regarded as autoinflammatory in origin and classified in the spectrum of the so-called neutrophilic dermatoses, which are a group of conditions hallmarked by accumulation of mature neutrophils in the skin (4–6). Albeit rarely, in this disease almost any organ system can be involved by sterile neutrophilic infiltrates, with the lungs being the most commonly affected site (3, 4). This condition may be idiopathic or associated with underlying disorders, notably inflammatory bowel diseases, rheumatological forms or neoplasms, particularly of lymphoreticular origin (3, 4). PG is typically accompanied by a skin hyperreactivity leading to the pathergy phenomenon, which is the occurrence of disease manifestations at sites of traumas, either accidental or surgical ones (3, 7).

Herein, we report an extraordinary case of a female patient with PG manifesting as classic ulcerative skin lesions associated with a mass in an empty thyroid bed after total thyroidectomy for PTC. This extracutaneous infiltrate mimicked a recurrence of PTC on ultrasound (US) examination, making challenging the diagnosis and management of this unique case.

MATERIALS AND METHODS

Serum thyroglobulin (Tg) levels were measured by electrochemiluminescence sandwich immunoassay (ECLIA, Elecsys Tg II, Roche®, Mannheim, Germany) with an analytic sensitivity of 0.04 ng/ml. Serum anti-Tg antibodies levels were measured by fluorescence enzyme immunoassay (EliA; Thermo Fisher Scientific, Life Technologies Italia®, Monza, Italy; normal <40 IU/ml). Thyroid ultrasound was performed at each time of follow-up using a 14–16-MHz linear probe by the same endocrinologist.

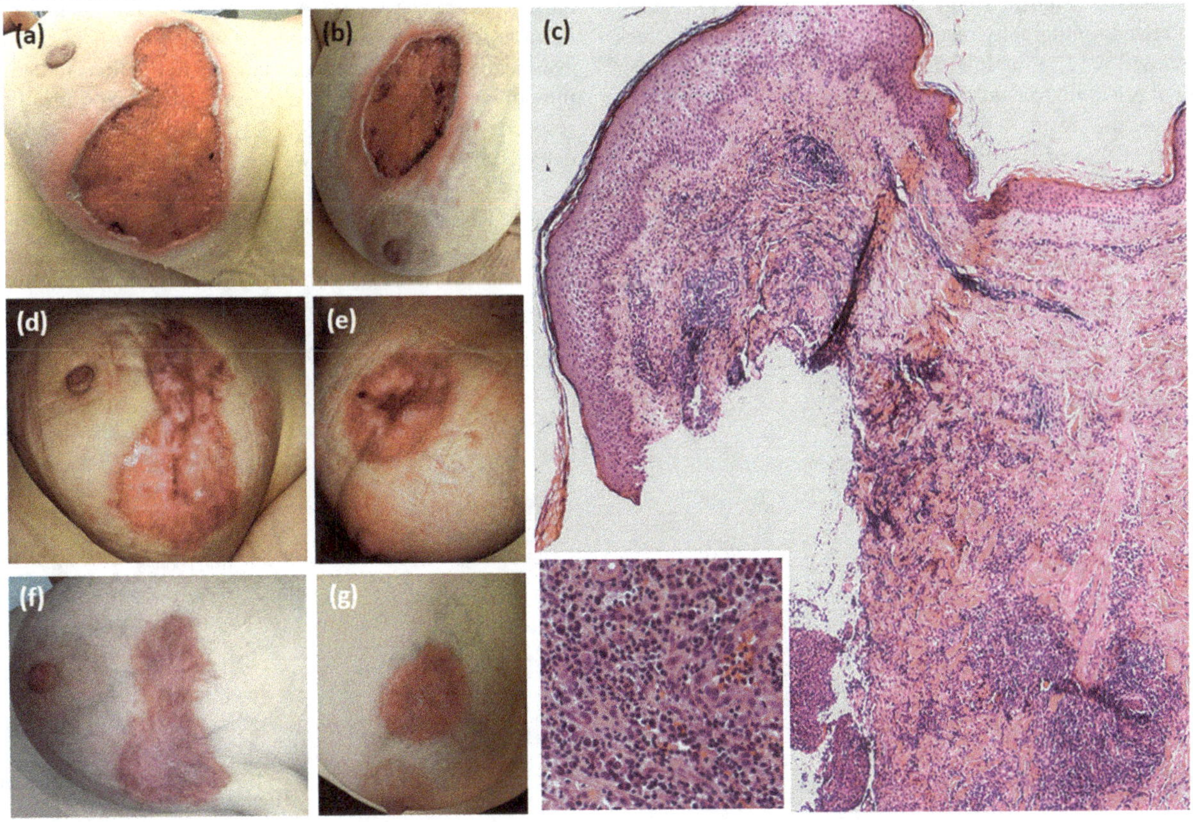

FIGURE 1 | Dermatological and histopathological characteristics of pyoderma gangrenosum. **(a,b)** Ulcerative lesions showing necrotic base and erythematous-violaceous undermined borders on the right and left breast, respectively; **(c)** Skin histology revealing epidermal necrosis and a dermal-hypodermal inflammatory infiltrate mainly consisting of neutrophils (haematoxylin-eosin, original magnification ×100) (in the box, a magnified detail of the inflammatory infiltrate); **(d,e)** Partial healing after therapy with pulsed intravenous methylprednisolone, followed by the combination of prednisone and cyclosporine given orally; **(f,g)** Complete healing with hypertrophic aspects.

Skin biopsy including both the edge and bed of the ulcer was performed. The skin specimen was fixed in 10% buffered formalin, embedded in paraffin, and sectioned into 3-μm sections that were stained with haematoxylin-eosin.

Written informed consent was obtained from the patient for the publication of this case report and any potentially-identifying images and/or information.

CASE DESCRIPTION

A 51-year-old woman was hospitalized for the occurrence of two bilateral painful skin ulcers with undermined, erythematous-violaceous edges in the mammary region, which had begun 6 months before and had rapidly developed from pustular lesions (**Figures 1a,b**). The skin lesions were refractory to antiseptic and antibiotic therapies which had been administered in another dermatology department.

Skin biopsy showed a dermal-hypodermal neutrophilic infiltrate, suggesting PG (**Figure 1c**). Laboratory work-up ruled out any underlying inflammatory condition. Pulse-therapy with intravenous methylprednisolone 125 mg daily for 5 consecutive days was given with clinical improvement, followed and followed by prednisone at progressively tapering dosages in combination with cyclosporine 300 mg daily, inducing progressive healing of the lesions (**Figures 1d–g**). During hospitalization, chest computerized tomography revealed a multinodular goiter. Neck US disclosed a 12.4 mm solid hypoechoic nodule in the upper pole of the left thyroid lobe, and another 8.5 mm hypoechoic nodule in the lower pole of the same lobe. Fine-needle aspiration (FNA) of the dominant nodule was performed, and the cytological exam resulted in Tir4 category according to 2014 SIAPEC (Società Italiana di Anatomia Patologica) classification, equivalent to "suspicious for thyroid carcinoma" (8). A total thyroidectomy was performed, and the histological examination was consistent with multicentric classical PTC, with focal extension to extra-thyroidal soft tissues and surgical resection margins. Histopathologic stadium was pT3(m)Nx according to AJCC (American Joint Committee on Cancer) TNM VII Edition Staging System (9).

Postoperatively, she received radioactive iodine ablation treatment with 3700 MBq under human recombinant α-thyrotropin stimulation (Thyrogen®). The post-treatment Whole Body Scan showed no uptake outside the thyroid bed. The stimulated Tg serum value was 2.6 ng/ml.

Given these findings, the patient was classified at intermediate risk of recurrence according to 2015 ATA score system. Due to the neoplasm, cyclosporine was replaced by immunomodulating therapy with dapsone, without recurrence of skin manifestations.

As shown in **Table 1**, at the 6-month follow-up examination, there was no clinical, biochemical or US evidence of tumor persistence or recurrence. Serum Tg concentrations were undetectable during replacement thyroxine therapy (unstimulated Tg measured several times by an high-sensitive assay always <0.04 ng/mL) in the absence of interfering anti-Tg antibodies. However, US examination of the neck performed 12 months after thyroid surgery revealed two hard hypoechoic avascular areas with irregular margins in the thyroid bed, which measured 16 mm and 15 mm in their maximum diameter, respectively (**Figure 2**). No suspicious lymph nodes were detected. Serum Tg levels were still undetectable, with negative

TABLE 1 | Laboratory tests and neck ultrasound scans performed during the follow-up.

Time-point	TSH (mIU/L)	Tg (ng/mL)	Anti-Tg antibodies (IU/mL)	ESR (mm)	CRP (mg/dL)	Absolute neutrophil count ($\times 10^9$/L)	Neck ultrasound scan
6 months after radioiodine ablation	2.1	<0.04	<12	N/A	N/A	N/A	No suspicious lesions in the thyroid bed, no suspicious lymph nodes
12 months after radioiodine ablation	0.89	<0.04	<12	60	1.17	3.22	Two hypoechoic avascular areas with irregular margins in the thyroid bed, 16 mm and 15 mm in their maximum diameter, respectively; no suspicious lymph nodes
One week after pulse intravenous methylprednisolone	0.085	<0.04	<12	28	0.6	7.02	The two hypoechoic avascular areas in the thyroid bed reduced to 10.9 mm and 15 mm in their maximum diameter, respectively; no suspicious lymph nodes
One month after pulse intravenous methylprednisolone	N/A	N/A	N/A	Normal	Normal	Normal	The two hypoechoic areas furtherly reduced to 8.6 mm and 9.2 mm in their maximum diameter, respectively; no suspicious lymph nodes
Ten months after pulse intravenous methylprednisolone[a]	1.59	<0.04	<12	N/A	N/A	N/A	The two hypoechoic areas are no more visible in the thyroid bed; no suspicious lymph nodes

TSH, Thyroid Stimulating Hormone; Tg, thyroglobulin, analytic sensitivity 0.04 ng/ml; Anti-Tg antibodies, anti-thyroglobulin antibodies, analytic sensitivity 12 IU/mL; ESR, Erythrocyte Sedimentation Rate, normal values <20 mm; CRP, C-Reactive Protein, normal values < 0.5 mg/dl; N/A, not available.

[a]*During current therapy with oral prednisone and cyclosporine.*

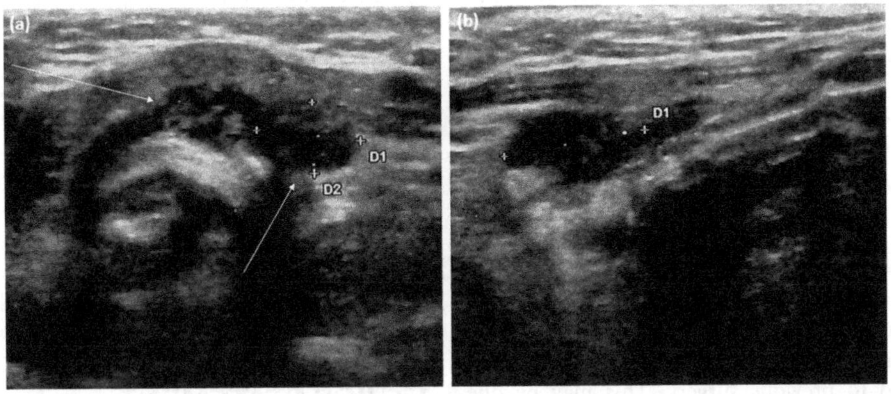

FIGURE 2 | Neck ultrasonography performed at 12-month follow-up visit after thyroidectomy. **(a)** Transversal scan shows two adjacent left paratracheal lesions (arrows). These marked hypoechoic areas have ill-defined margins but not microcalcifications; **(b)** Longitudinal scan depicts the elongated shape of the paratracheal lesion (lateral one) and its parallel orientation to the dermis without deformation of surrounding tissues, unlike true focal masses.

anti-Tg antibodies. FNA of the two above-mentioned lesions was performed under the impression of PTC recurrence; the cytologic specimen revealed numerous neutrophils, together with scattered erythrocytes, lymphocytes, histiocytes, and few thyrocytes without cytological alterations. Gram staining as well as bacterial and mycobacterial cultures of the FNA specimen were negative. Blood exams revealed increased inflammatory markers and neutrophilia.

The clinical, biochemical and cytological clues were consistent with PG infiltration of the thyroid bed. Therefore, the patient underwent again pulse therapy with intravenous methylprednisolone under a strict US follow-up. Following steroid treatment, the two cervical lesions appeared to be dramatically reduced on neck US (with one lesion passing from 10.9 mm in maximum diameter after the first week, to 8.6 mm after 1 month; the second cervical area passed from 15 to 9.2 mm in maximum diameter at the same time points). Both lesions mentioned above were no more visible after 10 months (**Figure 3**) confirming thyroid bed involvement by PG.

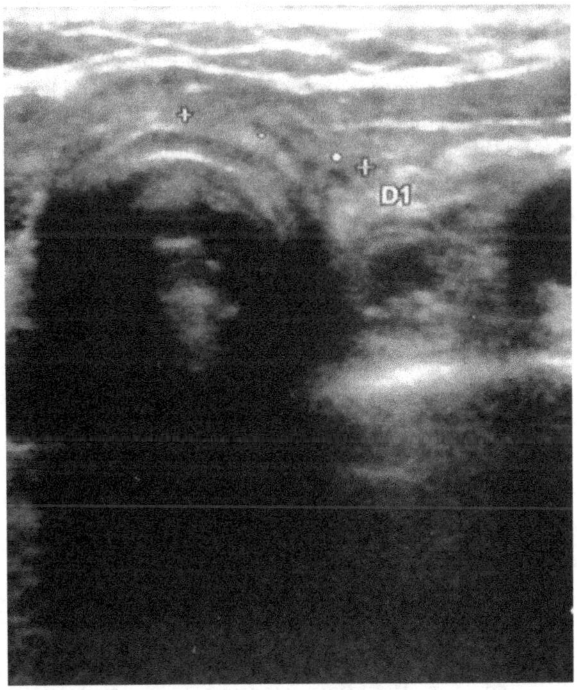

FIGURE 3 | Neck ultrasonography performed at 10-month follow-up visit after the second cycle of intravenous methylprednisolone treatment shows complete regression of the two hypoechoic areas in the thyroid bed.

DISCUSSION

Detecting a mass in the thyroid bed of a patient who had a past medical history of PG and thyroid cancer raises both the possibility of relapse of PG or local recurrence of PTC. PG of the thyroid bed has not been previously reported, and on ultrasound imaging the morphology of PG lesions appeared very similar to thyroid tissue. Essential clues for differentiating deep tissue localization of PG and a recurrence of PTC on US is the parallel orientation of the former, the absence of bright echogenic spots, the elongated and poorly defined borders and its proximity to a skin PG wound (7, 10).

To explain the exceptional association of these two different diseases, different pathogenetic hypotheses may be postulated. Firstly, PG can be a paraneoplastic manifestation of an underlying tumor, particularly haematolymphoid malignancies (11). However, DTC is rarely related to paraneoplastic syndromes (12, 13), and in the present case PG relapsed upon reaching complete remission of PTC, thus making the relation between PG and PTC unlike in our patient.

Common genetic basis may alternatively be involved. Germline mutations in different genes involved in the innate immune response have been identified in autoinflammatory diseases (4). Similarly, a number of somatic mutations have been found to occur in DTC (14). However, the cellular pathways involved in the two conditions look different, and it is difficult to support a common monogenic basis. Nevertheless, dedicated studies in this field are lacking, and we cannot definitely exclude that a polygenic background may eventually predispose to both conditions.

Finally, a conceivable hypothesis to explain the occurrence of PG at the thyroid bed following surgery for PTC is represented by the *pathergy* phenomenon. Pathergy consists in the development of new skin lesions or the aggravation of existing ones after trauma (15). Pathergy has a pivotal role in inducing new post-surgical *skin* PG in patients with a preexisting diagnosis of PG. However, while *cutaneous* PG has been frequently reported after surgical procedures involving the skin, especially breast surgery (16), visceral PG involvement is usually not related to previous surgery. This may be due to the fact that visceral PG is a very rare condition and its diagnosis may be difficult to reach. On the other hand, cases of visceral PG secondarily involving the skin have been reported, as in a patient with lung PG mimicking a lung carcinoma who, 3 months after a sleeve lobectomy and chest-wall resection, developed skin PG ulcers at the site of the surgical wound (17).

Therefore, we suppose that pathergy phenomenon may have contributed to the development of post-surgical visceral PG, even though its exact pathogenesis is still elusive. This case report reinforces the concept that PG may be regarded as a neutrophilic systemic disease, which may be associated with infiltration of sterile neutrophilic infiltration of internal organs (4). The rare extracutaneous neutrophilic involvement in PG (18), has been mainly described as culture-negative pulmonary lesions, but also bone, joint, central nervous system, spleen, kidney, and digestive tract involvements have been reported (18).

A role for radioiodine therapy in this context is not defined, as no specific association between PG and radioiodine has been reported so far.

There have been many reports of non-thyroidal lesions which can be mistaken for thyroid lesions on US (10). However, although it has never been reported that a PG asymptomatic localization might mimic a recurrent thyroidal lesion, establishing the correct diagnosis is crucial, since PG could be exacerbated by an unnecessary surgical intervention potentially leading to pathergy. On the other hand, surgery or radioactive iodine ablation would have been the first-choice treatments if a thyroid cancer recurrence had been ascertained.

In conclusion, a multidisciplinary approach is needed to correctly diagnose and manage these rare cases of extracutaneous PG.

ETHICS STATEMENT

This study was exempt from ethical approval procedures being a case report that describes the clinical course and outcome of a single patient who was referred to our outpatient clinic.

PATIENT CONSENT

The patient provided written consent to have her case published for the purpose to improve the medical knowledge.

AUTHOR CONTRIBUTIONS

AD, MA, and AM performed patient follow-up, clinical diagnosis, and manuscript preparation. RI, AD, and GG performed data interpretation and manuscript preparation. FD collected the patient's clinical information and contributed to manuscript preparation. AM and MA performed the critical revision of the manuscript. All authors approved the manuscript and this submission.

REFERENCES

1. Siegel RL, Miller KD, Jemal A. Cancer statistics, 2015. *CA Cancer J Clin.* (2015) 65:5–29. doi: 10.3322/caac.21254
2. Pellegriti G, Frasca F, Regalbuto C, Squatrito S, Vigneri R. Worldwide increasing incidence of thyroid cancer: update on epidemiology and risk factors. *J Cancer Epidemiol.* (2013) 2013:965212. doi: 10.1155/2013/965212
3. Maverakis E, Ma C, Shinkai K, Fiorentino D, Callen JP, Wollina U, et al. Diagnostic criteria of ulcerative pyoderma gangrenosum: a delphi consensus of international experts. *JAMA Dermatol.* (2018) 154:461–6. doi: 10.1001/jamadermatol.2017.5980
4. Marzano AV, Borghi A, Wallach D, Cugno M. A comprehensive review of neutrophilic diseases. *Clin Rev Allergy Immunol.* (2018) 54:114–30. doi: 10.1007/s12016-017-8621-8
5. Marzano AV, Cugno M, Trevisan V, Fanoni D, Venegoni L, Berti E, et al. Role of inflammatory cells, cytokines and matrix metalloproteinases in neutrophil-mediated skin diseases. *Clin Exp Immunol.* (2010) 162:100–7. doi: 10.1111/j.1365-2249.2010.04201.x
6. Marzano AV, Fanoni D, Antiga E, Quaglino P, Caproni M, Crosti C, et al. Expression of cytokines, chemokines and other effector molecules in two prototypic autoinflammatory skin diseases, pyoderma gangrenosum and Sweet's syndrome. *Clin Exp Immunol.* (2014) 178:48–56. doi: 10.1111/cei.12394
7. Binus AM, Qureshi AA, Li VW, Winterfield LS. Pyoderma gangrenosum: a retrospective review of patient characteristics, comorbidities and therapy in 103 patients. *Br J Dermatol.* (2011) 165:1244–50. doi: 10.1111/j.1365-2133.2011.10565.x
8. Nardi F, Basolo F, Crescenzi A, Fadda G, Frasoldati A, Palombini L, et al. Italian Consensus for the classification and reporting of thyroid cytology. *J Endocrinol Invest.* (2014) 37:593–9. doi: 10.1007/s40618-014-0062-0
9. Edge SB, Compton CC. The American Joint Committee on cancer: the 7th edition of the AJCC cancer staging manual and the future of TNM. *Ann Surg Oncol.* (2010) 17:1471–4. doi: 10.1245/s10434-010-0985-4
10. Choi SH, Kim EK, Kim SJ, Kwak JY. Thyroid ultrasonography: pitfalls and techniques. *Korean J Radiol.* (2014) 15:267–76. doi: 10.3348/kjr.2014.15.2.267
11. Wick MR, Patterson JW. Cutaneous paraneoplastic syndromes. *Semin Diagn Pathol.* (2019) doi: 10.1053/j.semdp.2019.01.001. [Epub ahead of print].
12. Gratwicke JP, Alli A, Rollin M, Vaz F, Rees J, Vincent A, et al. Paraneoplastic cerebellar syndrome and sensory ganglionopathy with papillary thyroid carcinoma. *J Neurol Sci.* (2014) 341:183–4. doi: 10.1016/j.jns.2014.03.042
13. Tavarelli M, Sarfati J, De Gennes C, Haroche J, Buffet C, Ghander C, et al. Hypertrophic osteoarthropathy and follicular thyroid cancer:

a rare paraneoplastic syndrome. *Eur Thyroid J.* (2015) 4:266–70. doi: 10.1159/000437052

14. Pstrag N, Ziemnicka K, Bluyssen H, Wesoły J. Thyroid cancers of follicular origin in a genomic light: in-depth overview of common and unique molecular marker candidates. *Mol Cancer.* (2018) 17:116. doi: 10.1186/s12943-018-0866-1
15. Kutlubay Z, Tüzün Y, Wolf R. The pathergy test as a diagnostic tool. *Skinmed.* (2017) 15:97–104.
16. Xia FD, Liu K, Lockwood S, Butler D, Tsiaras WG, Joyce C, et al. Risk of developing pyoderma gangrenosum after procedures in patients with a known history of pyoderma gangrenosum—A retrospective analysis. *J Am Acad Dermatol.* (2018) 78:310–4.e1. doi: 10.1016/j.jaad.2017.09.04
17. Field S, Powell FC, Young V, Barnes L. Pyoderma gangrenosum manifesting as a cavitating lung lesion. *Clin Exp Dermatol.* (2008) 33:418–21. doi: 10.1111/j.1365-2230.2008.02756.x
18. Prat L, Bouaziz JD, Wallach D, Vignon-Pennamen MD, Bagot M. Neutrophilic dermatoses as systemic diseases. *Clin Dermatol.* (2014) 32:376–88. doi: 10.1016/j.clindermatol.2013.11.004

15

A Surgeon-Centered Neuromuscular Block Protocol Improving Intraoperative Neuromonitoring Outcome of Thyroid Surgery

I-Cheng Lu[1,2], Chiung-Dan Hsu[1], Pi-Ying Chang[3], Sheng-Hua Wu[2,3], Tzu-Yen Huang[2,4], Yi-Chu Lin[4], How-Yun Ko[4], Gianlorenzo Dionigi[5,6], Young Jun Chai[7], Feng-Yu Chiang[8], Yi-Wei Kuo[9†] and Che-Wei Wu[2,4*†]*

[1] Department of Anesthesiology, Kaohsiung Municipal Siaogang Hospital, Kaohsiung Medical University Hospital, Kaohsiung Medical University, Kaohsiung, Taiwan, [2] Faculty of Medicine, College of Medicine, Kaohsiung Medical University, Kaohsiung, Taiwan, [3] Department of Anesthesiology, Kaohsiung Municipal Ta-Tung Hospital, Kaohsiung Medical University Hospital, Kaohsiung Medical University, Kaohsiung, Taiwan, [4] Department of Otorhinolaryngology, Kaohsiung Medical University Hospital, Kaohsiung Medical University, Kaohsiung, Taiwan, [5] Division of General Surgery, Endocrine Surgery Section, Istituto Auxologico Italiano IRCCS (Istituto di ricovero e cura a carattere scientifico), Milan, Italy, [6] Department of Pathophysiology and Transplantation, University of Milan, Milan, Italy, [7] Department of Surgery, Seoul National University College of Medicine, Seoul Metropolitan Government—Seoul National University Boramae Medical Center, Transdisciplinary Department of Medicine & Advanced Technology, Seoul National University Hospital, Seoul, South Korea, [8] Department of Otolaryngology, E-Da Hospital, I-Shou University, Kaohsiung, Taiwan, [9] Department of Anesthesiology, Kaohsiung Medical University Hospital, Kaohsiung Medical University, Kaohsiung, Taiwan

***Correspondence:**
Yi-Wei Kuo
harry.k101@msa.hinet.net
Che-Wei Wu
cwwu@kmu.edu.tw

[†]These authors have contributed equally to this work

Background: Neuromuscular blocking agents provide muscular relaxation for tracheal intubation and surgery. However, the degree of neuromuscular block may disturb neuromuscular transmission and lead to weak electromyography during intraoperative neuromonitoring. This study aimed to investigate a surgeon-friendly neuromuscular block degree titrated sugammadex protocol to maintain both intraoperative neuromonitoring quality and surgical relaxation during thyroid surgery.

Methods: A total of 116 patients were enrolled into two groups and underwent elective thyroid surgery with intraoperative neuromonitoring. All patients followed a standardized intraoperative neuromonitoring protocol with continuous neuromuscular transmission monitoring and received 0.6 mg/kg rocuronium for tracheal intubation. Patients were allocated into two groups according to the degree of neuromuscular block when the anterior surface of the thyroid gland was exposed. The neuromuscular block degree was assessed by the train-of-four (TOF) count and ratio. Patients in group I received sugammadex 0.25 mg/kg for non-deep neuromuscular block degree (TOF count = 1~4). Patients in group II were administered sugammadex 0.5 mg/kg for deep neuromuscular block degree (TOF count = 0). The quality of the intraoperative neuromonitoring was measured using the V_1 electromyography (EMG) amplitude. An amplitude less than 500 μV and greater than 500 μV was defined as weak and satisfactory, respectively.

Results: The quality of the intraoperative neuromonitoring was not different between groups I and II (satisfactory/weak: 75/1 vs. 38/2, P = 0.14). The quality of surgical relaxation was acceptable after sugammadex injection and showed no difference between groups [55/76 (72.3%) in group I vs. 33/40 (82.5%) in group II, P = 0.23].

Conclusions: This surgeon-centered sugammadex protocol guided by neuromuscular block degree (0.5 mg/kg for deep block and 0.25 mg/kg for others) showed comparably high intraoperative neuromonitoring quality and adequate surgical relaxation. The results expanded the practicality of sugammadex for precise neuromuscular block management during monitored thyroidectomy.

Keywords: intraoperative neuromonitoring (IONM), thyroid surgery, recurrent laryngeal nerve (RLN), neuromuscular block degree, sugammadex

INTRODUCTION

Intraoperative neuromonitoring (IONM) has gained increasing popularity during thyroid surgery in recent years. IONM is an adjunct tool for the identification and localization, detecting anatomical variations, differentiating mechanisms of injury, and predicting the postoperative function of the recurrent laryngeal nerve (RLN) (1–12). The goal of IONM is to diminish the occurrence of RLN injury and vocal cord paralysis associated with thyroid and parathyroid surgery.

Both good contact of surface electrodes (13–19) and adequate reversal of neuromuscular blockade (NMB) (20–27) are prerequisites for successful IONM of the RLN. For adequate relaxation to facilitate tracheal intubation and surgery, a profound or deep NMB is desirable. A proper reversal of the NMB is mandatory for functional IONM *via* evoked electromyogram (EMG) signals. Recently, sugammadex following rocuronium during anesthesia induction has been reported as an effective NMB regimen for successful IONM in animal and human clinical studies involving thyroid surgery (28–30).

Various sugammadex regimens have been reported. Low-dose sugammadex can enhance spontaneous neuromuscular functional recovery, while high-dose sugammadex can result in undesirable involuntary movement during surgery. In our previous report, sugammadex at a dose of 0.5 mg/kg induced NMB reversal from rocuronium 0.6 mg/kg and provided high-quality monitoring of the RLN for thyroid surgery (31). Chai et al. (32) demonstrated that sugammadex at either 1 or 2 mg/kg resulted in high-quality IONM. The bucking effect of sugammadex is dose-related, such that 2 mg/kg sugammadex was associated with up to 35% higher effects than 1 mg/kg sugammadex (32). However, the titration of sugammadex dosage according to the degree of NMB has not been investigated.

This study aimed to establish a surgeon-friendly protocol by titrating the sugammadex dose based on the degree of NMB before initial vagus nerve stimulation (V_1) to maintain both surgical relaxation and IONM quality during thyroid surgery. We hypothesized that sugammadex titrated at a dose of 0.25 mg/kg is effective for the reversal of rocuronium-induced moderate NMB and can provide effective IONM with sufficient surgical relaxation. We compared this protocol with 0.5 mg/kg sugammadex for deep NMB, which was routinely administered at our institution.

METHODS

Patient Data

This retrospective observational study was approved by the institutional review board of Kaohsiung Medical University Hospital [KMUHIRB-E(I)-20210070] and registered at ClinicalTrials.gov (NCT 04982185). Patients who underwent elective total thyroidectomy or total lobectomy with routine IONM were included between August 1, 2019, and July 31, 2020. Patients who met the following exclusion criteria were excluded from the study: age ≤20 years, American Society of Anesthesiologists (ASA) status of ≥4, vocal cord palsy, or previous thyroid surgery. All operations were performed by the same surgeon, and anesthesia was administered by two experienced anesthesiologists. The neuromonitoring setup, surgical procedures, and loss of signal algorithm followed the International Neural Monitoring Study Group Guidelines (1, 5, 11, 12).

Anesthesia

Upon arrival at the operating room, each patient was placed under standard physiological monitoring (oximetry, electrocardiography, non-invasive blood pressure, and capnography). Before anesthesia induction, a donut pad beneath the neck was placed for thyroidectomy. An oral endotracheal tube with a 7.0- and 7.5-mm internal diameter was placed for female and male patients, respectively.

The NMB degree was continuously monitored by the train-of-four (TOF) count and ratio derived from the adductor pollicis muscle. Anesthetic depth was assessed using the response entropy (RE) or bispectral index (BIS). Anesthesia induction was initiated with fentanyl (1 μg/kg), lidocaine (1 mg/kg), and propofol (1.5–2 mg/kg). When loss of consciousness was identified, rocuronium (0.6 mg/kg) was administered to induce

NMB in all patients. When the maximum NMB was achieved, the anesthesiologist performed tracheal intubation using a Trachway video intubating stylet (Biotronic Instrument Enterprise Ltd., Tai Chung, Taiwan). The position of the endotracheal tube was confirmed by end-tidal CO_2 and auscultation.

Anesthesia was maintained with sevoflurane and propofol target-controlled infusion with an Orchestra™ infusion pump (Fresenius Vial, France). The effect-site concentration of propofol was maintained at 1–1.5 μg/ml. Two registered nurse anesthetists followed the standardized anesthesia regimen according to our institution's protocol and adjusted the inhaled sevoflurane concentration to maintain an entropy or BIS value between 40 and 60. A bolus of fentanyl 0.5 μg/kg was administered before the skin incision.

Study Flowchart

The timing of sugammadex administration was decided by the surgeon after the initial surgical steps of subplatysmal flap creation and strap muscle separation to expose the anterior surface of the thyroid gland. Patients were allocated into two groups according to the degree of NMB before sugammadex administration. A TOF count of 0 was defined as deep NMB. A TOF count of 1–3 was defined as moderate neuromuscular block and 4 as recovery (33). Patients with non-deep NMB (group I) received sugammadex 0.25 mg/kg. Patients with deep NMB (group II) were administered sugammadex 0.5 mg/kg (**Figure 1**). All patients followed the standard anesthesia protocol for monitored thyroidectomy (**Table 1**).

Surgical Techniques and Intraoperative Neuromonitoring Setup

A lower neck skin incision was made along the skin crease. Subcutaneous fat and platysma were divided, and a subplatysmal dissection was made above the incision up to the level of the thyroid cartilage. The fascia between the strap muscles was divided, and the anterior surface of the thyroid gland was exposed. After resection of the pyramidal lobe, a pair of subdermal electrodes (length, 12.0 mm; diameter, 0.4 mm; Medtronic, Jacksonville, FL) was inserted into the subperichondrium of the thyroid cartilage lamina on both sides (34). The thyroid cartilage electrodes were connected to the nerve integrity monitoring (NIM). The elicited EMG signals with electrode leads were documented as channels 1 and 2 simultaneously. The NIM system generated stimuli with a time window set to 50 ms and an amplitude scale set to 0.2 mV/division. The pulsed stimuli were 100 μs in duration and 4 Hz in frequency. Event capture was activated at a threshold of 100 μV. The intraoperative standardized IONM protocol routinely followed the departmental guidelines. The highest EMG amplitudes were recorded. V_1 signal represents vagal stimulation before dissection, R_1 signal represents RLN stimulation at first identification, R_2 signal represents RLN stimulation after complete dissection, and V_2 signal represents repeat vagal stimulation after resection of the thyroid.

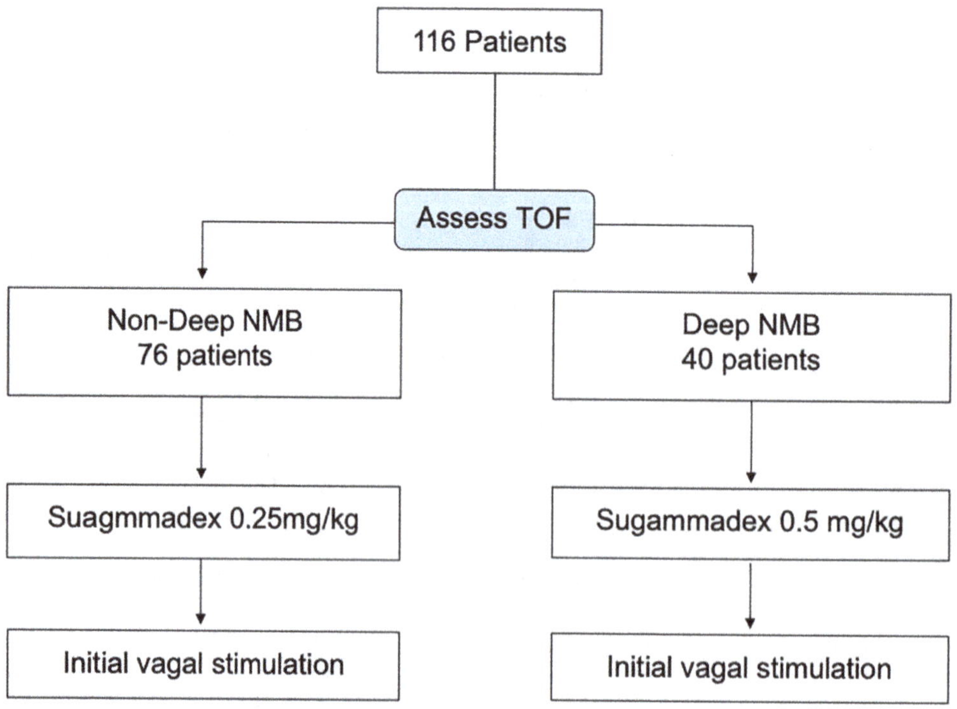

FIGURE 1 | Study flowchart of the 116 consecutive patients, 40 with deep neuromuscular block (NMB) are reversed by sugammadex 0.5 mg/kg. Another 76 patients with moderate NMB or recovery are reversed by sugammadex 0.25 mg/kg. TOF, train of four.

TABLE 1 | Departmental anesthesia protocol for intraoperative neuromonitoring during thyroid surgery.

Time courses	Remarks
Preoperative evaluation	ASA physical status and upper airway management assessment
Monitoring setup	Standard physical/neuromuscular/anesthesia depth monitors
Anesthesia induction	
Induction	Fentanyl 1 μg/kg, lidocaine 1 mg/kg, and propofol 1.5–2 mg/kg
NMBA	Rocuronium 0.6 mg/kg
Anesthesia maintenance	Avoid NMBA
Inhaled anesthetic	Sevoflurane 1%–4%
Intravenous anesthetic	Propofol TCI, effect-site concentration: 1~1.5 μg/kg
Anesthesia depth	Entropy or BIS between 40 and 60
Vasopressor	Ephedrine 8–10 mg if MAP reduction >20% mmHg
PONV prophylaxis	Dexamethasone 5 mg, avoid morphine
Inadequate relaxation	A bolus of fentanyl 0.5 μg/kg and propofol 20–30 mg
Neural monitoring	Low dose of sugammadex blockade
Placing TC electrodes	Sugammadex 0.5 mg/kg if TOF count = 0 (con) Sugammadex 0.25 mg/kg if TOF count = 1–4
V_1 and V_2 signal	EMG amplitude correlated with TOF ratio
Anesthesia emergency	
Extubation	Additional sugammadex up to 2.0 mg/kg Extubation when spontaneous breath with TOF ratio >0.95
Pain control	Parecoxib 40 mg or NSAID if not contraindicated Fentanyl 0.5 μg/kg
Postoperative visit	Anesthesia adverse events and satisfaction

ASA, American Society of Anesthesiologists; NMBA, neuromuscular blocking agent; TCI, target-controlled infusion; MAP, mean arterial pressure; BIS, bispectral index; PONV, postoperative nausea vomiting; TC, thyroid cartilage; V_1 and V_2, initial and final vagal stimulation; TOF, train-of-four mode of neuromuscular transmission monitoring; EMG, electromyography; NSAID, non-steroidal anti-inflammatory drug.

Outcome Measures

The primary outcomes of this study were the quality of the IONM and EMG amplitude of the V_1 signal. The quality of IONM was measured using the obtained V_1 amplitude. Satisfactory and weak signal was defined as a V_1 amplitude of >500 μV and <500 μV, respectively. The secondary outcome was the quality of surgical relaxation. The quality of relaxation was assessed by the number of free periods without any intraoperative limb movement, coughing, and swallowing events. The data of NMB, anesthesia depth, hemodynamics, postoperative adverse events, and surgical outcomes were also recorded and analyzed. All patients received preoperative and postoperative video recordings of vocal cord mobility by flexible laryngofiberoscopy. When asymmetric cord movement was found postoperatively, a comparison with the preoperative recording was performed.

Statistical Analysis

Continuous data were presented as mean ± standard deviation (SD) values, and nominal data are presented as number (%). The distribution of variables was tested using the Kolmogorov–Smirnov test. Statistical analysis of continuous variables with normal distribution between groups was compared using the unpaired t-test, while continuous variables without normal distribution were compared using the Mann–Whitney U test. All statistical tests were two-tailed. Categorical nominal variables were analyzed using the chi-square or Fisher exact test. Statistical significance was set at $P < 0.05$.

The sample size estimation was based on two similarly designed studies. To ensure adequate power for the study, a minimal sample size of 40 patients was used to measure the effect of 0.5 mg/kg sugammadex according to a previous study (31). One previous study showed satisfactory nerve monitoring (V_1 >500 μV) in 90% of patients when the vagus nerve was monitored after delivery of 1 mg/kg sugammadex (32). To establish a non-inferiority study in which 0.25 mg/kg sugammadex would not be less satisfactory, the case number required for the study was 38 patients per group with a 10% non-inferiority margin, an alpha of 0.05, and a beta of 0.2.

RESULTS

A total of 116 patients (24 men and 92 women; aged 21–88 years) were included in this study (**Figure 1**). Detailed patient characteristics are shown in **Table 2**. All tracheal intubations were successful after the first attempt, and no intubation-related upper airway trauma was noted. There was no difference between the two groups in terms of demographic data, physical status, disease diagnosis, vasopressor use, and surgical relaxation. The number of patients with complete surgical relaxation was significantly lower after sugammadex injection [71 (93.4%) to 55 (72.3%) in group I, $P < 0.01$, vs. 39 (97.5%) to 33 (82.5%) in group II, $P = 0.03$]. Overall, 193 nerves were at risk, and only one nerve had intraoperative loss of signal. This was a cancer patient who had postoperative temporary RLN palsy who recovered after 4 weeks.

Key time intervals for anesthesia, operation, and neuromonitoring did not differ significantly between the groups (**Table 3**). The average time from anesthesia induction (rocuronium) to sugammadex injection was 46.0 (± 9.1) min in group I and 43.4 (± 9.3) min in group II ($P = 0.14$). The average time from the surgeon's request to administer sugammadex to initial

TABLE 2 | Patient characteristics of 116 patients receiving monitored thyroidectomy.

	Group I (n = 76)	Group II (n = 40)	P value
Female gender	62 (81.5%)	30 (75%)	0.71
Age, mean (SD), years	51.2 (13.4)	55.6 (12.6)	0.82
Weight (kg)	60.0 (11.5)	57.8 (9.9)	0.29
Height (cm)	159.8 (7.7)	157.7 (7.3)	0.14
BMI (kg/m^2)	23.4 (3.6)	23.2 (3.5)	0.79
ASA status			
I	2 (2.6%)	1 (2.5%)	0.89
II	56 (73.7%)	31 (77.5%)	
III	18 (23.7%)	8 (20%)	
Diagnosis			0.75
Cancer	30 (39.5%)	16 (42.5%)	
Benign	46 (60.5%)	24 (57.5%)	
Vasopressor	7 (9.2%)	5 (12.5%)	0.58
Complete relaxation*			
Before sugammadex	71 (93.4%)	39 (97.5%)	0.35
After sugammadex	55 (72.3%)	33 (82.5%)	0.23
Nerve at risk (n)	122	71	
RLN signal loss#	1 (0.8%)	0 (0%)	0.44
Temporary palsy	1 (0.8%)	0 (0%)	0.44
Permanent palsy	0 (0%)	0 (0%)	1.0

*ASA status, American Society of Anesthesiologists Physical Status classification system; BMI, body mass index (calculated as weight in kilograms divided by height in meters squared); *Without any one event of limb movement, coughing, or swallowing; #signal loss was defined as an EMG amplitude decrease of more than 50% of the baseline value.*

vagal stimulation was as short as 5.4 (± 2.1) min in group I and 5.1 (± 2.1) min in group II ($P = 0.48$).

With respect to IONM quality, all patients showed a positive V_1 signal after sugammadex. The V_1 EMG amplitude was greater than 500 μV in most patients. There was no significant difference between the groups (satisfactory/weak: 75/1 in group I and 38/2 in group II, $P = 0.23$). The EMG amplitude and NMB degree were compared at V_1 and V_2 stimulations between the two groups. At the V_1 time point, group I demonstrated a higher EMG amplitude [1,926 (± 806) vs. 1,616 (± 939), $P = 0.06$] and a higher TOF ratio [36 (± 28) vs. 30 (± 32), $P = 0.29$] than group II, but the difference was not statistically significant (**Table 3**). Both the mean EMG amplitude and TOF ratio at the V_2 time point were comparable between the two groups (**Table 3**).

DISCUSSION

The present results revealed that both 0.5 mg/kg sugammadex for deep NMB and 0.25 mg/kg sugammadex for moderate NMB could be feasible for monitored thyroidectomy. Both groups were comparable in terms of surgical relaxation quality in terms of freedom from intraoperative limb movements, coughing, and swallowing. To the best of our knowledge, this is the first report evaluating the effects of sugammadex titrated

TABLE 3 | Time interval of procedures and quality of intraoperative neural monitoring comparison of neuromuscular blockade degree, neural monitoring recordings, and postoperative adverse events.

	Group I (n = 76)	Group II (n = 40)	P value
Time interval			
Anesthesia to skin incision	23.8 (7.2)	22.2 (7.3)	0.26
Skin incision to sugammadex	22.2 (6.2)	21.2 (5.4)	0.38
Sugammadex to V_1	5.4 (2.1)	5.1 (2.2)	0.48
Sugammadex to V_2	27.6 (12.7)	31.4 (12.6)	0.12
V_1 amplitude			0.23
<500 μV	1 (1.3%)	2 (5%)	
>500 μV	75 (98.7%)	38 (95%)	
V_1 stimulation			
EMG amplitude (μV)	1929 (806)	1616 (939)	0.06
TOF ratio (%)	36 (28)	30 (32)	0.29
V_2 stimulation			
EMG amplitude (μV)	2084 (972)	1868 (1070)	0.27
TOF ratio (%)	73 (24)	76 (19)	0.53

V_1, initial vagal stimulation; V_2, final vagal stimulation; EMG, electromyography; TOF, train of four.

according to the degree of NMB for IONM during thyroid surgery.

Two fundamental elements of successful neuromonitoring are a proper recording of electrode position and NMB recovery. With respect to electrode position, in this study, we used a pair of outer thyroid cartilage electrodes to ensure stable EMG signals (34–39) instead of electrodes of an EMG endotracheal tube, which was susceptible to rotational or depth changes (18, 38, 40). Regarding NMB management, several feasible regimens have been proposed to facilitate tracheal intubation and functional IONM (8). Sugammadex has gained increasing popularity in IONM during thyroid surgery. The reported dose of sugammadex that was effective for IONM ranged from 0.5 to 2.0 mg/kg (28, 29, 31, 32, 41, 42). There is a wide variation between patients in the spontaneous recovery time from rocuronium-induced NMB group. Hence, precise and timely titration of sugammadex dose according to different NMB doses could be more effective and practical during IONM.

Sugammadex at 0.5 mg/kg was reported to achieve a high EMG amplitude of 1,214 (± 623) μV at V_1 stimulation during thyroidectomy (31). Complete and early reversal of NMB was very effective for IONM, providing surgical relaxation. In clinical observations, vigorous movements might occur immediately after a dose of 1 or 2 mg/kg sugammadex. Chai et al. (32) also demonstrated that sugammadex at 2 mg/kg was associated with more bucking than 1 mg/kg (35% vs. 14%) during thyroid surgery with IONM. Since different sugammadex doses provided comparable high-quality EMG signals, this modified NMB protocol attempted to explore minimal sugammadex doses that could allow high-quality IONM signals. In a previous report, sugammadex at 0.5 mg/kg was effective for deep NMB, and sugammadex dose at 0.25 mg/kg provided moderate NMB or recovery. A reduction in sugammadex dose for a lower degree of NMB was found to be effective for high-quality IONM (V_1 amplitude >500 μV) in 98.7% (75/76) of patients. Although there was one patient with a V_1 signal of <500 μV (445 μV), typical EMG waveforms can be easily observed, and IONM was successfully performed without difficulty.

In addition to the dose of sugammadex, the timing of administration plays a key role in NMB management. Sugammadex has been developed to selectively bind to amino-steroidal NMBAs (i.e., rocuronium) selectively (43, 44). Sugammadex provides rapid and effective reversal of rocuronium-induced NMB not only for residual NMB after extubation but also for high-quality IONM signals during surgery. When considering the rapid time of onset, the interval between V_1 and sugammadex in this protocol was modified to be as short as possible. This study employed a team approach during IONM, wherein the anesthesiologist administered sugammadex per the surgeon's request after exposing the anterior surface of the thyroid gland and preparing for initial (V_1) vagal stimulation. The overall interval from sugammadex administration to V_1 stimulation was 5.32 (± 2.2) min.

There is a lack of consensus regarding sugammadex timing before vagal stimulation; several time points reported for administration were as follows: immediately after tracheal tube fixation, at skin incision, at 10 min after skin excision, and at exposure and identification of the vagus nerve. The interval from sugammadex to V1 stimulation was between 3 and 32 min (9, 12, 13, 22). In a selective protocol, sugammadex was used after V_1 stimulation when the EMG amplitude was absent or below 100 μV. However, a low initial V_1 amplitude limits the application of the IONM troubleshooting algorithm in case of signal loss (10). Sugammadex timing may affect the reversal of NMB. In this study, the mean TOF ratio was 30% at V_1 stimulation after sugammadex 0.5 mg/kg was administered before V_1 stimulation. In our previous report, the TOF ratio was 59% after sugammadex 0.5 mg/kg was administered 10 min after starting the operation (12). Both regimens were able to present comparable high-quality IONM signals during thyroid surgery.

There are several advantages to this surgeon-centered NMB degree titrated sugammadex protocol for monitored thyroidectomy. First, sugammadex titration based on NMB degree provided two effective rocuronium doses (0.6 mg/kg) to provide an excellent condition for tracheal intubation in most patients (9, 12). Second, sugammadex administration approximately 5 min before V_1 stimulation ensured an adequate onset time to reverse NMB. The protocol maximizes the sugammadex-free interval to avoid bucking or movement resulting from a lower degree of NMB (13). Finally, regarding IONM quality, a high EMG amplitude was noted in 97.4% (113/116) of patients. An initial high-quality V_1 signal is crucial to the signal loss algorithm because the initial EMG amplitude is a standard reference to be compared (1, 5, 45, 46) and to detect imminent nerve stress or injury (11, 12, 47–50).

In addition to the application of sugammadex, several alternative methods could be used for IONM during thyroid surgery. Since sugammadex is not available in all institutes because of its high cost, dose titration of neuromuscular blocking agents might also enable tracheal intubation and surgical relaxation. In a review of NMB management for IONM without using sugammadex, regimens including relaxant-free, succinylcholine, and low to standard dose of rocuronium (0.3~0.6 mg/kg) were all feasible with some clinical limitations (24, 27).

This study had several limitations. First, the study design lacked patient randomization and blinding regarding the administered sugammadex dose because of grouping based on the degree of NMB. Patients in both groups showed comparable demography, disease, and procedure profiles. Second, there might be a selection bias due to the high cost of sugammadex. This was a self-payment regimen; thus, patients who could afford sugammadex and had a high socioeconomic status were included. Third, this protocol was limited by the NMB monitoring equipment in addition to sugammadex. The NMB degree was measured by the TOF ratio generally *via* acceleromyography or kinemyography devices in Taiwan. However, both devices and sugammadex are not easily available for every institute. Finally, caution should be exercised when interpreting the outcomes in this trial. The outcomes were based on the close cooperation between the surgery and the anesthesia team with much clinical and laboratory experience in thyroid surgery with IONM. The IONM outcomes may be influenced by team members in various clinical backgrounds.

CONCLUSIONS

Before vagal stimulation, this surgeon-centered sugammadex protocol according to NMB degree allowed high IONM quality and adequate surgical relaxation. Both sugammadex 0.5 mg/kg for deep NMB and 0.25 mg/kg for moderate NMB or less showed comparable high EMG amplitude at V_1 stimulation. Sugammadex titration for reversal of NMB prevented undetectable or markedly low EMG amplitudes whenever nerve stimulation was required during thyroidectomy. Moreover, the flexibility of sugammadex administration timing based on the surgical procedure was also feasible for IONM during thyroid surgery. These initial positive results warrant further randomized controlled trials.

ETHICS STATEMENT

The studies involving human participants were reviewed and approved by the institutional review board of Kaohsiung Medical University Hospital, Kaohsiung Taiwan. Written informed consent for participation was not required for this study in accordance with the national legislation and institutional requirements.

AUTHOR CONTRIBUTIONS

C-WW had full access to all the data in the study and takes responsibility for the integrity of the data and the accuracy of the data analysis. Y-WK and C-WW contributed equally to this work. Concept and design: I-CL and C-WW. Acquisition, analysis, or interpretation of data: I-CL, C-DH, P-YC, GD, YJC, C-WW. Drafting of the article: I-CL, F-YC, Y-WK, C-WW. Critical revision of the article and final approval: All authors. Statistical analysis: I-CL, F-YC, Y-CL, C-WW. Obtained funding: I-CL, T-YH, C-WW. Administrative, technical, or material support: S-HW, T-YH, Y-CL, H-YK, and F-YC. Supervision: Y-WK and C-WW.

ACKNOWLEDGMENTS

The authors express gratitude to Hsiu-Ya Chen (nurse anesthetist, Department of Anesthesiology, KMUH, KMU), Hui-Chun Chen (clinical nurse specialist, Department of Nursing, KMUH, KMU), and Pao-Chu Hun (veterinarian, Laboratory Animal Center, KMU) for their excellent technical assistance.

REFERENCES

1. Randolph GW, Dralle H, Abdullah H, Barczynski M, Bellantone R, Brauckhoff M, et al. Electrophysiologic Recurrent Laryngeal Nerve Monitoring During Thyroid and Parathyroid Surgery: International Standards Guideline Statement. *Laryngoscope* (2011) 121(Suppl 1):S1–16. doi: 10.1002/lary.21119
2. Sanabria A, Kowalski LP, Nixon I, Angelos P, Shaha A, Owen RP, et al. Methodological Quality of Systematic Reviews of Intraoperative Neuromonitoring in Thyroidectomy: A Systematic Review. *JAMA Otolaryngol Head Neck Surg* (2019) 145(6):563–73. doi: 10.1001/jamaoto.2019.0092
3. Feng AL, Puram SV, Singer MC, Modi R, Kamani D, Randolph GW. Increased Prevalence of Neural Monitoring During Thyroidectomy: Global Surgical Survey. *Laryngoscope* (2020) 130(4):1097–104. doi: 10.1002/lary.28210
4. Genther DJ, Kandil EH, Noureldine SI, Tufano RP. Correlation of Final Evoked Potential Amplitudes on Intraoperative Electromyography of the Recurrent Laryngeal Nerve With Immediate Postoperative Vocal Fold Function After Thyroid and Parathyroid Surgery. *JAMA Otolaryngol Head Neck Surg* (2014) 140(2):124–8. doi: 10.1001/jamaoto.2013.6139
5. Wu CW, Randolph GW, Barczyński M, Schneider R, Chiang FY, Huang TY, et al. Training Courses in Laryngeal Nerve Monitoring in Thyroid and Parathyroid Surgery- The INMSG Consensus Statement. *Front Endocrinol (Lausanne)* (2021) 12:705346:705346. doi: 10.3389/fendo.2021.705346
6. Fundakowski CE, Hales NW, Agrawal N, Barczyński M, Camacho PM, Hartl DM, et al. Surgical Management of the Recurrent Laryngeal Nerve in Thyroidectomy: American Head and Neck Society Consensus Statement. *Head Neck* (2018) 40(4):663–75. doi: 10.1002/hed.24928
7. Vasileiadis I, Karatzas T, Charitoudis G, Karakostas E, Tseleni-Balafouta S, Kouraklis G. Association of Intraoperative Neuromonitoring With Reduced Recurrent Laryngeal Nerve Injury in Patients Undergoing Total Thyroidectomy. *JAMA Otolaryngol Head Neck Surg* (2016) 142(10):994–1001. doi: 10.1001/jamaoto.2016.1954
8. Patel KN, Yip L, Lubitz CC, Grubbs EG, Miller BS, Shen W, et al. The American Association of Endocrine Surgeons Guidelines for the Definitive Surgical Management of Thyroid Disease in Adults. *Ann Surg* (2020) 271(3): e21–93. doi: 10.1097/sla.0000000000003580
9. Al-Qurayshi Z, Randolph GW, Alshehri M, Kandil E. Analysis of Variations in the Use of Intraoperative Nerve Monitoring in Thyroid Surgery. *JAMA Otolaryngol Head Neck Surg* (2016) 142(6):584–9. doi: 10.1001/jamaoto.2016.0412
10. Abdelhamid A, Aspinall S. Intraoperative Nerve Monitoring in Thyroid Surgery: Analysis of United Kingdom Registry of Endocrine and Thyroid Surgery Database. *Br J Surg* (2021) 108(2):182–7. doi: 10.1093/bjs/znaa081
11. Schneider R, Randolph GW, Dionigi G, Wu CW, Marcin Barczynski M, Chiang FU, et al. International Neural Monitoring Study Group Guideline 2018 Part I: Staging Bilateral Thyroid Surgery With Monitoring Loss of Signal. *Laryngoscope* (2018) 128(Suppl 3):S1–17. doi: 10.1002/lary.27359
12. Wu CW, Dionigi G, Barczynski M, Chiang FY, Dralle H, Schneider R, et al. International Neuromonitoring Study Group Guidelines 2018: Part II: Optimal Recurrent Laryngeal Nerve Management for Invasive Thyroid Cancer-Incorporation of Surgical, Laryngeal, and Neural Electrophysiologic Data. *Laryngoscope* (2018) 128(Suppl 3):S18–27. doi: 10.1002/lary.27360
13. Lu IC, Chu KS, Tsai CJ, Wu CW, Kuo WR, Chen HY, et al. Optimal Depth of NIM EMG Endotracheal Tube for Intraoperative Neuromonitoring of the Recurrent Laryngeal Nerve During Thyroidectomy. *World J Surg* (2008) 32 (9):1935–9. doi: 10.1007/s00268-008-9549-1
14. Berkow L, Dackiw AP, Tufano RP. Use of the GlideScope for Placement of a Recurrent Laryngeal Nerve Monitoring Endotracheal Tube. *J Clin Anesth* (2011) 23(1):81–3. doi: 10.1016/j.jclinane.2009.12.013
15. Tsai CJ, Tseng KY, Wang FY, Lu IC, Wang HM, Wu CW, et al. Electromyographic Endotracheal Tube Placement During Thyroid Surgery in Neuromonitoring of Recurrent Laryngeal Nerve. *Kaohsiung J Med Sci* (2011) 27(3):96–101. doi: 10.1016/j.kjms.2010.08.002
16. Kanotra SP, Kuriloff DB, Lesser J, Rest-Flarer F. GlideScope-Assisted Nerve Integrity Monitoring Tube Placement for Intra-Operative Recurrent Laryngeal Nerve Monitoring. *J Laryngol Otol* (2012) 126(12):1271–3. doi: 10.1017/S0022215112002460
17. Cherng CH, Huang YH, Shih ML. Middle Fixation of Electromyographic

Endotracheal Tube for Intraoperative Recurrent Laryngeal Nerve Monitoring. *J Clin Anesth* (2014) 26(3):252–3. doi: 10.1016/j.jclinane.2014.01.009

18. Barber SR, Liddy W, Kyriazidis N, Cinquepalmi M, Brian M Lin BM, Modi R, et al. Changes in Electromyographic Amplitudes But Not Latencies Occur With Endotracheal Tube Malpositioning During Intraoperative Monitoring for Thyroid Surgery: Implications for Guidelines. *Laryngoscope* (2017) 127 (9):2182–8. doi: 10.1002/lary.26392
19. Huang JM, Hsu CD, Wu SH, Kuo YW, Huang TY, Wu CW, et al. Optimization of Electromyographic Endotracheal Tube Electrode Position by UEScope for Monitored Thyroidectomy. *Laryngoscope Investig Otolaryngol* (2021) 6(5):1214–19. doi: 10.1002/lio2.635
20. Marusch F, Hussock J, Haring G, Hachenberg T, Gastinger I. Influence of Muscle Relaxation on Neuromonitoring of the Recurrent Laryngeal Nerve During Thyroid Surgery. *Br J Anaesth* (2005) 94(5):596–600. doi: 10.1093/bja/aei110
21. Shi Y, Hou V, Tucker A, Cohen J. Changes of Extremity and Laryngeal Muscle Electromyographic Amplitudes After Intravenous Administration of Vecuronium. *Laryngoscope* (2008) 118(12):2156–60. doi: 10.1097/MLG.0b013e318184574e
22. Chu KS, Wu SH, Lu IC, Tsai CJ, Wu CW, Kuo WR, et al. Feasibility of Intraoperative Neuromonitoring During Thyroid Surgery After Administration of Nondepolarizing Neuromuscular Blocking Agents. *World J Surg* (2009) 33(7):1408–13. doi: 10.1007/s00268-009-0049-8
23. Chu KS, Tsai CJ, Lu IC, Tseng KY, Chau SW, Wu CW, et al. Influence of Nondepolarizing Muscle Relaxants on Intraoperative Neuromonitoring During Thyroid Surgery. *J Otolaryngol Head Neck Surg* (2010) 39(4):397–402.
24. Lu IC, Tsai CJ, Wu CW, Cheng KI, Wang FY, Tseng KY, et al. A Comparative Study Between 1 and 2 Effective Doses of Rocuronium for Intraoperative Neuromonitoring During Thyroid Surgery. *Surgery* (2011) 149(4):543–8. doi: 10.1016/j.surg.2010.11.006
25. Brunaud L, Fuchs-Buder T. In Reference to Reversal of Rocuronium-Induced Neuromuscular Blockade by Sugammadex Allows for Optimization of Neural Monitoring of the Recurrent Laryngeal Nerve. *Laryngoscope* (2017) 127(1): E50. doi: 10.1002/lary.25990
26. Lu IC, Lin IH, Wu CW, Chen HY, Lin YC, Chiang FY, et al. Preoperative, Intraoperative and Postoperative Anesthetic Prospective for Thyroid Surgery: What's New. *Gland Surg* (2017) 6(5):469–75. doi: 10.21037/gs.2017.05.02
27. Lu IC, Wu SH, Wu CW. Neuromuscular Blockade Management for Intraoperative Neural Monitoring. *Kaohsiung J Med Sci* (2020) 36(4):230–5. doi: 10.1002/kjm2.12153
28. Lu IC, Wu CW, Chang PY, Chen HY, Tseng KY, Randolph GW, et al. Reversal of Rocuronium-Induced Neuromuscular Blockade by Sugammadex Allows for Optimization of Neural Monitoring of the Recurrent Laryngeal Nerve. *Laryngoscope* (2016) 126(4):1014–9. doi: 10.1002/lary.25577
29. Empis de Vendin O, Schmartz D, Brunaud L, Fuchs-Buder T. Recurrent Laryngeal Nerve Monitoring and Rocuronium: A Selective Sugammadex Reversal Protocol. *World J Surg* (2017) 41(9):2298–303. doi: 10.1007/s00268-017-4004-9
30. Wu CW, Huang TY, Chen HC, Chen HY, Tsai TY, Chang PY, et al. Intra-Operative Neural Monitoring of Thyroid Surgery in a Porcine Model. *J Vis Exp* (2019) 144:e57919. doi: 10.3791/57919
31. Lu IC, Wu SH, Chang PY, Ho PY, Huang TY, Lin YC, et al. Precision Neuromuscular Block Management for Neural Monitoring During Thyroid Surgery. *J Invest Surg* (2020) 34(12):1389–96. doi: 10.1080/08941939.2020.1805055
32. Chai YJ, Lee JM, Won D, Jiwon Lee J, Hwang JY, Kim TK, et al. Comparison of Sugammadex Dose for Intraoperative Neuromonitoring in Thyroid Surgery: A Randomized Controlled Trial. *Laryngoscope* (2021) 131 (9):2154–9. doi: 10.1002/lary.29515
33. Fuchs-Buder T, Meistelman C, Raft J. Sugammadex: Clinical Development and Practical Use. *Korean J Anesthesiol* (2013) 65(6):495–500. doi: 10.4097/kjae.2013.65.6.495
34. Chiang FY, Wu CW, Chang PY, Wu SH, Chen HY, Lin YC, et al. Trans-Thyroid Cartilage Recording for Neural Monitoring of the Recurrent Laryngeal Nerve in Thyroid Surgery. *Laryngoscope* (2020) 130(4):E280–3. doi: 10.1002/lary.28049
35. Türk Y, Kıvratma G, Özdemir M, İçöz G, Makay Ö. The Use of Thyroid Cartilage Needle Electrodes in Intraoperative Neuromonitoring During Thyroidectomy: A Case-Control Study. *Head Neck* (2021) 43(11):3287–93. doi: 10.1002/hed.26810
36. Jung SM, Tae K, Song CM, Lee SH, Jeong JH, Ji YB. Efficacy of Transcartilaginous Electrodes for Intraoperative Neural Monitoring During Thyroid Surgery. *Clin Exp Otorhinolaryngol* (2020) 13(4):422–8. doi: 10.21053/ceo.2019.01529
37. Liddy W, Lawson BR, Barber SR, Kamani D, Shama M, Soylu S, et al. Anterior Laryngeal Electrodes for Recurrent Laryngeal Nerve Monitoring During Thyroid and Parathyroid Surgery: New Expanded Options for Neural Monitoring. *Laryngoscope* (2018) 128(12):2910–5. doi: 10.1002/lary.27362
38. Chiang FY, Lu IC, Chang PY, Dionigi G, Randolph GW, Sun H, et al. Comparison of EMG Signals Recorded by Surface Electrodes on Endotracheal Tube and Thyroid Cartilage During Monitored Thyroidectomy. *Kaohsiung J Med Sci* (2017) 33(10):503–9. doi: 10.1016/j.kjms.2017.06.014
39. Huang TY, Kim HY, Dionigi G, Lu IC, Chang PY, Chiang FY, et al. Laryngeal Neural Monitoring During Pediatric Thyroid Cancer Surgery—Is Transcartilage Recording a Preferable Method? *Cancers* (2021) 13(16):4051. doi: 10.3390/cancers13164051
40. Kim HY, Tufano RP, Randolph G, Marcin Barczyński M, Wu CW, Chiang FY, et al. Impact of Positional Changes in Neural Monitoring Endotracheal Tube on Amplitude and Latency of Electromyographic Response in Monitored Thyroid Surgery: Results From the Porcine Experiment. *Head Neck* (2016) 38 (Suppl 1):E1004–8. doi: 10.1002/hed.24145
41. Donmez T, Erdem VM, Sunamak O, Ozcevik H. Thyroid Surgery, Ionm and Sugammadex Sodium Relationships: Benefits in Sugammadex Sodium Use for Ionm. *Acta Endocrinol (Buchar)* (2019) 15(4):454–9. doi: 10.4183/aeb.2019.454
42. Gunes ME, Dural AC, Akarsu C, Guzey D, Sahbaz NA, Tulubas EK, et al. Effect of Intraoperative Neuromonitoring on Efficacy and Safety Using Sugammadex in Thyroid Surgery: Randomized Clinical Trial. *Ann Surg Treat Res* (2019) 97(6):282–90. doi: 10.4174/astr.2019.97.6.282
43. Kovac AL. Sugammadex: The First Selective Binding Reversal Agent for Neuromuscular Block. *J Clin Anesth* (2009) 21(6):444–53. doi: 10.1016/j.jclinane.2009.05.002
44. Yang LP, Keam SJ. Sugammadex: A Review of its Use in Anaesthetic Practice. *Drugs* (2009) 69(7):919–42. doi: 10.2165/00003495-200969070-00008
45. Chiang FY, Lu IC, Kuo WR, Lee KW, Chang NC, Wu CW. The Mechanism of Recurrent Laryngeal Nerve Injury During Thyroid Surgery–the Application of Intraoperative Neuromonitoring. *Surgery* (2008) 143(6):743–9. doi: 10.1016/j.surg.2008.02.006
46. Chiang FY, Lee KW, Chen HC, Chen HY, Lu IC, Kuo WR, et al. Standardization of Intraoperative Neuromonitoring of Recurrent Laryngeal Nerve in Thyroid Operation. *World J Surg* (2010) 34(2):223–9. doi: 10.1007/s00268-009-0316-8
47. Wu CW, Wang MH, Chen CC, Chen HC, Chen HY, Yu JY, et al. Loss of Signal in Recurrent Nerve Neuromonitoring: Causes and Management. *Gland Surg* (2015) 4(1):19–26. doi: 10.3978/j.issn.2227-684X.2014.12.03
48. Wu CW, Hao M, Tian M, Dionigi G, Tufano RP, Kim HY, et al. Recurrent Laryngeal Nerve Injury With Incomplete Loss of Electromyography Signal During Monitored Thyroidectomy-Evaluation and Outcome. *Langenbecks Arch Surg* (2017) 402(4):691–9. doi: 10.1007/s00423-016-1381-8
49. Wu CW, Dionigi G, Sun H, Liu X, Kim HY, Hsiao PJ, et al. Intraoperative Neuromonitoring for the Early Detection and Prevention of RLN Traction Injury in Thyroid Surgery: A Porcine Model. *Surgery* (2014) 155(2):329–39. doi: 10.1016/j.surg.2013.08.015
50. Schneider R, Randolph GW, Sekulla C, Phelan E, Thanh PN, Bucher M, et al. Continuous Intraoperative Vagus Nerve Stimulation for Identification of Imminent Recurrent Laryngeal Nerve Injury. *Head Neck* (2013) 35 (11):1591–8. doi: 10.1002/hed.23187

16

Thyroid Autoimmunity: Role of Anti-Thyroid Antibodies in Thyroid and Extra-Thyroidal Diseases

Eleonore Fröhlich[1,2] *and Richard Wahl*[1*]

[1] *Internal Medicine (Department of Endocrinology and Diabetology, Angiology, Nephrology and Clinical Chemistry), University of Tuebingen, Tuebingen, Germany,* [2] *Center for Medical Research, Medical University Graz, Graz, Austria*

Correspondence:
Richard Wahl
richard.wahl@med.uni-tuebingen.de

Autoimmune diseases have a high prevalence in the population, and autoimmune thyroid disease (AITD) is one of the most common representatives. Thyroid autoantibodies are not only frequently detected in patients with AITD but also in subjects without manifest thyroid dysfunction. The high prevalence raises questions regarding a potential role in extra-thyroidal diseases. This review summarizes the etiology and mechanism of AITD and addresses prevalence of antibodies against thyroid peroxidase, thyroid-stimulating hormone receptor (TSHR), and anti-thyroglobulin and their action outside the thyroid. The main issues limiting the reliability of the conclusions drawn here include problems with different specificities and sensitivities of the antibody detection assays employed, as well as potential confounding effects of altered thyroid hormone levels, and lack of prospective studies. In addition to the well-known effects of TSHR antibodies on fibroblasts in Graves' disease (GD), studies speculate on a role of anti-thyroid antibodies in cancer. All antibodies may have a tumor-promoting role in breast cancer carcinogenesis despite anti-thyroid peroxidase antibodies having a positive prognostic effect in patients with overt disease. Cross-reactivity with lactoperoxidase leading to induction of chronic inflammation might promote breast cancer, while anti-thyroid antibodies in manifest breast cancer might be an indication for a more active immune system. A better general health condition in older women with anti-thyroid peroxidase antibodies might support this hypothesis. The different actions of the anti-thyroid antibodies correspond to differences in cellular location of the antigens, titers of the circulating antibodies, duration of antibody exposure, and immunological mechanisms in GD and Hashimoto's thyroiditis.

Keywords: autoimmune thyroiditis, thyroid autoantibodies, thyroid peroxidase, thyroglobulin, thyroid-stimulating hormone receptor, Graves' orbitopathy

INTRODUCTION

Autoimmune diseases (AD) represent a spectrum of disorders caused by inflammation of organs due to production of antibodies against self-structures and cytotoxic action of T cells. Data from Europe, North America, Australia, New Zealand (defined as area 1) and Asia, Middle East, Caribbean, South America (defined as area 2) differ in the reported prevalence (cases/100,000 individuals) of the most frequent AD (1) as follows: Graves' disease (GD, area 1: 50–626, area 2: 20), Hashimoto's thyroiditis (HT, chronic autoimmune thyroiditis, autoimmune hypothyroidism, area 1: 300–2,980, area 2: 350), rheumatoid arthritis (RA, area 1: 310–810, area 2: 120–550), type 1 diabetes mellitus (T1DM, area 1: 310–570, area 2: no data), Crohn's disease (CRD, area 1: 28–201, area 2: 6–113), multiple sclerosis (MS, area 1: 177–358, area 2: 4–101), and Sjögren disease (SD, area 1: 93–3,500, area 2: 330–1,560). The disparity by sex is high in most of these diseases with a female preponderance of ≥85%; only in some childhood-onset AD, such as T1DM, is the risk equal in both sexes. There are three age peaks for AD onset, namely, 8–10 years (juvenile RA, T1DM), 33–50 years (myasthenia gravis, MS, systemic lupus erythematosus, scleroderma, GD), and 52–63 years (HT, SD, adult RA, etc.) (2).

Autoimmune thyroid diseases (AITDs) include several inflammatory thyroid diseases with GD and HT as most frequent forms (3).

FACTORS LINKED TO THYROID AUTOIMMUNITY

Autoimmune thyroid diseases are usually accompanied by the presence of anti-thyroid peroxidase (TPO), anti-thyroglobulin (Tg), and anti-thyroid-stimulating hormone receptor (TSHR) antibodies. Antibodies against thyroid antigens such as carbonic anhydrase 2, megalin, T3 and T4, sodium iodide symporter (NIS), and pendrin have also been detected, although rarely (4).

Antibodies to Thyroid Antigens

Table 1 provides a comparison of characteristics of anti-TSHR, anti-TPO, and anti-Tg antibodies.

Thyroid-Stimulating Hormone Receptor

After expression on the thyrocyte cell surface, the TSHR undergoes cleavage within the "hinge" region at two or more sites; loss of a C-peptide like region leads to an extracellular A-subunit linked by disulfide bonds to the B-subunit (comprising the remainder of the hinge region, transmembrane, and cytoplasmic tail). Subsequently, some A-subunits are shed. Substantial evidence suggests that the shed A-subunit (rather than the holoreceptor) is the autoantigen initiating and/or driving the autoimmune response to the TSHR in GD [for a recent review, see Ref. (5)]. As shown by crystallization, stimulating TSHR monoclonal antibody M22 and TSH blocking monoclonal antibody K1-70 (both of human origin) bind to closely overlapping epitopes at the amino terminus (6). In addition, neutral antibodies directed against the "hinge" region exist (7). These antibodies can induce generation of oxidative radicals and induce apoptosis. The balance between stimulating TSHR and neutral antibodies can provide a balance between thyrocyte proliferation and apoptosis. DNA released from apoptotic cells stimulates the immune response. Since shedding of A-subunits occurs in all humans, the presence of exogenous and endogenous factors (see Environmental (Exogenous) Factors and Endogenous Factors) is mandatory for the development of GD (5).

The biological action of autoantibodies against TSHR was the reason for their discovery by Adams and Purves (8). These authors were the first to identify a molecule with similar action to TSH and termed it long-acting thyroid stimulator (LATS) due to its prolonged effect. LATS was later identified as an immunoglobulin G and later found to be an antibody against TSHR.

Anti-TSHR antibodies are found in 90% of GD patients, 0–20% HT, and 10–75% of atrophic thyroiditis patients (9). Other studies noted TSHR antibodies in around 10% of HT patients

TABLE 1 | Characterization of different anti-thyroid antibodies.

Parameter	Antibodies		
	Anti-TSHR	**Anti-TPO**	**Anti-Tg**
Antigen location	Extracellular	Intracellular	Intrafollicular, low levels in blood circulation
Access of immune cells to antigen	Without tissue destruction	After thyrocyte destruction	With and without tissue destruction
Duration of antigen exposure	Short, low levels (normalization upon treatment)	Prolonged time, intermediate levels (pathologic levels also upon treatment)	Prolonged time, high levels (pathologic levels also upon treatment)
Type of antibody	Oligoclonal, different epitopes	Polyclonal, one domain immunodominant	Polyclonal, different epitopes
Class of antibody	Mainly IgG1, other subclasses to low extent	IgG1, IgG4 > IgG2, IgG3; low levels of IgA	IgG1, IgG4 > IgG2, IgG3; low levels of IgA and IgM (healthy individuals)
Action on neonate	Transplacental passage; transient hyperthyroidism or hypothyroidism with delayed development of thyroid gland	Transplacental passage; potential effects on cognitive development	Transplacental passage; potential effects on cognitive development
Prevalence in AITD	~90% GD; ~10% HT	>80% in GD and HT	>50% in GD and HT
Prevalence in other AD	Usually no expression, one study 18% in T1DM	16–37% RA; 40% T1DM; 12–30% CD	12–23% RA; 30% T1DM; 11–32% CD
Action of antibodies	Stimulating, blocking, apoptosis	Little action *per se*	No defined action
Extra-thyroidal targets	Few, defined effects (GO, GDP), partly known mechanism	Several, ill-defined actions (HE, breast cancer), mechanism of action not known	No specific targets identified
Action in breast cancer progression	No protective effect	Potential protective effects	Potential protective effects

TSHR, thyroid-stimulating hormone receptor; TPO, thyroid peroxidase; Tg, thyroglobulin; CD, celiac disease; GD, Graves' disease; GDP, Graves' dermopathy; GO, Graves' orbitopathy; HT, Hashimoto's thyroiditis; RA, rheumatoid arthritis; T1DM, type 1 diabetes mellitus; AITD, autoimmune thyroid disease; AD, autoimmune diseases; HE, Hashimoto's encephalopathy.

(10, 11). Stimulating antibodies can be oligoclonal and belong to IgG1 class, while blocking antibodies are polyclonal and not restricted to a specific subclass (12, 13). The pleiotropic action of anti-thyroid antibodies is typical for anti-TSHR antibodies. Stimulatory antibodies are detected in 73–100% and blocking anti-TSHR antibodies in 25–75% of GD patients (14–16). The variations in the detection appear to be linked to the type of assay that has been used. TRAb usually refers to any type of antibody interacting specifically with the TSHR. When assessed by competitive binding assay, the TSHR antibodies are called TSHR-binding inhibitory immunoglobulins. By contrast, cell-based bioassays measure either TSHR stimulatory antibodies or TSHR-stimulating immunoglobulins, or alternately TSHR-blocking antibodies (TBAb) or TSHR-blocking immunoglobulins (17). Although all studies support the higher prevalence of stimulatory antibodies [for instance, Ref. (18)], the presence of only blocking TSHR antibodies may cause myxedema (19). High TSHR antibodies at diagnosis and/or positive TSHR antibodies at cessation of therapy suggest a high likelihood of relapse, mostly within the first 2 years. The levels can help to identify patients that need definitive therapy (radioiodine or surgery) (20). Anti-TSHR antibodies can cross the placental barrier and may induce transient hyperthyroidism in the neonate (21). Since half-life of IgG is ~3 weeks, symptoms disappear gradually. Blocking antibodies may also cause transient hypothyroidism with delayed development of the neonate thyroid gland.

Thyroid Peroxidase

Thyroid peroxidase is a poorly glycosylated membrane-bound enzyme, responsible for iodine (I_2) oxidation and iodination of tyrosyl residues of the Tg molecule (22). It had been termed microsomal antigen based on its intracellular localization. Antibodies react against conformational epitopes at the surface of the molecules and against linear epitopes (23). Polyclonal antibodies from healthy individuals and patients are directed against the same epitopes. Anti-TPO antibodies from healthy subjects did not block TPO activity or interfere with the blocking activity of anti-TPO antibodies from AITD patients (24), while anti-TPO antibodies from AITD patients can fix complement, destroy thyrocytes, and act as competitive inhibitors of enzymatic activity (25). These antibodies can be of any class of IgG, although some studies indicated a higher prevalence of IgG1 (70%) and IgG4 (66.1%) compared to IgG2 (35.1%) and IgG3 (19.6%) (26). Low levels of IgA antibodies have also been reported (21). Anti-TPO antibodies are more common than anti-Tg antibodies and more indicative for thyroid disease (21). Anti-TPO antibodies are inductors of oxidative stress evidenced by decreased antioxidant potential, advanced glycosylation products and oxygen metabolites in blood (27). However, their contribution to thyroid damage compared to T cell and cytokine-mediated apoptosis is minor (28). Anti-TPO antibodies are detected in 90–95% of AITD patients, 80% of GD, and 10–15% of non-AITD patients (9). While anti-TPO antibodies may act cytotoxic on thyrocytes in HT they do not have an established role in GD (29). Anti-TPO antibodies are able to cross the placenta barrier to variable extent, but the effect on the neonate is unclear. Concerns on a potential negative effect on cognitive development of the offspring have not been confirmed so far (21).

Thyroglobulin

Thyroglobulin is a large (600 kDa) glycoprotein consisting of dimers and containing on average 2–3 molecules of T4 and 0.3 molecules T3. The molecule is heterogeneous regarding hormone content, glycosylation, and size. The production of antibodies against Tg can be induced by massive destruction of the thyroid gland, but high Tg levels in blood do not *per se* induce antibody production (4). Out of the 40 epitopes that have been identified, 6 according to some authors and 1–2 according to others are immunogenic (30, 31). Antibodies against Tg differ between healthy subjects and AITD patients in that polyclonal antibodies are seen in normal subjects and oligoclonal antibodies in AITD patients (4). Antibodies in healthy subjects and AITD patients differentially recognize mainly two conformational epitopes of the molecule (32). Pattern of anti-Tg antibodies are similar in GD and HT patients and similar in healthy individuals and patients with TC (33). In general, low levels of self-antigens induce tolerance (34). It has been hypothesized that normal blood levels of Tg induce self-tolerance in T cells but not in B cells. B cells that recognize Tg arrest their migration in the T cell zone of peripheral lymphoid tissues but do not interact with CD4 helper cells. The lack of interaction prevents the B cells from migrating out of the T cell zones into the follicles, and they undergo apoptosis. As a consequence of the B cell activity, healthy individuals have very low, usually below detection threshold levels of anti-Tg antibodies. In the presence of higher Tg levels after tissue damage, changed conformation of the Tg molecule due to high I_2 levels, and supernormal TSH levels, the anti-Tg antibody titers become abnormal (31). Administration of I_2 induced antibody production in 8–20% of subjects, together with intra-thyroidal lymphocyte infiltration in some of the patients (35). The proposed mechanisms are either antibody formation due to massive release of antigens following thyrocyte destruction or generation of new epitopes by a changed and more immunogenic conformation of the Tg molecule with high I_2 content. The effects of I_2 on immune responses of Tg and TPO antigens in thyroid autoimmunity might not be completely the same. On the basis that salt intake is the main source of I_2, universal salt iodization has been introduced as protective measure against goiter. Excessive I_2 intake, defined as table salt I_2 concentrations of 40–100 mg/kg for 5 years, increased thyroid autoimmunity (36).

Anti-Tg antibodies do not fix complement because the epitopes are too widely spaced to allow cross-linking. Furthermore, anti-Tg antibodies in GD belong mainly to the IgG4 class, which is not complement binding (37). Low levels of IgA antibodies have also been reported (21). IgM antibodies against Tg have been reported to 1% in healthy individuals. The functional consequence of anti-Tg antibodies is not clear as they do not cause thyroid cell destruction. Circulating antibodies could be detected in about 10% of healthy young subjects and 15% of people >60 years of age. Among HT patients, antibody prevalence was 60–80% and in 50–60% in GD patients. Another study identified anti-Tg antibodies in 70–80% of AITD patients, 30–40% of GD patients, and 10–15% of patients with non-thyroid immune disorders (9).

Anti-Tg antibodies can cross the placenta barrier, but the effect on the neonate is unclear (21).

The distribution among the classes of antibodies against Tg has been reported differently. IgG1 and IgG4 were the most important classes in GD and HT patients according to one study, while other authors reported distribution between IgG1, IgG2, and IgG4 classes. Interestingly, distribution differed between GD and HT patients; IgG4 class was dominant in patients with GD and IgG2 class in HT patients (37). This different distribution may reflect the different type of immune action taking place in the thyroid.

Other Thyroid Antigens

Antibodies against other thyroid autoantigens are not determined routinely since their incidence is much lower and their physiological role unclear. Data obtained by immunization of mice and binding of patient sera to stably transfected COS 7 cells expressing high levels of NIS indicate that the antibodies did not display marked inhibiting effect on iodide uptake (38). Macro-TSH is the result of the binding of anti-TSH antibodies to TSH and results in a high-molecular protein complex with low TSH bioreactivity. Incidence increases with age, and altered TSH antigenicity or decrease in autoimmune tolerance have been proposed as pathogenic mechanism (39).

In summary, prevalence of anti-TPO and anti-Tg antibodies is high in patients with GD and HT, while anti-TSHR antibodies are common in GD patients but relatively rare in patients with HT. This may suggest that anti-TSHR antibodies are produced under more specific situations than the other antibodies. This difference is also reflected in some factors that have opposite effects in GD and HT, like, for instance, smoking and stress (see Factors with Opposite Effects on GD and HT). There are additional differences in development and manifestation of the diseases. GD is usually characterized by rapid onset of the symptoms and is, except for elderly people with less typical symptoms, diagnosed and treated quite fast (40). Established treatments normalize titers of TSHR antibodies in adults within 2 years, while treatment of children and adolescents requires longer treatment times (41, 42). HT develops gradually over months and years with very high antibody titers in some patients (43). Symptoms can be mild, and patients might not seek medical advice. Even when treatment has been initiated, titers of anti-TPO antibodies decrease only slowly (e.g., over 5 years) upon treatment with levothyroxine, and anti-TPO antibody titers remain in the pathological range (44). Normal anti-thyroid antibody titers are lower for anti-TSHR antibodies than for anti-TPO and anti-Tg antibodies. Exact values cannot be compared directly since sensitivities of the assays differ, but the range of >1.75 U/ml for anti-TSHR, >35 U/l for anti-TPO, and >20 U/l for anti-Tg according to most laboratories (45) can serve as approximate indication that titers are markedly different.

Environmental (Exogenous) Factors

Exogenous and endogenous factors contribute to the risk of developing AITDs. Major exogenous causative factors are infections, intake of particular substances, and radiation, while endogenous factors are mainly sex and genetic disposition (**Figure 1**). Other factors have opposite effects in the development of GD and HT or protect rather than promote the manifestation of AITD.

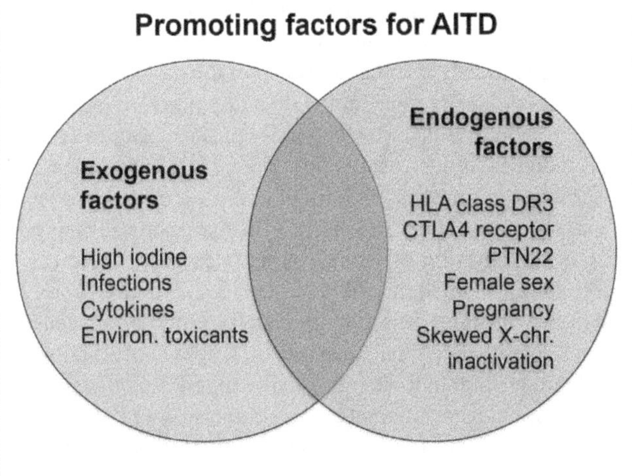

FIGURE 1 | Promoting factors in Hashimoto's and Graves' disease. Abbreviations: chr., chromosome; CTLA4, cytotoxic T-lymphocyte-associated protein 4; Environ., environmental; PTN22, protein tyrosine phosphatase, non-receptor type 22.

Factors with Opposite Effects on GD and HT

Exogenous factors include *smoking*, which has a protective effect on HT incidence by lowering anti-Tg and anti-TPO antibody levels, while favoring the development of GD (odd's ratio, OR 3.3). Opposing effects in AD affecting the same organs have also been reported for inflammatory bowel diseases. Smoking protects against ulcerative colitis but induces worsening of CRD. Recent studies suggest that smoking acts through modulation of the phenotype of dendritic cells, which are involved in the activation and differentiation of T cells (46). It might be speculated that a similar mechanism also causes the different effect of smoking on HT and GD. *Stress* or major life events can increase the prevalence of GD, but not of HT (47).

Protective Factors

Alcohol intake, which protects against several AD, also decreases the incidence of GD and of HT; abstainers have a 2.17 higher risk than non-abstainers (48, 49). High doses of alcohol consumption can directly suppress immune responses, and alcohol abuse is associated with an increased incidence of a number of infectious diseases (50). Moderate alcohol consumption seems to have a beneficial impact on the immune system compared to alcohol abuse or abstinence, but the mechanisms behind the protective effect are not clear. *Selenium* supplementation does not consistently decrease anti-TPO antibody levels, which might be due to different baseline concentrations of both selenium and anti-TPO antibodies (51). *Vitamin D* supplementation has the reputation of improving immunological function, but studies on vitamin D in AITDs are not conclusive (52); insufficient matching of all patients' parameters was suspected to potentially hide an existing correlation.

Promoting (Worsening) Factors

High oral I_2 intake (~400–600 μg/day) increases the immunogenicity of Tg by creating new epitopes or unmasking cryptic epitopes. These levels, on the other hand, are lower than the short-term treatment for thyrotoxicosis with 250 mg every 6–8 h (53). Iodine usually refers to any form of the molecule including molecular I_2, I_2 salts, sodium iodide and potassium iodide (NaI and KI), sodium iodate ($NaIO_3$), and lipids or proteins containing I_2 moieties (iodotyrosin, iodolactone) (54). The human body on the average contains 25–50 mg I_2, 50–70% of which is stored in extra-thyroidal tissues, especially in the gastrosalivary pool. $NaIO_3$ is dissolved in the stomach and releases I_2, which can be absorbed in the small intestine. In the blood, I_2 is transported as iodide and can enter cells that express NIS. Only certain cells, for example, breast cancer cells, can take up I_2 by facilitated diffusion. I_2 and iodide differ in their antioxidant properties; I_2 has a 10-fold greater antioxidant potential than ascorbic acid and 50-fold that of iodide (55). Common supplements contain either iodide alone or a mixture of I_2 and iodide. While the salt carries a great risk for interference with thyroid function, I_2 is more effective in breast pathologies, such as fibrocystic syndrome and mastalgia. Lugol's solution (5% I_2/10% kalium iodide) has a net anti-estrogenic effect. Natural food, fish, and seaweed contain mainly I_2, but the contents may vary between 1.6 μg/g and 2.9 mg/g. Despite their different physiological effects, all forms of I_2 have the potential to induce or exacerbate autoantibody formation. In addition, increased I_2 concentrations can also induce oxidative stress by increased activation of TPO (56). Membrane damage by oxidative stress can cause release of intracellular thyroid antigen and lead to the expression of intercellular adhesion molecule 1 (ICAM-1) by thyrocytes. Furthermore, excess iodide may promote apoptosis by tumor necrosis factor-related apoptosis-inducing ligand and death receptor (DR) 5 expression. Other effects of I_2 include augmentation of dendritic cell maturation, increase of T cells and antibody production by B cells, and increasing cytokine secretion (28). Iodinization increased the prevalence of anti-TPO antibodies in the population from 14.3 to 23.8% and for anti-Tg antibodies from 13.7 to 19.9% (57). It also increased apoptosis induction *via* the Fas-mediated pathway and downregulation of Bcl-2, $CD8^+$ T cell-mediated cytotoxicity by enhanced ICAM-1 expression increasing cell–cell binding, and gap junction changes by downregulation of connexin 43. In the latter case, gap junctions become less tight due to the downregulation of the protein, and TPO antibodies can access TPO at the apical plasma membrane of the thyrocytes and activate complement.

Infection with viruses, such as hepatitis C (HCV), hepatitis E, parvovirus, rubella, herpes simplex, Epstein–Barr, or human T lymphotropic virus type 1 (HLTV1), could be involved in the pathogenesis of AITDs (58). The release of IL-8 by thyroid cells infected with HCV as pathogenic mechanism has been demonstrated in cell culture (59). Gut microbiota can trigger HT, and enteroviruses have been identified in thyroid tissues. *Yersinia enterocolitica* antibody cross-reactions with TSHR are assumed to induce GD symptoms (57). This effect has been explained by molecular mimicry, which is defined as the phenomenon whereby exposure to a particular peptide epitope in the environment stimulates antibody production against an endogenous antigen containing the identical amino acid sequences (60). The role of commensal bacteria to the development of HT is not yet proven. Enteropathy (leaky gut syndrome) with increased intestinal permeability and intraepithelial lymphocyte infiltration may also increase the risk for developing thyroid autoimmunity, but further studies are needed (61). Infection with HLTV1 and with *Helicobacter pylori* have been linked to AITD by either thyrocyte damage or cytokine secretion (62). Animal experiments proved the mediator role of interferon-alpha in the induction of inflammatory thyroid destruction (63). Pathways associated with apoptosis and autophagy were not induced. Although contact with specific pathogenic and commensal viruses and bacteria can trigger the manifestation of GD and HT, lack of infections (termed "hygiene hypothesis") also increases the risk for allergies and AD, such as AITD (64).

Specific *cytokines* such as interferon-gamma (IFN-γ), IL-2, and granulocyte–macrophage colony-stimulating factor promote the development of AITD (65). In a similar way, treatment with the anti-programmed death 1 receptor monoclonal antibody pembrolizumab interfered with thyroid function causing elevation of anti-thyroid antibodies accompanied by AITDs resulting in either hypo- or hyperthyroidism (66).

Epidemiological studies showed that individuals exposed to *environmental toxicants*, such as polyaromatic hydrocarbons, including polychlorinated biphenyls and polyhalogenated biphenyls, had elevated circulating antibody levels against TPO and Tg (67). Furthermore, drugs, like, for instance, lithium in the treatment of bipolar mood disorders, precipitate AITD (68). *Radiation* (therapeutically or environmental) may induce thyrocyte damage and stimulate the development of AITD by release of thyroid antigens (69).

A broad panel of exogenous factors may contribute to the manifestation of AITDs. Some of these thyroiditis forms are also regarded as separate entities, such as radiation-induced (radioactive iodine, beam radiation) thyroiditis and drug-induced (amiodarone, lithium, interferon-α, cytokines) thyroiditis.

Endogenous Factors

Genetic effects can explain 79% of the manifestations of GD, and anti-thyroid antibody formation is positively correlated at a level of 73% in twins (70). Human leukocyte antigen (HLA) class II antigens are thought to contribute 20% of these genetic risk factors. Association with GD was around 30% for cytotoxic T-lymphocyte-associated protein 4 (CTLA4). CD40 can increase HLA and CTLA4 risk. Protein tyrosine phosphatase, non-receptor type 22 (PTN22), was associated with AITDs with an OR of 1.41–3.65 depending on geographic region and race (71). Some *HLA alleles* have a higher affinity for autoantigenic thyroid peptides than others. Polymorphisms in HLA class II DR3 predispose to GD, while for HT various HLA alleles have been reported such as DR3, DR5, DQ7, DQB1, DQw7, and others. Together with the binding of the T cell receptor to the HLA–antigen complex, activation of the T cell immune response requires binding of co-stimulatory ligands such as B7 on antigen-presenting cells (APC) to the CD28 receptor on the T cell. However, B7 also binds the *CTLA4* (*CD28*), which inhibits T cell proliferation to control rampant immune responses; several CTLA4 polymorphisms have been identified in HT and GD patients, mostly single nucleotide polymorphism (SNP). SNPs are also associated with antibody production (28). Certain of these CTLA4 polymorphisms result in a greater proliferative response of the T cells, which might explain associations with AD. SNPs in the *PTN22 gene* enable efficient inhibition of T cell activation and impaired thymic deletion of autoreactive T cells in combination with inhibition of regulatory T cells. This was suggested as reason why this might lead to AD. Additional SNPs have been identified in Tg genes, the vitamin D receptor, IL-4, transforming growth factor-beta (TGF-β), FoxP3, and the tumor necrosis factor-alpha (TNF-α) gene. Genomic imprinting (the activation of maternal or paternal genes) has not been well studied in AD, but the Tg promoter appears to be a candidate for epigenetic effects (silencing or activation of genes) in AITDs (72).

Female preponderance is seen in all AD. AITD is one example where this is very pronounced, and many studies aimed to understand the underlying mechanisms focusing first on differences in the immune system. Females have similar numbers of lymphocytes but higher antibody production by B cells. In addition to that, females have stronger humoral and cellular immune responses, higher $CD4^+$ T cell levels after immunization, and lower susceptibility to various bacterial infections (73). Typically, only herpes simplex type 2 infections are more common in females than in males. One reason for the observed differences might be the prominent immune modulatory effects of estrogens. Immune cells carry receptors for estrogen, testosterone, and progesterone (74). Estrogen decreases the $CD4^+/CD8^+$ T cell ratio and TNF-α cytotoxicity in T cells and increases immunoglobulin secretion, B cell survival, and polyclonal activation of B cells as well as IgG and IgM production in peripheral blood mononuclear cells. High estrogen levels decrease Th1 pro-inflammatory pathways and increase Th2 anti-inflammatory pathways. Progesterone in general acts in an anti-inflammatory manner by inhibition of macrophage activation, nitric oxide production, and IFN-γ production by NK cells (75).

The higher prevalence of AD in patients with structural X-chromosome defects and monosomy implied a crucial role of the X-chromosome in autoimmune reactions. In women, one of the two X-chromosomes is inactivated in every cell. Usually, the ratio of inactivation is 50:50 for paternal and maternal X-chromosomes. However, in some women a skewed inactivation is seen that could lead to insufficiently high levels of specific antigens to induce self-tolerance. Consistent with this idea *skewed X-chromosome inactivation* has been preferentially detected in women with AITD with a correlation of OR 2.54 for GD and 2.40 for HT (57). The correlation of skewed X-chromosome inactivation and TPO antibody level was stronger in dizygotic than in monozygotic twin supporting the assumption that the inactivation is more important for the manifestation of the disease than the genes themselves. The Y-chromosome is less important for survival because it harbors only a few genes. Nevertheless, loss of the Y-chromosome has been identified in GD and HT patients and is accompanied by reduced testosterone levels. The few genes not related to male fertility are X-chromosome homologs with relevant roles in immune function (76). The loss could cause haplo-insufficiency similar to X-chromosome loss, and an imbalance for the alleles shared with the X-chromosome could emerge. An additional reason might be the relationship between thyroid and testosterone *via* regulation of sex-hormone binding globulin (77). High thyroid hormone levels increase the levels of free testosterone with subsequent physiological effects. Alterations in hormone levels such as increases in testosterone in females with polycystic ovary syndrome increase the prevalence of AITDs (78).

Pregnancy has a marked impact on AD, whereby the number of regulatory T cells is increased in gravidity and levels of anti-thyroid antibodies decreased. This decrease is usually transient, and a rebound effect of the antibody levels is seen 6 weeks post-partum (28). The postpartum period is a risk for onset of GD, and postpartum thyroiditis may lead to HT. Postpartum thyroiditis is defined as destructive thyroiditis within 1 year of parturition. The disease is characterized by transient hypothyroidism or hyper-thyroidism or hyperthyroidism followed by hypothyroidism. Patients often recover, but there is up to a 50% risk of developing permanent thyroid disease with time (79). Previous pregnancy as a risk factor for AITD could be due to fetal microchimerism, i.e., the phenomenon that fetal cells and antigens are transferred to the mother. Fetal microchimeric cells have been found particularly in AITD patients. The fetal cells were cytotoxic T cells able to mitigate graft-versus-host reactions (75). The more fetal cells show similarities with the maternal cells, the more likely they have the potential to mediate such reactions. Although pregnancies ≥ 1 have an OR of 1.1–1.8 for AITD compared to nulliparous women there is still no proof for the hypothesis that fetal microchimerism causes HT (80). Furthermore, parity is not linked to increased antibody levels in all studies.

Immunologic Processes in AITD

The basic differences between the two most common AITDs, HT and GD, is the reaction to the deregulated immune system. Several excellent reviews are available on the mechanisms of AITD [examples are Ref. (57, 72, 81), which will be only presented in cursory way in this review in **Figure 2**]. Presentation of autoantigens *via* MHC complex/self-peptide complexes by APC and recognized in the periphery by thymus-selected autoreactive $CD4^+$ T cells is the initial step in the pathogenesis of AITDs (82). Reduction of immune tolerance by various mechanisms and changes in the thyroid microenvironment are contributing factors in the development of GD and HT. Despite intense research, the exact mechanism of HT is not completely clear, but the following mechanisms are proposed (83). Decreased function of regulatory T cells, increased activity of follicular T helper cells, release of DNA fragments, and alteration in miRNA profile initiate and perpetuate HT. The number of regulatory T cells plays an important role, and their number increases upon levothyroxine treatment. The hypothesized mechanism of regulatory T cells is the suppression of lymphocyte differentiation to Th1 cells (84). Th17 cells are a newly identified $CD4^+$ subgroup of T helper cells, which were found to be increased in the blood of children with untreated HT but not in GD patients. Double-stranded DNA released from the nuclei of damaged thyrocytes is actively taken up or leak into neighboring cells. Extra-chromosomal histone (H2B) recognizes the misplaced DNA and induces the release of pro-inflammatory cytokines *via* translocation of interferon regulatory transcription factor and nuclear factor "kappa-light-chain-enhancer" of activated B cells (NFκB) into the nucleus. As a result of the release of the cytokine/chemokine MHC expression by thyrocytes and lymphocytes infiltration takes place. Activated

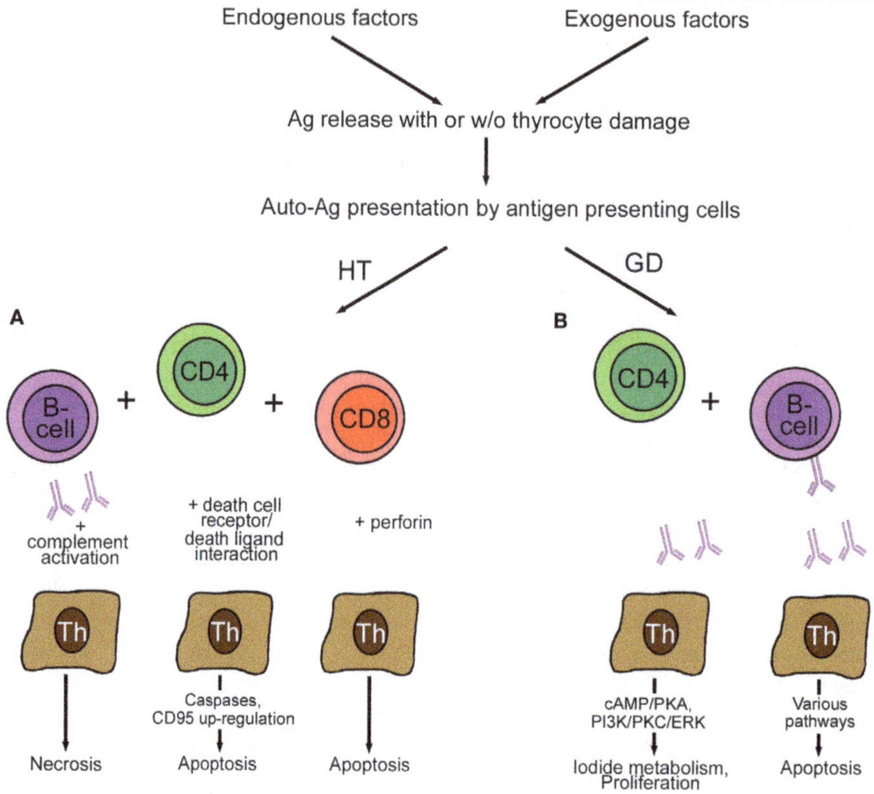

FIGURE 2 | Pathogenesis of Hashimoto's disease (A) and GD (B). **(A)** Autoreactive CD4⁺ T cells in HT induce antibody production by B cells. The antibodies bind to the basal membrane of the thyroid follicle, activate complement, and induce necrosis of thyrocytes. The activation of cytotoxic CD8⁺ T cells leads to the induction of apoptosis by action of perforin. Finally, the expression of Fas (CD95) and FasL (CD95L) by thyrocytes perpetuates HT. **(B)** Autoreactive CD4⁺ T cells in GD induce only anti-thyroid-stimulating hormone receptor antibody-producing B cells. These antibodies act stimulatory by increasing I_2 metabolism (cAMP/PKA) and promoting proliferation and survival (PI3K/PKC/ERK) of thyrocytes. Blocking antibodies are characterized by lack of effect (not shown), and neutral antibodies activate various pathways, such as PI3K/Akt, mTOR/p70S6K, and MAPK/ERK1/2 and induce thyrocyte apoptosis. Abbreviations: GD, Graves' disease; HT, Hashimoto's thyroiditis; ERK, extracellular signal-regulated kinase; MAPK, mitogen-activated protein kinase; p70S6K, ribosomal protein S6 kinase beta-1; PKC, protein kinase C; PI3K, phosphatidylinositol 3,4,5, triphosphate kinase; PKA, protein kinase; mTOR, mammalian target of rapamycin.

T and B cells and DR-mediated apoptosis initiate and perpetuate the autoimmune reaction in HT (85). Self-reactive $CD4^+$ T cells recruit $CD8^+$ cytotoxic T cells, which cause thyrocyte death by release of granzyme and perforin (**Figure 2**). Antibodies secreted by B cells are deposited at the basal membrane of the thyroid follicle, activate complement system, and thereby induce necrosis. Increased levels of the cytokines IFN-γ and IL-12 (Th1 cytokines) induce TNF-α, IL-1β, IL-2, and CD40L, which cause apoptosis of thyrocytes but not of infiltrating lymphocytes. Apoptotic death of thyrocytes can occur in a paracrine way by expression of cell DR (Fas, apoptosis protein 1, CD95) and death ligands (FasL, CD95L).

In contrast to HT, self-reactive $CD4^+$ lymphocytes in GD recruit only TSH-reactive B cells. Secretion of IL-4 (a Th2 cytokine) together with IL-5, IL-6, IL-10, IL-13, and CD40L causes apoptosis of the infiltrating lymphocytes and proliferation of thyrocytes resulting in GD. Lymphocytes resident in the thyroid, not lymphocytes in lymphoid organs, produce the anti-thyroid antibodies. Usually, when the thyroid is removed, the production of autoantibodies ceases.

Antibodies reach the blood stream *via* transepithelial transport by uptake combined with megalin (receptor) and release into the extracellular space or by disruption of the thyroid follicles. Alternatively, secretion by transformed thyrocytes may occur (4). The nature of the immune reaction differs in different AITDs with mainly T cell-mediated autoimmunity in HT and primary humoral response in GD (86). In reality, there are mixed Th1/Th2 responses in both GD and HT and, although the diseases have different phenotypes, GD and HT may coexist in the same thyroid gland, and some individuals progress from one to the other. The transition from GD to hypothyroidism due to HT can occur, while the development of GD from HT is rare (87).

ANTI-THYROID ANTIBODY TYPES: THE KEY TO THE DIAGNOSIS

Increased levels of anti-thyroid antibodies usually accompany AITDs, and their detection may support its diagnosis. Manifestations of the main AITDs are described in the following sections.

Hashimoto's Thyroiditis

Hashimoto's thyroiditis may lead to manifest hypothyroidism, but most patients have subclinical hypothyroidism with increased TSH and normal thyroid hormone levels. There are different variants of HT, termed fibrous, fibrous atrophic (Ord's disease), or goitrous forms, and IgG4 thyroiditis (88). Based on debates that Riedel thyroiditis is not primarily a thyroid disease but rather a manifestation of the systemic disorder multifocal fibrosclerosis, this variant is no longer classified as a variant of HT. Conversely, IgG4-related thyroiditis is now recognized as new entity of AITD (89). IgG4-related thyroiditis is associated with more frequent subclinical hypothyroidism and with higher levels of thyroid autoantibodies compared to the non-IgG4 thyroiditis group. In contrast to the other AITD forms there is a male preponderance (90). In long course of HT mainly IgG4 autoantibodies are produced (91), which trigger the development of IgG4-related disease (IgG4-RD). IgG4-RD can affect a variety of tissues (pancreas, skin, salivary glands, lacrimal glands, etc.), and the hallmarks are lymphoplasmacytic infiltrations with predominance of IgG4-positive plasma cells and fibrosis in the affected tissue. The atrophic form is more common than HT with enlargement of the thyroid gland (92). Although both forms lead to hypothyroidism, they have been reported as distinct diseases, differing in immunological background (associated with different HLA alleles), involvement of autoantibodies, and type of immune response (humoral versus cellular). The hypothesis that Ord's disease was the end stage of HT could not be confirmed in follow-up studies (93). Thyroid autoantibody levels differ between goitrous and atrophic thyroiditis in that inhibitory TSHR antibodies are higher in Ord's thyroiditis. These antibodies block cAMP production as well as TSH-induced DNA synthesis and iodide uptake (94). It has been hypothesized that antibody production promotes progression to hypothyroidism because higher levels of antibodies against Tg and TPO accompany deterioration of thyroid function (95). Destruction of the thyroid gland >90% leads to hypothyroidism (4). In the case of overt hypothyroidism, patients experience fatigue, weight gain, increased sensitivity to cold, difficulty concentrating, dry skin, nails, and hair, constipation, drowsiness, muscle soreness, and increased menstrual flow. HT is much more frequent in individuals affected by another AD. Although high anti-thyroid antibody titers may provide an indication of the likelihood of overt hypothyroidism, no correlation of antibody titer and risk for hypothyroidism has been found so far (96).

Graves' Disease

Symptoms often become manifest after emotional trauma and symptoms of hyperthyroidism arise with weight loss, weakness, dyspnea, palpitations, increased hunger and thirst, hyperdefecation, sweating, sensitivity to heat, tremor, irritability, and menstrual irregularity. Thyroid metabolism is accelerated with faster plasma turnover, higher TPO activity, excess Tg release, increased clearance of iodide from the plasma and decreased retention of iodide in the thyroid, and usually increased gland volume (97). Administration of high doses of I_2 (1–2 mg) temporarily inhibits iodide uptake, trapping, organification, and hormone release in addition to reduction of thyroidal blood flow (98). Organification of I_2 presumably is decreased by the blocking action of an oxidized iodide intermediate or depressed H_2O_2 generation. Although the blocking of I_2 organification, reduced iodide uptake, and hormone release is a physiological reaction of the thyroid (Wolff–Chaikoff effect), it is more pronounced in GD patients than in healthy controls.

Anti-thyroid Antibodies and Non-Thyroid Immunological Diseases

Circulating antibodies against thyroid antigens are not restricted to AITDs but were also detected in other common AD like RA, T1DM, and celiac disease (CD). Anti-TPO and anti-Tg antibodies were identified in 37 and 22.9% of RA patients, respectively. The authors detected anti-TPO in 13% and anti-Tg antibodies in 11.5% of healthy controls (99). In other studies lower prevalence of 16 and 12.3% in RA patients was detected, while the prevalence of anti-thyroid antibodies in healthy controls (8%) was similar (100, 101). Around 39.6% of T1DM patients had anti-TPO, and 30% had anti-Tg antibodies in one study, but other studies reported variations of 7–40% for anti-TPO and around 15% for anti-Tg antibodies (102, 103). This relatively high incidence in T1DM patients could not be explained by the fact that glycosylation of the Tg protein increased antigenicity or immunogenicity of the protein (104). Circulating anti-TPO and anti-Tg antibodies in CD patients have been detected in 11.7–30.5% (TPO) and 11.2–32% (Tg) (105) of patients. Other studies reported anti-thyroid antibodies in 26.2–41.1% of CD patients (106). The close interaction between CD and AITD was evidenced by the decrease of thyroid disorders and anti-thyroid antibodies after switching to a gluten-free diet. The link to other immune pathologies is further demonstrated by the fact that anti-TPO antibodies were also detected in patients affected by non-AD such as asthma patients. The antibodies were detected in 27.3% of subjects in one study and 15% of subjects in the other, compared to 10 and 8.3% in the controls (107, 108). Also 10–29% of idiopathic urticarial patients possessed anti-TPO antibodies, rather as an epiphenomenon than as cause of the disease (109). While the presence of anti-thyroid antibodies in other immune diseases is relatively frequent, patients with AITD produce antibodies against extra-thyroidal organs less frequently (10–15%) although comorbidities with other AD, such as vitiligo, may occur (110). It appears that subjects with deregulated immune systems are most prone to anti-thyroid antibody production. The prevalence of anti-TPO antibodies in AD is slightly higher than that of anti-Tg antibodies. In contrast to that, anti-TSHR antibodies have rarely been reported in non-thyroid immunological diseases. No expression of anti-TSHR antibodies was seen in RA patients while one study detected the antibodies in 18% of T1DM patients (111, 112). According to other authors, anti-TSHR antibodies are only seen in AITDs (21). The reason why anti-TSHR antibodies are specific for GD and antibodies against TPO and Tg also seen in other AD appears to suggest that HT and AD are more similar than GD and HT.

The link of specific pathological changes to anti-thyroid antibody titers in patients with other AD is complicated by the multifaceted manifestation of the diseases. Effects of anti-thyroid antibodies are best studied in subjects without AD or manifest thyroid dysfunction.

Anti-thyroid Antibodies in Extra-Thyroidal Pathologies

Extra-thyroidal effects of anti-TSHR, anti-Tg, and anti-TPO antibodies are shown in **Figure 3**.

Anti-TSHR Antibodies

Extra-thyroidal manifestation of GD include swelling of the orbital tissue and of the skin, termed as *Graves' orbitopathy* (*GO*) and *Graves' dermopathy*. The term ophthalmopathy is also being used, but orbitopathy is preferred because it describes the pathological alterations more correctly. *GO* affects about 25% of GD patients (113) and results in dysmobility of extraocular muscles and optic nerve compression. It represents also the only extra-thyroidal pathology where the role of anti-thyroid antibodies is relatively well known. Target cells are infiltrating autoreactive T cells and fibroblasts resident between the extra-orbital muscles. These cell types interact *via* cytokine secretion and mutually stimulate each other. Both cell types express TSHR and IGF-1 receptors, which form a functional complex on orbital fibroblasts. Activated fibroblasts may either differentiate into myofibroblasts or adipocytes, or they may secrete hyaluronic acid and prostaglandin E2 (**Figure 4**). Major cytokines secreted by T cells include IL-1, IL-4, IL-6, TGF-β, leukoregulin, and IGF-1, while orbital fibroblasts release IL-1, IL-6, IL-8, IL-10, IL-12, MCP-1, and TNF-α (114). Inflammation and increased hyaluronic acid cause an increase in volume and lead to exopthalmos (115). Anti-TSHR antibody levels correlate with severity of GO and are predictive for the later development. By contrast, no correlation between severity of GO and hormone levels has been identified (116, 117). This finding highlights the role of TSHR antibodies as promoters of GO.

Graves' dermopathy is an extra-thyroidal manifestation exclusively found in GD patients. Dermopathy develops in the presence of high TSHR antibody levels and is, with a frequency of 15%, a less common extra-thyroidal manifestation of GD (118). The main localization is pretibial and is associated with acropachy (digital clubbing, swelling of digits and toes, and periosteal reaction of extremity bones) in 20% of patients. TSHR is expressed in skin fibroblasts and abundant mucin deposition, possessing gel-like properties, separates the collagen fibers. Stimulation of fibroblasts by anti-TSHR antibodies along with mechanical factors and venous stasis causes accumulation of mucin. Trauma and injury may lead to the activation of T cells and the initiation of an antigen specific response, in this case the activation of fibroblasts and production of glucosaminoglycans (GAGs) (119).

Anti-TPO Antibodies

Hashimoto's encephalopathy (*HE*) with confusion, agitation, seizures, status epilepticus, cognitive decline, and psychiatric symptoms appears to be independent of the state of the thyroid (120). HE is believed to be an immune-mediated disorder rather than representing the direct effect of an altered thyroid state on the central nervous system. Hypotheses include autoimmune vasculitis or other inflammatory processes, which may lead to disruption of the cerebral microvasculature. Although the presence of anti-TPO antibodies is the most common feature, a

Antibodies against

TSHR	TPO	Tg

• Graves' Orbitopathy
• Graves' Dermatopathy
• Cancer incidence:
  • Breast
  • Colon,
  • Kidney
  • Uterus
  • Ovary
	• Hashimoto's encephalitis
	• Infertility
	• Vasculo-placental complications
	• Health in aged women
	• Cancer incidence:
	  • Breast
	  • Colon
	  • Kidney
	  • Uterus
	• Survival breast cancer patients
		• Infertility
		• Cancer incidence:
		  • Breast
		  • Colon
		  • Kidney
		  • Uterus
		• Survival breast cancer patients

FIGURE 3 | Overview of extra-thyroidal effects of anti-thyroid antibodies.

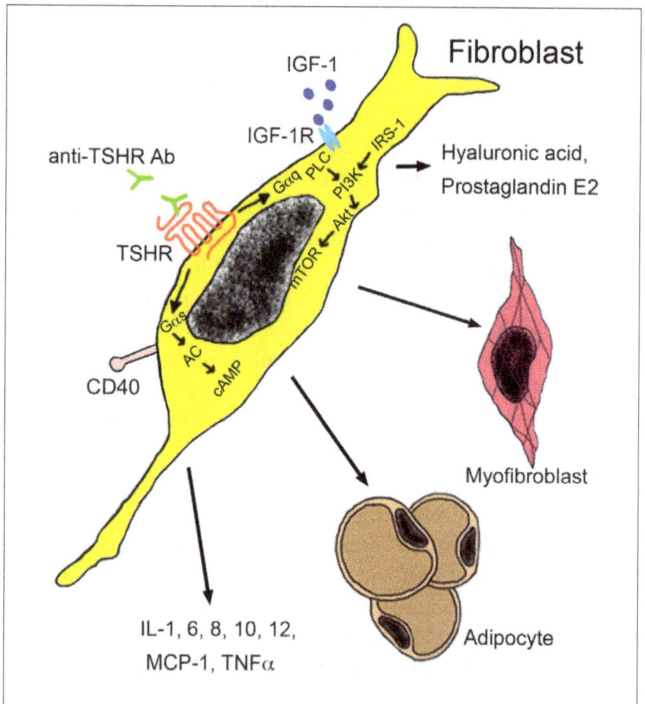

FIGURE 4 | Autoantibodies in the pathogenesis of Graves' orbitopathy. Anti-TSHR antibodies bind to the TSHR on orbital fibroblasts, which initiate signaling through Gαs and Gαq subunits. The Gαs complex initiates signaling by the protein kinase A through generation of cAMP by adenylyl kinase (AC). The Gαq pathway mediates activation of phospholipase C (PLC) and leads to activation of phosphatidylinositol 3,4,5 triphosphate by phosphatidylinositol 3,4,5 triphosphate kinase (PI3K) under the influence of insulin receptor substrate 1 (IRS-1). Akt activation results in mammalian target of rapamycin (mTOR) signaling with proliferation and secretion of cytokines, hyaluronic acid, and adipogenesis. Activation of orbital fibroblasts by T cells occurs *via* binding of the CD154 molecule on the T cell surface to the CD40 on the fibroblast surface. Abbreviations: IGF-1, insulin growth factor 1; IGF-1R, insulin growth factor 1 receptor; MCP-1, monocyte chemotactic protein 1; TNF-α, tumor necrosis factor-alpha; TSHR, thyroid-stimulating hormone receptor.

pathogenic role of anti-thyroid antibodies could not be identified (121). Further concerns about the relevance of anti-thyroid antibodies are linked to the use of assays that have not been validated for liquor as matrix. Matrix differences may play a role because liquor samples, due to the lower antibody levels that are expected, are usually tested in less diluted form than serum or plasma samples [for example, Ref. (122)]. Anti-TPO antibodies were shown to bind to cerebellar astrocytes, but their pathogenic role is unclear (123). Furthermore, α-enolase has been suggested as the true antigen for antibodies in HE (88). HT is also related to dysfunction of the vestibular system, which can be identified by abnormal caloric test and vestibular-evoked myogenic potential. The dysfunction was linked to increased anti-TPO antibodies without identification of the pathogenic mechanism (124).

Correlations of anti-thyroid antibody production with *decreased fertility* is suspected but was not confirmed in a recent study (125), which was performed in a highly selected study collective of predominantly very healthy and well educated women, and might not be representative for all women. The rate of miscarriage and preterm delivery was increased in women with anti-TPO and anti-Tg antibodies who underwent *in vitro* fertilization/intracytoplasmic sperm injection (IVF/ICSI). However, no difference was noted in the number of retrieved oocytes or success of IVF/ICSI (126). Anti-TPO antibodies are suspected to cause *vasculo-placental* complications, such as hypertonia, pre-eclampsia, preterm placenta abruption, postpartum hemorrhage, and postpartum thyroiditis (127). Since anti-thyroid antibodies can cross the placental barrier, they are able to induce hypothyroidism in the newborns. Women with high anti-TPO antibody titers display an impaired thyroidal response to human chorionic gonadotropin, and this may explain the higher risk of premature delivery in these women (128).

Positive *health effects* have been identified in older women. Women with anti TPO antibodies were less frail, defined as weight loss >10% of body weight between 60 years and age at the evaluation, exhaustion, slowness, weakness, and low energy expenditure (129). The authors did not find any indications of deficient immune function in the non-seropositive (frailer) women. In contrast, they emphasized the concept of beneficial autoimmunity, which proposes that natural autoantibodies have a role in broadening the B-cell repertoire. Although this idea appears attractive, anti-thyroid antibodies do not fit into this classification because they do not bind any pro-inflammatory or cytotoxic mediators.

In summary, anti-TSHR antibodies affect eye and skin as part of GD, and the mechanisms of anti-TSHR antibody action is relatively well known, while effects of anti-TPO antibodies are more varied and affect central nervous system, female reproductive organs, and female health. The underlying mechanisms are largely unknown. Anti-Tg antibodies were often determined together with anti-TPO antibodies, but independent effects have been identified so far.

AITD AND CANCER

The risk of development of differentiated thyroid cancer (DTC) following AITD is still under debate. HT patients had a three times higher risk to develop papillary thyroid cancer according to some studies, while other studies did not report an increased incidence in HT patients (33). Differences in methodology, especially the use of fine needle biopsy versus thyroidectomy sections, might contribute to the contradictory results (130). While an increased risk has been identified based on evaluation of thyroidectomy samples [hazard ratio (HR) 1.15–4.16], fine needle analysis did not show such a link (HR 0.39–1.00). GD was associated with DTC with an adjusted HR of 10.4 for TC and explained by the stimulating activity of TSHR antibodies (131). Synchronicity of breast and thyroid cancer formation was found with the breast cancer growing faster (132).

Thyroid diseases, benign and malignant, presented an increased risk for extra-thyroidal cancers, particularly for breast, colon, melanoma, hematologic malignancies, uterus, kidney, and ovary (133). GD was associated with breast cancer with an HR of 1.54 (131). The main link between thyroid and breast cancer appears to occur *via* thyroid hormones. Breast cells possess dysregulated thyroid hormone receptors, and thyroid hormones can activate estrogen receptors, which correlate with breast cancer risk (133). High thyroid hormone levels were linked to breast cancer incidence, suggesting that the antibodies themselves were not important in the pro-cancer action. The study itself was conducted carefully, and the rate of mammography was not different between the groups. However, family history, smoking activity, and socioeconomic status were not evaluated. The coexistence of HT and TC has been reported at a rate of 1–23%, while correlation of lung and colon cancer and HT were reported only inconsistently. AITD was correlated to DTC risk, parathyroid tumors, oral, and breast cancer. Incidence of colon cancer, melanoma, and non-Hodgkin lymphoma was decreased (134, 135). Breast cancer prevalence was significantly higher in patients with thyroid diseases versus healthy controls (6.11 versus 2.07%). There was, however, no significant difference in the risk between type of thyroid disease or antibody status (136). AITD has been correlated with breast cancer prevalence in some cross-sectional studies (137–139). However, a correlation of thyroid diseases and breast cancer was documented in only 6 of 13 analyzed studies. Summarizing all studies, Sarlis et al. computed a relative risk for patients with thyroid diseases of 1.07 (140). The debate on the relationship of AITD and breast cancer is still not resolved, and indications of a higher percentage of thyroid dysfunction in breast cancer patients than in the general population are reported by some groups but not by others [for instance, Ref. (141–143)]. A major disadvantage of the cross-sectional studies is that breast cancer is already present, and an effect of breast cancer on thyroid physiology cannot be excluded. The best way to exclude such an influence is to analyze thyroid parameters and breast cancer incidence in prospective studies. Such studies have identified an association of high free thyroxine (fT4) and breast cancer incidence (144, 145). Elevated T3 levels were also correlated with a higher incidence of breast cancer as well as shorter survival time (HR 2.80) but not with increased overall cancer mortality (HR 1.09) (146, 147). In contrast, studies on free triiodothyronine (fT3) yielded discordant results on the link to breast cancer (145), and the authors advised that, due to the short half-life of fT3, either total T3 or fT4 were more suitable parameters for these analyses.

Role of Anti-thyroid Antibodies

Cancer Incidence

The combination of high TSH levels, anti-TPO, and anti-Tg antibodies was identified as a risk factor for DTC (148), but seropositivity for Tg antibodies has not been reported consistently. An increased prevalence of melanoma, colon cancer, breast cancer, and hematological malignancies in patients suffering from GD or HT has been identified, but the overall risk for breast, colon, kidney, and uterine cancer was lower in patients with anti-TPO and anti-Tg antibodies than without (133). Prevalence of breast, colon, kidney, uterine, and ovarian cancer was increased in AITD patients with high titer anti-TSHR antibodies, but numbers were too low for statistical analysis. The authors identified a protective effect of anti-TPO and anti-Tg antibodies for breast cancer in this study and a previous study on the association of benign thyroid diseases and cancer (149). This correlation appears consistent with the finding that anti-TPO-positive breast cancer patients had better survival and longer disease-free intervals (150). Surprisingly, the beneficial action of anti-TPO antibody on breast cancer was restricted to women with thyroid volume (10–18 ml) in the normal range of between 10.7 and 17.5 ml (151–153). Several studies specifically investigated the role of anti-thyroid antibodies in breast cancer. In one study anti-TPO and anti-Tg seropositive patients had a higher risk of developing breast cancer than the antibody-negative group (154), while another study did not find such a correlation (136). Anti-TSHR antibody levels were higher in breast cancer patients than in women with benign tumors or healthy controls (155), but a pathogenic role of anti-TSHR antibodies in breast cancer is not expected because breast tissue does not express TSHR (156). According to time-dependency, antibody generation preceded the manifestation of breast cancer, making antibody production as an epiphenomenon of breast cancer unlikely (157). Seropositivity for TPO, but not for Tg, was linked to breast cancer prevalence, while no correlation was identified between the presence of anti-thyroid antibodies and tumor estrogen and progesterone receptor status (158, 159). A recent meta-analysis of eight studies reported higher anti-TPO and anti-Tg antibodies as well as higher T3 and T4 levels in breast cancer patients than in controls (160).

It might be speculated that inflammation initiated by anti-thyroid antibodies play an important role in promoting tumorigenesis. The fact that colon cancer is more frequent in patients with inflammatory bowel diseases than in controls supports the link of chronic inflammation and transformation (161). A causative role of chronic inflammation might also be deduced in breast cancer development since anti-TPO antibodies are able to cross-react with lactoperoxidase and initiate the inflammatory process. Cross-reactivity of anti-TPO antibodies with lactoperoxidase and myeloperoxidase as has been shown by Rapoport and McLachlan, and some anti-TPO antibodies actually inhibited peroxidase activity (162). Anti-TPO antibodies could also cause direct effects on neutrophilic granulocytes since its cross-reactivity with myeloperoxidase was observed in a subgroup of patients with vasculitic disorders and AITDs (163). Another study, however, failed to identify cross-reactivity of anti-TPO antibodies from AITD patients with myeloperoxidase (164).

In summary, a promoting role of anti-TSHR antibodies on breast cancer has been shown, while the role of anti-Tg and anti-TPO is unclear.

Breast Cancer Survival

The stronger link of thyroid disease to breast malignancies than to other cancers can be explained by the specific connection between these tissues. Twenty-eight percent of patients with benign fibrocytic mastopathy have anti-TPO antibodies, and 80% have thyroid hypertrophy. It is possible that generation of oxidative stress upon iodination of proteins may promote transformation of mammary cells and promote breast cancer development. On the other hand, I_2 may have a beneficial role in tumor development; reduction of lipidperoxidation and formation of anti-proliferative lipids, iodolactones, has been reported (165). The intake of moderately high I_2 concentrations (0.05% I_2/kalium iodide) reduced mammary fibrosis in women by suppression of NIS, pendrin, TPO, and deiodinase type 1, but metabolism of I_2 was found to be independent of TPO (166). Molecular I_2 caused apoptosis in human breast cancer cells and reduced cancer growth in rat models (167). Consistent with this hypothesis, I_2 levels in breast cancer were lower than in normal breast tissue (168).

Many studies recorded incidence without distinguishing between early and advanced breast cancer. In the study by Kuijpens et al., high TSH and anti-TPO antibody levels were not correlated with the risk of breast cancer (169). When patients were grouped into early and advanced stages, with the exception of an early study in 1976, thyroiditis was not linked to advanced breast cancer (138, 139, 170). When focusing on advanced stages of breast cancer, Fiore et al. identified a favorable effect of anti-TPO and/or anti-Tg antibodies on survival (171). Jiskra et al., on the other hand, found no influence of anti-thyroid antibodies on breast cancer survival (172). Thyroid hormones *per se* have an impact on breast cells by potentiating the growth-promoting effect of estrogen (173). Therefore, the presence of increased thyroid hormone levels impairs the identification of potential protective effects caused by anti-thyroid antibodies. A higher incidence of breast cancer in seropositive women could be explained by the fact that, due to the thyroid disease, these women received better medical care or had more frequent medical examinations, resulting in an earlier diagnosis of breast cancer. Since routine mammography has already been introduced in most countries, an earlier diagnosis due to stricter adherence to mammography would have to be suggested. There are, however, no indications that this could be the case (145). Studies on patients with newly diagnosed breast cancer reported that anti-TPO antibodies were linked to lower incidence of metastasis and less lymph node involvement (174–176). This finding might be explained by a better immune response against tumor tissue. On the other hand, longer survival of breast cancer patients with anti-thyroid antibodies could be due to the fact that these women are taking additional medications that might be beneficial for breast cancer.

There are currently no hypotheses as to how anti-thyroid antibodies can inhibit breast cancer progression. Despite correlations with lower proliferation rates and lower numbers of affected axillary lymph nodes, anti-TPO antibodies have not yet been proven to engage in interaction with receptors located on cancerous breast tissue (176). Therefore, it is assumed that they are simply indicators for a more active immune system, and that an active immune system may also limit progression of breast cancer. In contrast to that, anti-TSHR antibodies do not appear to have a positive effect in manifest breast cancer.

CONCLUSION

There are currently only a few indications for a specific role of anti-thyroid antibodies in extra-thyroidal pathologies. Anti-TSHR antibodies differ from anti-TPO and anti-Tg antibodies in many respects (localization of the antigen, class, action, duration of increased levels, and prevalence of the antibody), which are indicated in **Table 1**. Most importantly, action of anti-TSHR antibodies appears relatively well defined and restricted to specific targets (skin, eye), while action of the other anti-thyroid antibodies is less well known and less specific. The role of thyroid diseases and anti-TPO and anti-Tg antibodies in the development of breast cancer has been investigated in numerous studies with still controversial results. Reasons for this include the use of cross-sectional studies where breast cancer was diagnosed and a potential influence of breast cancer cannot be ruled out. Anti-TPO antibodies might initiate chronic inflammation and destruction of mammary cells *via* cross-reactivity with lactoperoxidase, but generation of oxidative stress by lactoperoxidase activity alone might also promote breast cancer. Due to the known interaction of thyroid hormones and estrogen on breast cells, abnormal hormone levels in manifest AITD may aggravate or mask the effect of anti-thyroid antibodies. Anti-thyroid antibodies may also display an effect on cancer progression, but early and advanced breast cancers in several studies were not analyzed separately. More precise data on the promoting or protecting action of anti-thyroid antibodies have been obtained by prospective studies and by distinguishing between early and advanced breast cancer. These studies appear to indicate that anti-TPO antibodies might have a beneficial effect in manifest breast cancer. In addition to other factors, these results are influenced by different time points of blood sampling, either before or after breast surgery, and recruitment of patients in third level oncologic centers (143). However, different effects of anti-thyroid antibodies in both cancer development and progression could explain the contradictory findings. Such behavior has already been shown for autophagy in breast cancer (177). Autophagy is reduced in the development of breast cancer but increased in tumor progression when nutrients and oxygen supply become limiting factors for growth. Anti-thyroid antibodies in breast cancer may not have a beneficial action *per se* but may be indicators for a more active immune system. The finding that older women with anti-thyroid antibodies are less fragile than the seronegative control group may support this theory.

Although GD and HT belong both to AITD, they have different pathogenic mechanisms. The absence of cytotoxicity in GD is a major difference to HT and other AD. Location and immunogenicity of the antigen (178) and dominant class of the antibodies may contribute to these differences. Surprisingly, most of the contributing factors (**Figure 1**) are similar for both AITDs.

AUTHOR CONTRIBUTIONS

EF and RW planned the review outline and wrote the manuscript.

ACKNOWLEDGMENTS

The authors are grateful to Dr. Graham Pawelec for his help with English language.

REFERENCES

1. Cooper GS, Bynum ML, Somers EC. Recent insights in the epidemiology of autoimmune diseases: improved prevalence estimates and understanding of clustering of diseases. *J Autoimmun* (2009) 33:197–207. doi:10.1016/j.jaut.2009.09.008
2. Cooper GS, Stroehla BC. The epidemiology of autoimmune diseases. *Autoimmun Rev* (2003) 2:119–25. doi:10.1016/S1568-9972(03)00006-5
3. McLeod DS, Cooper DS. The incidence and prevalence of thyroid autoimmunity. *Endocrine* (2012) 42:252–65. doi:10.1007/s12020-012-9703-2
4. Marcocci C, Marino M. Thyroid-directed antibodies. In: Braverman LE, Utiger R, editors. *Part II Laboratory Assessment of Thyroid Function*. Philadelphia, PA: Lippincott Williams and Wilkins (2005). p. 360–72.
5. Rapoport B, McLachlan SM. TSH receptor cleavage into subunits and shedding of the A-subunit; a molecular and clinical perspective. *Endocr Rev* (2016) 37:114–34. doi:10.1210/er.2015-1098
6. Furmaniak J, Sanders J, Rees Smith B. Blocking type TSH receptor antibodies. *Auto Immun Highlights* (2013) 4:11–26. doi:10.1007/s13317-012-0028-1
7. Morshed SA, Ando T, Latif R, Davies TF. Neutral antibodies to the TSH receptor are present in Graves' disease and regulate selective signaling cascades. *Endocrinology* (2010) 151:5537–49. doi:10.1210/en.2010-0424
8. Adams D, Purves H. Abnormal responses in the assay of thyrotrophin. *Proc Univ Otago Med Sch* (1956) 34:11–2.
9. de Carvalho G, Perez C, Ward L. The clinical use of thyroid function tests. *Arq Bras Endocrinol Metabol* (2013) 57:193–204. doi:10.1590/S0004-27302013000300005
10. Kamijo K. TSH-receptor antibody measurement in patients with various thyrotoxicosis and Hashimoto's thyroiditis: a comparison of two two-step assays, coated plate ELISA using porcine TSH-receptor and coated tube radioassay using human recombinant TSH-receptor. *Endocr J* (2003) 50:113–6. doi:10.1507/endocrj.50.113
11. Macchia E, Concetti R, Borgoni F, Cetani F, Fenzi GF, Pinchera A. Assays of TSH-receptor antibodies in 576 patients with various thyroid disorders: their incidence, significance and clinical usefulness. *Autoimmunity* (1989) 3:103–12. doi:10.3109/08916938909019959
12. Weetman AP, Yateman ME, Ealey PA, Black CM, Reimer CB, Williams RC Jr, et al. Thyroid-stimulating antibody activity between different immunoglobulin G subclasses. *J Clin Invest* (1990) 86:723–7. doi:10.1172/jci114768
13. Kraiem Z, Cho BY, Sadeh O, Shong MH, Pickerill P, Weetman AP. The IgG subclass distribution of TSH receptor blocking antibodies in primary hypothyroidism. *Clin Endocrinol* (1992) 37:135–40. doi:10.1111/j.1365-2265.1992.tb02297.x
14. Tada H, Izumi Y, Watanabe Y, Takano T, Fukata S, Kuma K, et al. Blocking type anti-TSH receptor antibodies detected by radioreceptor assay in Graves' disease. *Endocr J* (2001) 48:703–10. doi:10.1507/endocrj.48.703
15. Kim WB, Chung HK, Park YJ, Park DJ, Tahara K, Kohn LD, et al. The prevalence and clinical significance of blocking thyrotropin receptor

antibodies in untreated hyperthyroid Graves' disease. *Thyroid* (2000) 10: 579–86. doi:10.1089/thy.2000.10.579

16. Roti E, Braverman L, DeGroot L. TSH receptor antibody measurement in the diagnosis and management of Graves' disease is rarely necessary. *J Clin Endocrinol Metab* (1988) 83:3781–4. doi:10.1210/jcem.83.11.5056-2
17. Kahaly G, Diana T. TSH receptor antibody functionality and nomenclature. *Front Endocrinol* (2017) 8:28. doi:10.3389/fendo.2017.00028
18. Laurberg P, Nygaard B, Andersen S, Carle A, Karmisholt J, Krejbjerg A, et al. Association between TSH-receptor autoimmunity, hyperthyroidism, goitre, and orbitopathy in 208 Patients included in the remission induction and sustenance in Graves' disease study. *J Thyroid Res* (2014) 2014:165487. doi:10.1155/2014/165487
19. Konishi J, Iida Y, Kasagi K, Misaki T, Nakashima T, Endo K, et al. Primary myxedema with thyrotrophin-binding inhibitor immunoglobulins. Clinical and laboratory findings in 15 patients. *Ann Intern Med* (1985) 103:26–31. doi:10.7326/0003-4819-103-1-26
20. Tun N, Beckett G, Zammitt N, Strachan M, Seckl J, Gibb F. Thyrotropin receptor antibody levels at diagnosis and after thionamide course predict Graves' disease relapse. *Thyroid* (2016) 26:1004–9. doi:10.1089/thy.2016.0017
21. Balucan FS, Morshed SA, Davies TF. Thyroid autoantibodies in pregnancy: their role, regulation and clinical relevance. *J Thyroid Res* (2013) 2013:182472. doi:10.1155/2013/182472
22. McLachlan SM, Rapoport B. The molecular biology of thyroid peroxidase: cloning, expression and role as autoantigen in autoimmune thyroid disease. *Endocr Rev* (1992) 13:192–206. doi:10.1210/edrv-13-2-192
23. Le Fourn V, Ferrand M, Franc JL. Endoproteolytic cleavage of human thyroperoxidase: role of the propeptide in the protein folding process. *J Biol Chem* (2005) 280:4568–77. doi:10.1074/jbc.M408042200
24. Kohno Y, Yamaguchi F, Saito K, Niimi H, Nishikawa T, Hosoya T. Anti-thyroid peroxidase antibodies in sera from healthy subjects and from patients with chronic thyroiditis: differences in the ability to inhibit thyroid peroxidase activities. *Clin Exp Immunol* (1991) 85:459–63. doi:10.1111/j.1365-2249.1991.tb05749.x
25. Kaczur V, Vereb G, Molnar I, Krajczar G, Kiss E, Farid NR, et al. Effect of anti-thyroid peroxidase (TPO) antibodies on TPO activity measured by chemiluminescence assay. *Clin Chem* (1997) 43:1392–6.
26. Xie LD, Gao Y, Li MR, Lu GZ, Guo XH. Distribution of immunoglobulin G subclasses of anti-thyroid peroxidase antibody in sera from patients with Hashimoto's thyroiditis with different thyroid functional status. *Clin Exp Immunol* (2008) 154:172–6. doi:10.1111/j.1365-2249.2008.03756.x
27. Ruggeri RM, Vicchio TM, Cristani M, Certo R, Caccamo D, Alibrandi A, et al. Oxidative stress and advanced glycation end products in Hashimoto's thyroiditis. *Thyroid* (2016) 26:504–11. doi:10.1089/thy.2015.0592
28. Zaletel K, Gaberscek S. Hashimoto's thyroiditis: from genes to the disease. *Curr Genomics* (2011) 12:576–88. doi:10.2174/138920211798120763
29. DeGroot LJ. Graves' disease and the manifestations of thyrotoxicosis. In: De Groot LJ, Chrousos G, Dungan K, Feingold KR, Grossman A, Hershman JM, et al., editors. *Endotext*. South Dartmouth, MA: MDText. Com, Inc (2000).
30. Latrofa F, Ricci D, Grasso L, Vitti P, Masserini L, Basolo F, et al. Characterization of thyroglobulin epitopes in patients with autoimmune and non-autoimmune thyroid diseases using recombinant human monoclonal thyroglobulin autoantibodies. *J Clin Endocrinol Metab* (2008) 93:591–6. doi:10.1210/jc.2007-1199
31. Volpe R. Immunology of human thyroid disease. In: Volpe R, editor. *Autoimmune Diseases of the Endocrine System*. Boca Raton, FL: CRC Press (1990). p. 73–240.
32. Prentice L, Kiso Y, Fukuma N, Horimoto M, Petersen V, Grennan F, et al. Monoclonal thyroglobulin autoantibodies: variable region analysis and epitope recognition. *J Clin Endocrinol Metab* (1995) 80:977–86. doi:10.1210/jcem.80.3.7533775
33. Lazarus J. Chapter 83: Chronic (Hashimoto's) thyroiditis. In: De Groot LJ, Jameson JL, editors. *Endocrinology Adult and Pediatric: The Thyroid Gland E-Book*. Philadelphia, PA: Elsevier Saunders (2010). p. 1583–94.
34. Janeway CJ, Travers P, Walport M, Shlomchik M. Chapter 13: Autoimmunity and transplantation. In: Janeway CJ, Travers P, Walport M, Shlomchik M, editors. *The Immune System in Health and Disease*. New York, NY: Garland Science (2001).
35. Cyriac T, Chellappa P, Sinnet P, Anish I. Prevalence of hypothyroidism and its association with anti-thyroid peroxidase antibody among adult sea food consuming population attending a tertiary health care centre in Kerala. *Int J Biomed Adv Res* (2015) 6:648–55. doi:10.7439/ijbar
36. Camargo RY, Tomimori EK, Neves SC, Rubio GS I, Galrão AL, Knobel M, et al. Thyroid and the environment: exposure to excessive nutritional iodine increases the prevalence of thyroid disorders in Sao Paulo, Brazil. *Eur J Endocrinol* (2008) 159:293–9. doi:10.1530/eje-08-0192
37. Caturegli P, Kuppers RC, Mariotti S, Burek CL, Pinchera A, Ladenson PW, et al. IgG subclass distribution of thyroglobulin antibodies in patients with thyroid disease. *Clin Exp Immunol* (1994) 98:464–9. doi:10.1111/j.1365-2249.1994.tb05514.x
38. Chin HS, Chin DK, Morgenthaler NG, Vassart G, Costagliola S. Rarity of anti-Na+/I- symporter (NIS) antibody with iodide uptake inhibiting activity in autoimmune thyroid diseases (AITD). *J Clin Endocrinol Metab* (2000) 85:3937–40. doi:10.1210/jcem.85.10.6884
39. Hattori N, Ishihara T, Matsuoka N, Saito T, Shimatsu A. Anti-thyrotropin autoantibodies in patients with macro-thyrotropin and long-term changes in macro-thyrotropin and serum thyrotropin levels. *Thyroid* (2017) 27:138–46. doi:10.1089/thy.2016.0442
40. Ginsberg J. Diagnosis and management of Graves' disease. *CMAJ* (2003) 168:575–85.
41. Laurberg P, Wallin G, Tallstedt L, Abraham-Nordling M, Lundell G, Torring O. TSH-receptor autoimmunity in Graves' disease after therapy with anti-thyroid drugs, surgery, or radioiodine: a 5-year prospective randomized study. *Eur J Endocrinol* (2008) 158:69–75. doi:10.1530/eje-07-0450
42. Smith J, Brown RS. Persistence of thyrotropin (TSH) receptor antibodies in children and adolescents with Graves' disease treated using antithyroid medication. *Thyroid* (2007) 17:1103–7. doi:10.1089/thy.2007.0072
43. Mariotti S, Caturegli P, Piccolo P, Barbesino G, Pinchera A. Antithyroid peroxidase autoantibodies in thyroid diseases. *J Clin Endocrinol Metab* (1990) 71:661–9. doi:10.1210/jcem-71-3-661
44. Schmidt M, Voell M, Rahlff I, Dietlein M, Kobe C, Faust M, et al. Long-term follow-up of antithyroid peroxidase antibodies in patients with chronic autoimmune thyroiditis (Hashimoto's thyroiditis) treated with levothyroxine. *Thyroid* (2008) 18:755–60. doi:10.1089/thy.2008.0008
45. Elhomsy G. In: Staros E, editor. *Antithyroid Antibody*. Laboratory Medicine (2014).
46. Ueno A, Jijon H, Traves S, Chan R, Ford K, Beck PL, et al. Opposing effects of smoking in ulcerative colitis and Crohn's disease may be explained by differential effects on dendritic cells. *Inflamm Bowel Dis* (2014) 20:800–10. doi:10.1097/mib.0000000000000018
47. Swain M, Swain T, Mohanty BK. Autoimmune thyroid disorders-an update. *Indian J Clin Biochem* (2005) 20:9–17. doi:10.1007/BF02893034
48. Carle A, Bulow Pedersen I, Knudsen N, Perrild H, Ovesen L, Rasmussen LB, et al. Graves' hyperthyroidism and moderate alcohol consumption: evidence for disease prevention. *Clin Endocrinol* (2013) 79:111–9. doi:10.1111/cen.12106
49. Carle A, Pedersen IB, Knudsen N, Perrild H, Ovesen L, Rasmussen LB, et al. Moderate alcohol consumption may protect against overt autoimmune hypothyroidism: a population-based case-control study. *Eur J Endocrinol* (2012) 167:483–90. doi:10.1530/eje-12-0356
50. Romeo J, Warnberg J, Nova E, Diaz LE, Gomez-Martinez S, Marcos A. Moderate alcohol consumption and the immune system: a review. *Br J Nutr* (2007) 98(Suppl 1):S111–5. doi:10.1017/s0007114507838049
51. Wichman J, Winther KH, Bonnema SJ, Hegedus L. Selenium supplementation significantly reduces thyroid autoantibody levels in patients with chronic autoimmune thyroiditis: a systematic review and meta-analysis. *Thyroid* (2016) 26:1681–92. doi:10.1089/thy.2016.0256
52. Weetman A, DeGroot LJ. Autoimmunity to the thyroid gland. *Thyroid Disease Manager*. (2016). Available from: http://www.thyroidmanager.org/chapter/autoimmunity-to-the-thyroid-gland/
53. Carroll R, Matfin G. Endocrine and metabolic emergencies: thyroid storm. *Ther Adv Endocrinol Metab* (2010) 1:139–45. doi:10.1177/2042018810382481
54. Kaczor T. *Iodine and Cancer: A Summary of the Evidence to Date*. (2014). Available from: http://www.naturalmedicinejournal.com/journal/2014-06/iodine-and-cancer
55. Winkler R. Iodine – a potential antioxidant and the role of iodine/iodide in health and disease. *Nat Sci* (2015) 7:548–57. doi:10.4236/ns.2015.712055

56. Zarkovic M. The role of oxidative stress on the pathogenesis of Graves' disease. *J Thyroid Res* (2012) 2012:302537. doi:10.1155/2012/302537
57. Effraimidis G, Wiersinga WM. Mechanisms in endocrinology: autoimmune thyroid disease: old and new players. *Eur J Endocrinol* (2014) 170:R241–52. doi:10.1530/EJE-14-0047
58. Desailloud R, Hober D. Viruses and thyroiditis: an update. *Virol J* (2009) 6:5. doi:10.1186/1743-422x-6-5
59. Blackard JT, Kong L, Huber AK, Tomer Y. Hepatitis C virus infection of a thyroid cell line: implications for pathogenesis of hepatitis C virus and thyroiditis. *Thyroid* (2013) 23:863–70. doi:10.1089/thy.2012.0507
60. Wolf MW, Misaki T, Bech K, Tvede M, Silva JE, Ingbar SH. Immunoglobulins of patients recovering from *Yersinia enterocolitica* infections exhibit Graves' disease-like activity in human thyroid membranes. *Thyroid* (1991) 1:315–20. doi:10.1089/thy.1991.1.315
61. Mori K, Nakagawa Y, Ozaki H. Does the gut microbiota trigger Hashimoto's thyroiditis? *Discov Med* (2012) 14:321–6.
62. de Luis DA, Varela C, de La Calle H, Canton R, de Argila CM, San Roman AL, et al. *Helicobacter pylori* infection is markedly increased in patients with autoimmune atrophic thyroiditis. *J Clin Gastroenterol* (1998) 26:259–63. doi:10.1097/00004836-199806000-00008
63. Akeno N, Smith EP, Stefan M, Huber AK, Zhang W, Keddache M, et al. IFN-alpha mediates the development of autoimmunity both by direct tissue toxicity and through immune cell recruitment mechanisms. *J Immunol* (2011) 186:4693–706. doi:10.4049/jimmunol.1002631
64. Davies TF. Infection and autoimmune thyroid disease. *J Clin Endocrinol Metab* (2008) 93:674–6. doi:10.1210/jc.2008-0095
65. Hoekman K, von Blomberg-van der Flier BM, Wagstaff J, Drexhage HA, Pinedo HM. Reversible thyroid dysfunction during treatment with GM-CSF. *Lancet* (1991) 338:541–2. doi:10.1016/0140-6736(91)91103-2
66. de Filette J, Jansen Y, Schreuer M, Everaert H, Velkeniers B, Neyns B, et al. Incidence of thyroid-related adverse events in melanoma patients treated with pembrolizumab. *J Clin Endocrinol Metab* (2016) 101(11):4431–9. doi:10.1210/jc.2016-2300
67. Bahn AK, Mills JL, Snyder PJ, Gann PH, Houten L, Bialik O, et al. Hypothyroidism in workers exposed to polybrominated biphenyls. *N Engl J Med* (1980) 302:31–3. doi:10.1056/nejm198001033020105
68. Kibirige D, Luzinda K, Ssekitoleko R. Spectrum of lithium induced thyroid abnormalities: a current perspective. *Thyroid Res* (2013) 6:3. doi:10.1186/1756-6614-6-3
69. Hancock SL, Cox RS, McDougall IR. Thyroid diseases after treatment of Hodgkin's disease. *N Engl J Med* (1991) 325:599–605. doi:10.1056/NEJM199108293250902
70. Hansen PS, Brix TH, Iachine I, Kyvik KO, Hegedus L. The relative importance of genetic and environmental effects for the early stages of thyroid autoimmunity: a study of healthy Danish twins. *Eur J Endocrinol* (2006) 154:29–38. doi:10.1530/eje.1.02060
71. Luo L, Cai B, Liu F, Hu X, Wang L. Association of protein tyrosine phosphatase nonreceptor 22 (PTPN22) C1858T gene polymorphism with susceptibility to autoimmune thyroid diseases: a meta-analysis. *Endocr J* (2012) 59:439–45. doi:10.1507/endocrj.EJ11-0381
72. Tomer Y. Mechanisms of autoimmune thyroid diseases: from genetics to epigenetics. *Annu Rev Pathol* (2014) 9:147–56. doi:10.1146/annurev-pathol-012513-104713
73. Fairweather D, Frisancho-Kiss S, Rose NR. Sex differences in autoimmune disease from a pathological perspective. *Am J Pathol* (2008) 173:600–9. doi:10.2353/ajpath.2008.071008
74. Zandman-Goddard G, Peeva E, Shoenfeld Y. Gender and autoimmunity. *Autoimmun Rev* (2007) 6:366–72. doi:10.1016/j.autrev.2006.10.001
75. Ngo ST, Steyn FJ, McCombe PA. Gender differences in autoimmune disease. *Front Neuroendocrinol* (2014) 35:347–69. doi:10.1016/j.yfrne.2014.04.004
76. Persani L, Bonomi M, Lleo A, Pasini S, Civardi F, Bianchi I, et al. Increased loss of the Y chromosome in peripheral blood cells in male patients with autoimmune thyroiditis. *J Autoimmun* (2012) 38:J193–6. doi:10.1016/j.jaut.2011.11.011
77. Meikle AW. The interrelationships between thyroid dysfunction and hypogonadism in men and boys. *Thyroid* (2004) 14(Suppl 1):S17–25. doi:10.1089/105072504323024552
78. Janssen OE, Mehlmauer N, Hahn S, Offner AH, Gartner R. High prevalence of autoimmune thyroiditis in patients with polycystic ovary syndrome. *Eur J Endocrinol* (2004) 150:363–9. doi:10.1530/eje.0.1500363
79. Groer M, Jevitt C. Symptoms and signs associated with postpartum thyroiditis. *J Thyroid Res* (2014) 2014:531969. doi:10.1155/2014/531969
80. Klintschar M, Schwaiger P, Mannweiler S, Regauer S, Kleiber M. Evidence of fetal microchimerism in Hashimoto's thyroiditis. *J Clin Endocrinol Metab* (2001) 86:2494–8. doi:10.1210/jcem.86.6.7540
81. Cogni G, Chiovato L. An overview of the pathogenesis of thyroid autoimmunity. *Hormones* (2013) 12:19–29.
82. Mikos H, Mikos M, Obara-Moszynska M, Niedziela M. The role of the immune system and cytokines involved in the pathogenesis of autoimmune thyroid disease (AITD). *Endokrynol Pol* (2014) 65:150–5. doi:10.5603/ep.2014.0021
83. Ajjan RA, Weetman AP. The pathogenesis of Hashimoto's thyroiditis: further developments in our understanding. *Horm Metab Res* (2015) 47:702–10. doi:10.1055/s-0035-1548832
84. Pyzik A, Grywalska E, Matyjaszek-Matuszek B, Rolinski J. Immune disorders in Hashimoto's thyroiditis: what do we know so far? *J Immunol Res* (2015) 2015:979167. doi:10.1155/2015/979167
85. Kawashima A, Tanigawa K, Akama T, Yoshihara A, Ishii N, Suzuki K. Innate immune activation and thyroid autoimmunity. *J Clin Endocrinol Metab* (2011) 96:3661–71. doi:10.1210/jc.2011-1568
86. Fountoulakis S, Tsatsoulis A. On the pathogenesis of autoimmune thyroid disease: a unifying hypothesis. *Clin Endocrinol* (2004) 60:397–409. doi:10.1046/j.1365-2265.2004.01978.x
87. De Luca F, Santucci S, Corica D, Pitrolo E, Romeo M, Aversa T. Hashimoto's thyroiditis in childhood: presentation modes and evolution over time. *Ital J Pediatr* (2013) 39:8. doi:10.1186/1824-7288-39-8
88. Hiromatsu Y, Satoh H, Amino N. Hashimoto's thyroiditis: history and future outlook. *Hormones* (2013) 12:12–8.
89. Kottahachchi D, Topliss DJ. Immunoglobulin G4-related thyroid diseases. *Eur Thyroid J* (2016) 5:231–9. doi:10.1159/000452623
90. Li Y, Nishihara E, Hirokawa M, Taniguchi E, Miyauchi A, Kakudo K. Distinct clinical, serological, and sonographic characteristics of Hashimoto's thyroiditis based with and without IgG4-positive plasma cells. *J Clin Endocrinol Metab* (2010) 95:1309–17. doi:10.1210/jc.2009-1794
91. Minamino H, Inaba H, Ariyasu H, Furuta H, Nishi M, Yoshimasu T, et al. A novel immunopathological association of IgG4-RD and vasculitis with Hashimoto's thyroiditis. *Endocrinol Diabetes Metab Case Rep* (2016) 2016:160004. doi:10.1530/edm-16-0004
92. Davies TF. Ord-Hashimoto's disease: renaming a common disorder – again. *Thyroid* (2003) 13:317. doi:10.1089/105072503321669776
93. Carle A, Pedersen IB, Knudsen N, Perrild H, Ovesen L, Jorgensen T, et al. Thyroid volume in hypothyroidism due to autoimmune disease follows a unimodal distribution: evidence against primary thyroid atrophy and autoimmune thyroiditis being distinct diseases. *J Clin Endocrinol Metab* (2009) 94:833–9. doi:10.1210/jc.2008-1370
94. Jara L, Vera-Lastra O, Medina G. V. Endocrine and reproductive autoimmune diseases. Atrophic thyroiditis. In: Shoenfeld Y, Cervera R, Gershwin M, editors. *Diagnostic Criteria in Autoimmune Diseases*. Totowa, NJ: Humana Press (2008). p. 221–6.
95. Cappa M, Bizzarri C, Crea F. Autoimmune thyroid diseases in children. *J Thyroid Res* (2010) 2011:675703. doi:10.4061/2011/675703
96. Garber JR, Cobin RH, Gharib H, Hennessey JV, Klein I, Mechanick JI, et al. Clinical practice guidelines for hypothyroidism in adults: cosponsored by the American Association of Clinical Endocrinologists and the American Thyroid Association. *Endocr Pract* (2012) 18:988–1028. doi:10.4158/ep12280.gl
97. Weetman AP. Graves' disease. *N Engl J Med* (2000) 343:1236–48. doi:10.1056/NEJM200010263431707
98. Arntzenius AB, Smit LJ, Schipper J, van der Heide D, Meinders AE. Inverse relation between iodine intake and thyroid blood flow: color Doppler flow imaging in euthyroid humans. *J Clin Endocrinol Metab* (1991) 73:1051–5. doi:10.1210/jcem-73-5-1051
99. Cardenas Roldan J, Amaya-Amaya J, Castellanos-de la Hoz J, Giraldo-Villamil J, Montoya-Ortiz G, Cruz-Tapias P, et al. Autoimmune thyroid disease in rheumatoid arthritis: a global perspective. *Arthritis* (2012) 2012:864907. doi:10.1155/2012/864907
100. Yavasoglu I, Senturk T, Coskun A, Bolaman Z. Rheumatoid arthritis and anti-thyroid antibodies. *Autoimmunity* (2009) 42:168–9. doi:10.1080/08916930802428114

101. Przygodzka M, Filipowicz-Sosnowska A. Prevalence of thyroid diseases and antithyroid antibodies in women with rheumatoid arthritis. *Pol Arch Med Wewn* (2009) 119:39–43.
102. Ali O. Part V diabetes syndromes. Type 1 diabetes mellitus: epidemiology, genetics, pathogenesis, and clinical manifestations. In: Poretsky L, editor. *Principles of Diabetes Mellitus*. New York, NY: Springer Science + Business Media (2010). p. 181–202.
103. Sharifi F, Ghasemi L, Mousavinasab N. Thyroid function and anti-thyroid antibodies in Iranian patients with type 1 diabetes mellitus: influences of age and sex. *Iran J Allergy Asthma Immunol* (2008) 7:31–6. doi:07.01/ijaai.3136
104. Hatzioannou A, Kanistras I, Mantzou E, Anastasiou E, Peppa M, Sarantopoulou V, et al. Effect of advanced glycation end products on human thyroglobulin's antigenicity as identified by the use of sera from patients with Hashimoto's thyroiditis and gestational diabetes mellitus. *Int J Endocrinol* (2015) 2015:849615. doi:10.1155/2015/849615
105. Ch'ng CL, Jones MK, Kingham JG. Celiac disease and autoimmune thyroid disease. *Clin Med Res* (2007) 5:184–92. doi:10.3121/cmr.2007.738
106. Kalyoncu D, Urganci N. Antithyroid antibodies and thyroid function in pediatric patients with celiac disease. *Int J Endocrinol* (2015) 2015:276575. doi:10.1155/2015/276575
107. El-Aziz M, Rafaat M, Sabry I, Yousef M, Mandour A. Study of thyroid auto-antibodies in patients with bronchial asthma and allergic rhinitis. *Thyroid Sci* (2010) 5:CLS1–5.
108. Fekri M, Shokoohi M, Gozashti M, Esmailian S, Jamshidian N, Shadkam-Farokhi M, et al. Association between anti-thyroid peroxidase antibody and asthma in women. *Iran J Allergy Asthma Immunol* (2012) 11:241–5. doi:10.1016/j.ejcdt.2015.08.018
109. Bansal AS, Hayman GR. Graves disease associated with chronic idiopathic urticaria: 2 case reports. *J Investig Allergol Clin Immunol* (2009) 19:54–6.
110. Nakamura H, Usa T, Motomura M, Ichikawa T, Nakao K, Kawasaki E, et al. Prevalence of interrelated autoantibodies in thyroid diseases and autoimmune disorders. *J Endocrinol Invest* (2008) 31:861–5. doi:10.1007/BF03346432
111. Koszarny A, Majdan M, Suszek D, Wielosz E, Dryglewska M. Relationship between rheumatoid arthritis activity and antithyroid antibodies. *Pol Arch Med Wewn* (2013) 123:394–400.
112. Unnikrishnan AG, Kumaravel V, Nair V, Rao A, Jayakumar RV, Kumar H, et al. TSH receptor antibodies in subjects with type 1 diabetes mellitus. *Ann N Y Acad Sci* (2006) 1079:220–5. doi:10.1196/annals.1375.034
113. Bartalena L, Fatourechi V. Extrathyroidal manifestations of Graves' disease: a 2014 update. *J Endocrinol Invest* (2014) 37:691–700. doi:10.1007/s40618-014-0097-2
114. Shan SJ, Douglas RS. The pathophysiology of thyroid eye disease. *J Neuroophthalmol* (2014) 34:177–85. doi:10.1097/wno.0000000000000132
115. Hiromatsu Y, Yang D, Bednarczuk T, Miyake I, Nonaka K, Inoue Y. Cytokine profiles in eye muscle tissue and orbital fat tissue from patients with thyroid-associated ophthalmopathy. *J Clin Endocrinol Metab* (2000) 85:1194–9. doi:10.1210/jcem.85.3.6433
116. Lytton SD, Ponto KA, Kanitz M, Matheis N, Kohn LD, Kahaly GJ. A novel thyroid stimulating immunoglobulin bioassay is a functional indicator of activity and severity of Graves' orbitopathy. *J Clin Endocrinol Metab* (2010) 95:2123–31. doi:10.1210/jc.2009-2470
117. Woo YJ, Jang SY, Lim TH, Yoon JS. Clinical association of thyroid stimulating hormone receptor antibody levels with disease severity in the chronic inactive stage of Graves' orbitopathy. *Korean J Ophthalmol* (2015) 29:213–9. doi:10.3341/kjo.2015.29.4.213
118. Reddy SV, Gupta SK, Jain M. Dermopathy of Graves' disease: clinico-pathological correlation. *Indian J Endocrinol Metab* (2012) 16:460–2. doi:10.4103/2230-8210.95714
119. Dhali TK, Chahar M. Thyroid dermopathy – a diagnostic clue of hidden hyperthyroidism. *Dermatoendocrinol* (2014) 6:e981078. doi:10.4161/19381980.2014.981078
120. Promberger R, Hermann M, Ott J. Hashimoto's thyroiditis in patients with normal thyroid-stimulating hormone levels. *Expert Rev Endocrinol Metab* (2012) 7:175–9. doi:10.1586/eem.12.3
121. Kothbauer-Margreiter I, Sturzenegger M, Komor J, Baumgartner R, Hess CW. Encephalopathy associated with Hashimoto thyroiditis: diagnosis and treatment. *J Neurol* (1996) 243:585–93. doi:10.1007/BF00900946
122. Sekisui Virotech GmbH. *CSF-Standards*. Rüsselsheim (2014).
123. Leyhe T, Mussig K. Cognitive and affective dysfunctions in autoimmune thyroiditis. *Brain Behav Immun* (2014) 41:261–6. doi:10.1016/j.bbi.2014.03.008
124. Chiarella G, Tognini S, Nacci A, Sieli R, Costante G, Petrolo C, et al. Vestibular disorders in euthyroid patients with Hashimoto's thyroiditis: role of thyroid autoimmunity. *Clin Endocrinol* (2014) 81:600–5. doi:10.1111/cen.12471
125. Plowden TC, Schisterman EF, Sjaarda LA, Zarek SM, Perkins NJ, Silver R, et al. Subclinical hypothyroidism and thyroid autoimmunity are not associated with fecundity, pregnancy loss or live birth. *J Clin Endocrinol Metab* (2016) 101(6):2358–65. doi:10.1210/jc.2016-1049
126. Busnelli A, Paffoni A, Fedele L, Somigliana E. The impact of thyroid autoimmunity on IVF/ICSI outcome: a systematic review and meta-analysis. *Hum Reprod* (2016) 22(6):775–90. doi:10.1093/humupd/dmw034
127. Seror J, Amand G, Guibourdenche J, Ceccaldi PF, Luton D. Anti-TPO antibodies diffusion through the placental barrier during pregnancy. *PLoS One* (2014) 9:e84647. doi:10.1371/journal.pone.0084647
128. Korevaar TI, Steegers EA, Pop VJ, Broeren MA, Chaker L, de Rijke YB, et al. Thyroid autoimmunity impairs the thyroidal response to hCG: two population-based prospective cohort studies. *J Clin Endocrinol Metab* (2016) 102(1):69–77. doi:10.1210/jc.2016-2942
129. Wang GC, Talor MV, Rose NR, Cappola AR, Chiou RB, Weiss C, et al. Thyroid autoantibodies are associated with a reduced prevalence of frailty in community-dwelling older women. *J Clin Endocrinol Metab* (2010) 95:1161–8. doi:10.1210/jc.2009-1991
130. Jankovic B, Le KT, Hershman JM. Clinical review: Hashimoto's thyroiditis and papillary thyroid carcinoma: is there a correlation? *J Clin Endocrinol Metab* (2013) 98:474–82. doi:10.1210/jc.2012-2978
131. Amiri-Kordestani L, Luchenko VL, Peer CJ, Ghafourian K, Reynolds J, Draper D, et al. Phase I trial of a new schedule of romidepsin in patients with advanced cancers. *Clin Cancer Res* (2013) 19(16):4499–507. doi:10.1158/1078-0432.CCR-13-0095
132. Nio Y, Iguchi C, Itakura M, Toga T, Hashimoto K, Koike M, et al. High incidence of synchronous or metachronous breast cancer in patients with malignant and benign thyroid tumor or tumor-like disorders. *Anticancer Res* (2009) 29:1607–10.
133. Prinzi N, Sorrenti S, Baldini E, De Vito C, Tuccilli C, Catania A, et al. Association of thyroid diseases with primary extra-thyroidal malignancies in women: results of a cross-sectional study of 6,386 patients. *PLoS One* (2015) 10:e0122958. doi:10.1371/journal.pone.0122958
134. Chen YK, Lin CL, Chang YJ, Cheng FT, Peng CL, Sung FC, et al. Cancer risk in patients with Graves' disease: a nationwide cohort study. *Thyroid* (2013) 23:879–84. doi:10.1089/thy.2012.0568
135. Shu X, Ji J, Li X, Sundquist J, Sundquist K, Hemminki K. Cancer risk in patients hospitalised for Graves' disease: a population-based cohort study in Sweden. *Br J Cancer* (2010) 102:1397–9. doi:10.1038/sj.bjc.6605624
136. Muller I, Pinchera A, Fiore E, Belardi V, Rosellini V, Giustarini E, et al. High prevalence of breast cancer in patients with benign thyroid diseases. *J Endocrinol Invest* (2011) 34:349–52. doi:10.3275/7141
137. Rasmusson B, Feldt-Rasmussen U, Hegedus L, Perrild H, Bech K, Hoier-Madsen M. Thyroid function in patients with breast cancer. *Eur J Cancer Clin Oncol* (1987) 23:553–6. doi:10.1016/0277-5379(87)90319-1
138. Giani C, Fierabracci P, Bonacci R, Gigliotti A, Campani D, De Negri F, et al. Relationship between breast cancer and thyroid disease: relevance of autoimmune thyroid disorders in breast malignancy. *J Clin Endocrinol Metab* (1996) 81:990–4. doi:10.1210/jcem.81.3.8772562
139. Turken O, NarIn Y, DemIrbas S, Onde ME, Sayan O, KandemIr EG, et al. Breast cancer in association with thyroid disorders. *Breast Cancer Res* (2003) 5:R110–3. doi:10.1186/bcr609
140. Sarlis NJ, Gourgiotis L, Pucino F, Tolis GJ. Lack of association between Hashimoto thyroiditis and breast cancer: a quantitative research synthesis. *Hormones* (2002) 1:35–41. doi:10.14310/horm.2002.1152
141. Freitas PA, Vissoci GM, Pinto RM, Lajolo PP, Jorge PT. Study of the prevalence of autoimmune thyroid disease in women with breast cancer. *Endocr Pract* (2016) 22:16–21. doi:10.4158/ep14445.or
142. Hajtmanova E, Murin P, Kinclova I, Hajtman A, Pec M, Kostkova L, et al. Thyroid disorders in women with breast cancer. *Klin Onkol* (2012) 25:124–9.
143. Sisti G, Di Tommaso M. Commentary on 'study of the prevalence of autoimmune thyroid disease in women with breast cancer'. *Endocr Pract* (2016) 22:114–6. doi:10.4158/ep151035.co

144. Brandt J, Borgquist S, Manjer J. Prospectively measured thyroid hormones and thyroid peroxidase antibodies in relation to risk of different breast cancer subgroups: a Malmo Diet and Cancer Study. *Cancer Causes Control* (2015) 26:1093–104. doi:10.1007/s10552-015-0602-8
145. Tosovic A, Becker C, Bondeson AG, Bondeson L, Ericsson UB, Malm J, et al. Prospectively measured thyroid hormones and thyroid peroxidase antibodies in relation to breast cancer risk. *Int J Cancer* (2012) 131:2126–33. doi:10.1002/ijc.27470
146. Tosovic A, Bondeson AG, Bondeson L, Ericsson UB, Malm J, Manjer J. Prospectively measured triiodothyronine levels are positively associated with breast cancer risk in postmenopausal women. *Breast Cancer Res* (2010) 12:R33. doi:10.1186/bcr2587
147. Tosovic A, Bondeson AG, Bondeson L, Ericsson UB, Manjer J. Triiodothyronine levels in relation to mortality from breast cancer and all causes: a population-based prospective cohort study. *Eur J Endocrinol* (2013) 168:483–90. doi:10.1530/eje-12-0564
148. Qin J, Yu Z, Guan H, Shi L, Liu Y, Zhao N, et al. High thyroglobulin antibody levels increase the risk of differentiated thyroid carcinoma. *Dis Markers* (2015) 2015:648670. doi:10.1155/2015/648670
149. Prinzi N, Baldini E, Sorrenti S, De Vito C, Tuccilli C, Catania A, et al. Prevalence of breast cancer in thyroid diseases: results of a cross-sectional study of 3,921 patients. *Breast Cancer Res Treat* (2014) 144:683–8. doi:10.1007/s10549-014-2893-y
150. Smyth PP, Shering SG, Kilbane MT, Murray MJ, McDermott EW, Smith DF, et al. Serum thyroid peroxidase autoantibodies, thyroid volume, and outcome in breast carcinoma. *J Clin Endocrinol Metab* (1998) 83:2711–6. doi:10.1210/jcem.83.8.5049
151. Hegedus L, Perrild H, Poulsen LR, Andersen JR, Holm B, Schnohr P, et al. The determination of thyroid volume by ultrasound and its relationship to body weight, age, and sex in normal subjects. *J Clin Endocrinol Metab* (1983) 56:260–3. doi:10.1210/jcem-56-2-260
152. Ivanac G, Rozman B, Skreb F, Brkljacic B, Pavic L. Ultrasonographic measurement of the thyroid volume. *Coll Antropol* (2004) 28:287–91.
153. Şeker S, Taş I. Determination of thyroid volume and its relation with isthmus thickness. *Eur J Gen Med* (2010) 7:125–9.
154. Hardefeldt PJ, Eslick GD, Edirimanne S. Benign thyroid disease is associated with breast cancer: a meta-analysis. *Breast Cancer Res Treat* (2012) 133:1169–77. doi:10.1007/s10549-012-2019-3
155. Ditsch N, Liebhardt S, Von Koch F, Lenhard M, Vogeser M, Spitzweg C, et al. Thyroid function in breast cancer patients. *Anticancer Res* (2010) 30:1713–7.
156. Davies TF, Ando T, Lin RY, Tomer Y, Latif R. Thyrotropin receptor-associated diseases: from adenomata to Graves disease. *J Clin Invest* (2005) 115:1972–83. doi:10.1172/JCI26031
157. Kandi S, Pinnelli V, Rao P, Ramana K. Effect of anti-thyroperoxidase on thyroid gland and breast tissue: a comprehensive review. *Am J Med Stud* (2014) 2:34–7. doi:10.12691/ajms-2-2-2
158. Giustarini E, Pinchera A, Fierabracci P, Roncella M, Fustaino L, Mammoli C, et al. Thyroid autoimmunity in patients with malignant and benign breast diseases before surgery. *Eur J Endocrinol* (2006) 154:645–9. doi:10.1530/eje.1.02108
159. Michalaki V, Kondi-Pafiti A, Gennatas S, Antoniou A, Primetis H, Gennatas C. Breast cancer in association with thyroid disorders. *J BUON* (2009) 14:425–8.
160. Shi XZ, Jin X, Xu P, Shen HM. Relationship between breast cancer and levels of serum thyroid hormones and antibodies: a meta-analysis. *Asian Pac J Cancer Prev* (2014) 15:6643–7. doi:10.7314/APJCP.2014.15.16.6643
161. Mattar MC, Lough D, Pishvaian MJ, Charabaty A. Current management of inflammatory bowel disease and colorectal cancer. *Gastrointest Cancer Res* (2011) 4:53–61.
162. Rapoport B, McLachlan S. Thyroid peroxidase as an autoantigen in autoimmune thyroid disease: update 1994. In: Negro-Vilar A, Braverman L, Refetoff S, editors. *Endocrine Review Monographs 3. Clinical and Molecular Aspects of Diseases of the Thyroid*. Bethesda, MD: The Endocrine Society (1994). p. 96–102.
163. Haapala AM, Hyoty H, Parkkonen P, Mustonen J, Soppi E. Antibody reactivity against thyroid peroxidase and myeloperoxidase in autoimmune thyroiditis and systemic vasculitis. *Scand J Immunol* (1997) 46:78–85. doi:10.1046/j.1365-3083.1997.d01-90.x
164. Freire BA, Paula ID, Paula F, Kallenberg CG, Limburg PC, Queluz TT. Absence of cross-reactivity to myeloperoxidase of anti-thyroid microsomal antibodies in patients with autoimmune thyroid diseases. *Am J Med Sci* (2001) 321:109–12. doi:10.1097/00000441-200102000-00001
165. Aceves C, Anguiano B, Delgado G. Is iodine a gatekeeper of the integrity of the mammary gland? *J Mammary Gland Biol Neoplasia* (2005) 10:189–96. doi:10.1007/s10911-005-5401-5
166. Anguiano B, Garcia-Solis P, Delgado G, Aceves Velasco C. Uptake and gene expression with antitumoral doses of iodine in thyroid and mammary gland: evidence that chronic administration has no harmful effects. *Thyroid* (2007) 17:851–9. doi:10.1089/thy.2007.0122
167. Shrivastava A, Tiwari M, Sinha RA, Kumar A, Balapure AK, Bajpai VK, et al. Molecular iodine induces caspase-independent apoptosis in human breast carcinoma cells involving the mitochondria-mediated pathway. *J Biol Chem* (2006) 281:19762–71. doi:10.1074/jbc.M600746200
168. Szychta P, Szychta W, Gesing A, Lewinski A, Karbownik-Lewinska M. TSH receptor antibodies have predictive value for breast cancer – retrospective analysis. *Thyroid Res* (2013) 6:8. doi:10.1186/1756-6614-6-8
169. Kuijpens JL, Nyklictek I, Louwman MW, Weetman TA, Pop VJ, Coebergh JW. Hypothyroidism might be related to breast cancer in post-menopausal women. *Thyroid* (2005) 15:1253–9. doi:10.1089/thy.2005.15.1253
170. Mittra I, Perrin J, Kumaoka S. Thyroid and other autoantibodies in British and Japanese women: an epidemiological study of breast cancer. *Br Med J* (1976) 1:257–9. doi:10.1136/bmj
171. Fiore E, Giustarini E, Mammoli C, Fragomeni F, Campani D, Muller I, et al. Favorable predictive value of thyroid autoimmunity in high aggressive breast cancer. *J Endocrinol Invest* (2007) 30:734–8. doi:10.1007/bf03350810
172. Jiskra J, Barkmanova J, Limanova Z, Lanska V, Smutek D, Potlukova E, et al. Thyroid autoimmunity occurs more frequently in women with breast cancer compared to women with colorectal cancer and controls but it has no impact on relapse-free and overall survival. *Oncol Rep* (2007) 18:1603–11.
173. Hall LC, Salazar EP, Kane SR, Liu N. Effects of thyroid hormones on human breast cancer cell proliferation. *J Steroid Biochem Mol Biol* (2008) 109:57–66. doi:10.1016/j.jsbmb.2007.12.008
174. Kemal Y, Demirag G, Ekiz K, Yucel I. Antithyroid peroxidase antibody positivity is associated with lower incidence of metastasis in breast cancer. *Mol Clin Oncol* (2015) 3:629–32. doi:10.3892/mco.2015.521
175. Farahati J, Roggenbuck D, Gilman E, Schutte M, Jagminaite E, Seyed Zakavi R, et al. Anti-thyroid peroxidase antibodies are associated with the absence of distant metastases in patients with newly diagnosed breast cancer. *Clin Chem Lab Med* (2012) 50:709–14. doi:10.1515/cclm.2011.819
176. Özmen T, Güllüoglu B, Yegen C, Soran A. Autoimmune thyroid disease and breast cancer prognosis. *J Breast Health* (2015) 11:67–71. doi:10.5152/tjbh.2015.2462
177. Berardi DE, Campodonico PB, Diaz Bessone MI, Urtreger AJ, Todaro LB. Autophagy: friend or foe in breast cancer development, progression, and treatment. *Int J Breast Cancer* (2011) 2011:595092. doi:10.4061/2011/595092
178. Fröhlich E, Wahl R. Chapter 12: Differentiation therapy in thyroid carcinoma. In: Fahey T, editor. *Updates in the Understanding and Management of Thyroid Cancer*. Rijeka: InTech (2015). p. 251–82.

17

Transient thyroiditis after surgery for tertiary hyperparathyroidism

*Yasser Ali Hakami**

Obesity, Endocrine and Metabolism Center, King Fahad Medical City, Riyadh, Saudi Arabia

Correspondence:
Yasser Ali Hakami,
Obesity, Endocrine and Metabolism Center, King Fahad Medical City, Aldabab Street, P.O. Box 59046, Riyadh 11525, Saudi Arabia
dr.yasser.ali@hotmail.com

Parathyroid (PTH) exploration surgery carries the risk of developing post-operative thyroiditis due to vigorous manual manipulation of the thyroid gland during surgery. Post-operative thyroiditis has a wide spectrum of clinical manifestations. However, it remains underreported. Here, we describe a case of post-operative transient thyroiditis in a 33-year-old male who developed 3 days after parathyroidectomy for PTH hyperplasia. We review the limited literature regarding this interesting entity.

Keywords: thyroiditis, thyroid function tests, hyperparathyroidism, post-operative period, parathyroidectomy, adrenergic beta-antagonists

Introduction

Post-operative thyroiditis is one cause of iatrogenic thyrotoxicosis. It usually occurs after vigorous manual manipulation of the thyroid gland during neck or parathyroid (PTH) exploratory surgery. It has a wide spectrum of clinical manifestations, varying from asymptomatic hyperthyroxinemia to a severe overt thyrotoxic state (1).

However, this disorder remains underestimated and only a few cases have been reported. In current clinical practice, this condition is likely more common and important than previously thought.

Case Report

A 33-year-old male came to the clinic complaining of generalized bone pain associated with progressive weakness over the last year. The patient had been diagnosed with end-stage renal disease secondary to glomerulonephritis 11 years before his presentation and had been on hemodialysis three times per week for the last 10 years. The patient had no past history of thyroid disorders. There was no goiter on physical examination.

The patient's serum corrected-calcium level was 2.79 mmol/L (normal range, 2.19–2.54 mmol/L), his serum phosphate level was 1.29 mmol/L (normal range, 0.7–1.5 mmol/L), his vitamin D25-OH level was normal, his serum creatinine level was 756 μmol/L (normal range, 53–106.1 μmol/L), his serum urea was 17.2 mmol/L (normal range, 2.9–8.2 mmol/L), and his serum PTH level was 489.5 pmol/L (normal range, 1.6–6.8 pmol/L).

At our clinic, the patient was diagnosed with tertiary hyperparathyroidism and renal osteodystrophy as complications from his chronic kidney disease. His pre-operative serum thyroid-stimulating hormone (TSH) level was within normal parameters (1.1 mIU/L; normal range, 0.35–5.0 mIU/L). A dual-phase PTH scan revealed two foci located below the lower poles of both thyroid lobes with intact thyroid uptake compatible with PTH adenomas (**Figure 1**). Diagnostic computed tomography (CT) or magnetic resonance imaging (MRI) scans were necessary for the final reading, which involved fusion of the available axial cuts of the PTH scan with structural imaging data. Neck MRI

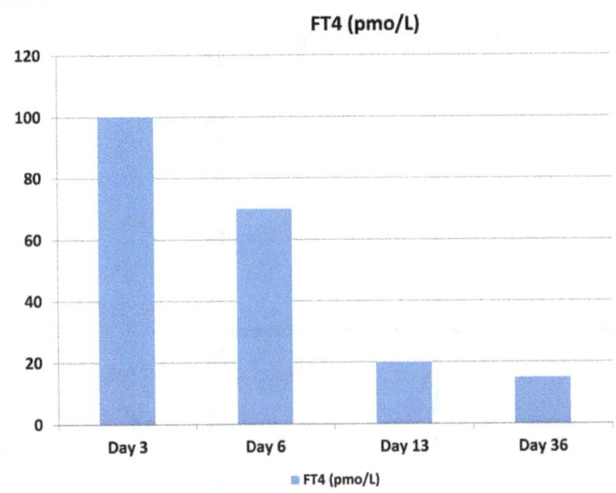

FIGURE 1 | The patient's FT4 levels peaked on post-operative day 3. Reference values are the following: free thyroxine (FT4): 9.1–23.8 pmol/L.

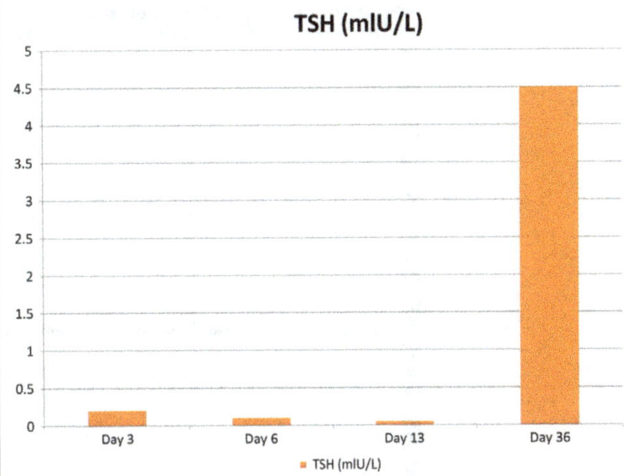

FIGURE 2 | The patient's TSH levels following surgery. Reference values are the following: thyroid-stimulating hormone (TSH): 0.35–5.0 mIU/L.

revealed four PTH masses posterior and inferior to the normal thyroid gland, with two masses on each side, suggesting PTH adenomas. Fine-needle aspiration (FNA) of the right PTH masses was performed, and pathological examination revealed PTH cells consistent with hyperplastic proliferation. Therefore, the patient was diagnosed with PTH hyperplasia.

The patient underwent parathyroidectomy to remove his PTH glands. He was brought to the operating room under general anesthesia. A transverse incision 6-cm long and 3-cm superior to the sternal angle was made. The strap muscle was separated, and the dissection was continued until the surgeon reached the thyroid gland. Retraction of the thyroid gland on the right side was successful, and the recurrent laryngeal nerve was identified. The superior right PTH gland was anterior to the nerve and was dissected successfully. The inferior right PTH gland was deep and near the sternum. It was difficult to separate the inferior right PTH gland from the thyroid gland surgically because they were firmly attached, so the attached part of the thyroid gland was taken as a resection margin along with the inferior right PTH gland. Subcapsular dissection of the thyroid gland was done on the left side also, and the left recurrent laryngeal nerve was identified. The superior left PTH gland, posterior to the nerve, was identified and separated successfully. The left inferior PTH gland was located, dissected from around the gland, and extracted. All of the PTH glands were resected. The duration of the surgery was 78 min.

The intra-operative serum PTH level was 414.2 pmol/L and had declined to 22.4 pmol/L 1 h after surgery. One day after surgery, it was 4.2 pmol/L. The resected part of the thyroid gland was normal on pathological examination. The pathological examination of the resected PTH glands revealed nodular hyperplasia involving all glands confirming the PTH hyperplasia diagnosis. There were no complications during surgery. However, the patient developed hypocalcemia that was normalized with calcium replacement therapy.

Three days after the surgery, the patient presented with new symptoms of palpitation, anxiety, and hand tremors. A complete examination revealed mild, diffuse, non-tender goiter, and fine tremor, with stable vital signs. Serum thyroid function tests revealed that his TSH level was 0.171 mIU/L and that his free thyroxine (FT4) level was 97.6 pmol/L (normal range, 9.1–23.8 pmol/L), consistent with primary hyperthyroidism (**Figures 2** and **3**). Technetium-99m (Tc-99m) pertechnetate scintigraphy revealed generalized reduced tracer uptake in the thyroid gland, a finding that is compatible with thyroiditis (**Figure 4**). Autoimmune markers were normal, including thyroglobulin (Tg) antibodies (2.08 IU/mL; normal range, 0–80 IU/mL), thyroid peroxidase (TPO) antibodies (0.3 IU/mL; normal range, 0–20 IU/mL), and TSH receptor antibodies (negative). However, inflammatory markers were elevated including C-reactive protein (CRP) (8.8 mg/L; normal range, 1.0–3.0 mg/L) and erythrocyte sedimentation rate (ESR) (78 mm/H; normal range, 0.0–20.0 mm/H). There was no clinical evidence of sepsis. The patient did not receive iodinated contrast agents; he did not receive lithium or amidarone nor medication that might have affected his thyroid function tests. Other possible causes of thyroiditis have been ruled out, specifically, viral thyroiditis, bacterial thyroiditis, autoimmune thyroiditis, radiation thyroiditis, or drug-induced thyroiditis. Therefore, he was diagnosed with post-operative thyroiditis and given oral Bisoprolol. He did not receive an antithyroid agent.

His condition improved over the following weeks. After 3 weeks, he made a complete recovery and had no persistent clinical or biochemical manifestations of thyroid disease. Bisoprolol was withdrawn. The patient was examined in the clinic after 6 months. At this time, he was clinically and biochemically euthyroid, with no indication of hypothyroidism.

A definitive diagnosis of post-operative transient thyroiditis secondary due to manual manipulation of the thyroid gland during surgery was made.

Discussion

The incidence of post-operative thyroiditis is unknown as it is underreported. There are no data in the literature pertaining to

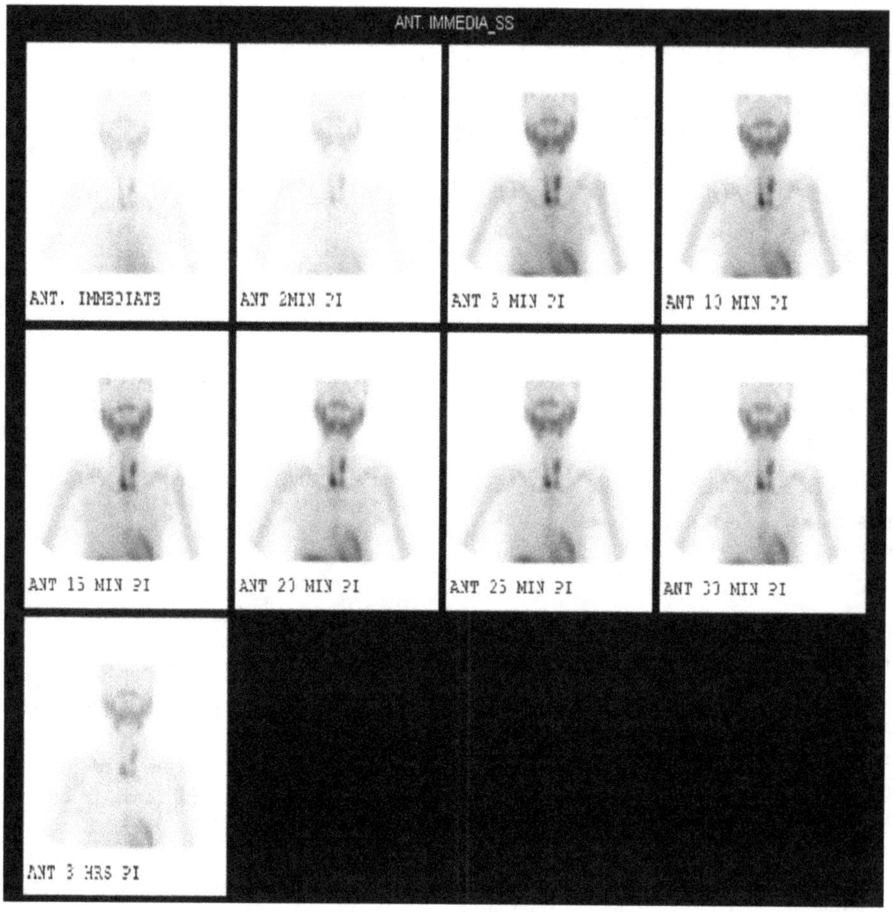

FIGURE 3 | 99m TcMIBI (sestamibi) dual-phase parathyroid scintigraphy revealed two foci located below the lower poles of both thyroid lobes with intact thyroid uptake compatible with parathyroid adenomas.

complications of parathyroidectomy on the prevalence of post-operative transient thyroiditis. This is likely because most patients are asymptomatic or have mild non-specific symptoms.

In 2005, Stang et al. examined pre- and post-operative thyroid function and outcomes in 199 patients who had PTH exploratory surgery for primary sporadic hyperparathyroidism. They found that the incidence of TSH suppression below the lower limits of normal levels was 29% (58/199) (1). Akira et al. reported a type of thyrotoxicosis that occurred after needle aspiration of thyroid cysts. The incidence of post-aspiration thyrotoxicosis was 0.9% (1 of 115) (2). In two small studies, the rate of post-operative hyperthyroidism after parathyroidectomy was 20% (3, 4). Reported causes of iatrogenic thyrotoxicosis include use of medication that can affect the thyroid gland, such as lithium and amiodarone, recent radioiodine ablation, thyroid hormone replacement therapy, iodine excess, immunotherapy, external irradiation, and manipulation of the thyroid gland during surgery.

The exact mechanism of post-operative thyroiditis is unclear. In the past, hyperthyroidism arising after PTH surgery has been thought to be transient and relate to retraction of the thyroid gland for exposure during surgery.

In 1975, Carney et al. described an association between vigorous thyroid lobe palpations under pentobarbital anesthesia with the histological finding of granulomatous thyroid folliculitis in massaged thyroid lobes in dogs. Noting that similar multifocal inflammatory changes usually were present in resected human thyroid lobes. It is suggested that manipulation of the thyroid gland was sufficient to cause transient inflammatory reactions in both humans and dogs, which they termed as palpation thyroiditis and multifocal granulomatous folliculitis (5).

In 1992, Walfish et al. reported on three patients who had undergone resection of PTH adenoma, which occurred after routine transection of the superior thyroid pole and vessels and developed thyrotoxicosis post-operatively. They concluded that the thyroid disruption caused post-operative hyperthyroidism. They were the first to suggest evidence of a clinical syndrome of trauma-induced thyroiditis in those patients (6). On the contrary, in Stang et al. study, they treat the thyroid gland as gently as possible, but there data supported a causative role of operative trauma to the thyroid lobe, since bilateral exploration was associated with the development of post-operative hyperthyroidism (1).

In Akira et al. study, the mechanism of post-aspiration thyrotoxicosis is unknown; however, they speculated that the combination of thyroiditis and leakage of thyroid contents into the cyst might have triggered thyroid hormone release into circulation after needle aspiration of thyroid cysts (2). In Bergenfelz et al.

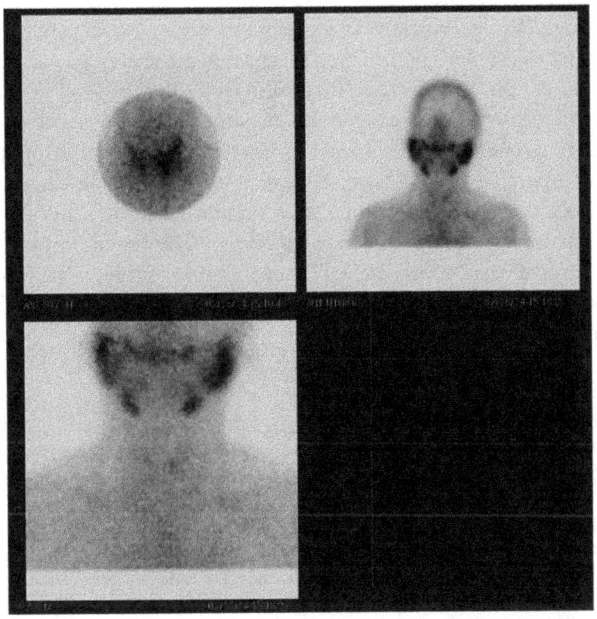

FIGURE 4 | Technetium-99m (Tc-99m) pertechnetate scintigraphy of the patient's thyroid gland is faintly observed with generalized reduced tracer uptake in the thyroid gland. There is increased background tracer activity in the salivary glands. These findings are compatible with thyroiditis.

prospective study of 20 patients undergoing operation for primary hyperparathyroidism, compared with 6 patients undergoing laparoscopic cholecystectomy. Four patients (20%) developed biochemical hyperthyroidism, but serum antithyroid antibody levels did not increase. Control patients experienced a slight increase in mean TSH post-operatively, and the authors concluded that post-parathyroidectomy hyperthyroidism was related to metabolic derangement intrinsic to the primary hyperparathyroidism itself (3).

In Lindblom et al. report, they examined post-parathyroidectomy hyperthyroidism in 26 patients undergoing operation for primary hyperparathyroidism, but with more detail about anesthetic and operative factors and with a different control group of 11 patients undergoing breast cancer surgery. Post-operative levels of T4 and T3 were higher after PTH operation than after breast operation. The investigator concluded that manipulation of the thyroid gland was most likely the major contributing factor to post-operative hyperthyroidism. However, it may not be the sole explanation, since there data suggest a more multifactorial scenario (4).

Rudofsky et al. reported a case of transient symptomatic thyrotoxicosis following PTH surgery for tertiary hyperparathyroidism in a 33-year-old woman; they presumed that it was caused by a traumatic thyroiditis as a result of manipulation of the thyroid gland during surgery (7).

Calle and Cohen reported on a patient who developed transient thyroiditis following total laryngopharyngoesophagectomy with gastric pull-up for a right hypopharynx tumor with preservation of the thyroid gland (8).

In the Stang et al. study cited above, the incidence of post-operative hyperthyroidism was independent of age, gender, the pre-operative and intra-operative PTH levels, and adenoma weight. There was no relationship between the type of PTH pathology, that is, multi-glandular disease versus solitary adenoma, the presence of goiter, or prior thyroiditis. None of the following indicators of operative trauma were predictive of post-operative thyroiditis: time that the operation took, incision length, difficulty in making the dissection, thyroid nodulectomy, thyroidectomy for intrathyroidal PTH adenoma, retropharyngeal adenoma, concurrent cervical thymectomy, the degree of perithyroidal inflammation, or whether or not a drain was placed (1).

Stang et al. identified three surgical variables associated with post-parathyroidectomy hyperthyroidism. These were bilateral exploration, the absence of concurrent thyroid lobectomy, and performance of the operation at community hospitals. When patients were cared for at the community hospitals, exploration had to be done bilaterally because the intra-operative PTH could not be monitored. The use of lithium was observed to be an independent risk factor for post-operative hyperthyroidism. This may be because lithium provides a persistent toxic insult to thyroid tissue, rendering it more sensitive to manipulation during neck surgery. Patients who underwent complete thyroid lobectomy were less likely to have post-operative thyroiditis (1).

Post-operative thyroiditis has a wide clinical presentation spectrum, ranging from asymptomatic hyperthyroxinemia to severe hyperthyroidism. In addition, a few cases of thyroiditis following neck surgery that caused the onset of atrial fibrillation have been reported (9, 10). McDermott et al. reported a case of transient thyroiditis secondary to surgical manipulation of the thyroid in a 76-year-old man, which caused significant tachyarrhythmia following total laryngectomy for a subglottic tumor with preservation of thyroid gland (11).

In the Stang et al. study, hyperthyroidism symptoms were reported in 19 of 125 (15%) patents with pre-operatively normal serum TSH levels. Of these, five patients (4%) were found to be overtly thyrotoxic. The duration for complete biochemical resolution ranged from 12 days to 90 days post-operation, whether or not there was medical management (1). The finding that there was spontaneous resolution of the condition within 6 weeks in the majority of the patients supports the hypothesis that manipulation of the gland during parathyroidectomy is a major contributing factor in its development. Development of thyrotoxicosis with more prolonged hyperthyroxinemia later than 6 weeks after surgery may be caused by other factors, including lithium therapy or a predisposition to Grave's disease (12). It is not clear that permanent hypothyroidism is common in these cases, as there are few data on this question. There is also little information on how an abnormal thyroid status will affect the development of post-operative thyroiditis compared to patients with a normal thyroid. Nonetheless, it would appear to be prudent to follow up patients who suffered post-operative thyroiditis for permanent hypothyroidism. In all cases, symptomatic treatment should be applied until spontaneous resolution of symptoms.

We speculate that there is an association between vigorous manual manipulation of the thyroid gland during PTH exploration surgery and the incidence of post-operative transient thyroiditis.

Further retrospective and prospective studies should be conducted to confirm the association between vigorous manual manipulation of the thyroid gland during PTH exploration surgery and the incidence of post-operative thyroiditis. They should also address identification of the risk factors and the patients who should undergo additional testing. This would be important to enhance our understanding of the disease process, and establish the clinical criteria for accurate diagnosis and early treatment.

Post-operative thyroiditis can cause significant clinical problems that can be easily missed. Clinicians should have an increased awareness of the clinical consequences and complications.

Establishing the risks inherent to PTH exploration surgery should enable clinicians to develop strategies for effective risk reduction, such as minimizing the extent of surgery.

Based on the current literature data, the authors recommend pre-operative counseling as well as routine biochemical and clinical surveillance for hyperthyroidism during the post-operative period. Although diagnosis should be early and expectant, treatment should be symptomatic as allowed by spontaneous resolution of symptoms. Continued efforts to minimize the extent of PTH exploration surgery, if possible, may reduce the potential morbidity of thyrotoxicosis after surgery.

References

1. Stang MT, Yim JH, Challinor SM, Bahl S, Carty SE. Hyperthyroidism after parathyroid exploration. *Surgery* (2005) **138**:1058–65. doi:10.1016/j.surg.2005.09.011
2. Kobayashi A, Kuma K, Matsuzuka F, Hirai K, Fukata S, Sugawara M. Thyrotoxicosis after needle aspiration of thyroid cyst. *J Clin Endocrinol Metab* (1992) **75**:21–4. doi:10.1210/jc.75.1.21
3. Bergenfelz A, Ahren B. Hyperthyroxinemia after surgery for primary hyperparathyroidism. *Langenbecks Arch Chir* (1994) **379**:178–81. doi:10.1007/BF00680115
4. Lindblom P, Valdemarsson S, Westerdahl J, Tennvall J, Bergenfelz A. Hyperthyroidism after surgery for primary hyperparathyroidism. *Langenbecks Arch Surg* (1999) **384**:568–75. doi:10.1007/s004230050245
5. Carney JA, Moore SB, Northcutt RC, Woolner LB, Stillwell GK. Palpation thyroiditis (multifocal granulomatous folliculitis). *Am J Clin Pathol* (1975) **64**:639–47.
6. Walfish PG, Caplan D, Rosen IB. Postparathyroidectomy transient thyrotoxicosis. *J Clin Endocrinol Metab* (1992) **75**:224–7. doi:10.1210/jcem.75.1.1619014
7. Rudofsky G Jr, Grafe IA, Metzner C, Leowardi C. Transient post-operative thyrotoxicosis after parathyroidectomy. *Med Sci Monit* (2009) **15**(3):CS41–3.
8. Calle RA, Cohen KL. Transient thyroiditis due to surgical trauma. *Am J Med* (1993) **95**:546–8. doi:10.1016/0002-9343(93)90342-M
9. Mai V, Glister B, Clyde P. Palpation thyroiditis causing new-onset atrial fibrillation. *Thyroid* (2008) **18**:571–3. doi:10.1089/thy.2007.0246
10. Blenke EJ, Vernham GA, Ellis G. Surgery-induced thyroiditis following laryngectomy. *J Laryngol Otol* (2004) **118**:313–4. doi:10.1258/002215504323012111
11. McDermott A, Onyeaka CV, Macnamara M. Surgery-induced thyroiditis: fact or fiction? *Ear Nose Throat J* (2002) **81**:408–10.
12. McGown DM, Vaswani A, Shperling I. Coexisting hyperparathyroidisim with thyrotoxicosis. *J Endocrinol Invest* (1991) **14**:305–10. doi:10.1007/BF03346819

18

Prognostic Indicators of Non-Transection Nerve Injury and Vocal Fold Motion Impairment after Thyroid Surgery – Correlation between Intraoperative Neuromonitoring Findings and Perioperative Voice Parameters

Tzu-Yen Huang[1,2,3], *Wing-Hei Viola Yu*[1], *Feng-Yu Chiang*[4,5], *Che-Wei Wu*[1,6], *Shih-Chen Fu*[7,8], *An-Shun Tai*[7,8], *Yi-Chu Lin*[1], *Hsin-Yi Tseng*[1], *Ka-Wo Lee*[1,9] *and Sheng-Hsuan Lin*[7,8,10,11*]

***Correspondence:**
Sheng-Hsuan Lin
shenglin@nctu.edu.tw

[1] International Thyroid Surgery Center, Department of Otolaryngology-Head and Neck Surgery, Kaohsiung Medical University Hospital, Faculty of Medicine, College of Medicine, Kaohsiung Medical University, Kaohsiung, Taiwan, [2] Department of Biological Science and Technology, National Yang Ming Chiao Tung University, Hsinchu, Taiwan, [3] Department of Biological Science and Technology, National Chiao Tung University, Hsinchu, Taiwan, [4] Department of Otolaryngology-Head and Neck Surgery, E-Da Hospital, Kaohsiung, Taiwan, [5] School of Medicine, College of Medicine, I-Shou University, Kaohsiung, Taiwan, [6] Department of Otolaryngology-Head and Neck Surgery, Kaohsiung Municipal Siaogang Hospital, Kaohsiung Medical University Hospital, Faculty of Medicine, College of Medicine, Kaohsiung Medical University, Kaohsiung, Taiwan, [7] Institute of Statistics, National Yang Ming Chiao Tung University, Hsinchu, Taiwan, [8] Institute of Statistics, National Chiao Tung University, Hsinchu, Taiwan, [9] Department of Otolaryngology-Head and Neck Surgery, Kaohsiung Municipal Tatung Hospital, Kaohsiung Medical University Hospital, Faculty of Medicine, College of Medicine, Kaohsiung Medical University, Kaohsiung, Taiwan, [10] Institute of Data Science and Engineering, National Yang Ming Chiao Tung University, Hsinchu, Taiwan, [11] Institute of Data Science and Engineering, National Chiao Tung University, Hsinchu, Taiwan

Objectives: In patients with recurrent laryngeal nerve (RLN) injury after thyroid surgery, unrecovered vocal fold motion (VFM) and subjective voice impairment cause extreme distress. For surgeons, treating these poor outcomes is extremely challenging. To enable early treatment of VFM impairment, this study evaluated prognostic indicators of non-transection RLN injury and VFM impairment after thyroid surgery and evaluated correlations between intraoperative neuromonitoring (IONM) findings and perioperative voice parameters.

Methods: 82 adult patients had postoperative VFM impairment after thyroidectomy were enrolled. Demographic characteristics, RLN electromyography (EMG), and RLN injury mechanism were compared. Multi-dimensional voice program, voice range profile and Index of voice and swallowing handicap of thyroidectomy (IVST) were administered during I-preoperative; II-immediate, III-short-term and IV-long-term postoperative periods. The patients were divided into R/U Group according to the VFM was recovered/unrecovered 3 months after surgery. The patients in U Group were divided into U1/U2 Group according to total IVST score change was <4 and ≥4 during period-IV.

Results: Compared to R Group (42 patients), U Group (38 patients) had significantly more patients with EMG >90% decrease in the injured RLN ($p<0.001$) and thermal injury as the RLN injury mechanism ($p=0.002$). Voice parameter impairments were more severe in U Group compared to R Group. Compared to U1 group (19 patients), U2 Group (19 patients) had a significantly larger proportion of patients with EMG decrease >90% in the injured RLN ($p=0.022$) and thermal injury as the RLN injury mechanism ($p=0.017$). A large pitch range decrease in period-II was a prognostic indicator of a moderate/severe long-term postoperative subjective voice impairment.

Conclusion: This study is the first to evaluate correlations between IONM findings and voice outcomes in patients with VFM impairment after thyroid surgery. Thyroid surgeons should make every effort to avoid severe type RLN injury (e.g., thermal injury or injury causing EMG decrease >90%), which raises the risk of unrecovered VFM and moderate/severe long-term postoperative subjective voice impairment. Using objective voice parameters (e.g., pitch range) as prognostic indicators not only enables surgeons to earlier identify patients with low voice satisfaction after surgery, and also enable implementation of interventions sufficiently early to maintain quality of life.

Keywords: thyroid surgery, intraoperative neuromonitoring (IONM), vocal fold motion, recurrent laryngeal nerve (RLN), index of voice and swallowing handicap of thyroidectomy (IVST), subjective/objective voice analysis

INTRODUCTION

Recurrent laryngeal nerve (RLN) injury during thyroid surgery is the most common etiology of vocal fold motion (VFM) impairment (1) and morbidity after this procedure and a leading cause of medico-legal litigation after thyroid surgery (2). To avoid RLN injury during thyroid surgery, adjunct use of intraoperative neuromonitoring (IONM) has gained widespread use for identifying the RLN early in thyroid surgery and for elucidating nerve injury mechanism (3–6). The incidence of RLN paralysis may be underestimated if VFM is not routinely examined (7). Previous works report that permanent RLN palsy occurs in 1–3% of thyroid surgeries and that temporary RLN palsy occurs in 1.4-38% of these procedures (8, 9). For comprehensive evaluation of RLN function before and after thyroid surgery, current practice guidelines recommend performing pre- and post-operative laryngofiberscopy routinely (6, 10).

Patients who had a RLN injury during thyroid surgery are expected to have VFM impairment after surgery and may also experience severe dysphonia, dyspnea, and aspiration (11). In patients with temporary RLN palsy caused by a non-transection RLN injury, Chiang et al. (12) reported that VFM usually recovers within 3 days to 4 months (mean, 30.7 days) after surgery. However, the course of VFM recovery depends on the nerve injury mechanism (13). Thermal injuries are associated with a long recovery time and severe histological disturbance in the endoneurium whereas mechanical injuries are associated with distorted epineuria and perineuria (13, 14). After RLN injury, natural neuromuscular compensation mechanisms may yield outcomes that are acceptable to the patient, including RLN function outcomes and voice outcomes (15). However, early assessment of voice performance is important for deciding subsequent voice intervention (16). There is evidence that voice interventions 3 months after RLN injury can greatly improve voice outcome after thyroid surgery (10, 17, 18).

Impaired VFM after thyroid surgery is considered evidence of RLN injury. Unrecovered VFM and subjective voice impairment degrade quality of life and satisfaction with treatment, which causes extreme distress in patients. For surgeons, treating these poor outcomes is also extremely challenging. To enable early identification and treatment of VFM impairment and to improve patient satisfaction with surgery outcomes, this study evaluated prognostic indicators of non-transection RLN injury and VFM impairment after thyroid surgery. Correlations between IONM findings and perioperative voice parameters were also investigated.

MATERIALS AND METHODS

The subjects of this study were adult patients who had received IONM-assisted primary thyroid surgery by "IONM team" at a single institution (Kaohsiung Medical University Hospital, Taiwan) from June, 2013, to June, 2019. All patients had normal and symmetric VFM before surgery and had VFM impairment within 2 weeks after surgery. The total number of surgeries performed in this period was 1033, and the number of surgeries without VFM impairment was 951. The analysis included 82 (7.9%) patients after exclusion of one oral cancer patient who had received cancer surgery combined with lateral neck dissection and one nasopharyngeal carcinoma patient who had received radiation therapy in the neck region. The flowchart in **Figure 1** depicts the procedure for inclusion and exclusion of

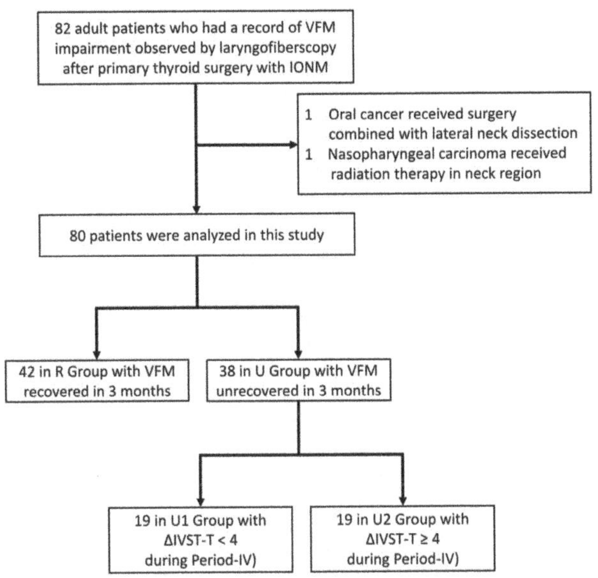

FIGURE 1 | Flow diagram for inclusion and exclusion of patients. VFM, vocal fold motion; IONM, intraoperative neuromonitoring; IVST, Index of Voice and Swallowing Handicap of Thyroidectomy.

patients in this study. Ethical approval of this study was obtained from the Kaohsiung Medical University Hospital Institutional Review Board (KMUHIRB-E(I)-20200359). In all patients, vagus nerve function and RLN function were routinely evaluated using the standard four-step vagus nerve and RLN stimulation (V1-R1-R2-V2) procedure under IONM and the evoked electromyography (EMG) amplitudes were obtained and recorded (3, 19). The RLN EMG decrease was defined and calculated as the decrease in the EMG amplitude of the post-dissection R2 signal from the EMG amplitude of the pre-dissection R1 signal. No patient who had received bilateral thyroidectomy in this study had RLN signal >50% decreases on both sides. All exposed RLNs, including injury mechanisms (transection, mechanical, or thermal), were documented by photograph. Mechanical injury was classified as type 1 (segmental injury) or type 2 (global injury) according to the criteria proposed by Chiang et al. (3) and the INMSG (6). All patients received surgery by "IOINM team" routinely received a VFM survey. Laryngofiberscopy was documented by video in all patients before surgery and within 2 weeks after surgery. All patients with VFM impairment 2 weeks after surgery underwent additional monthly examinations until VFM recovery. Patients were divided into two groups according to VFM recovery: a recovered VFM group (R Group) and an unrecovered VFM group (U Group). The R Group criterion was laryngofiberscopic evidence of VFM impairment recovery within 3 months after thyroidectomy; the U group criterion was persistent VFM impairment more than 3 months after thyroidectomy. Patient information, including gender, age, surgery type (unilateral versus bilateral), and pathology results (benign versus malignant) was recorded and compared between groups.

Objective and Subjective Voice Analysis

All patients underwent both subjective and objective voice analyses in four periods: period-I (preoperative period, within 2 months before surgery), period-II (immediate postoperative period, median duration of 3 days, range of 1-7 days), period-III (short-term postoperative period, median duration of 12 days, range of 7-30 days), and period-IV (long-term postoperative period, median duration of 40 days, range of 30-90 days).

All objective voice analyses in all subjects were performed by a single experienced speech-language pathologist (WHV. Y) using the Multidimensional Voice Program (model 5105, version 3.1.7; KayPENTAX, USA) and the Voice Range Profile (model 4326, version 3.3.0; KayPENTAX, USA). Multidimensional Voice Program analyses included mean fundamental frequency (mean F0), jitter, shimmer and noise-to-harmonic ratio whereas Voice Range Profile analyses included maximum pitch frequency (Fmax), minimum pitch frequency (Fmin), and pitch range (PR). The PR was defined as the number of semitones between Fmax and Fmin.

All preoperative and postoperative subjective voice analyses were performed using the 10-item Index of Voice and Swallowing Handicap of Thyroidectomy (IVST) (**Supplemental Table 1**), which provides an index of the main symptoms observed in the patient. Each item in this subjective assessment is scored from 0-2 (never, sometimes, and always), respectively. The two domains of the IVST are the voice domain (IVST-V; items 1-7; score range 0-14) and the swallowing domain (IVST-S; items 8-10; score range 0-6). Thus, the score range for the total IVST (IVST-T) is 0 to 20.

The equation for calculating postoperative change in objective voice analysis data was $\Delta = (B - A)/A$, and the equation for calculating postoperative change in subjective voice analysis data was $\Delta = B - A$, where A and B are preoperative and postoperative values, respectively.

Long-term postoperative subjective voice impairment was also evaluated in patients with unrecovered VFM (U Group). The U group was divided into patients with no/mild subjective voice impairment (ΔIVST-T < 4) in Period-IV (U1 Group) and patients with moderate/severe subjective voice impairment (ΔIVST-T ≥ 4) in Period-IV (U2 Group).

Statistical Analysis

To analyze the variables, independent t test and Pearson chi-square test were performed using R software (version-3.4). A two-tailed p value less than 0.05 was considered statistically significant.

RESULTS

Demographic Characteristics of R Group and U Group

Table 1 compares the 42 (52.5%) patients in R Group and the 38 (47.5%) patients in U Group. Age, gender, surgical extent, and pathology results did not significantly differ between groups. The proportions of patients with <50%, 50-90%, >90% EMG decreases in the injured RLN were 0.0%, 83.3%, and 16.7% in

TABLE 1 | Demographic characteristics of Recovered VFM Group (R Group) and Unrecovered VFM Group (U Group).

	R Group	U Group	p value
Number (%)	42 (52.5%)	38 (47.5%)	
Age (mean ± SD)	50.7 ± 13.7	52.7 ± 12.4	0.497
Gender			0.073
Male (%)	11 (26.2%)	5 (13.2%)	
Female (%)	31 (73.8%)	33 (86.8%)	
Surgical extent			0.086
Unilateral (%)	7 (16.7%)	1 (2.6%)	
Bilateral (%)	35 (83.3%)	37 (97.4%)	
Pathology			0.069
Benign (%)	24 (57.1%)	14 (36.8%)	
Malignant (%)	18 (42.9%)	24 (73.2%)	
EMG decrease in the injured RLN			<0.001
<50% decreased (%)	0 (0.0%)	0 (0.0%)	
50-90% decreased (%)	35 (83.3%)	17 (44.7%)	
>90% decreased(%)	7 (16.7%)	21 (55.3%)	
RLN Injury mechanism and type			0.002
Transection (%)	0 (0.0%)	0 (0.0%)	
Mechanical (%)	42 (100.0%)	30 (78.9%)	
Type 1	33	27	
Type 2	9	3	
Thermal (%)	0 (0.0%)	8 (21.1%)	
Subjective voice impairment during period-IV			0.028*
No/Mild (ΔIVST-T <4) (%)	31 (73.8%)	19 (50.0%)	
Moderate/Severe (ΔIVST-T ≥4) (%)	11 (26.2%)	19 (50.0%)	
RLN reinnervation or nerve grafting	0 (0.0%)	0 (0.0%)	

VFM, vocal fold motion; SD, standard deviation; EMG, electromyography; RLN, recurrent laryngeal nerve; IVST, Index of Voice and Swallowing Handicap of Thyroidectomy; IVST-T, Total IVST score; period IV, Long-term postoperative period (range of 30-90 days).
**p value <0.05, showed significant difference.*

R Group, respectively; the corresponding proportions in U Group were 0.0%, 44.7%, and 55.3%, respectively. That is, the proportions of patients with >90% EMG decreases were significantly larger in U Group compared to R Group (p<0.001).

No patients had transection injury in either the R Group or the U Group. All 42 (100.0%) patients in the R Group had mechanical injury (type 1 in 33 patients and type 2 in 9 patients). Among the 38 patients in U Group, 30 (78.9%) patients had mechanical injury, 27 had type 1 injury, 3 had type 2 injury; and 8 (21.1%) had thermal injury. The percentage of patients with thermal injury was significantly higher in U Group compared to R Group (p=0.002). The proportions of patients with no/mild (ΔIVST-T <4) and moderate/severe (ΔIVST-T ≥4) subjective voice impairment in period-IV were 73.8% and 26.2% in R Group, respectively, versus 50.0% and 50.0% in U Group, respectively. In period-IV, U group also had significantly more patients with moderate/severe subjective voice impairment compared to R Group (p=0.028). No patients in this study had received RLN reinnervation or nerve grafting.

Voice Parameter Changes (Δ) Associated With Different VFM Outcomes

In **Supplemental Table 2**, the detailed voice parameters, voice parameter changes (Δ), and p values are compared between R Group and U Group in each follow-up period. Voice parameter comparisons between the two groups revealed significant differences in preoperative Fmax and preoperative PR. Postoperative parameters did not significantly differ. To minimize the influence of preoperative differences, voice parameter changes (Δ) were calculated and compared. In period-IV the U group had a ΔIVST-T score of 7.1 ± 6.8.

Figure 2 compares voice parameter changes (Δ) between the R Group and the U Group in each follow-up period. Due to large standard deviations, the two groups did not significantly differ in objective or subjective voice parameters in all follow-up periods. However, U Group showed larger impairments of voice parameters compared to R Group, especially in ΔFmax, ΔPR, ΔJitter, ΔIVST-T, ΔIVST-V, and ΔIVST-S.

Demographic Characteristics and Objective Voice Parameter Changes (Δ) in U Group According to Severity of Subjective Voice Impairment in Long-Term Postoperative Period

To evaluate the wide range of subjective voice impairment within U Group, **Table 2** shows the demographic characteristics of the U1 Group (no/mild subjective voice impairment) and U2 Group (moderate/severe subjective voice impairment). Compared to the U1 Group the U2 Group had significantly larger proportions of patients with EMG decrease >90% in the injured RLN (p=0.022) and patients with thermal injury as the primary RLN injury mechanism (p=0.017). **Figure 3** compares objective voice parameter changes (Δ) in the U1 Group and U2 Group in each follow-up period. In all postoperative periods, impairments in objective voice parameters were much larger in U2 Group compared to the U1 group. In period-II, ΔPR significantly p=0.007) differed between the U1 and U2 groups. In period-III, ΔFmax (p=0.013) and ΔPR (p=0.004) differed between the U1 and

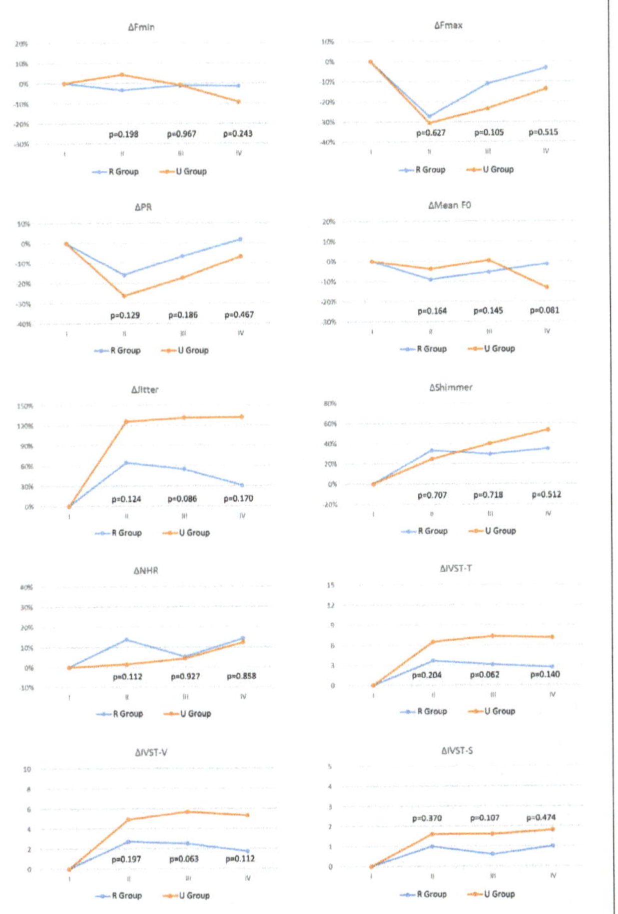

FIGURE 2 | Voice parameter changes (Δ) with different vocal cord movement (VFM) outcomes: R Group (Blue line) and U Group (Red line). Fmax, Maximum pitch frequency; Fmin, Minimum pitch frequency; PR, Pitch range; Mean F0, mean fundamental frequency; NHR, noise-to-harmonic ratio; IVST, Index of Voice and Swallowing Handicap of Thyroidectomy; IVST-T, Total IVST score; IVST-V, IVST score of voice domain score; IVST-S, IVST score of swallowing domain. period I, Preoperative period (within 2 months before surgery); period II, Immediate postoperative period (median duration of 3 days; range of 1-7 days); period III, Short-term postoperative period (median duration of 12 days; range of7-30 days); period IV, Long-term postoperative period (median duration of 40 days, range of 30-90 days). The equation for calculating postoperative change in objective voice analysis (Fmax, Fmin, PR, Mean F0, Jitter, Shimmer, NHR) data was Δ= (B - A)/A, the unit is %; the equation for calculating postoperative change in subjective voice analysis (IVST-T, IVST-V, IVST-S) data was Δ= B – A, the unit is score. Where A and B are preoperative and postoperative values, respectively. The preoperative Δ is 0 in all the voice parameter. p value <0.05, showed significant difference.

U2 groups; ΔJitter and ΔShimmer were larger in U2 Group compared to U1 Group. In period-IV, ΔPR (p=0.006) also significantly differed between groups; ΔFmax, ΔJitter, and ΔShimmer were larger in U2 Group compared to U1 Group.

DISCUSSION

This study is the first to investigate correlations between IONM findings and voice outcomes in patients with impaired VFM after thyroid surgery. This analysis showed that, compared to the R Group, the U Group (particularly the U2 Group) had larger proportions of patients with EMG decrease >90% in the injured RLN and patients with thermal injury as the RLN injury mechanism (**Tables 1**, **2**). Voice parameter changes were much larger in the U Group compared to the R Group, but the change did not reach statistical significance (**Figure 2**). A large pitch range decrease in period-II is a prognostic indicator of moderate/severe long-term postoperative subjective voice impairment (**Figure 3**). Therefore, surgeons should make every effort to avoid severe type RLN injury during thyroid surgery and should utilize voice analysis to enable early identification of patients who may be experiencing distress and low satisfaction caused by poor surgical outcomes and to enable early initiation of intervention therapy to maintain quality of life in these patients.

The EMG data in revealed four interesting findings regarding injury mechanisms and postoperative VFM outcomes (**Table 1**). 1) No patient with EMG <50% decrease had postoperative asymmetric VFM. This finding indicates that preserving RLN function during surgery is the key factor in VFM preservation after surgery. Accurately recording all data for asymmetric VFM before surgery is also essential for avoiding misjudgment of vocal cord function and potential legal liability (20). 2) Patients with EMG 50-90% decrease in the injured RLN may not achieve total recovery from asymmetric VFM. Using continuous IONM can minimize complications by avoiding surgical procedures that can cause mechanical injury (21). Continuous IONM prevents most mechanical injuries with visually intact RLN, thereby enabling modification of injury-causing surgical procedures in 80% of cases (22). The advancement of continuous IONM technology can make a breakthrough in VFM evaluation after thyroidectomy (23). 3) All patients with thermal RLN injury in this study had unrecovered VFM (U Group). RLN thermal injury is difficult to be detected visually and the risk of permanent palsy is high, surgeons should maintain vigilance in modern thyroid surgery that increases the use of energy-based devices (24). Compared to relatively mild mechanical injuries, thermal injuries sustained during surgery may require earlier voice intervention (25) performed under comprehensive postoperative laryngofiberscopy and voice analysis. 4) The R Group and the U Group in this study did not significantly differ in Type 1 and Type 2 mechanical injury. In severe Type 2 (global) mechanical injury, VFM may have chance to be unrecovered.

In current study, patients in U group had higher proportion of malignant pathologic report than patients in R group (73.2% vs. 42.9%). For malignant disease, surgeons tend to dissect a longer segment in proximal end of RLN and perform central neck dissection; and tend to dissect the most distal end of RLN near laryngeal entry to decrease the tissue remnant in malignant disease. According to a large international registry database study with 1,000 RLNs at risks enrolled, the abnormal RLN trajectory (23%) was higher than surgeon expected, and 34% of RLN with loss of signal following an abnormal trajectory, for instance, fixed/splayed/entrapped RLN at the ligament of Berry,

TABLE 2 | Demographic characteristic of patients in U Group with different subjective voice outcomes during long-term postoperative period (Period-IV).

	U1 Group (ΔIVST-T < 4 during Period-IV)	U2 Group (ΔIVST-T ≥ 4 during Period-IV)	p value
Case number	19 patients (50.0%)	19 patients (50.0%)	
Age	50.5 ± 10.9	54.9 ± 11.8	0.240
Gender			0.150
Male (%)	4 (21.1%)	1 (5.3%)	
Female (%)	15 (78.8%)	18 (94.7%)	
Surgical extent			0.311
Unilateral (%)	1 (5.3%)	0 (0.0%)	
Bilateral (%)	18 (94.7%)	19 (100.0%)	
Pathology			0.179
Benign (%)	5 (26.3%)	9 (47.4%)	
Malignant (%)	14 (73.7%)	10 (52.6%)	
EMG decrease in the injured RLN			0.022*
50-90% decreased (%)	12 (63.2%)	5 (26.3%)	
>90% decreased (%)	7 (36.8%)	14 (73.7%)	
RLN injury mechanism			0.017*
Mechanical (%)	18 (94.7%)	12 (63.2%)	
Thermal (%)	1 (5.3%)	7 (36.8%)	

IVST, Index of Voice and Swallowing Handicap of Thyroidectomy; IVST-T, Total IVST score; EMG, electromyography; RLN, recurrent laryngeal nerve.
Period IV (range of 30-90 days).
**p value <0.05, showed significant difference.*

extensive RLN dissection, cases of cancer invasion or when lateral lymph node dissection (26). In this manner, the risk of RLN mechanical and thermal injury rate can be higher in malignant disease.

Some of the patients who revealed asymmetric VFM under laryngofiberscopy still had good subjective voice performance, which has been mentioned previously (27, 28). Reiter et al. (29) reported that voice parameters did not significantly differ between patients with and patients without recovery from vocal cord paralysis at the end of a 12-month follow up. In the current study, the R Group and the U Group did not significantly differ in objective or subjective voice parameters in all follow-up periods. However, U Group had much larger impairments compared to R Group, especially in ΔFmax, ΔPR, ΔJitter, ΔIVST-T, ΔIVST-V, and ΔIVST-S in **Figure 2**. The likely explanation for the lack of significant between-group differences was the large within-group differences in subjective voice outcomes. As **Table 2** indicates, the U1 and U2 Groups significantly differed in the incidence of severe RLN injury (i.e., EMG >90% decrease in injured RLN) and in RLN injury mechanism (thermal injury). Therefore, thyroid surgeons should make every effort to avoid severe type RLN injury. In the literature, several technical maneuvers had been reported for rescuing RLN function, including intravenous steroid (30), nimodipine (31), cold dextrose solution irrigation (32), etc., but the effectiveness of these methods remain uncertain. Besides of RLN factors, sufficient neuromuscular compensation plays an important role in reducing voice impairment after thyroid surgery (15, 33). Therefore, for good long-term postoperative voice outcomes after thyroid surgery, surgeons should prioritize restoration of neuromuscular compensation. Achieving the maximum neuromuscular compensation requires a multidisciplinary approach, especially with the participation of a speech-language pathologist to perform speech and dysphagia therapy (34). Other advanced interventions such as augmentation laryngoplasty and nerve reinnervation also have important rehabilitative roles in patients with voice recovery failure (35, 36).

In many institutions, the clinical practice environment may not include a thyroid surgeon with a laryngology background and may not have well-established procedures for routine cooperation between surgeons and speech-language pathologists (34). Under these conditions, compensation for voice impairment after thyroid surgery may not occur until long after surgery, which complicates detection of complications and other outcomes. Inadequate personnel and practices such as these may also mislead surgeons to believe that follow-up laryngofiberscopy and voice analysis are unnecessary. Early identification of voice impairment caused by VFM asymmetry can reduce the number of patient consultations needed to address psychological distress caused by poor voice outcomes and related concerns. It is worth mentioning that the voice impairment related to external branch of superior laryngeal nerve (EBSLN) injury is less significant than that of iatrogenic RLN injury. However, the stable EBSLN IONM (37) and careful analysis of high-pitched voice change (16) after thyroidectomy will largely improve life quality of the patients.

In terms of screening and interpreting voice outcomes, subjective voice analysis using IVST still has advantages over objective voice analysis. First, since a normal range of objective voice parameters has not been established, objective voice analysis requires time-consuming calculations of voice parameter changes (Δ) in individual patients whereas subjective voice analysis avoids this limitation. Second, for classifying patients with a wide range of long-term postoperative subjective voice impairments, e.g., the U Group in this study, IVST-T is simpler and more acceptable than objective voice parameters. Nevertheless, comprehensive objective voice analysis is still preferable for collecting and analyzing detailed voice data and for using these data as prognostic indicators of subjective voice impairment (**Figure 3**). Third, in patients with vocal cord paralysis, change in voice quality and loudness are

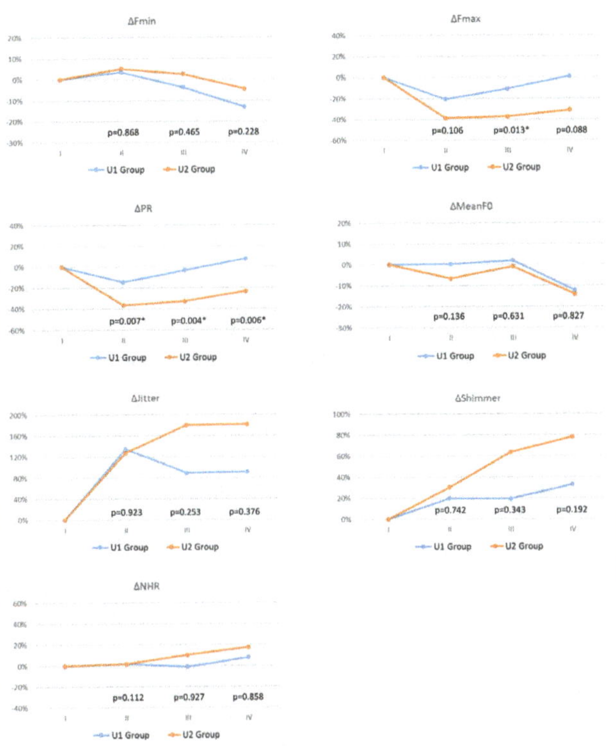

FIGURE 3 | Objective voice parameter changes (Δ) with different subjective voice outcomes during long-term postoperative period (Period-IV): U1 Group (Blue line, ΔIVST-T< 4 during Period-IV) and U2 Group (Red line, ΔIVST-T ≥ 4 during Period-IV). The abbreviations of objective/subjective voice parameters, the definition of follow-up periods (I/II/III/IV), and the equation for calculating postoperative change in objective voice analysis are same in **Figure 2**. The preoperative Δ is 0 in all the voice parameter. p value <0.05, showed significant difference.

among the most common complaints (38). Since objective voice recording method was used in the current study, loudness adjustments were made during recording, which limited objective assessments of loudness changes. Such changes could only be represented by IVST scores.

Several limitations of this study should be mentioned. First, demographic characteristics that may affect preoperative objective voice parameters differed between R Group and U Group. Future research may investigate novel preoperative objective voice parameters with less demographic variation and define "normal" ranges for such parameters. Second, no system for classifying nerve reinnervation or grafting has been established. Therefore, future works should consider how to account for the wide variation in nerve function outcomes after these procedures. Last, a longer observation time (e.g., 1 year) may be needed to observe voice compensation processes. However, the current data were sufficient for initial identification of trends in voice parameter changes after thyroidectomy. A future long-term post-thyroidectomy voice study should discuss and compare voice interventions (e.g., voice therapy, augmentation laryngoplasty, and medialization thyroplasty) and their effects.

CONCLUSION

This study is the first to evaluate correlations between IONM findings and voice outcomes in patients with VFM impairment after thyroid surgery. In addition to assessing EMG status and RLN injury mechanisms, thyroid surgeons should routinely include laryngofiberscopy and subjective/objective voice analyses as standard tools for evaluation and diagnosis before and after thyroid surgery. Thyroid surgeons should also make every effort to avoid severe type (EMG >90% decrease, thermal-related) RLN injury, which is associated with a high risk of unrecovered VFM and with a high risk of moderate-to-severe long-term postoperative subjective voice impairment. Using objective voice parameters (e.g., pitch range) as prognostic indicators only enables surgeons to earlier identify patients who have low voice satisfaction after surgery, it also enables early implementation of intervention therapy (e.g., speech therapy, augmentation laryngoplasty, and nerve reinnervation), which can maximize neuromuscular compensation in these patients and maintain their quality of life.

ETHICS STATEMENT

Ethical approval of this study was obtained from the Kaohsiung Medical University Hospital Institutional Review Board (KMUHIRB-E(I)-20200359). The patients/participants provided their written informed consent to participate in this study.

AUTHOR CONTRIBUTIONS

Supervision – F-YC, C-WW, K-WL, and S-HL. Materials – T-YH, W-HY, F-YC, and C-WW. Data Collection and Processing – T-YH, W-HY, and S-HL. Analysis and Interpretation- T-YH, S-CF, A-ST, and S-HL. Literature Search - T-YH, W-HY, Y-CL, H-YT, and S-HL. Writing Manuscript – All authors. All authors have read and agreed to the published version of the manuscript.

FUNDING

This study was supported by grants from Kaohsiung Medical University Hospital, Kaohsiung Medical University (KMUH109-9M44), Kaohsiung Municipal Siaogang Hospital/Kaohsiung Medical University Research Center grants (KMHK-DK(C)

110009, I-109-04, H-109-05, I-108-02), and Ministry of Science and Technology (MOST 108-2628-B-037-006, MOST 109-2628-B-037-014, MOST 110-2636-B-009-008, MOST 110-2314-B-037-104-MY2, MOST 110-2314-B-037-120), Taiwan.

ACKNOWLEDGMENTS

The authors would like to thank all authors of the papers included in this study, as well as participants in the contributing studies.

REFERENCES

1. Rosenthal LHS, Benninger MS, Deeb RH. Vocal Fold Immobility: A Longitudinal Analysis of Etiology Over 20 Years. *Laryngoscope* (2007) 117 (10):1864–70. doi: 10.1097/MLG.0b013e3180de4d49
2. Dralle H, Lorenz K, Machens A. Verdicts on Malpractice Claims After Thyroid Surgery: Emerging Trends and Future Directions. *Head Neck* (2012) 34(11):1591–6. doi: 10.1002/hed.21970
3. Chiang FY, Lu IC, Kuo WR, Lee KW, Chang NC, Wu CW. The Mechanism of Recurrent Laryngeal Nerve Injury During Thyroid Surgery–the Application of Intraoperative Neuromonitoring. *Surgery* (2008) 143(6):743–9. doi: 10.1016/j.surg.2008.02.006
4. Snyder SK, Lairmore TC, Hendricks JC, Roberts JW. Elucidating Mechanisms of Recurrent Laryngeal Nerve Injury During Thyroidectomy and Parathyroidectomy. *J Am Coll Surg* (2008) 206(1):123–30. doi: 10.1016/j.jamcollsurg.2007.07.017
5. Chiang FY, Lee KW, Chen HC, Chen HY, Lu IC, Kuo WR, et al. Standardization of Intraoperative Neuromonitoring of Recurrent Laryngeal Nerve in Thyroid Operation. *World J Surg* (2010) 34(2):223–9. doi: 10.1007/s00268-009-0316-8
6. Randolph GW, Dralle H, Abdullah H, Barczynski M, Bellantone R, Brauckhoff M, et al. Electrophysiologic Recurrent Laryngeal Nerve Monitoring During Thyroid and Parathyroid Surgery: International Standards Guideline Statement. *Laryngoscope* (2011) 121 Suppl 1:S1–16. doi: 10.1002/lary.21119
7. Jeannon JP, Orabi A, Bruch G, Abdalsalam H, Simo R. Diagnosis of Recurrent Laryngeal Nerve Palsy After Thyroidectomy: A Systematic Review. *Int J Clin Pract* (2009) 63(4):624–9. doi: 10.1111/j.1742-1241.2008.01875.x
8. Leow C, Webb A. The Lateral Thyroid Ligament of Berry. *Int Surg* (1998) 83 (1):75–8.
9. Yang S, Zhou L, Lu Z, Ma B, Ji Q, Wang Y. Systematic Review With Meta-Analysis of Intraoperative Neuromonitoring During Thyroidectomy. *Int J Surg* (2017) 39:104–13. doi: 10.1016/j.ijsu.2017.01.086
10. Chandrasekhar SS, Randolph GW, Seidman MD, Rosenfeld RM, Angelos P, Barkmeier-Kraemer J, et al. Clinical Practice Guideline: Improving Voice Outcomes After Thyroid Surgery. *Otolaryngology—Head Neck Surg* (2013) 148(6_suppl):S1–S37. doi: 10.1177/0194599813487301
11. Crumley RL. Unilateral Recurrent Laryngeal Nerve Paralysis. *J voice* (1994) 8 (1):79–83. doi: 10.1016/S0892-1997(05)80323-6
12. Chiang F-Y, Wang L-F, Huang Y-F, Lee K-W, Kuo W-R. Recurrent Laryngeal Nerve Palsy After Thyroidectomy With Routine Identification of the Recurrent Laryngeal Nerve. *Surgery* (2005) 137(3):342–7. doi: 10.1016/j.surg.2004.09.008
13. Dionigi G, Wu C-W, Kim HY, Rausei S, Boni L, Chiang F-Y. Severity of Recurrent Laryngeal Nerve Injuries in Thyroid Surgery. *World J Surg* (2016) 40(6):1373–81. doi: 10.1007/s00268-016-3415-3
14. Wu CW, Dionigi G, Sun H, Liu X, Kim HY, Hsiao PJ, et al. Intraoperative Neuromonitoring for the Early Detection and Prevention of RLN Traction Injury in Thyroid Surgery: A Porcine Model. *Surgery* (2014) 155(2):329–39. doi: 10.1016/j.surg.2013.08.015
15. Dewan K, Vahabzadeh-Hagh A, Soofer D, Chhetri DK. Neuromuscular Compensation Mechanisms in Vocal Fold Paralysis and Paresis. *Laryngoscope* (2017) 127(7):1633–8. doi: 10.1002/lary.26409
16. Huang T-Y, Yu W-HV, Chiang F-Y, Wu C-W, Fu S-C, Tai A-S, et al. Correlation Between Objective and Subjective High-Pitched Voice Impairment in Patients After Thyroid Surgery. *Front Endocrinol* (2021) 12:788878(1514). doi: 10.3389/fendo.2021.788878
17. Friedman AD, Burns JA, Heaton JT, Zeitels SM. Early Versus Late Injection Medialization for Unilateral Vocal Cord Paralysis. *Laryngoscope* (2010) 120 (10):2042–6. doi: 10.1002/lary.21097
18. Yung KC, Likhterov I, Courey MS. Effect of Temporary Vocal Fold Injection Medialization on the Rate of Permanent Medialization Laryngoplasty in Unilateral Vocal Fold Paralysis Patients. *Laryngoscope* (2011) 121(10):2191–4. doi: 10.1002/lary.21965
19. Chiang F-Y, Lu I-C, Chen H-C, Chen H-Y, Tsai C-J, Hsiao P-J, et al. Anatomical Variations of Recurrent Laryngeal Nerve During Thyroid Surgery: How to Identify and Handle the Variations With Intraoperative Neuromonitoring. *Kaohsiung J Med Sci* (2010) 26(11):575–83. doi: 10.1016/S1607-551X(10)70089-9
20. Heuer RJ, Sataloff RT, Emerich K, Rulnick R, Baroody M, Spiegel JR, et al. Unilateral Recurrent Laryngeal Nerve Paralysis: The Importance of "Preoperative" Voice Therapy. *J voice* (1997) 11(1):88–94. doi: 10.1016/S0892-1997(97)80028-8
21. Dionigi G, Donatini G, Boni L, Rausei S, Rovera F, Tanda ML, et al. Continuous Monitoring of the Recurrent Laryngeal Nerve in Thyroid Surgery: A Critical Appraisal. *Int J Surg* (2013) 11:S44–S6. doi: 10.1016/S1743-9191(13)60014-X
22. Schneider R, Randolph GW, Barczynski M, Dionigi G, Wu C-W, Chiang F-Y, et al. Continuous Intraoperative Neural Monitoring of the Recurrent Nerves in Thyroid Surgery: A Quantum Leap in Technology. *Gland Surg* (2016) 5 (6):607. doi: 10.21037/gs.2016.11.10
23. Kim DH, Kim SW, Hwang SH. Intraoperative Neural Monitoring for Early Vocal Cord Function Assessment After Thyroid Surgery: A Systematic Review and Meta-Analysis. *World J Surg* (2021) 45(11):3320–7. doi: 10.1007/s00268-021-06225-x
24. Liu C-H, Wang C-C, Wu C-W, Lin Y-C, Lu I, Chang P-Y, et al. Comparison of Surgical Complications Rates Between LigaSure Small Jaw and Clamp-And-Tie Hemostatic Technique in 1,000 Neuro-Monitored Thyroidectomies. *Front Endocrinol* (2021) 12:313. doi: 10.3389/fendo.2021.638608
25. Leclerc A-A, Smith LJ. Early Management of Unilateral Vocal Fold Paralysis. In: Amin M, Johnson M, (eds). *Decision Making in Vocal Fold Paralysis* (2019) 29–39. doi: 10.1007/978-3-030-23475-1_3
26. Liddy W, Wu C-W, Dionigi G, Donatini G, Giles Senyurek Y, Kamani D, et al. Varied RLN Course Is Associated With Increased Risk of Nerve Dysfunction During Thyroidectomy: Results of the Surgical Anatomy of the RLN in Thyroid Surgery (SAR) Study, an International Multicenter Prospective Anatomic and Electrophysiologic Study of 1000 Monitored Nerves at Risk From the International Neural Monitoring Study Group (INMSG). *Thyroid* (2021) 31(11):1730–40. doi: 10.1089/thy.2021.0155
27. Christakis I, Klang P, Talat N, Galata G, Schulte K-M. Long-Term Quality of Voice Is Usually Acceptable After Initial Hoarseness Caused by a Thyroidectomy or a Parathyroidectomy. *Gland Surg* (2019) 8(3):226. doi: 10.21037/gs.2018.09.02
28. Sorensen JR, Printz T, Iwarsson J, Grøntved ÅM, Døssing H, Hegedüs L, et al. The Impact of Post-Thyroidectomy Paresis on Quality of Life in Patients With Nodular Thyroid Disease. *Otolaryngology–Head Neck Surg* (2019) 161 (4):589–97. doi: 10.1177/0194599819855379
29. Reiter R, Heyduck A, Hoffmann TK, Brosch S, Buchberger MA, Schorer K, et al. Quality of Voice and Prognostic Markers for the Recovery of Vocal Fold Paralysis After Thyroid Surgery. *Ann Otol Rhinol Laryngol* (2019) 128 (12):1104–10. doi: 10.1177/0003489419858629
30. Wang L-F, Lee K-W, Kuo W-R, Wu C-W, Lu S-P, Chiang F-Y. The Efficacy of Intraoperative Corticosteroids in Recurrent Laryngeal Nerve Palsy After Thyroid Surgery. *World J Surg* (2006) 30(3):299–303. doi: 10.1007/s00268-005-0399-9
31. Hydman J, Björck G, Persson JK, Zedenius J, Mattsson P. Diagnosis and Prognosis of Iatrogenic Injury of the Recurrent Laryngeal Nerve. *Ann Otol Rhinol Laryngol* (2009) 118(7):506–11. doi: 10.1177/000348940911800709
32. Chung SR, Baek JH, Choi YJ, Lee JH. Management Strategy for Nerve Damage During Radiofrequency Ablation of Thyroid Nodules. *Int J Hyperthermia* (2019) 36(1):203–9. doi: 10.1080/02656736.2018.1554826
33. Borel F, Christou N, Marret O, Mathonnet M, Caillard C, Bannani S, et al. Long-Term Voice Quality Outcomes After Total Thyroidectomy: A

Prospective Multicenter Study. *Surgery* (2018) 163(4):796–800. doi: 10.1016/j.surg.2017.09.023

34. Wu C-W, Hao M, Tian M, Dionigi G, Tufano RP, Kim HY, et al. Recurrent Laryngeal Nerve Injury With Incomplete Loss of Electromyography Signal During Monitored Thyroidectomy—Evaluation and Outcome. *Langenbeck's Arch Surg* (2017) 402(4):691–9. doi: 10.1007/s00423-016-1381-8
35. Lee SW, Kim JW, Chung CH, Mok JO, Shim SS, Koh YW, et al. Utility of Injection Laryngoplasty in the Management of Post-Thyroidectomy Vocal Cord Paralysis. *Thyroid* (2010) 20(5):513–7. doi: 10.1089/thy.2009.0397
36. Lee SW, Park KN. A Long-Term Comparative Prospective Study Between Reinnervation and Injection Laryngoplasty. *Laryngoscope* (2018) 128(8):1893–7. doi: 10.1002/lary.27140
37. Zhang D, Pino A, Caruso E, Dionigi G, Sun H. Neural Monitoring in Thyroid Surgery Is Here to Stay. *Gland Surg* (2020) 9(Suppl 1):S43. doi: 10.21037/gs.2019.10.24
38. Siu J, Tam S, Fung K. A Comparison of Outcomes in Interventions for Unilateral Vocal Fold Paralysis: A Systematic Review. *Laryngoscope* (2016) 126(7):1616–24. doi: 10.1002/lary.25739

19

Thyroid Function in Preterm/Low Birth Weight Infants: Impact on Diagnosis and Management of Thyroid Dysfunction

*Stephen H. LaFranchi**

Department of Pediatrics, Doernbecher Children's Hospital, Oregon Health & Sciences University, Portland, OR, United States

***Correspondence:** Stephen H. LaFranchi lafrancs@ohsu.edu*

Maternal thyroid hormone crosses the placenta to the fetus beginning in the first trimester, likely playing an important role in fetal development. The fetal thyroid gland begins to produce thyroid hormone in the second trimester, with fetal serum T4 levels gradually rising to term. Full maturation of the hypothalamic-pituitary-thyroid (HPT) axis does not occur until term gestation or the early neonatal period. Postnatal thyroid function in preterm babies is qualitatively similar to term infants, but the TSH surge is reduced, with a corresponding decrease in the rise in T4 and T3 levels. Serum T4 levels are reduced in proportion to the degree of prematurity, representing both loss of the maternal contribution and immaturity of the HPT axis. Other factors, such as neonatal drugs, e.g., dopamine, and non-thyroidal illness syndrome (NTIS) related to co-morbidities contribute to the "hypothyroxinemia of prematurity". Iodine, both deficiency and excess, may impact thyroid function in infants born preterm. Overall, the incidence of permanent congenital hypothyroidism in preterm infants appears to be similar to term infants. However, in newborn screening (NBS) that employ a total T4-reflex TSH test approach, a higher proportion of preterm babies will have a T4 below the cutoff, associated with a non-elevated TSH level. In NBS programs with a primary TSH test combined with serial testing, there is a relatively high incidence of "delayed TSH elevation" in preterm neonates. On follow-up, the majority of these cases have transient hypothyroidism. Preterm/LBW infants have many clinical manifestations that might be ascribed to hypothyroidism. The question then arises whether the hypothyroxinemia of prematurity, with thyroid function tests compatible with either non-thyroidal illness syndrome or central hypothyroidism, is a physiologic or pathologic process. In particular, does hypothyroxinemia contribute to the neurodevelopmental impairment common to preterm infants? Results from multiple studies are mixed, with some randomized controlled trials in the most preterm infants born <28 weeks gestation appearing to show benefit. This review will summarize fetal and neonatal thyroid physiology, thyroid disorders specific to preterm/LBW infants and their impact on NBS for congenital hypothyroidism, examine treatment studies, and finish with comments on unresolved questions and areas of controversy.

Keywords: thyroid function, preterm, low birth weight, newborn screening, congenital hypothyroidism, iodine

INTRODUCTION

Thyroid hormone plays a significant role in development and function of every organ system in the body. The presence of triiodothyronine (T3) occupied nuclear receptors in the fetal brain demonstrated by 10 weeks of gestation provides evidence that thyroid hormone has a critical role in brain development (1). Infants born preterm have lower serum thyroid hormone levels as compared to term infants, a reflection of reduced thyroid stimulating hormone (TSH) surge following birth, immature postnatal pituitary-thyroid function, and loss of the maternal contribution. Preterm/low birth weight (LBW) infants are at increased risk for co-morbidities, leading to changes in serum thyroid hormone levels typical of non-thyroidal illness syndrome (NTIS), but which may be difficult to separate from central hypothyroidism. To properly interpret thyroid function tests, newborn screening programs need to be cognizant of these perturbations in T4 and TSH levels in preterm/LBW infants. Clinicians who are consulted for evaluation of potential thyroid dysfunction need to be aware of these dynamic changes to make appropriate management decisions. This review will describe fetal and neonatal thyroid physiology, thyroid dysfunction specific to preterm/LBW infants and their impact on newborn screening (NBS) for congenital hypothyroidism, examine treatment studies, and finish with comments on unresolved questions and areas of controversy.

MATERNAL-FETAL THYROID RELATIONSHIPS

Evidence supports the notion that thyroid hormone present in the fetus in the first trimester is the result of transplacental transfer of maternal hormone (2). This is primarily T4; fetal T3 levels are low as a result of increased placental deiodinase type 3 activity which converts T4 to reverse T3 (RT3). At term, approximately one-third to one-half of cord blood T4 levels are of maternal origin (3). Increased maternal iodine intake during pregnancy is required to keep both mother and fetus iodine sufficient. The recommended dietary allowance (RDA) increases from 150 mcg daily to 250-300 mcg daily with pregnancy (4). As a subgroup, women of reproductive age in the U.S. are borderline iodine deficient (5). Insufficient maternal iodine intake may be a significant factor contributing to lower serum thyroid hormone levels in preterm infants. Maternal hypothyroidism (and maternal iodine deficiency) also are risk factors for preterm birth (6). In addition, excess iodine exposure during pregnancy may also be associated with neonatal hypothyroidism (the Wolff-Chaikoff effect, resulting in temporary decreased production of thyroid hormone). This is a particular problem for preterm/LBW infants, as they are slow to "escape" from this down regulation and may not recover to normal thyroid hormone production for several weeks. Other drug treatment during pregnancy may also affect neonatal thyroid hormone levels. Treatment with steroids or dopaminergic drugs may decrease TSH secretion, resulting in lower neonatal T4 levels.

Abbreviations: LBW, low birth weight; VLBW, very low birth weight; L-T4, levothyroxine; NBS, newborn screening; NTIS, non-thyroidal illness syndrome; RDA, recommended daily allowance; RT3, reverse T3; TBG, thyroxine binding globulin; T3, triiodothyronine; T4, thyroxine; TSH, thyroid stimulating hormone.

MATURATION OF FETAL THYROID FUNCTION

The thyroid gland starts development at the foramen cecum, migrating to its normal location over the thyroid cartilage. The bilobed thyroid shape is evident by 7 weeks gestation, and thyroid follicles containing colloid are seen histologically by 10 weeks. Thyroglobulin synthesis is detected by 4 weeks, iodine trapping by 8 to 10 weeks, and T4 production by 12 weeks. Significant production of thyroid hormone does not begin until the second trimester (7). Fetal serum T4 concentrations rise from approximately 2 ug/dl (26 nmol/L) at 12 weeks to 10 ug/dL (128 nmol/L) at term (8, 9). Parallel changes are seen in fetal serum free T4 concentrations, rising from approximately 0.1 ng/dL (1.3 pmol/L) at 12 weeks to 2 ng/dL (25.7 pmol/L) at term. As noted above, fetal serum T3 concentrations are low as compared to infant levels, rising from approximately 6 ng/dL (0.09 nmol/L) at 12 weeks to 45 ng/dL (0.68 nmol/L) at term. Thyrotropin releasing hormone (TRH) is present in hypothalamic neurons by 6-8 weeks gestation, and TSH secretion can be detected by 12 weeks. Fetal serum TSH concentrations rise from approximately 4 mIU/L at 12 weeks gestation to 8 mIU/L at term (8, 9). Maturation of the hypothalamic-pituitary-thyroid axis occurs in the second half of gestation, but normal feedback relationships are not mature until term gestation.

POSTNATAL THYROID FUNCTION IN PRETERM/LOW BIRTH WEIGHT INFANTS

The dramatic rise in serum TSH 30 to 60 minutes following delivery is reduced in preterm infants as compared to term infants, generally in proportion to their degree of prematurity (10). The peak approximates 30 to 50 mIU/L in preterm infants vs. 60 to 80 mIU/mL in term infants (**Figure 1**). Cord blood T4 levels are lower in infants born preterm, again generally in proportion to the degree of prematurity (**Table 1**). In response to the dramatic TSH rise, serum T4 and T3 levels are elevated at 24 hours following birth in term infants, gradually falling back to "normal" infant ranges around 5 to 7 days of age. In contrast, in the most preterm infants born at 23 to 27 weeks gestation, serum total T4 levels actually decrease in the first week of life, are "level" in infants born at 28 to 30 weeks gestation, while only those babies born >30 weeks gestation show a rise in total T4 in the first week (**Figure 2**). The differences in total T4 concentrations in term *vs.* preterm babies is explained by a combination of immature thyroid hormone production from the thyroid gland, decreased binding proteins (primarily thyroxine binding globulin [TBG]) by the liver,

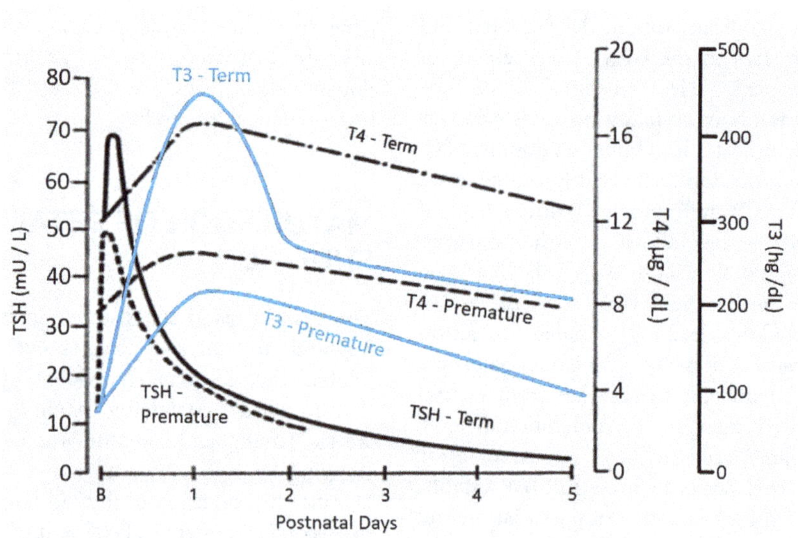

FIGURE 1 | Changes in serum TSH, T4, and T3 following birth in term as compared to preterm newborn infants. Figure developed (with permission) from Fisher DA Thyroid system immaturities in very low birth weight premature infants. Semin Perinatol 2008; 32:387-397.

and the effects of NTIS. Postnatal serum free T4 levels are also lower in the first weeks of life, though proportionally not as low as total T4 levels (**Table 1**, **Figure 3**). Serum total T3 levels follow a pattern similar to total T4, though the levels are proportionally even lower in the most preterm babies, likely a reflection of the impact of NTIS (sometimes referred to as the "low T3 syndrome") (**Table 1**). Administration of certain drugs used to manage co-morbidities in preterm infants may affect thyroid hormone levels; glucocorticoids and dopaminergic agents may inhibit TSH secretion, while excess iodine may inhibit thyroid hormone production.

UNIQUE PATTERNS OF THYROID DYSFUNCTION IN PRETERM/LOW BIRTH WEIGHT INFANTS

Hypothyroxinemia of Prematurity

Serum total T4, and to a lesser extent free T4 concentrations are decreased in proportion to the degree of prematurity, generally without elevation of serum TSH levels, findings described as "hypothyroxinemia of prematurity". In otherwise healthy preterm infants, serum T4 levels gradually rise, such that by 37

TABLE 1 | Concentrations of free T4, T4, T3, and TSH in preterm and term infants in cord blood at birth, and at 7, 14, and 28 days of age (mean +/- 1 SD).

Gestation (weeks)	Age of Infant	Free T4 (ng/dL)	T4 (µg/dL)	T3 (ng/dL)	TSH (mU/L)
23-27 weeks	Cord	1.28 ± 0.4	5.4 ± 2.0	20 ± 15	6.8 ± 2.9
	7d	1.47 ± 0.6	4.0 ± 1.8	33 ± 20	3.5 ± 2.6
	14d	1.45 ± 0.5	4.7 ± 2.6	41 ± 25	3.9 ± 2.7
	28d	1.50 ± 0.4	6.1 ± 2.3	63 ± 27	3.8 ± 4.7
28-30 weeks	Cord	1.45 ± 0.4	6.3 ± 2.0	29 ± 21	7.0 ± 3.7
	7d	1.82 ± 0.7	6.3 ± 2.1	56 ± 24	3.6 ± 2.5
	14d	1.65 ± 0.4	6.6 ± 2.3	72 ± 28	4.9 ± 11.2
	28d	1.71 ± 0.4	7.5 ± 2.3	87 ± 31	3.6 ± 2.5
31-34 weeks	Cord	1.49 ± 0.3	7.6 ± 2.3	35 ± 23	7.9 ± 5.2
	7d	2.14 ± 0.6	9.4 ± 3.4	92 ± 36	3.6 ± 4.8
	14d	1.98 ± 0.4	9.1 ± 3.6	110 ± 41	3.8 ± 9.3
	28d	1.88 ± 0.5	8.9 ± 3.0	120 ± 40	3.5 ± 3.4
≥37 weeks	Cord	1.41 ± 0.3	9.2 ± 1.9	60 ± 35	6.7 ± 4.8
	7d	2.70 ± 0.6	12.7 ± 2.9	148 ± 50	2.6 ± 1.8
	14d	2.03 ± 0.3	10.7 ± 1.4	167 ± 31	2.5 ± 2.0
	28d	1.65 ± 0.3	9.7 ± 2.2	176 ± 32	1.8 ± 0.9

T4, thyroxine; T3, triiodothyronine; TSH, thyroid stimulating hormone.

Adapted with permission from: Williams FL, Simpson J, Delahunty C, et al. Developmental trends in cord and postpartum serum thyroid hormones in preterm infants. J Clin Endocrinol Metab 2004; 89:5314-20 (9).

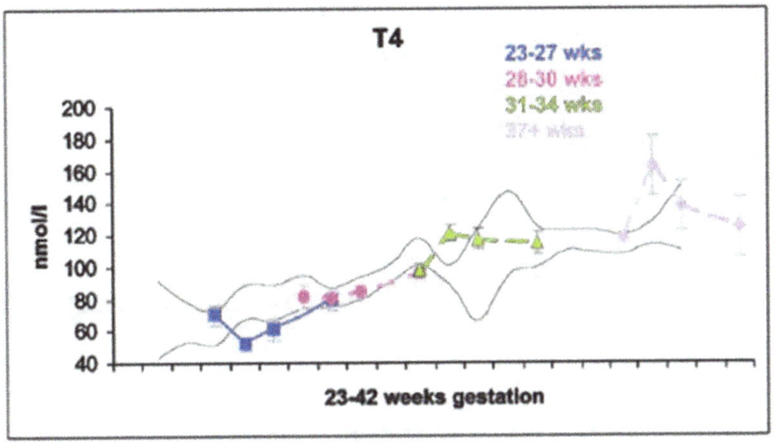

FIGURE 2 | Serum T4 levels in cord blood, and at 7, 14 and 28 days of life in neonates of 23-27, 28-30, 31-34, and 37+ weeks gestation. With permission from Williams FL, Simpson J, Delahunty C, et al. Developmental trends in cord and postpartum serum thyroid hormones in preterm infants. J Clin Endocrinol Metab 2004; 89:5314-5320 (9).

weeks gestation they overlap levels seen in term infants (9). In preterm infants born <28 weeks gestation, serum TSH may rise into the 6 to 15 mIU/L range around 2 to 3 weeks of age (11) (**Figure 4**), a transient elevation speculated to play a role in stimulating the immature thyroid gland to normal T4 production, so compensating for the loss of maternal T4 contribution. Common co-morbidities associated with preterm birth, such as respiratory distress syndrome, sepsis, intraventricular hemorrhage, etc. are associated with thyroid function tests typical of NTIS: normal or low total T4, low total T3, elevated reverse T3, and normal to low serum TSH (12). Serum free T4 concentrations measured by the more common analog assay method may be low in this setting, while free T4 measured by the more accurate equilibrium dialysis method tends to be in the normal range (13).

Delayed TSH Elevation

Some preterm/LBW infants manifest serum TSH concentrations greater than the 15 mIU/L "compensatory" rise described above. The New England NBS program reported an incidence of delayed TSH elevation >20 mUI/mL on the dried blood spot of 1:294 VLBW infants (1000-1500 g) and 1:1878 LBW infants (1501-2500 g), as compared to 1:77,280 in term babies (>2500 g) (14). The delayed TSH elevation occurred at a peak age of 58 days of life (range 11 to 176 days). In even lower birth weight infants, the Wisconsin NBS program reported an incidence of

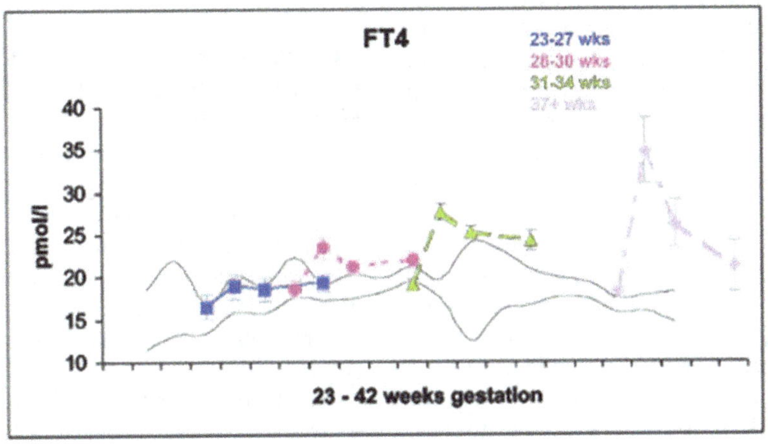

FIGURE 3 | Serum free T4 levels in cord blood, and at 7, 14 and 28 days of life in neonates of 23-27, 28-30, 31-34, and 37+ weeks gestation. With permission from Williams FL, Simpson J, Delahunty C, et al. Developmental trends in cord and postpartum serum thyroid hormones in preterm infants. J Clin Endocrinol Metab 2004; 89:5314-5320 (9).

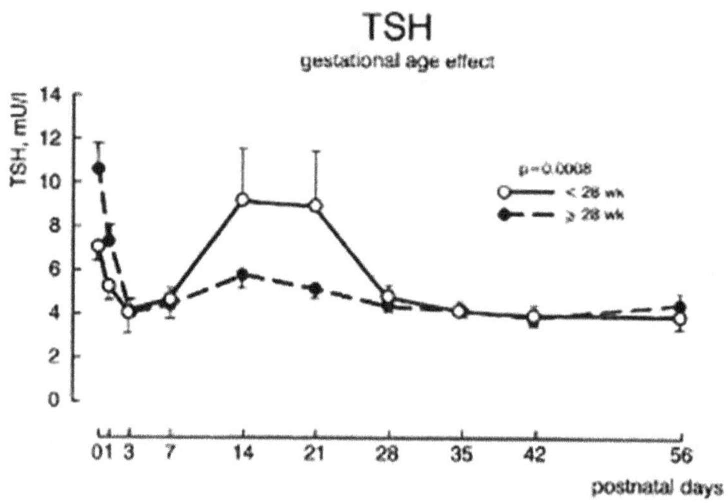

FIGURE 4 | Plasma TSH concentrations ± SEM during the first 8 weeks after birth in infants of 28-30 week gestation and <28 weeks gestation. With permission from van Wassenaer AG, Kok JH, Dekker FW de Vijlder JJ. Thyroid function in very preterm infants: influences of gestational age and disease. Pediatr Res 1997; 42:604-9 (11).

delayed TSH elevation in 1:13 in babies <500 g, 1:28.5 in babies 500 – 1000 g, 1:330 babies 1000-1500 g, and 1:737 babies 1500-2500 g (15). In infants with higher TSH elevation >100 mIU/L, the TSH elevation occurred earlier, ~3 weeks, while those with milder TSH elevation >20 mIU/L occurred later, ~8 weeks of age. Follow-up serum testing has shown that most cases of delayed TSH elevation are transient, particularly if the TSH elevation is mild. In a report from the Rhode Island NBS program, of 19 preterm babies with delayed TSH elevation, three with TSH >50 mIU/L were treated with l-thyroxine, while the other 16 infants monitored without treatment recovered to normal thyroid function between 8 and 58 days of life (16).

Role of Iodine: Too Little, Too Much

Although universal salt iodization has greatly improved the status of iodine sufficiency (17), worldwide iodine deficiency remains one of the most common preventable causes of intellectual disability (18). Preterm infants are particularly vulnerable to iodine deficiency, a result of a combination of loss of the maternal contribution, relatively low levels of iodine in preterm formulas, and near absence of iodine in most parenteral nutritional preparations (19). A study of iodine balance in 27 to 30 week gestational age infants showed that they were in negative iodine balance for the first two weeks of life, and they did not reach the RDA of 30 mcg/kg/day until 120 days of age (20). Lower iodine intake was correlated with lower serum free T4 and T3 and higher TSH levels. If present, iodine deficiency would be a significant factor contributing to slow recovery from hypothyroxinemia of prematurity.

Exposure to excess iodine has also been demonstrated to cause thyroid dysfunction in preterm infants. Excess iodine results in down regulation of thyroid hormone production (the Wolff-Chaikoff effect), thought to be a mechanism to protect against development of hyperthyroidism. Normal thyroid function is maintained by "escape" from this down regulation; however, preterm infants are slow to escape and so may become hypothyroid. Common sources of iodine exposure include iodinated contrast agents and topical iodine antiseptics. Infants with congenital heart disease (CHD) are frequently exposed to such sources; in a study of 183 infants with CHD, one-quarter manifested elevation of serum TSH levels, ranging from 9 to >100 mIU/mL (21). About half were treated with thyroid hormone, while others recovered to euthyroidism after discontinuation of excess iodine exposure. This study involved primarily term infants; likely the effect of excess iodine would apply to preterm/LBW infants.

Impact of Preterm Birth/Low Birth Weight on Newborn Screening for Congenital Hypothyroidism

Several NBS programs from Europe and North America report that the incidence of congenital hypothyroidism is higher in preterm infants. As compared to an incidence of approximately 1:1,500 to 1:2,000 in term infants (22, 23), the incidence in preterm infants approximates 1:900 (24). The incidence is even higher in NBS programs that undertake repeat screening in preterm babies, from 1:300 in LBW to 1:50 in VLBW babies (14, 16).

In NBS programs that employ a primary T4-reflex TSH test strategy, preterm/LBW infants make up a higher percentage of cases that fall below the T4 cutoff (typically the 10th percentile), while the screening TSH is not elevated. These NBS programs must then decide whether to follow-up cases with low T4-non-elevated TSH levels. In some programs, lack of an abnormal TSH elevation is the end of screening. However, most NBS programs now collect a 2nd dried blood specimen at 2 to 4 weeks of life in infants born <32 weeks gestation or <1500 g birth weight (25). In the very preterm babies <28 weeks gestation, several NBS programs collect a 3rd dried blood specimen at 6 to 8 weeks of life, which is typically around 37 weeks or term gestation. In the majority of preterm/LBW babies, the screening T4 will reach the range seen in term infants by the 2nd or 3rd specimen (5). Collection of the 2nd and 3rd specimens allows detection of preterm babies with delayed TSH elevation, described above.

A few preterm infants will not normalize total T4 by term gestation; such results could be explained by low binding protein levels or NTIS, although central hypothyroidism cannot be ruled out. In these cases, NBS programs recommend serum thyroid function tests, including TSH, total and free T4. In the presence of low binding proteins or NTIS, serum free T4 is most accurately measured by equilibrium dialysis. A normal free T4 and TSH rule out hypothyroidism, while a low free T4 and low or normal range TSH is compatible with central hypothyroidism, leading to evaluation for other pituitary hormone deficiencies. Such cases in preterm infants are rare, likely with an incidence matching term infants:!:25,000 (26).

In NBS programs that employ a primary TSH test approach, otherwise healthy preterm babies will fall below the dried blood TSH cutoff, typically <25 mIU/L (serum units). As described for T4-reflex TSH test programs, most primary TSH test programs collect a 2nd dried blood specimen at 2 to 4 weeks of life in infants born <32 weeks gestation or <1500 g birth weight, and many collect a 3rd dried blood specimen at 6 to 8 weeks of life in preterm babies born <28 weeks gestation. Collection of the 2nd and 3rd specimens allows detection of preterm babies with delayed TSH elevation, whereas stopping screening with a normal TSH on the 1st test risks missing infants with delayed TSH elevation. Re evaluation after age 2 to 3 years of age shows that many have transient hypothyroidism (27–29).

Unique patterns of Thyroid Dysfunction in Preterm/Low Birth Weight Infants: Physiologic or Pathologic?

Preterm/LBW infants manifest clinical features that might be ascribed to thyroid dysfunction, such as temperature instability, apnea with immature pulmonary function and low surfactant levels, bradycardia, slow to feed with sluggish gut motility, edema, hypotonia, and slow growth and development. Several observational studies demonstrate a correlation between low serum T4 levels and these clinical manifestations (30, 31). As these babies typically have low serum T4-non-elevated TSH levels, clinicians face the dilemma as to whether these features are caused by central hypothyroidism and so might improve with thyroid hormone treatment. However, randomized, placebo-controlled trials using either T4 or a combination of T4 and T3 generally do not show an effect on objective measures, such as O2 requirements, incidence of respiratory distress syndrome, requirement for inotropic agents, progression from parenteral to oral feedings, weight gain, length, or head circumference measurements, or on mortality (32–34). A Cochrane Database Review in 2007 also found no benefit of thyroid hormone treatment in this situation (35).

A more compelling question asks whether deficits in neurodevelopment in preterm infants are a consequence of the hypothyroxinemia. Several studies report an increased odds ratio for endpoints such as disabling cerebral palsy (36), reduced attention span (37), vision disturbances (38), and overall lower IQ (39). However, owing to "confounding variables" common to preterm infants, it is difficult to establish a causal relationship with the hypothyroxinemia alone. In a study of preterm infants <1500 g, a comparison of outcome in infants with and without hypothyroxinemia did not find any significant differences in neurodevelopmental, vision or hearing impairment at 5 years of age (40).

What about treatment trials? A randomized, placebo-controlled trial of T4 treatment in 200 infants less than 30 weeks gestational age with multiple assessments of neurodevelopment over time was carried out by the Dutch. Half were treated with l-T4 8 mcg/kg/d, half with placebo for the first 6 weeks of life. In the first assessment at 24 months of age, there were no differences in the Bayley Infant Scales of Mental and Motor Development (41). However, subgroup analysis showed that the Bayley Mental Developmental Index (MDI) score was 18 points higher in the T4-treated group ≤27 weeks gestation, ($p<.05$), but 10 points lower in the T4-treated group ≥27 weeks gestation (42) (**Table 2**). Re-evaluation at school age (5.7 years) showed that the MDI score had narrowed to 10 points, now not statistically significant (43). Survey of study families at 10 years of age showed that in subjects ≤27 weeks gestation treated with T4, there was a trend toward a lower percentage needing special education, whereas in subjects at 29 weeks gestation, the opposite was true, though only the latter reached statistical significance (**Table 2**). In subjects ≤28 weeks gestation treated with T4, again there was a trend toward better motor outcome as compared to control subjects, but this difference did not reach statistical significance (44). To try and resolve the question of potential benefit in infants born <28 weeks, a more recent trial of thyroid supplementation was undertaken in Amsterdam, Madrid and New York (45). This trial included six treatment arms to investigate different modalities of thyroid hormone administration, combination T4 and T3 treatment, one iodine treatment arm, and one placebo arm. Testing at 36 months of age did not find any differences in neurodevelopmental index scores among the eight groups (**Table 2**). Finally, in a double-blind, randomized, placebo-controlled trial in preterm babies <28 weeks gestation from the United Kingdom, evaluation at 42 months by the Bayley III Mental and Psychomotor Developmental Indices showed statistically better motor, language, and cognitive domains in the group treated with thyroid hormone (46). In summary, the randomized, placebo-controlled trials show mixed results, with potentially some benefit of T4 treatment in infants <28 weeks but potential harm in infants >28 weeks gestation.

TABLE 2 | Summary of studies investigating l-T4 treatment v placebo on neurocognitive outcome in preterm infants.

Study (Ref)	Age at Evaluation	Total Group T4 Rx v Placebo	25/26 weeks T4 Rx v Placebo	27 weeks T4 Rx v Placebo	28 weeks T4 Rx v Placebo	29 weeks T4 Rx v Placebo	>27 weeks T4 Rx v Placebo
van Wassenaer (41, 42)	24 mo Bayley Mental	92 v 95 P = 0.62	93 v 75 P= 0.01	90 v 100 P = 0.37	97 v 102 P = 0.49	92 v 102 P = 0.36	92 v 102 P = 0.08
	Bayley Psychomotor	92 v 88 P = 0.39	80 v 70 P = 0.11	81 v 84 P = 0.35	98 v 90 P = 0.29	86 v 91 P = 0.90	90 v 90 P = 0.90
Briet et al. (43)	5.7 years	93.6 ± 16.2 v 95.7 ± 20.4 P = NS	94.2v 84.7 P = 0.11	90 v 92 P = 0.77	98 v 96 P = 0.58	90.6 v 105.2 P = 0.01	
van Wassenaer [Questionaire only] (44)	10.5 years	School outcome, motor function, behavior: T4 Rx v placebo P = NS	Percent in Special Ed T4 Rx =10% placebo=28% P=0.07	Motor Im-pairment T4 Rx=12% placebo=28% P = 0.23		Percent in Special Ed T4 Rx=30% placebo=5% P = 0.05	
van Wassenaer (45)	36 months	**Bayley III Cognitive** T4 Rx v placebo 99.2 11.3 v 105.5 ± 12.3 P= NS		**Bayley III Gross Motor** T4 Rx v placebo 9.3 ± 2.8 v 11.0 ± 2.8 P=NS		**Bayley III Fine Motor** T4 Rx v placebo 11.1 ± 2.2 v 11.8 ± 2.4 P=NS	
Ng et al. (46)	42 months	**Bayley III Cognitive** T4 Rx v placebo 91 ± 10 v 85 ± 13 P = .045		**Bayley III Motor** T4 Rx v placebo 84 ± 12 v 77 ± 13 P = .034		**Bayley III Language** T4 Rx v placebo 92 ± 13 v 83 ± 20 P = .041	

T4 Rx, l-thyroxine treated group.
NS, non-significant.

CONCLUSION: UNRESOLVED QUESTIONS AND AREAS OF CONTROVERSY

Much has been learned over the last few decades about fetal and neonatal thyroid physiology; thyroid function is different in babies born preterm/LBW as compared to term infants. As such, there remain unresolved questions and areas of controversy regarding management of thyroid issues in preterm infants. The following section highlights a few of these areas.

At What Gestational Age Can the Postnatal HPT Axis Compensate for Loss of Maternal T4 Quickly Enough to Avert Untoward Effects of Thyroid Hormone Deficiency?

A reasonable goal for serum T4 or free T4 levels after birth in preterm babies might be to either match *in utero* concentrations present at a similar gestational age or levels in term infants by 1-2 weeks after birth. Evidence suggests that infants born <28 weeks gestation have serum T4 (and to a lesser extent free T4) concentrations that take up to 4 to 6 weeks to overlap the range seen in term infants. The transient rise in serum TSH to the 6-15 mU/L range between 2 and 4 weeks of age in babies born <28 weeks gestation (but not in babies ≥28 weeks gestation) supports the notion that the thyroid gland in babies born <28 weeks gestation requires increased TSH stimulation to normalize thyroid hormone production. Slow recovery of normal thyroid physiology might impact any organ system, e.g., maturation of lung function, but most importantly it could impact neurodevelopment.

Should Iodine Supplementation Be Routine in Preterm Infants?

Most preterm infant formulas do not contain enough iodine to allow these babies to meet the RDA of 30 mcg I/kg/d, and many parenteral nutritional preparations lack iodine completely. A recent Cochrane database review did not show benefit of iodine supplementation in preterm infants on morbidity, mortality, or neurodevelopmental outcome (47). Despite this report, given the known effect of iodine to prevent "endemic cretinism", routine supplementation of preterm formulas and parenteral nutritional preparations would seem important to achieve T4 production matching term infants. Sufficient iodine intake is equally important for nursing mothers. At the same time, care should be taken to avoid exposure to excess iodine.

Do Infants With "Delayed TSH Elevation" Benefit From Detection and Treatment?

Studies show that the majority of preterm babies with delayed TSH elevation will recover to normal TSH levels without treatment. However, the average age at peak TSH elevation is approximately 8 weeks, with a range from 11 to 176 days of life (14). The TSH elevation likely reflects inadequate thyroid hormone production. Although babies recover to normal thyroid function, are there consequences from low T4 levels, present over several weeks? Few studies have been carried out to address this issue. The study from Rhode Island showed developmental scores were similar to control infants, although the incidence of infants with head circumference <10th percentile was higher in the delayed TSH elevation group (16). It would seem prudent to treat infants with elevated serum TSH and low free T4 levels until recovery to normal thyroid function; since this is difficult to judge without stopping l-thyroxine, most babies are treated until age 2-3 years and then re-evaluated.

Does T4 Treatment Improve Morbidity/ Mortality and Neurodevelopmental Outcome in Preterm Infants <28 Weeks Gestation?

While it is difficult to separate out the effects of co-morbidities from hypothyroxinemia on neurodevelopmental outcome, there are now two randomized, placebo controlled trials in preterm infants <28 weeks gestation that report higher scores in the T4-treated group (42, 46). As noted above, there may be some "physiological" support for this finding, as thyroid function in infants born <28 weeks gestation may be too immature to quickly replace the lost maternal thyroid hormone contribution. That said, the follow-up studies by the Dutch showed that the higher neurodevelopmental scores in the treated group tended to approach the placebo group over time (44). While the more recent trial from Amsterdam, Madrid, and New York did not show benefit of thyroid hormone treatment, the investigators cautioned that "power was insufficient to detect any but very large differences". With these mixed results, as the saying goes, more randomized controlled trials are needed before such treatment becomes standard of care.

AUTHOR CONTRIBUTIONS

SL undertook focused literature review and writing of the manuscript.

REFERENCES

1. Bernal J, Pekonen F. Ontogenesis of the Nuclear 3,5,3'-Triiodothyronine Receptor in the Human Fetal Brain. *Endocrinology* (1984) 114:677–9. doi: 10.1210/endo-114-2-677
2. Obregon MJ, Calvo RM, Del Rey FE, de Escobar GM. Ontogenesis of Thyroid Function and Interactions With Maternal Function. *Endocr Dev* (2007) 10:86. doi: 10.1159/000106821
3. Vulsma T, Gons MH, de Vijlder JJ. Maternal-Fetal Transfer of Thyroxine in Congenital Hypothyroidism Due to A Total Organification Defect or Thyroid Agenesis. *N Engl J Med* (1989) 321:13. doi: 10.1056/NEJM198907063210103
4. Alexander EK, Pearce EN, Brent GA, Brown RS, Chen H, Dosiou C, et al. 2017 Guidelines of the American Thyroid Association for the Diagnosis and Management of Thyroid Disease During Pregnancy and the Postpartum. *Thyroid* (2017) 27:315. doi: 10.1089/thy.2016.0457
5. Herrick KA, Perrine CG, Aoki Y, Caldwell KL. Iodine Status and Consumption of Key Iodine Sources in the U.S. Population With Special Attention to Reproductive Age Women. *Nutrients* (2018) 10:874. doi: 10.3390/nu10070874
6. Sheehan PM, Nankervis A, Araujo Júnior E, Da Silva Costa F. Maternal Thyroid Disease and Preterm Birth: Systematic Review and Meta-Analysis. *J Clin Endocrinol Metab* (2015) 100:4325–31. doi: 10.1210/jc.2015-3074
7. Thorpe-Beeston JG, Nicolaides KH, McGregor AM. Fetal Thyroid Function. *Thyroid* (1992) 2:207. doi: 10.1089/thy.1992.2.207
8. Thorpe-Beeston JG, Nicolaides KH, Felton CV, Butler J, McGregor AM. Maturation of the Secretion of Thyroid Hormone and Thyroid-Stimulating Hormone in the Fetus. *N Engl J Med* (1991) 324:532. doi: 10.1056/NEJM199102213240805
9. Williams FL, Simpson J, Delahunty C, Ogston SA, Bongers-Schokking JJ, Murphy N, et al. Developmental Trends in Cord and Postpartum Serum Thyroid Hormones in Preterm Infants. *J Clin Endocrinol Metab* (2004) 89:5314. doi: 10.1210/jc.2004-0869
10. Murphy N, Hume R, van Toor H, Matthews TG, Ogston SA, Wu S-Y, et al. The Hypothalamic-Pituitary-Thyroid Axis in Preterm Infants; Changes in the First 24 Hours of Postnatal Life. *J Clin Endocrinol Metab* (2004) 89:2824. doi: 10.1210/jc.2003-030317
11. Van Wassenaer AG, Kok JH, Dekker FW, de Vijlder JJ. Thyroid Function in Very Preterm Infants: Influences of Gestational Age and Disease. *Pediatr Res* (1997) 42:604–9. doi: 10.1203/00006450-199711000-00009
12. Simpson J, Williams FL, Delahunty C, van Toor H, Wu S-Y, Ogston SA, et al. Serum Thyroid Hormones in Preterm Infants and Relationships to Indices of Severity of Intercurrent Illness. *J Clin Endocrinol Metab* (2005) 90:1271. doi: 10.1210/jc.2004-2091
13. Deming DD, Rabin CW, Hopper AO, Peverini RL, Vyhmeister NR, Nelson JC. Direct Equilibrium Dialysis Compared With Two Non-Dialysis Free T4 Methods in Premature Infants. *J Pediatr* (2007) 151:404. doi: 10.1016/j.jpeds.2007.03.046
14. Mandel SJ, Hermos RJ, Larson CA, Prigozhin AB, Rojas DA, Mitchell ML. Atypical Hypothyroidism and the Very Low Birthweight Infant. *Thyroid* (2000) 10:693. doi: 10.1089/10507250050137770
15. Kaluarachchi DC, Allen DB, Eickhoff JC, Dawes JT, Baker MW. Increased Congenital Hypothyroidism Detection in Preterm Infants With Serial Newborn Screening. *J Pediatr* (2019) 207:220. doi: 10.1016/j.jpeds.2018.11.044
16. Woo HC, Lizarda A, Tucker R, Mitchell ML, Vohr B, Oh W, et al. Congenital Hypothyroidism With a Delayed Thyroid-Stimulating Hormone Elevation in Very Premature Infants: Incidence and Growth and Developmental Outcomes. *J Pediatr* (2011) 158:538. doi: 10.1016/j.jpeds.2010.10.018
17. Lazarus JH. Role of the Iodine Global Network in Elimination of Iodine Deficiency. *Recent Pat Endor Metab Immune Drug Discovery* (2017) 10:119–22. doi: 10.2174/1872214811666170330152202
18. Cao XY, Jiang XM, Dou ZH, Rakeman MA, Zhang ML, O'Donnell K, et al. Timing of Vulnerability of the Brain to Iodine Deficiency in Endemic Cretinism. *N Engl J Med* (1994) 331(26):1739–44. doi: 10.1056/NEJM199412293312603
19. Belfort MB, Pearce EN, Braverman LE, He X, Brown RS. Low Iodine Content in the Diets of Hospitalized Preterm Infants. *J Clin Endocrinol Metab* (2012) 97:E632–6. doi: 10.1210/jc.2011-3369
20. Ares S, Escobar-Morreale HF, Quero J, Durán S, Presas MJ, Herruzo R, et al. Neonatal Hypothyroxinemia: Effects of Iodine Intake and Premature Birth. *J Clin Endocrinol Metab* (1997) 82:1704–12. doi: 10.1210/jcem.82.6.4019
21. Thaker VV, Galler MF, Marshall AC, Almodovar MC, Hsu H-W, Addis CJ, et al. Hypothyroidism in Infants With Congenital Heart Disease Exposed to Excess Iodine. *J Endocrin Soc* (2017) 1:1067–78. doi: 10.1210/js.2017-00174
22. Hinton CF, Harris KB, Borgfeld L, Drummond-Borg M, Eaton R, Lorey F, et al. Trends Incidence Rates of Congenital Hypothyroidism Related to Select Demographic Factors: Data From the United States, California, Massachusetts, New York, and Texas. *Pediatrics* (2010) 125:Suppl 2:S37–47. doi: 10.1542/peds.2009-1975D
23. Corbetta C, Weber G, Cortinovis F, Calebrio D, Passoni A, Vigone MC, et al. A 7-Year Experience With Low Blood TSH Cutoff Levels for Neonatal Screening Reveals an Unsuspected Frequency of Congenital Hypothyroidism (CH). *Clin Endocrinol* (2009) 71:739–45. doi: 10.1111/j.1365-2265.2009.03568.x

24. Cavarzere P, Camilot M, Popa FI, Lauriola S, Teofoli F, Gaudino R, et al. Congenital Hypothyroidism With Delayed TSH Elevation in Low-Birth-Weight Infants: Incidence, Diagnosis and Management. *Eur J Endocrinol* (2016) 175:395–402. doi: 10.1530/EJE-15-1233
25. van Trotsenburg AS, Stoupa A, Léger J, Rohrer T, Peters C, Fuggazzola L, et al. Congenital Hypothyroidism: A 2020 Consensus Guidelines Update An ENDO-EUROPEAN REFERENCE NETWORK (ERN) Initiative Endorsed by the European Society for Pediatric Endocrinology and the European Society for Endocrinology. *Thyroid* (2021) 31:387–419. doi: 10.1089/thy.2020.0333
26. Naafs JC, Verkerk JC, Fliers E, van Trotsenburg ASP, Zwaveling-Soonawala N. Clinical and Genetic Characteristics of Dutch Children With Central Congenital Hypothyroidism, Early Detected by Neonatal Screening. *Eur J Endocrinol* (2020) 183:627–36. doi: 10.1530/EJE-20-0833
27. Mitchell ML, Hsu H-W, Sahai I. And the Massachusetts Pediatric Endocrine Work Group. The Increased Incidence of Congenital Hypothyroidism: Fact or Fancy? *Clin Endocrinol* (2011) 75:806–10. doi: 10.1111/j.1365-2265.2011.04128.x
28. Srinivasan R, Harigopal S, Turner S, Cheetham T. Permanent and Transient Congenital Hypothyroidism in Preterm Infants. *Acta Paediatr* (2012) 101: e179–82. doi: 10.1111/j.1651-2227.2011.02536.x
29. Vigone MC, Caiulo S, Di Fenna M, Ghirardello S, Corbetts C, Mosca F, et al. Evolution of Thyroid Function in Preterm Infants Detected by Screening for Congenital Hypothyroidism. *J Pediatr* (2014) 164:1296–302. doi: 10.1016/j.jpeds.2013.12.048
30. Hadeed AJ, Asay LD, Klein AH, Fisher DA. Significance of Transient Postnatal Hypothyroxinemia in Premature Infants With and Without Respiratory Distress Syndrome. *Pediatrics* (1981) 68:494.
31. Mercado M, Szymonowicz W, Yu VY, Gold H. Symptomatic Hypothyroxinemia With Normal TSH Levels in Preterm Infants. *Clin Pediatr (Phila)* (1987) 26:343. doi: 10.1177/000992288702600704
32. Chowdhry P, Scanlon JW, Auerbach R, Abbassi V. Results of Controlled Double-Blind Study of Thyroid Replacement in Very Low-Birth-Weight Premature Infants With Hypothyroxinemia. *Pediatrics* (1984) 73:301.
33. Ng SM, Turner MA, Gamble C, Didi M, Victors S, Manning D, et al. An Explanatory Randomized Placebo Controlled Trial of Levothyroxine Supplementation for Babies Born <28 Weeks' Gestation: Results of the TIPIT Trial. *Trials* (2013) 14:211. doi: 10.1186/1745-6215-14-211
34. Valerio PG, van Wassenaer AG, de Vijlder JJ, Kok JH. A Randomized, Masked Study of Triiodothyronine Plus Thyroxine Administration in Preterm Infants Less Than 28 Weeks of Gestational Age: Hormonal and Clinical Effects. *Pediatr Res* (2004) 55:248. doi: 10.1203/01.PDR.0000104153.72572.F5
35. Osborn DA, Hunt RW. Prophylactic Postnatal Thyroid Hormones for Prevention of Morbidity and Mortality in Preterm Infants. *Cochrane Database Syst Rev* (2007), CD005948. doi: 10.1002/14651858.CD005948.pub2
36. Reuss ML, Paneth N, Pinto-Martin JA, Lorenz JM, Susser M. The Relation of Transient Hypothyroxinemia in Preterm Infants to Neurologic Development At Two Years of Age. *N Engl J Med* (1996) 334:821. doi: 10.1056/NEJM199603283341303
37. Simic N, Asztalos EV, Rovet J. Impact of Neonatal Thyroid Hormone Insufficiency and Medical Morbidity on Infant Neurodevelopment and Attention Following Preterm Birth. *Thyroid* (2009) 19:395. doi: 10.1089/thy.2008.0282
38. Simic N, Westall C, Astzalos EV, Rovet J. Visual Abilities at 6 Months in Preterm Infants: Impact of Thyroid Hormone Deficiency and Neonatal Medical Morbidity. *Thyroid* (2010) 20:309. doi: 10.1089/thy.2009.0128
39. Den Ouden AL, Kok JH, Verkerk PH, Brand R, Verloove-Vanhorick SP. The Relation Between Neonatal Thyroxine Levels and Neurodevelopmental Outcome at Age 5 and 9 Years in a National Cohort of Very Preterm and/or Very Low Birth Weight Infants. *Pediatr Res* (1996) 39:142. doi: 10.1203/00006450-199601000-00021
40. Tan LO, Tan MG, Poon WB. Lack of Association Between Hypothyroxinemia of Prematurity and Transient Thyroid Abnormalities With Adverse Long-Term Neurodevelopmental Outcome in Very Low Birth Weight Infants. *PloS One* (2019) 14:e0222018. doi: 10.1371/journal.pone.0222018
41. van Wassenaer AG, Kok JH, de Vijlder JJ, Briet JM, Smit BJ, Tamminga P, et al. Effects of Thyroxine Supplementation on Neurologic Development in Infants Born at Less Than 30 Weeks' Gestation. *N Engl J Med* (1997) 336:21. doi: 10.1056/NEJM199701023360104
42. Van Wassenaer AG, Kok JH, Briët JM, van Baer AL, De Vijlder JJ. Thyroid Function in Preterm Newborns; Is T4 Treatment Required in Infants < 27 Weeks' Gestational Age? *Exp Clin Endocrinol Diabetes* (1997) 105 Suppl 4:12. doi: 10.1055/s-0029-1211925
43. Briët JM, van Wassenaer AG, Dekker FW, de Vijlder JJ, van Baer A, Kok JH. Neonatal Thyroxine Supplementation in Very Preterm Children: Developmental Outcome Evaluated at Early School Age. *Pediatrics* (2001) 107:712. doi: 10.1542/peds.107.4.712
44. van Wassenaer AG, Westera J, Houtzager BA, Kok JH. Ten-Year Follow-Up of Children Born at <30 Weeks' Gestational Age Supplemented With Thyroxine in the Neonatal Period in A Randomized, Controlled Trial. *Pediatrics* (2005) 116:e613. doi: 10.1542/peds.2005-0876
45. van Wassenaer-Leemhuis A, Ares S, Golombek G, Kok J, Paneth N, Kase J, et al. Thyroid Hormone Supplementation in Preterm Infants Born Before 28 Weeks Gestational Age and Neurodevelopmental Outcome at Age 36 Weeks. *Thyroid* (2014) 24:1162–9. doi: 10.1089/thy.2013.0618
46. Ng SM, Turner MA, Weindling M. Neurodevelopmental Outcomes at 42 Months After Thyroxine Supplementation in Infants Below 28 Weeks' Gestation: A Randomized Controlled Trial. *Thyroid* (2020) 30:948. doi: 10.1089/thy.2019.0293
47. Walsh V, Brown JVE, McGuire W. Iodine Supplementation for the Prevention of Mortality and Adverse Neurodevelopmental Outcomes in Preterm Infants. *Cochrane Database Systemic Rev* (2019) 2(2):CD005253. doi: 10.1002/14651858.CD005253.pub3

20

Management of Unilateral Vocal Fold Paralysis after Thyroid Surgery with Injection Laryngoplasty

Li-Jen Liao[1,2] *and Chi-Te Wang*[1,2,3]*

[1]*Department of Otolaryngology Head and Neck Surgery, Far Eastern Memorial Hospital, Taipei, Taiwan,* [2]*Department of Electrical Engineering, Yuan Ze University, Taoyuan, Taiwan,* [3]*Department of Special Education, University Of Taipei, Taipei, Taiwan*

***Correspondence:**
Chi-Te Wang
drwangct@gmail.com

Background: Unilateral vocal fold paralysis (UVFP) after thyroid surgery often leads to significant morbidity including dysphonia, dysphagia, and aspiration. Injection laryngoplasty (IL) is an effective treatment of UVFP with numerous readily available materials. However, few studies focus on IL for UVFP following thyroidectomy.

Objectives: This review aims to critically review current literature to determine the timing, materials, methods and outcomes of IL for UVFP after thyroid surgery.

Type of Review: Literature review.

Methods: A literature review was performed using the Pubmed, Medline and EMBASE databases. All relevant articles published in English addressing the effect of IL in post thyroid surgery related UVFP were analyzed. Studies using IL for UVFP of multiple etiologies were excluded. Meta-analysis was conducted using fixed and random effect model.

Results: Five original studies were identified, including 214 patients received IL for UVFP following thyroid surgery. Two studies injected autologous fat via direct suspension laryngoscope under general anesthesia, while the other 3 studies injected polyacrylamide, hyaluronic acid, and polymethyl methacrylate from cricothyroid membrane under local anesthesia. All 5 studies reported improved voice outcomes of IL for post-thyroidectomy UVFP. Meta-analysis showed MPT increased for 3.18 s (95% CI: 2.40–3.96, fix effect model) after IL. Another common acoustic parameter, jitter (%) also improved for 1.46 (95% CI: 0.73–2.19, random effects model) after IL for post-thyroidectomy UVFP.

Conclusions: This review supported that IL can improve the voice outcome for post-thyroidectomy UVFP. Autologous fat remains a good augmentation material with a potential longer lasting effect. More research and long-term surveys are needed to document the safety and longevity of other synthetic materials.

Keywords: vocal cord paralysis, injection laryngoplasty, dysphonia, larynx, review

BACKGROUND

The synonymous term of unilateral vocal fold paralysis (UVFP) includes vocal cord palsy, vagal paralysis and recurrent laryngeal neuropathy. Iatrogenic injury is now the prevailing etiologies for UVFP (1) and thyroid surgery related recurrent laryngeal nerve injury is one of the most common cause for iatrogenic UVFP. The an average incidence of transient and permanent UVFP following thyroid surgeries were 9.8 and 2.3%, respectively (2). UVFP often leads to significant morbidity that may include dysphonia, dysphagia, aspiration, or even pneumonia after thyroid surgery, especially in elder patients (3). Several modalities had been introduced for post-thyroidectomy UVFP, e.g., voice therapy, medialization thyroplasty, and injection laryngoplasty (IL).

The first IL was reported by Dr. Bruening in 1911 using liquid paraffin (4). Unfortunately, this material is not tissue compatible and resulted in chronic granuloma formation and material extrusion (5). Later on, IL using Teflon paste was re-introduced in 1960's (6). Although short-term effectiveness was satisfactory, Teflon paste was gradually noted to cause serious long-term sequel, i.e., Teflon granuloma, owing to profound foreign body reaction (7). After the frustrating experience with paraffin and Teflon (8), subsequent study shifted to more histologically compatible materials, i.e. homologous and autologous collagen (9–11), and bovine / porcine collagen (12, 13). Since 2000s, other synthetic compatible materials had been introduced to clinical use during IL (14), e.g. carboxymethylcellulose (15), hyaluronic acid (13, 16), and calcium hydroxylappatite (17).

Compared with other treatment modalities for post-thyroidectomy UVFP, IL has several advantages. IL can be performed in the office under local anesthesia. Real-time feedback of voice improvement can also be conducted. Most-importantly, patient did not need another open-surgery (e.g. thyroplasty) to correct UVFP resulting from prior thyroid surgeries. From our clinical experience, IL is well tolerated in the office and most patients exhibit stable hemodynamics throughout the procedure (18). Although IL is effective for UVFP, most of the existing studies included a mixture of different etiologies of UVFP (e.g., iatrogenic, neoplastic, idiopathic). Only a few studies focused on IL in the management of post-thyroidectomy related UVFP. Accordingly, we conducted this literature review to summarize the state of art practice and evidence in this specific clinical scenario.

MATERIAL AND METHOD

A literature review was performed using the Pubmed, Medline and EMBASE database. The following keywords and MeSH Terms were applied: vocal fold palsy OR vocal cord palsy AND injection therapy. All relevant articles published in English addressing the effect of injection laryngoplasty in UVFP were reviewed. We limit the literatures into IL for UVFP after thyroidectomy. Studies including multiple etiologies of UVFP were excluded. We evaluated the risk of bias in recruited studies using Risk of Bias in Non-Randomized Studies of Interventions (ROBINS-I) (19).

Retrieved information include the number of patients, injected material, injection approach, and treatment outcomes before and after injection laryngoplasty. Owing to different reporting timeline across each studies, outcomes of the longest follow-up period was selected for subsequent meta-analysis (R software, version 4.1.2, with packages for meta-analysis (20). We adapted results from either fixed or random effect model for statistical inference based on the significance of potential heterogeneity among the recruited research.

RESULTS

The flow chart of the study selection process is shown in **Figure 1**. We identified 5 original articles summarized in **Table 1**. Totally 214 patients received IL after thyroid surgery related UVFP were reported. Fang et al. (21) reported acoustic outcomes of 27 patients with autologous fat injection and follow-up the residual fat volume with 3-dimensional imaging. The mean residual fat volume remained consistent after 26-month follow-up. The maximal phonation time (MPT), s/z ratio, jitter, and noise-to-harmonic ratio (NHR) were significantly improved during follow-up.

Lee et al. (22) reported 34 patients received polyacrylamide hydrogel (PAAG (Aquamid®) for permanent UVFP and Hyaluronic acid (Rofilan®) for temporary UVFP after thyroidectomy. Acoustic and perceptual parameters (GRBAS),

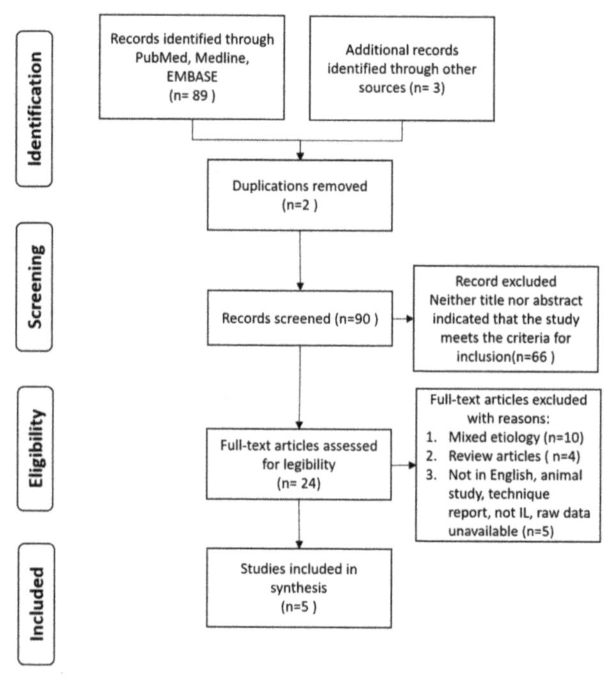

FIGURE 1 | PRISMA flow diagram depicts the process of literature searching.

TABLE 1 | Summary for the literatures focus on the management of UVFP after thyroid surgery with IL.

	Authors	Main findings
1	Fang et al. (21)	27 patients with autologous **fat injection** MPT, s/z ratio, jitter, and harmonic-to-noise ratio were significantly improved. Mean residual fat volume remained consistent after 26-month follow-up.
2	Lee et al. (22)	34 patients with **PAAG (PAAG (Aquamid®) and Hyaluronic acid (Rofilan®) injection** Acoustic and perceptual parameters (overall GBRAS), MPT, jitter, and shimmer, voice handicap index, and grades of mucosal waves and glottic closure were significantly improved and remained stable over 6 months
3	Jang et al. (23)	55 patients (24 early, 31 late injection) with **PMMA (polymethyl methacrylate, ArteSense™)** and early voice rehabilitation All tested voice parameters were significantly improved in both the early and late groups. The amount of voice improvement was significantly larger in the early injection group, especially jitter % ($P = 0.02$) and shimmer % ($P = 0.03$).
4	Chun et al. (24)	25 patients received IL using **hyaluronic acid**, comparing with 23 patients received voice therapy Greater improvement in UVFP patients who underwent IL then voice therapy
5.	Lin et al. (25)	73 patients underwent **autologous fat injection** Gender and age may stand as significant categories on analysis voice indicators

GBRAS, grade of hoarseness, roughness, breathiness, asthenia, and strain.
S/Z ratio, the maximal length when pronouncing "S", divided by the maximal length when pronouncing "Z".

MPT, jitter, and shimmer, voice handicap index, and grades of mucosal waves and glottic closure were all significantly improved after the injection and remained stable over 6 months.

Jang et al. (23) reported 55 patients injected with PMMA (polymethyl methacrylate, ArteSense™, a relatively long-lasting injectable substance for soft-tissue augmentation) for UVFP after thyroidectomy. The authors further divided these patients into 24 early injection (within 3 months between IL and thyroid surgery) and 31 late injection (IL at longer than 3 months after thyroidectomy). All of the measured objective and subjective voice parameters were significantly improved in both the early and late groups. The degree of voice improvement was significantly larger in the early injection group, especially jitter % ($P = 0.02$) and shimmer % ($P = 0.03$) improvement.

Chun et al. (24) reported 25 patients of post-thyroidectomy with aspiration symptoms receiving injection laryngoplasty using hyaluronic acid (Rofilan), and another 23 patients without aspiration receiving only voice therapy. They found greater improvement in thyroidectomy-related voice questionnaire, GRBAS scale, jitter, shimmer and NHR in patients who underwent injection laryngoplasty comparing to voice therapy alone.

Lin et al. (25) reported 73 patients underwent autologous fat injection for UVFP after thyroid surgery. They reported a significant improvement of multi-dimensional voice parameters 1 year after lipoinjection. This study also found that patients under 60 years old presented better improvement of MPT then the other patient older than 60 years. BMI did not alter post-operative voice parameters, whereas sex may present differently upon acoustic analysis.

The numerical outcomes were summarized in **Table 2**. We also evaluated the risk of bias in the recruited studies using ROBINS-I tool as shown in **Table 3**. Most of recruited studies reveal low risk of bias, 2 studies have moderate concern of missing data bias due to short follow-up time; one study has moderate concern of bias in selection of the main reported result (lack of MPT outcomes); and the other one study had moderate bias in participant selection (vague description of inclusion criteria).

We combined the result of these studies for subsequent meta-analysis. The first outcome parameter iS MPT, reported

TABLE 2 | Compare the effects of ILs for post thyroid surgery UVFP with different injection material.

	Pre-treatment	3–6 month	12-month	Post-treatment
MPT (seconds)				
Fat (Fang et al. (21))	**4.9 ± 2.9**	9.3 ± 3.1	9.9 ± 2.5	**10 ± 3.2**
PAAG &HA (Lee et al. (22))	**4.7 ± 2.9**		8.8 ± 4.5	**7.8 ± 5.4**
TVFP	7.8 ± 4.9	12.1 ± 4.4		
PVFP	4.3 ± 1.9	8.2 ± 3.6		
PMMA (Jang et al. (23))				
Early IL	**5.60 ± 3.19**	**7.93 ± 3.29**		
Late IL	**5.41 ± 3.68**	**7.61 ± 3.77**		
Fat (Lin et al. (25))	**5.95 ± 4.15**		8.77 ± 4.92	
Jitter (%)				
Fat (Fang et al. (21))	**3.1 ± 1.7**	1.2 ± 0.6	1.2 ± 0.7	**1.0 ± 0.4**
PAAG &HA (Lee et al. (22))	**2.9 ± 1.1**		3.0 ± 2.7	**2.2 ± 0.6**
TVFP	3.8 ± 1.0	1.3 ± 0.3		
PVFP	3.6 ± 2.6	2.7 ± 0.8		
PMMA (Jang et al. (23))				
Early IL	**5.12 ± 4.81**	**2.22 ± 1.80**		
Late IL	**3.89 ± 2.34**	**3.10 ± 4.18**		
HA (Chun et al. (24))	**3.36 ± 2.05**	2.12 ± 1.38	**1.85 ± 1.23**	

MPT, Maximal phonation time; PAAG, PAAG (Aquamid®); HA, Hyaluronic acid (Rofilan®); TVFP, transient vocal fold paralysis; PVFP, permanent vocal fold paralysis; IL, injection laryngoplasty.
The bold values are used in meta-analysis.

among 4 studies. Because the heterogeneity test showed non-significance (I square = 46%, $p = 0.11$), we adapted the results of fixed effect model (**Figure 2**). Meta-analysis showed an increased MPT of 3.18s (95% CI: 2.40–3.96) after IL. The second outcome parameter was jitter (%), which was also reported in 4 studies. Considering significant heterogeneity among the recruited research (I square = 75%, $p < 0.01$), we adapted results of random effect model which showed an improvement of 1.46 (95% CI: 0.73–2.19).

TABLE 3 | Evaluating the risk of bias in recruited studies using ROBINS-I (19).

Publications	D1	D2	D3	D4	D5	D6	D7
Fang et al. (21)	L	L	L	L	L	L	L
Lee et al. (22)	L	L	L	L	L	L	L
Jang et al. (23)	L	L	L	L	M	L	L
Chun et al. (24)	L	L	L	L	L	L	M
Lin et al. (25)	L	M	L	L	M	L	L

Domains included in ROBINS-I.
D1: Bias due to confounding.
D2: Bias in selection of participants into the study.
D3: Bias in classification of interventions.
D4: Bias due to deviations from intended interventions.
D5: Bias due to missing data.
D6: Bias in measurement of outcomes.
D7: Bias in selection of the reported result.
Judgement: Low risk of bias: ***L****; Moderate risk of bias:* ***M****; Serious risk of bias:* ***S****; Critical risk of bias: C; No information: NA.*

DISCUSSION

UVFP often leads to significant morbidity that may include dysphonia, swallowing problems and aspiration after thyroid surgery. Conservative treatment via voice therapy may ameliorate part of the symptoms of UVFP (26, 27). For patients not responding to voice therapy, surgical correction include injection laryngoplasty, medialization thyroplasty, arytenoid adduction and reinnervation of recurrent laryngeal nerve (28). Chen et al. (29) conduct a meta-analysis for management of UVFP, they recommend absorbable material injection laryngoplasty during the first year and reinnervation after 12 months. According to another systematic review for UVFP management, earlier IL is suggested to decrease the necessary of subsequent medialization thyroplasty (30). Considering IL for UVFP after thyroid surgery, Jang et al. (23) reported that the amount of voice improvement was significantly larger in the early injection group, especially in jitter (%) ($P = 0.02$) and shimmer (%) ($P = 0.03$). Therefore, earlier IL is suggested for post thyroid surgery related UVFP.

Despite continual reports show that IL is effective and are available for treatment of UVFP (16, 28–31), most of the

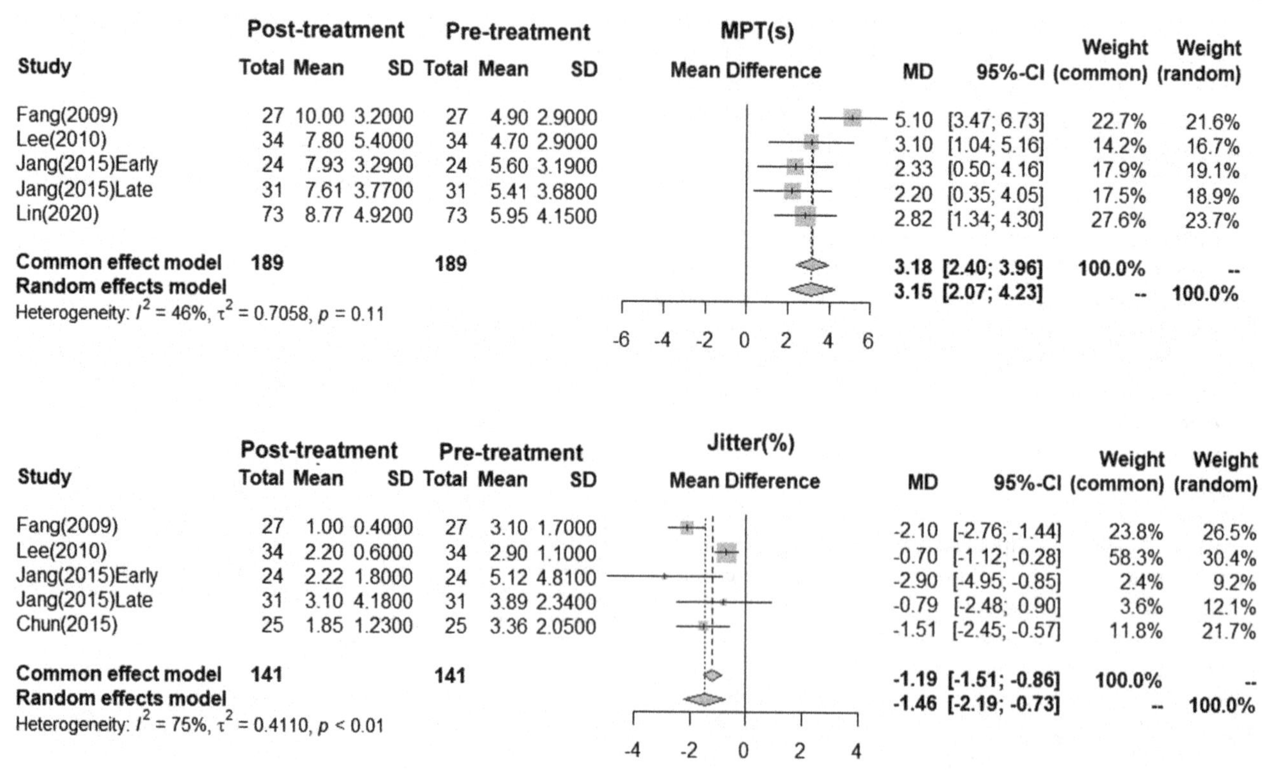

FIGURE 2 | Forest plots show the results of meta-analysis from the included research. Fixed effect (i.e., common effect) model was selected for statistical inference when heterogeneity between research was non-significant, whereas random effects model was applied in presence of significant heterogeneity.

published literature mixed with different etiologies of UVFP. Considering the prevalence of thyroid neoplasm and the high incidence of thyroidectomy-related UVFP (2), this review specifically retain only original papers reporting IL for UVFP after thyroid surgeries. Considering the potential heterogeneity when pooling the effectiveness of IL, we adapted the results from either fixed effect or random effect model. Our literatures review supported that IL is an effective management for post-thyroidectomy related UVFP. Further meta-analysis showed IL could increase MPT for 3.18 (2.40–3.96) seconds and decrease Jitter (%) for 1.46 (0.73–2.19), both results were statistically significant (**Figure 2**).

Different injection material for IL were noticed in this literature review and may be further divided into temporary versus permanent intentions. Temporary material as hyaluronic acid and permanent material as autologous fat are the most common injection materials for IL. In the report by Fang et al, CT scan showed that injected autologous fat remained in situ with a mean interval of 26 ± 13 months after initial IL. The parameters from acoustic analyses also revealed stable results after 12 months, indicating that autologous fat may be a potential long-term filler. Similar results had also been reported by Umeno et al. (32), which showed that only a minimum patients (<5%) needs secondary IL following autologous fat injection. Nevertheless, controversial findings from other studies showed higher failure rates ranged from 30% to 41%, and patients may need further revision fat injection after 12 to 24 months (33, 34). Possible explanations for such a great diversity include different donor site of adipose tissues, harvesting techniques (e.g., liposuction vs. mincing), additive insulin, centrifugation, size of the injection needle, and pressurized instrument (35–38).

Another advantage of IL is that it could be performed under local anesthesia with multiple injection routes (39). In this review, 3 article performed transcutaneous injection route from cricothyoid membrane (**Figure 3**) (22–24). Other methods include ultrasound guided (40) or EMG guided (41, 42) injection. Otherwise, IL may also be performed under routine general anesthesia with direct laryngoscope suspension, similar to the 2 studies using autologous fat for IL in this review (21, 25). With regarding to the voice outcome, in our opinion, no technique is superior to other approaches. The choice of guiding and injection technique depends on the patient's preference and the operator's experience.

The long-term effect of IL remains undetermined. The recruited studies did not report the percentage of patients who need repeated IL or laryngeal framework surgery. Limited by varying reported parameters (2 studies using VHI-30 (22, 23) while another study use VHI-10 (25), we cannot perform a meta-analysis using patient-reported outcomes in this study. In addition, some of these studies were conducted retrospectively via chart review (23, 25) and may present some degree of bias. Further prospective study is still necessary to confirm the longer effect of IL for post-thyroidectomy related UVFP.

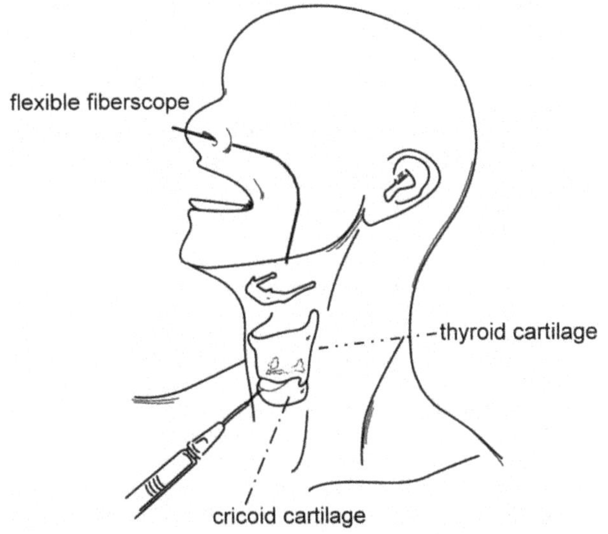

FIGURE 3 | IL performed under local anesthesia with flexible fiberscope guidance via cricothyroid membrane.

CONCLUSION

This review supported that IL could improve the voice outcome for post-thyroidectomy UVFP. Autologous fat remains a good augmentation material with a potential longer lasting effect. More research and long-term survey might be needed to document the safety and longevity of other synthetic materials.

AUTHOR CONTRIBUTIONS

L-JL: Study conceptualization, Data extracting, Statistical Analysis, Manuscript drafting. C-TW: Manuscript drafting, Article proof-reading. All authors contributed to the article and approved the submitted version.

ACKNOWLEDGEMENTS

We thank CH Lee for drawing the pictures illustrating injection method.

REFERENCES

1. Merati AL, Shemirani N, Smith TL, Toohill RJ. Changing trends in the nature of vocal fold motion impairment. *Am J Otolaryngol.* (2006) 27:106–8. doi: 10.1016/j.amjoto.2005.07.020
2. Tolley NS, Chaidas K, Bergenfelz A. Rates of RLN and SLN injury: Data from national quality registries and the literature. In: GW Randolph, editor. *The recurrent and superior laryngeal nerves.* Switzerland: Springer (2016). p. 1–16.
3. Tsai M-S, Yang Y-H, Liu C-Y, Lin M-H, Chang G-H, Tsai Y-T, et al. Unilateral vocal fold paralysis and risk of pneumonia: a nationwide population-based cohort study. *Otolaryngol Head Neck Surg.* (2018) 158:896–903. doi: 10.1177/0194599818756285
4. Cantarella G, Viglione S, Forti S, Pignataro L. Voice therapy for laryngeal hemiplegia: the role of timing of initiation of therapy. *J Rehabil Med.* (2010) 42:442–6. doi: 10.2340/16501977-0540
5. O'Leary MA, Grillone GA. Injection laryngoplasty. *Otolaryngol Clin North Am.* (2006) 39:43–54. doi: 10.1016/j.otc.2005.10.008
6. Arnold GE. Vocal rehabilitation of paralytic dysphonia: IX. Technique of intracordal injection. *Arch Otolaryngol.* (1962) 76:358–68. doi: 10.1001/archotol.1962.00740050368013
7. Varvares MA, Montgomery WW, Hillman RE. Teflon granuloma of the larynx: etiology, pathophysiology, and management. *Annals of Otology, Rhinol Laryngol.* (1995) 104:511–5. doi: 10.1177/000348949510400702
8. Kwon TK, Buckmire R. Injection laryngoplasty for management of unilateral vocal fold paralysis. *Curr Opin Otolaryngol Head Neck Surg.* (2004) 12:538–42. doi: 10.1097/01.moo.0000144393.40874.98
9. Remacle M, Lawson G, Keghian J, Jamart J. Use of injectable autologous collagen for correcting glottic gaps: initial results. *J Voice.* (1999) 13:280–8. doi: 10.1016/S0892-1997(99)80033-2
10. Courey MS. Homologous collagen substances for vocal fold augmentation. *Laryngoscope.* (2001) 111:747–58. doi: 10.1097/00005537-200105000-00001
11. Ford CN, Staskowski PA, Bless DM. Autologous collagen vocal fold injection: a preliminary clinical study. *Laryngoscope.* (1995) 105:944–8. doi: 10.1288/00005537-199509000-00014
12. Ford CN, Martin DW, Warner TF. Injectable collagen in laryngeal rehabilitation. *Laryngoscope.* (1984) 94:513–8. doi: 10.1288/00005537-198404000-00016
13. Wen MH, Cheng PW, Liao LJ, Chou HW, Wang CT. Treatment outcomes of injection laryngoplasty using cross-linked porcine collagen and hyaluronic acid. *Otolaryngol Head Neck Surg.* (2013) 149:900–6. doi: 10.1177/0194599813508082
14. Carroll TL. Ideal Material Selection for Vocal Fold Augmentation. In: BJ Lee, TK Kown, CA Rosen, editors. *Vocal fold injection.* Singapore: Springer (2021). p. 73–8.
15. Kwon T-K, Rosen CA, Gartner-Schmidt J. Preliminary results of a new temporary vocal fold injection material. *J Voice.* (2005) 19:668–73. doi: 10.1016/j.jvoice.2005.01.009
16. Wang C-C, Wu S-H, Tu Y-K, Lin W-J, Liu S-A. Hyaluronic acid injection laryngoplasty for unilateral vocal fold paralysis—a systematic review and meta-analysis. *Cells.* (2020) 9:2417. doi: 10.3390/cells9112417
17. Carroll TL, Rosen CA. Long-term results of calcium hydroxylapatite for vocal fold augmentation. *Laryngoscope.* (2011) 121:313–9. doi: 10.1002/lary.21258
18. Wang CT, Liao LJ, Lo WC, Huang TW, Cheng PW. Effects of comorbidity and medication use on the haemodynamic status during office-based laryngeal procedures: a prospective cohort study. *Clin Otolaryngol.* (2018) 43:124–30. doi: 10.1111/coa.12909
19. Sterne JA, Hernán MA, Reeves BC, Savović J, Berkman ND, Viswanathan M, et al. ROBINS-I: a tool for assessing risk of bias in non-randomised studies of interventions. *BMJ.* (2016) 355:i4919. doi: 10.1136/bmj.i4919
20. Balduzzi S, Rücker G, Schwarzer G. How to perform a meta-analysis with R: a practical tutorial. *Evid Based Ment Health.* (2019) 22:153–60. doi: 10.1136/ebmental-2019-300117
21. Fang TJ, Lee LA, Wang CJ, Li HY, Chiang HC. Intracordal fat assessment by 3-dimensional imaging after autologous fat injection in patients with thyroidectomy-induced unilateral vocal cord paralysis. *Surgery.* (2009) 146:82–7. doi: 10.1016/j.surg.2009.02.005
22. Lee SW, Kim JW, Chung CH, Mok JO, Shim SS, Koh YW, et al. Utility of injection laryngoplasty in the management of post-thyroidectomy vocal cord paralysis. *Thyroid.* (2010) 20:513–7. doi: 10.1089/thy.2009.0397
23. Jang JY, Lee G, Ahn J, Son YI. Early voice rehabilitation with injection laryngoplasty in patients with unilateral vocal cord palsy after thyroidectomy. *Eur Arch Otorhinolaryngol.* (2015) 272:3745–50. doi: 10.1007/s00405-015-3720-8
24. Chun BJ, Bae JS, Chae BJ, Park JO, Nam IC, Kim CS, et al. The therapeutic decision making of the unilateral vocal cord palsy after thyroidectomy using thyroidectomy-related voice questionnaire (TVQ). *Eur Arch Otorhinolaryngol.* (2015) 272:727–36. doi: 10.1177/0194599814541629a139
25. Lin WY, Chang WD, Ko LW, Tsou YA, Chen SH. Impact of patient-related factors on successful autologous fat injection laryngoplasty in thyroid surgical treated related unilateral vocal fold paralysis- observational study. *Medicine (Baltimore).* (2020) 99:e18579. doi: 10.1097/MD.0000000000019406
26. Schindler A, Bottero A, Capaccio P, Ginocchio D, Adorni F, Ottaviani F. Vocal improvement after voice therapy in unilateral vocal fold paralysis. *J Voice.* (2008) 22:113–8. doi: 10.1016/j.jvoice.2006.08.004
27. D'Alatri L, Galla S, Rigante M, Antonelli O, Buldrini S, Marchese MR. Role of early voice therapy in patients affected by unilateral vocal fold paralysis. *J Laryngol Otol.* (2008) 122:936–41. doi: 10.1017/S0022215107000679
28. Siu J, Tam S, Fung K. A comparison of outcomes in interventions for unilateral vocal fold paralysis: a systematic review. *Laryngoscope.* (2016) 126:1616–24. doi: 10.1002/lary.25739
29. Chen X, Wan P, Yu Y, Li M, Xu Y, Huang P, et al. Types and timing of therapy for vocal fold paresis/paralysis after thyroidectomy: a systematic review and meta-analysis. *J Voice.* (2014) 28:799–808. doi: 10.1016/j.jvoice.2014.02.003
30. Vila PM, Bhatt NK, Paniello RC. Early-injection laryngoplasty may lower risk of thyroplasty: a systematic review and meta-analysis. *Laryngoscope.* (2018) 128:935–40. doi: 10.1002/lary.26894
31. Chang W-D, Chen S-H, Tsai M-H, Tsou Y-A. Autologous fat injection laryngoplasty for unilateral vocal fold paralysis. *J Clin Med.* (2021) 10:5034. doi: 10.3390/jcm10215034
32. Umeno H, Shirouzu H, Chitose S-I, Nakashima T. Analysis of voice function following autologous fat injection for vocal fold paralysis. *Otolaryngol Head Neck Surg.* (2005) 132:103–7. doi: 10.1016/j.otohns.2004.09.016
33. Laccourreye O, Papon JF, Kania R, Crevier-Buchman L, Brasnu D, Hans S. Intracordal injection of autologous fat in patients with unilateral laryngeal nerve paralysis: long-term results from the patient's perspective. *Laryngoscope.* (2003) 113:541–5. doi: 10.1097/00005537-200303000-00027
34. McCulloch TM, Andrews BT, Hoffman HT, Graham SM, Karnell MP, Minnick C. Long-term follow-up of fat injection laryngoplasty for unilateral vocal cord paralysis. *Laryngoscope.* (2002) 112:1235–8. doi: 10.1097/00005537-200207000-00017
35. Erdim M, Tezel E, Numanoglu A, Sav A. The effects of the size of liposuction cannula on adipocyte survival and the optimum temperature for fat graft storage: an experimental study. *J Plast Reconstr Aesthet Surg.* (2009) 62:1210–14. doi: 10.1016/j.bjps.2008.03.016
36. de Souza Kruschewsky L, de Mello-Filho FV, dos Santos AC, Rosen CA. Autologous fat graft absorption in unilateral paralyzed canine vocal folds. *Laryngoscope.* (2007) 117:96–100. doi: 10.1097/01.mlg.0000245013.98844.30
37. Shiffman MA, Mirrafati S. Fat transfer techniques: the effect of harvest and transfer methods on adipocyte viability and review of the literature. *Dermatol Surg.* (2001) 27:819–26. doi: 10.1046/j.1524-4725.2001.01062.x
38. Butterwick KJ, Nootheti PK, Hsu JW, Goldman MP. Autologous fat transfer: an in-depth look at varying concepts and techniques. *Facial Plast Surg Clin.* (2007) 15:99–111. doi: 10.1016/j.fsc.2006.10.003
39. Lee BJ, Kwon T-K, Rosen CA. *Vocal fold injection.* Singapore: Springer (2021).
40. Carrillo A, Garcia-Del-Salto L, Vaca M. Injection laryngoplasty under ultrasonographic control. *Eur Arch Otorhinolaryngol.* (2021) 278:2143–6. doi: 10.1007/s00405-021-06666-z
41. Wang CC, Chang MH, Jiang RS, Lai HC, De Virgilio A, Wang CP, et al. Laryngeal electromyography-guided hyaluronic acid vocal fold injection for unilateral vocal fold paralysis: a prospective long-term follow-up outcome report. *JAMA Otolaryngol Head Neck Surg.* (2015) 141:264–71. doi: 10.1001/jamaoto.2014.3466

21

New Developments in Anterior Laryngeal Recording Technique During Neuromonitored Thyroid and Parathyroid Surgery

Cheng-Hsin Liu[1,2], *Tzu-Yen Huang*[1,3], *Che-Wei Wu*[1,4], *Jia Joanna Wang*[1,2], *Ling-Feng Wang*[1,4], *Leong-Perng Chan*[1,4,5], *Gianlorenzo Dionigi*[6,7], *Feng-Yu Chiang*[8,9], *Hsin-Yi Tseng*[1*] *and Yi-Chu Lin*[1*]

[1] *International Thyroid Surgery Center, Department of Otolaryngology-Head and Neck Surgery, Kaohsiung Medical University Hospital, Faculty of Medicine, College of Medicine, Kaohsiung Medical University, Kaohsiung, Taiwan,* [2] *Department of Otolaryngology-Head and Neck Surgery, Kaohsiung Municipal Siaogang Hospital, Kaohsiung Medical University Hospital, Faculty of Medicine, College of Medicine, Kaohsiung Medical University, Kaohsiung, Taiwan,* [3] *Department of Biological Science and Technology, National Yang Ming Chiao Tung University, Hsinchu, Taiwan,* [4] *Center for Liquid Biopsy and Cohort Research, Faculty of Medicine, College of Medicine, Kaohsiung Medical University, Kaohsiung, Taiwan,* [5] *Department of Otolaryngology-Head and Neck Surgery, Kaohsiung Municipal Tatung Hospital, Kaohsiung Medical University Hospital, Faculty of Medicine, College of Medicine, Kaohsiung Medical University, Kaohsiung, Taiwan,* [6] *Division of Surgery, Istituto Auxologico Italiano IRCCS, Piazzale Brescia, Milan, Italy,* [7] *Department of Pathophysiology and Transplantation, University of Milan, Milan, Italy,* [8] *Department of Otolaryngology-Head and Neck Surgery, E-Da Hospital, Kaohsiung, Taiwan,* [9] *School of Medicine, College of Medicine, I-Shou University, Kaohsiung, Taiwan*

***Correspondence:**
Hsin-Yi Tseng
sycatlovestar@gmail.com
Yi-Chu Lin
yichulin.ent@gmail.com

A recurrent laryngeal nerve (RLN) injury resulting in vocal fold paralysis and dysphonia remains a major source of morbidity after thyroid and parathyroid surgeries. Intraoperative neural monitoring (IONM) is increasingly accepted as an adjunct to the standard practice of visual RLN identification. Endotracheal tube (ET) surface recording electrode systems are now widely used for IONM; however, the major limitation of the clinical use of ET-based surface electrodes is the need to maintain constant contact between the electrodes and vocal folds during surgery to obtain a high-quality recording. An ET that is malpositioned during intubation or displaced during surgical manipulation can cause a false decrease or loss of electromyography (EMG) signal. Since it may be difficult to distinguish from an EMG change caused by a true RLN injury, a false loss or decrease in EMG signal may contribute to inappropriate surgical decision making. Therefore, researchers have investigated alternative electrode systems that circumvent common causes of poor accuracy in ET-based neuromonitoring. Recent experimental and clinical studies have confirmed the hypothesis that needle or adhesive surface recording electrodes attached to the thyroid cartilage (transcartilage and percutaneous recording) or attached to the overlying neck skin (transcutaneous recording) can provide functionality similar to that of ET-based electrodes, and these recording methods enable access to the EMG response of the vocalis muscle that originates from the inner surface of the thyroid cartilage. Studies also indicate that, during surgical manipulation of the trachea, transcartilage, percutaneous, and transcutaneous anterior laryngeal (AL) recording electrodes could be more stable than ET-based surface electrodes and could be equally accurate in depicting RLN stress during IONM. These findings show that these AL electrodes have potential applications in future designs of recording electrodes and support the use of IONM as a high-quality quantitative tool in thyroid and parathyroid surgery. This article reviews the major recent developments of newly emerging transcartilage, percutaneous, and transcutaneous AL recording techniques used in IONM and evaluates their contribution to improved voice outcomes in modern thyroid surgery.

Keywords: voice, vocal fold paralysis, thyroid surgery, intraoperative neural monitoring (IONM), recurrent laryngeal nerve (RLN), laryngeal electromyography (EMG), anterior laryngeal recording, thyroid cartilage recording

INTRODUCTION

Neural Monitoring for Improving Voice Outcomes After Thyroid Surgery

Although thyroid surgery is among the most common and safe interventions in endocrine surgery, the risk of complications is still evitable due to the unique anatomical structure and physiological function of the thyroid gland (1). Recurrent laryngeal nerve (RLN) paralysis remains a common thyroid surgery complication that can cause dysphonia, aspiration, and, in some cases, interference with breathing. Therefore, RLN paralysis is a common cause of litigation after thyroid surgery in the current era in which quality of life change is included in assessment of surgical outcome (2, 3). One major change in the past two decades is the growing acceptance of intraoperative neural monitoring (IONM) as a tool for minimizing surgical risk by assisting surgeons in the early localization and identification of the RLN and as a tool for assisting clinical decision-making by enabling real-time monitoring of evoked electrophysiologic laryngeal electromyography (EMG) responses during thyroid surgery.

Advantages and Disadvantages of EMG Endotracheal Tube Recording for IONM

Currently, EMG recording during neuromonitored thyroid surgery is almost always performed using endotracheal tube (ET) surface electrodes placed in contact with vocal folds during intubation for general anesthesia because of the advantages including their noninvasiveness, wide commercial availability, and capacity to monitor larger areas of the target muscle (4, 5). However, maintaining consistent and stable contact between the ET-based surface electrodes and vocal folds during surgery has become the major clinical challenge to obtain a high-quality recording. Improper positioning of the ET during intubation is not uncommon and may result from an ET that is undersized, rotated, or inserted to the incorrect depth (6, 7). During surgical manipulation, an ET may be displaced by tracheal and neck extension, which inevitably raises the possibility of rotation or depth change (8–10). Both malpositioning and displacement can cause a false decrease or loss of EMG signal. Since false signals may be difficult to distinguish from EMG signal changes caused by true RLN injuries, they may lead to inappropriate surgical decision making. During IONM with ET recording, a malpositioned or displaced ET requires adjustment by the anesthesiologist, which can be troublesome and time-consuming. Intraoperative adjustment of the ET is particularly disruptive in remote thyroid surgery and is virtually impossible in procedures such as transoral robotic approach (11). Additionally, EMG changes have a larger impact in continuous IONM (C-IONM) compared to conventional intermittent IONM (I-IONM) because unstable or shifting baseline EMG cause a C-IONM system malfunction and limit its use for early identification of RLN lesions (12, 13). In addition to the above issues of malpositioning or displacement that may occur during surgical manipulation, other disadvantages of ET include its high expense, the potential for accumulation of saliva to interfere with signal acquisition, and its limited use in pediatric patients and patients with airway abnormality.

Alternative Electrode Systems That Circumvent the Factors Affecting ET Recording

To avoid the time-consuming processes of verifying and readjusting the ET position during neuromonitored thyroid surgery and to minimize the safety hazard of signal inconsistency and instability. Regarding the basis of anatomy, there are many innovative hypotheses and possible solutions including novel electrodes designs have been proposed. For example, many experimental (14–18) and clinical studies (19–28) have confirmed the hypothesis that needle or adhesive surface recording electrodes attached to the thyroid cartilage (transcartilage or percutaneous recordings) or attached to the overlying neck skin (transcutaneous recording) can function like ET electrodes by enabling access to the EMG response of the vocal fold muscles (vocalis muscle and thyroarytenoid muscle) originating from the inner TC surface (**Table 1, Figure 1**). These studies have also demonstrated that transcutaneous or transcartilage anterior laryngeal (AL) recording electrodes are as accurate as ET-based surface electrodes in depicting RLN stress during IONM. However, transcutaneous or transcartilage AL recording electrodes could be more stable than ET-based surface electrodes during surgical manipulation on the trachea. These findings indicate that AL electrodes have potential applications in future designs of recording electrodes and support the use of IONM as a high-quality quantitative tool in thyroid and parathyroid surgery. This article reviews recent studies of new and emerging transcutaneous or transcartilage AL recording techniques used during IONM and compares these

TABLE 1 | Current published papers on AL EMG recording technique during neuromonitored thyroid and parathyroid surgery.

Technique	Study design	Author, year	Electrode form	Number of subject	Highlights
Transcartilage	Experimental	Wu et al. 2018 (14)	Two disposable adhesive pre-gelled ECG surface electrode on bilateral TC	Porcine model(12 pigs and 24 RLNs at risk)	A proof of concept for transcartilage technique. Confirm the stability and accuracy by trachea displacement and traction injury experiments.
		Zhao et al. 2019 (16)	Two disposable paired subdermal needle electrode (12-mm long, uninsulated) on bilateral TC	Porcine model(4 pigs and 8 RLNs at risk)	Test and identify an optimal site for placement of needle electrodes.
		Zhao et al. 2021 (18)	Two disposable adhesive pre-gelled ECG surface electrode on bilateral TC	Porcine model(4 pigs and 8 RLNs at risk)	Determine the optimal placement locations and sizes of adhesive electrodes.
	Clinical	Chiang et al. 2017 (19)	Two disposable single subdermal needle electrode (12-mm long, uninsulated) on bilateral TC	Comparative Study. Open thyroidectomy(110 patients, 205 RLNs at risk)	First clinical study on needle transcartilage approach and report it obtain higher and more stable EMG signals as well as fewer false EMG results as compared to ET recording.
		Liddy et al. 2018 (20)	One disposable paired adhesive laryngeal EMG surface electrode on bilateral TC	Comparative Study. Open thyroidectomy and parathyroidectomy (15 patients, 20 RLNs at risk)	Demonstrate the transcartilage technique is useful and offer significantly more robust monitoring of the EBSLN.
		Van Slycke et al., 2019 (21)	One disposable paired laryngeal EMG surface electrode suture fixed on bilateral TC	Comparative Study. Open thyroidectomy (25 patients, 25 RLNs at risk)	Confirm the transcartilage technique can obtain higher amplitudes after stimulating RLN and also EBSLN.
		Chiang et al., 2020 (22)	Two disposable paired subdermal needle electrode (12-mm long, uninsulated) on bilateral TC	Case series. Open thyroidectomy (100 patients, 200 RLNs at risk)	Report an optimal technique of needle placement by inserting into the TC subperichondrium from the anterior margin of the thyrohyoid muscle with a slope of 10 to 15 degree.
		Jung et al., 2020 (23)	One disposable paired twisted subdermal needle electrode (22-mm, uninsulated) on bilateral TC	Comparative Study. Open thyroidectomy (38 patients, 54 RLNs at risk)	Report the positive predictive values of loss of signal in ET and TC electrodes were 40% and 100%, respectively.
		Lee et al., 2021 (24)	One disposable paired subdermal needle electrode (12-mm long, uninsulated) on ipsilateral TC	Case series. Unilateral hemithyroidectomy (34 patients, 34 RLNs at risk)	Introduce an alternative method with the advantage of minimal exposure of the TC lamina during unilateral hemithyroidectomy.
		Türk et al., 2021 (27)	One disposable paired twisted subdermal needle electrode (22-mm, uninsulated) on bilateral TC	Case-control study. Open thyroidectomy (885 patients, 1717 RLNs at risk)	The first case-control study to compare ET and TC electrodes, and concluded that TC electrodes are an inexpensive and efficient alternative to ET electrodes.
		Huang et al. (28)	Two disposable paired subdermal needle electrode (12-mm long, uninsulated) on bilateral TC	Comparative Study. Open thyroidectomy (33 pediatric patients, 58 RLNs at risk)	First pediatric study. TC electrodes show excellent stability and quality of EMG signals, and can be a preferable monitoring method for pediatric thyroid surgery
Percutaneous	Experimental Clinical	Huang et al., 2020 (17)	Two disposable paired subdermal needle electrodes (25 and 38-mm long, insulated to within 5 mm of tip) percutaneously inserted to TC	Porcine model. (4 pigs, 8 RLNs at risk), 1 case of Transoral robotic thyroidectomy	A proof of concept for percutaneous technique in remote endoscopic or robotic thyroidectomy without neck incision wound.
	Clinical	Li et al., 2020 (25)	Two disposable paired subdermal needle electrode (12-mm long, uninsulated) percutaneously inserted to TC	Case series. Minimally invasive unilateral parathyroidectomy (20 patients, 20 RLNs at risk)	Verify this technique is a feasible, convenient, reliable, and inexpensive method for thyroid or parathyroid surgery with small incision wound.
Transcutaneous	Experimental	Wu et al., 2018 (15)	Two disposable adhesive pre-gelled ECG surface electrode	Porcine model (12 pigs, 24 RLNs at risk)	A proof of concept for transcutaneous technique. Confirm the stability and accuracy by trachea displacement and traction injury experiments.
	Clinical	Lee et al., 2020 (26)	Two disposable adhesive pre-gelled EMG surface electrode	Comparative Study. Open thyroidectomy (30 patients, 39 RLNs at risk)	The first published clinical study verifies the usefulness of transcutaneous technique using adhesive skin electrodes.

(Continued)

TABLE 1 | Continued

Technique	Study design	Author, year	Electrode form	Number of subject	Highlights
	Experimental Clinical	Shin et al., 2021 (29)	Two disposable adhesive pre-gelled EMG surface electrode	Porcine model (4pigs, 8 RLNs at risk) Comparative study. Open thyroidectomy (78 patients, 115 RLNs at risk)	Adhesive skin electrode was feasible in both animal models and human patients. Adhesive skin electrode was suggested to the lateral side of the thyroid cartilage lamina closer to the cricoarytenoid joint.

AL, anterior laryngeal; EMG, electromyography; ECG, Electrocardiography; TC, thyroid cartilage; ET, endotracheal tube; RLN, recurrent laryngeal nerve.

techniques in terms of their contribution to improved voice outcomes after modern thyroid surgery.

TRANSCARTILAGE ANTERIOR LARYNGEAL RECORDING

The trans-cartilage recording system has yielded many novel surgical applications of IONM technology in recent years. Since vocal fold muscles are innervated only by the RLN and are attached to the anterior inner surface of the thyroid cartilage (TC), surface recording electrodes placed on the outer surface of TC should enable access to EMG signals evoked in vocal fold muscles during IONM (**Figure 1** and **Figure 2A)** (14). To test this hypothesis, Wu et al. (14) performed an animal study using 12 male piglets under standard IONM settings. Adhesive pre-gelled EMG electrodes were attached to the outer surface of the TC for transcartilage AL recording. Evoked EMG signals detected by TC electrodes were compared with those detected by ET electrodes. Typical evoked laryngeal EMG waveforms for the vagus nerve (VN) and RLN were obtained under 1 mA stimulation. Experimental displacements and surgical manipulations of the trachea confirmed the stability and consistency of transcartilage method. Additionally, RLN traction experiments confirmed that transcartilage method accurately reflected neurophysiologic events (14). Zhao et al. (18) investigated the feasibility, EMG stability, and optimal location and size of adhesive surface arrays attached to the TC for use in IONM. Their experiments confirmed that, during surgical manipulations, EMG profiles obtained by transcartilage

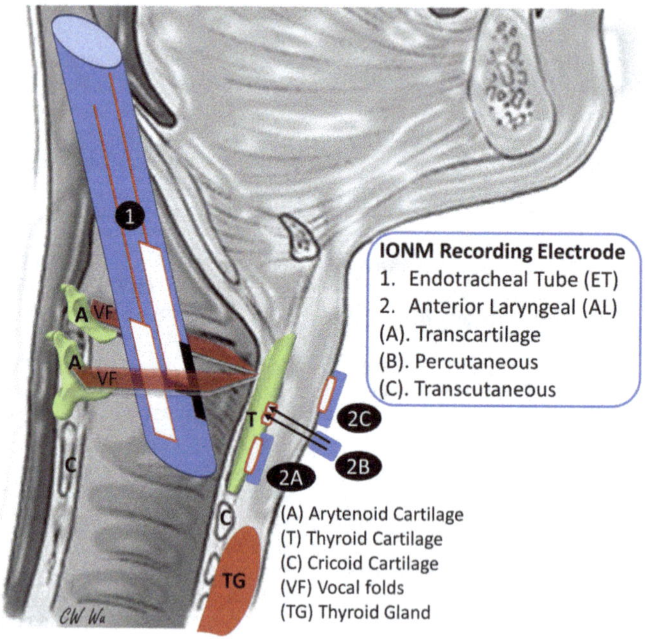

FIGURE 1 | Anatomic relationship between the thyroid cartilage (TC) - vocal folds and intraoperative neural monitoring (IONM) recording electrode placement in different electromyography (EMG) recording techniques used in thyroid and parathyroid surgery. The vocal fold (VF, vocalis and thyroarytenoid muscle) originates from the inner surface of the TC and inserts to the arytenoid cartilage (A). Conventional endotracheal tube (ET) surface electrodes are designed to be placed in contact with vocal folds during intubation for general anesthesia. However, potential displacement of the ET electrode during surgery may affect signal quality and stability. Recent studies have confirmed that anterior laryngeal (AL) transcartilage, percutaneous, and transcutaneous surface recording electrodes placed on the TC outer surface also enable access to the EMG response of the vocal folds and can circumvent factors that negatively affect ET electrode performance.

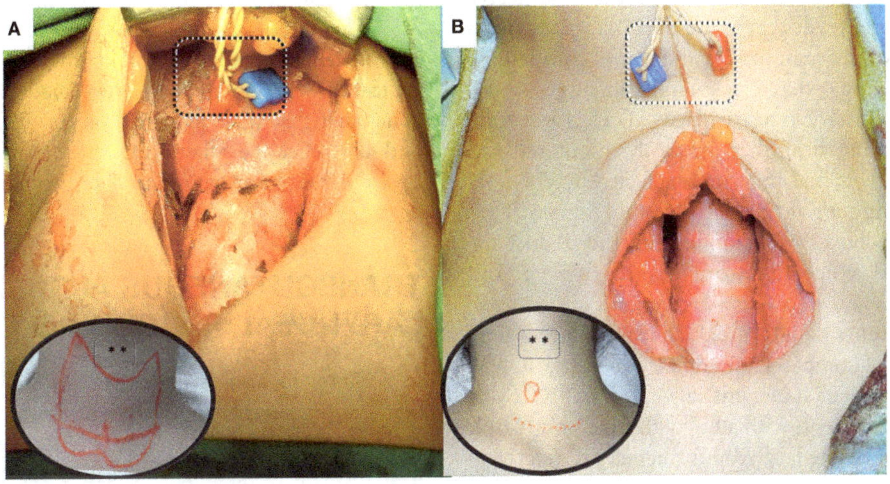

FIGURE 2 | Anterior laryngeal (AL) recording electrode placement for intraoperative neural monitoring. **(A)** Transcartilage Anterior Laryngeal Recording: Skin flaps are elevated superiorly to expose the thyroid cartilage. Needle electrodes are placed onto the subperichondrium layer of thyroid lamina. Inserting the needle at the anterior margin of the thyrohyoid muscle with a 10- to 15-degree angle from the surface of lamina. **(B)** Percutaneous Anterior Laryngeal Recording: The needle electrodes are percutaneously inserted and fixed onto the perichondrium layer of thyroid cartilage. It may be applied in surgeries with lower/smaller incision wound or in remote surgery. However, excessive traction may cause percutaneous needle displacement during the surgery.

recording method were more stable than those obtained by ET recording method.

Similarly, Zhao et al. (16) performed an experimental porcine model to test the transcartilage recording by placing needle electrodes on the TC in a porcine model. They confirmed that a perichondral needle electrode can be safely inserted into the avascular area of the TC. Comparing to ET electrodes, TC electrodes registered earlier changes in EMG amplitudes when the nerve is in traction injury. Additionally, TC electrodes obtained higher and more stable EMG amplitudes. Their findings indicate that transcartilage recording electrodes have superior function, easier placement, and lower cost compared to ET electrodes (16). Researchers are increasingly discussing clinical applications of transcartilage AL recording in IONM, and several methods of affixing electrodes to the TC have been reported. For example, one proposed method is to perform transcartilage AL recording using a commercially available 12mm subdermal single needle electrode. Chiang et al. (19) analyzed 205 at-risk RLNs in 110 patients in a clinical comparison of EMG signals recorded by ET and TC surface electrodes in the standardized monitored thyroidectomy. A pair of one-channel electrodes were inserted into the perichondrium of the TC lamina on bilateral side. According to their comparisons, transcartilage AL recording and ET recording had comparable efficacy and reliability during monitored thyroidectomy. In contrast with the complicated and time-consuming procedures for adjusting ET electrodes and verifying their proper position, the setup procedure for transcartilage AL electrodes can be performed quicker (approximately 2 minutes) and easier. Additionally, compared to ET recording, transcartilage AL recording obtains higher and more stable EMG signals during IONM as well as fewer false EMG results. Chiang et al. (22) developed a technique for using two-channel paired subdermal needle electrodes for transcartilage AL recording. Based on their experience in performing the technique in 100 consecutive monitored total thyroidectomies, the authors concluded that, in clinical practice, the technique can be performed without ET electrodes and that it provides high sensitivity and stability of EMG signals. Therefore, it improves the safety and reliability of thyroid surgery and is particularly suitable for use in C-IONM. Another recent study by Jung et al. (23) reported the efficacy of transcartilage recording during standardized monitored thyroidectomy. A pair of 22-mm twisted needle electrodes was attached to the TC in 38 patients with 54 at-risk RLNs. The positive predictive values of loss of signal were 40% and 100% for ET and TC electrodes, respectively. In 2021, Lee et al. (24) reported the advantage of minimizing exposure of one side of the TC by applying a single ipsilateral transcartilage needle electrode during unilateral monitored hemithyroidectomy. Additionally, Türk et al. (27) reported the first case-control study to compare ET and TC electrodes and concluded that TC electrodes are an inexpensive and effective alternative to ET electrodes.

In a prospective clinical cohort study of 25 patients, Van Slycke et al. (21) affixed electrodes directly to the TC perichondrium with two stitches. Compared to ET electrodes, the TC electrodes obtained higher EMG amplitudes induced by stimulation of the VN, RLN and external branch of the superior laryngeal nerve (EBSLN). Liddy et al. (20) proposed and evaluated the use of adhesive dragonfly bipolar surface electrodes (Neurovision Medical, Inomed, Medtronic & Stryker) in 15 consecutive patients undergoing monitored thyroid and parathyroid surgery. Their approach entailed cutting the adhesive electrode in half to create two recording surfaces and then positioning the electrodes over the TC on either side of the midline. The electrodes were then secured by suturing them to the perichondrium. Their experiments again demonstrated that, compared to ET electrodes, adhesive transcartilage AL electrodes provide EMG signals with comparable stability and amplitude and have comparable sensitivity in recording evoked responses during IONM. Additionally, since adhesive transcartilage AL electrodes are accessible in the operative field, they are easily monitored and controlled by the surgeon, and they are unaffected by potential ET displacement during surgery (20). Finally, since transcartilage AL electrodes enable robust EBSLN monitoring, they reduce the risk of high-pitched voice function loss in thyroid and parathyroid surgery (30).

In pediatric patients, anatomical characteristics, e.g., smaller RLN diameter compared to adults, can make IONM challenging. One consensus statement suggested that IONM is beneficial in pediatric patients with a bulky thyroid and lymph node disease (31). Since the larynx and trachea are relatively small in pediatric patients, the limited selection of commercially available ET electrode sizes combined with the increased difficulty of confirming ET electrode position in pediatric patients may result in unstable and inconsistent contact between the ET electrode and the vocal fold (28, 32). Huang et al. (28) compared electrode types in 33 pediatric patients who had received neuromonitored thyroid surgery and concluded that, compared to EMG signals obtained by ET electrodes, signals obtained by TC electrodes had superior amplitude, stability, and quality, which greatly facilitates the meticulous RLN dissection required in pediatric thyroidectomies, especially in pediatric patients with thyroid cancer.

PERCUTANEOUS ANTERIOR LARYNGEAL RECORDING

The feasibility of using TC perichondral needle electrodes as recording electrodes and their good signal stability have been well established in many animal and clinical studies. However, these electrodes require a standard neck incision for open exposure of the TC. That is, TC perichondral needle electrodes are inapplicable when invasiveness must be minimized and in remotely-performed endoscopic or robotic thyroidectomy. To overcome this limitation, Huang et al. (17) designed a novel IONM percutaneous recording method for remotely performed thyroid surgery (**Figure 1** and **Figure 2B**) in which pairs of insulated needle electrodes (lengths, 25 mm and 38 mm) were inserted percutaneously into the TC perichondrium to within 5 mm of the tip. The four most widely used remote thyroidectomy techniques (bilateral axillary-breast, transoral, transaxillary, and retroauricular approaches) were evaluated in animal experiments and in their initial case series. They concluded that percutaneous TC recording technique is feasible and can be modified according to the approach used for remote access. This technique reduces interruption of the surgical procedure while still providing reliable EMG signals (17).

Percutaneous AL recording during IONM in minimally invasive parathyroidectomy was recently reported by Li, et al. (25). The authors used paired 12mm long needle electrodes for percutaneous recording in 20 patients and successfully detected typical EMG signals. Based on their findings, the authors concluded that their technique is feasible, convenient, reliable, and cost-effective when IONM is used to assist minimally invasive thyroid or parathyroid surgery (25).

TRANSCUTANEOUS ANTERIOR LARYNGEAL RECORDING

In addition to transcartilage AL recording, transcutaneous AL recording is another innovative procedure that is proposed for modern IONM technology (15). **Figure 1** shows that transcartilage recording is effective for evaluating vocal fold muscle function and RLN function in TC, and transcutaneous recording may be effective for the same purpose.

Technical advances in epidermal electronics now enable fabrication of sensors in the ideal form can be affixed as an electronic second skin. In 2018, Wu et al. used a porcine model with well-established applicability in IONM research to verify the hypothesis of transcutaneous AL recording. Electrically evoked EMGs were recorded from surface electrodes attached to the ET and from adhesive pre-gelled surface electrodes (Neotrode II®-ConMed) attached to the anterior neck skin. In their experiments, ET electrodes and neck adhesive skin electrodes successfully recorded typical evoked laryngeal EMG waveforms from RLNs and VNs under 1 mA stimulation. Additionally, both electrode types accurately detected adverse EMG events under experimentally induced RLN traction stress. Under experimentally induced tracheal displacement, however, EMG signals obtained by ET electrodes widely varied whereas EMG signals obtained by transcutaneous electrodes were stable (15). Although this proof-of-concept study confirmed the stability and accuracy of EMG signals obtained by transcutaneous approach, it also revealed the need for new electrode designs that provide more consistent and accurate EMG amplitudes before practical clinical application of this approach.

In 2020, Lee et al. (26) performed the first clinical study to evaluate the efficacy of transcutaneous AL recording during monitored thyroidectomy. A disposable pre-gelled adhesive surface electrode (1.5 cm x 2.0 cm x 2.5 cm; DSE3125; Medtronic Xomed; Jacksonville, FL, USA) was attached to each of the two upper margins of the TC surface. The setup time for the skin electrodes was less than 1 minute in all cases. Their experimental results confirmed the effectiveness of IONM for recording evoked biphasic EMG signals of acceptable quality in all at-risk nerves.

Recently, Shin et al. (29) investigated the optimal attachment location of transcutaneous adhesive skin electrodes for IONM. In porcine animal model, the mean amplitude obtained using laterally attached transcutaneous electrodes was significantly higher than that obtained using medially attached skin surface electrodes. However, there was no significant difference in amplitude according to vertical levels (upper/middle/lower). In human patients, they reported that the ET electrode (716.25 ± 543.35 μV) showed a significantly higher mean amplitude than laterally attached transcutaneous electrodes (258.48 ± 77.31 μV), and the laterally attached transcutaneous electrodes showed a significantly higher mean amplitude than the medially attached skin electrodes (185.22 ± 66.56 μV) on RLN stimulation. Therefore, they concluded that transcutaneous recording is feasible and the lateral side of the thyroid cartilage lamina may be better than the medial side for electrode attachment to obtain better EMG signals from the intrinsic laryngeal muscles.

DISCUSSION

Although thyroid surgery is now a commonly performed procedure worldwide, RLN injuries are still common complications and a major cause of low satisfaction with thyroid surgery outcomes and medical malpractice litigation. Use of IONM in thyroid surgery has become well established in the past two decades, and surgical applications of IONM are increasingly accepted throughout the world. Recent registry-based studies performed in Sweden (SQRTPA) (33), Europe (EUROCRINE®) (34), United Kingdom (UKRETS) (35), and other regions (36) provide insight into current IONM practices. Most studies agree that a large and growing majority of thyroid surgeons currently use IONM for anatomical identification of the RLN and for evaluating RLN injury. Another common motivation for using IONM is to reduce the risk of temporary and permanent RLN paralysis.

The most important issue when IONM is performed using an ETT as the recording side is that IONM has a high negative predictive value (92%-100%) but a relatively low and variable positive predictive value (10%-90%) (37). The IONM recording quality (i.e., stability and consistency) depends on the stability of contact between the ET electrodes and the vocal folds, and contact quality may vary widely during surgical manipulations. Therefore, alternative electrode types such as transcartilage, percutaneous, and transcutaneous AL recording electrodes have been extensively studied in recent years to minimize factors that negatively affect ET-IONM accuracy and efficacy. This article presents a complete overview of state-of-the-art transcartilage, percutaneous, and transcutaneous AL recording techniques used in IONM and compares their contribution to improved voice outcomes in modern thyroid surgery.

This is the first comprehensive review in the literature of IONM with transcartilage (14, 16, 18–24, 27, 28), percutaneous (17, 25), and transcutaneous (15, 26) AL recording electrodes. The techniques are illustrated (**Figure 1**), major findings of each study are summarized and highlighted (**Table 1**), and the pros and cons of each method are discussed and compared (**Figure 2**, **Figure 3** and **Table 2**). In comparison with conventional ET recording IONM, advantages of AL recording IONM reported in both animal and clinical studies include lower invasiveness, better quality and stability of EMG signals, and avoidance of time-consuming disturbances such as the need to verify the ET position. In addition, the high reliability and quality of EMG response making these recording methods not only useful during routine ordinary thyroid and parathyroid surgery, but also practical during thyroid surgery with small incision, remote access, and in specific (e.g., pediatric) populations. In addition to ensuring stable EMG signals, AL recording IONM has several advantages. First, the equipment setup is user-friendly; reported setup times approximate 2 minutes for transcartilage needle electrodes (19) and less than 1 minute for transcutaneous electrodes (26). Second, only a short setup time is required for rapid implementation when an unexpected need for IONM occurs during surgery. Third, dislodged electrodes can be identified and managed intraoperatively. Finally, AL electrodes are apparently more cost effective than ET electrodes (28). A pair of adhesive pre-gelled electrodes or needle electrodes can be purchased for the equivalent of less than 100 USD, which is at least five-fold lower than the cost of EMG ET electrodes.

Whereas these novel techniques are apparently practicable and have no major disadvantages in most clinical applications, disadvantages of transcartilage electrodes include the higher skin flap elevation required to expose the TC (**Figure 2A**), and the difficulty of manipulating the electrodes in procedures performed within a limited operative space, e.g., in endoscopic thyroidectomy or in procedures in which the size of the incision is minimized to improve cosmetic outcome. Additionally, a needle electrode insertion may be complicated by scar tissue caused by revision surgery or, in older adults, by calcified TC, both of which can substantially impair recording of compound muscle action potential responses (14). Finally, patients undergoing such procedures have a low but still risk of laryngeal hematoma, laceration, infection, or rupture of an endotracheal cuff, especially in procedures performed with needle electrodes. Therefore, the recommendation is to insert the needle gently into the subperichondrium of the middle thyroid lamina from the anterior margin of the thyrohyoid muscle with a 10- to 15-degree slope on each side (22).

Although percutaneous AL electrodes are applicable in small incision thyroid and parathyroid surgery and in remote thyroidectomy, insertion of needle electrodes into the TC should be performed with extreme caution to avoid inadvertent injury to the cricothyroid muscle or EBSLN, which can cause muscular hematoma or scar tissue formation and subsequent alterations in vocal pitch. Additionally, percutaneous needle recording electrodes can inadvertently record far field potentials. Therefore, the recommended practices are confirming the stimulation site and comparing corresponding VN, RLN, or EBSLN waveforms, and adjusting the current intensity to minimize recording of far field potentials. Finally, excessive skin retraction or the use of skin retraction for counter-traction during remote thyroidectomy (17) could cause percutaneous needle displacement (**Figure 2B**).

Although transcutaneous AL recording in IONM has proven feasible and reliable, further technical refinement is needed to address some technical flaws. The skin electrode could be affected by patient characteristics such as obese or short neck,

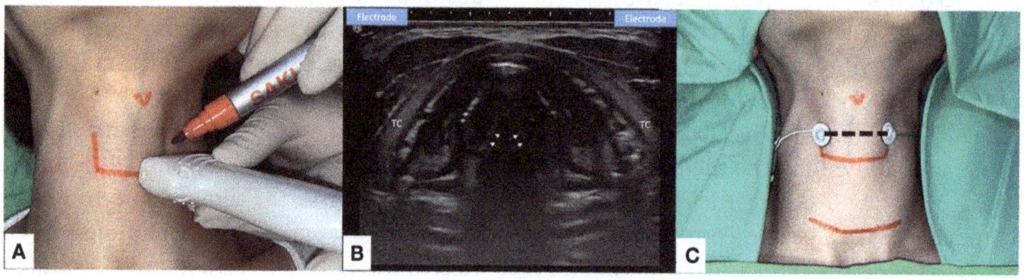

FIGURE 3 | Transcutaneous Anterior Laryngeal Recording electrode placement for Intraoperative neural monitoring. **(A)** Preoperative skin marking: lateral border of thyroid cartilage and the level of true vocal fold. Precise localization may be done with the application of ultrasound (US). **(B)** The axial view of true vocal folds (white arrow). Lateral side of the thyroid cartilage (TC) lamina is the optimal location to place the skin surface electrodes (US illustration). **(C)** Transcutaneous recording electrodes are placed at the level of true vocal fold (dotted line). Transcutaneous recording method is applicable in small incision wound or remote thyroid surgery. Skin flap beneath the surface electrodes should be avoided.

degree of subplatysmal flap elevation, and large tumor size. During surgery, subplatysmal flap and retraction of the strap muscle during dissection of the thyroid upper pole may hinder neural signal transmission. The EMG signals actually recorded after upper pole dissection might also be diminished (38). Therefore, this technique may not be useful in procedures that require a large incision or involve a large tumor size (15). Additionally, since both animal and clinical studies agree that low amplitude remains the major limitation of this technique, further research is needed to improve electrode designs and recording quality. Shin et al. (29) suggest that the lower amplitude could be overcome by attaching the skin electrodes more laterally and close to the cricoarytenoid joint. Therefore, the authors of this review suggest the surgeons may consider using ultrasonography to decide the optimal location of the AL electrodes preoperatively (**Figure 3**).

In summary, this review of the recent literature regarding the feasibility, stability, safety, and efficiency of new and emerging techniques for obtaining transcartilage, percutaneous, or transcutaneous AL recordings during IONM found that recently developed techniques increase the potential applications of IONM as a high-quality quantitative tool in thyroid and parathyroid surgery. However, this review also revealed that most clinical studies have enrolled a relatively small number of patients. Therefore, future prospective studies in larger populations are needed to explore and verify the applicability and benefits of these techniques. Several novel techniques that can further improve AL recordings have been recently reported in the literature. One study uses a nanosheet-based microneedle for EMG recording, which minimizes the risk of laryngeal injury caused by needle insertion (39). Instead of using electrophysiologic laryngeal EMG to evaluate muscle movement, several recent animal studies have also evaluated the use of novel devices that use a piezo-electric surface pressure sensor (40, 41) or an accelerometer sensor (42) to measure muscle twitch. Another interesting development is an "electronic skin" (e-skin) fabricated by embedding various serpentine sensors in a highly stretchable net sandwiched between two protective layers of equal thickness (43). Like a bandage, the device can be attached to the skin surface to acquire

TABLE 2 | The pros and cons of different AL EMG recording techniques during neuromonitored thyroid and parathyroid surgery.

Technique	Advantages	Disadvantages
Transcartilage	(1). EMG signal shows less affected by surgical manipulation and is comparable sensitive in reflecting a neurophysiologic event* (2). Cost-effectiveness and surgeon-friendly electrode setup* (3). Higher (needle electrode) or comparable (adhesive electrode) EMG amplitudes* (4). Enable of more robust EBSLN monitoring* (5). Suitable for pediatric and tracheostomy cases	(1). Requires an adequate skin flap elevation to expose the thyroid cartilage, limit of use in procedures with small or no neck incision wound. (2). Electrode (needle) insertion may be complicated by scar tissue caused by revision surgery or, in older adults, by calcified TC (3). Intralaryngeal penetration of (needle) electrode may cause laryngeal hematoma, laceration, infection, or rupture of an endotracheal cuff
Percutaneous	(1). and (2). same as Transcartilage method (3). High (needle electrode) EMG amplitudes recorded* (4). Feasible and useful for small incision and remote access procedures	(1). Longer electrode (needle) may be required according to different approach of remote access. (2). Electrode (needle) insertion may cause inadvertent injury to the cricothyroid or strap muscle, and can inadvertently record far field potentials. (3). Excessive skin retraction could cause percutaneous electrode displacement.
Transcutaneous	(1). and (2) same as Transcartilage/Percutaneous method (3). Biphasic EMG signals of acceptable quality recorded (adhesive skin electrode)	(1) The recorded EMG amplitude of skin electrode is relatively lower* (2) The electrode sensitivity could be affected by patient characteristics (short or obese neck), tumor size, and degree of subplatysmal flap elevation.

**as compared to EMG endotracheal tube recording.*

AL, anterior laryngeal; EMG, electromyography; TC, thyroid cartilage; EBSLN, external branch of superior laryngeal nerve.

physiological information that may be applicable in transcutaneous AL recording. In the future, these sensors may be integrated in various transcutaneous, transcartilage or ET-base surface electrode designs for IONM recording during thyroid surgery.

CONCLUSION

In the current era in which quality of life is increasingly included as a surgical outcome measure, voice outcome after thyroidectomy is an important consideration for both patients and any clinician involved in managing such patients. Several methods and technologies are being developed to overcome the limitations and disadvantages of the current IONM system that relies on EMG ET recording. This article reviews major recent developments and progress in new and emerging transcartilage, percutaneous, and transcutaneous AL recording techniques used during IONM. In comparison with the conventional ET recording method, many experimental and clinical studies have shown that these up-to-date AL recording methods have advantages of lower invasiveness, better EMG quality and stability, and avoidance of time-consuming disturbances for ET position verification. In addition, these methods are not only feasible for routine ordinary thyroid and parathyroid surgery, but also practical during thyroid or parathyroid surgery with a small incision, remote access, and in pediatric operations. Additional advantages of AL recordings include a cost-effective and surgeon-friendly set-up, allow for rapid implementation when an unexpected need, and the dislodged electrodes can be easily identified and managed intraoperatively. Although there are still some limitations of each recording method, we believe the continuous practical application and implementation of these developments will further optimize IONM to the ultimate benefit of thyroid surgery patients.

AUTHOR CONTRIBUTIONS

CL, TY-H, CW-W, and GD conceived and designed the study. Administrative support was obtained by LF-W, HY-T, and YC-L. Provision of study materials by JW, L-PC, H-YT, Y-CL had collected and assembled the data. Data analysis and interpretation was done by F-YC, T-YH, and CL. All authors contributed to the article and approved the submitted version.

FUNDING

This study was supported by grants from Kaohsiung Medical University Hospital (KMUH109-9M44), Kaohsiung Municipal Siaogang Hospital/Kaohsiung Medical University Research Center grants (KMHK-DK (C)110009, I-109-04, H-109-05, I-108-02) and Ministry of Science and Technology (MOST 108-2628-B-037-006, MOST 109-2628-B-037-014, MOST 110-2314-B-037-104-MY2, MOST 110-2314-B-037-120), Taiwan.

ACKNOWLEDGMENTS

The authors would like to thank all authors of the papers included in this study, as well as participants in the contributing studies.

REFERENCES

1. Jin S, Sugitani I. Narrative Review of Management of Thyroid Surgery Complications. *Gland Surg* (2021) 10(3):1135–46. doi: 10.21037/gs-20-859
2. Dralle H, Lorenz K, Machens A. Verdicts on Malpractice Claims After Thyroid Surgery: Emerging Trends and Future Directions. *Head Neck* (2012) 34(11):1591–6. doi: 10.1002/hed.21970
3. Gualniera P, Scurria S, Mondello C, Asmundo A, Sapienza D, Gianlorenzo D. Narrative Review of Proving the Causal Link of Recurrent Laryngeal Nerve Injury and Thyroidectomy: A Medico Legal Appraisal. *Gland Surg* (2020) 9 (5):1564–72. doi: 10.21037/gs-20-203
4. Randolph GW, Kamani D, Wu C-W, Schneider R. 36 - Surgical Anatomy and Monitoring of the Recurrent Laryngeal Nerve. In: Randolph GW, editor. *Surgery of the Thyroid and Parathyroid Glands, 3rd ed.* Boston: Elsevier (2021). p. 326–59.e10.
5. Randolph GW, Dralle H, Abdullah H, Barczynski M, Bellantone R, Brauckhoff M, et al. Electrophysiologic Recurrent Laryngeal Nerve Monitoring During Thyroid and Parathyroid Surgery: International Standards Guideline Statement. *Laryngoscope* (2011) 121(Suppl 1):S1–16. doi: 10.1002/lary.21119
6. Tsai CJ, Tseng KY, Wang FY, Lu IC, Wang HM, Wu CW, et al. Electromyographic Endotracheal Tube Placement During Thyroid Surgery in Neuromonitoring of Recurrent Laryngeal Nerve. *Kaohsiung J Med Sci* (2011) 27(3):96–101. doi: 10.1016/j.kjms.2010.08.002
7. Lu IC, Chu KS, Tsai CJ, Wu CW, Kuo WR, Chen HY, et al. Optimal Depth of NIM EMG Endotracheal Tube for Intraoperative Neuromonitoring of the Recurrent Laryngeal Nerve During Thyroidectomy. *World J Surg* (2008) 32 (9):1935–9. doi: 10.1007/s00268-008-9549-1
8. Wu CW, Wang MH, Chen CC, Chen HC, Chen HY, Yu JY, et al. Loss of Signal in Recurrent Nerve Neuromonitoring: Causes and Management. *Gland Surg* (2015) 4(1):19–26. doi: 10.3978/j.issn.2227-684X.2014.12.03
9. Kim HY, Tufano RP, Randolph G, Barczynski M, Wu CW, Chiang FY, et al. Impact of Positional Changes in Neural Monitoring Endotracheal Tube on Amplitude and Latency of Electromyographic Response in Monitored Thyroid Surgery: Results From the Porcine Experiment. *Head Neck* (2016) 38(Suppl 1):E1004–8. doi: 10.1002/hed.24145
10. Barber SR, Liddy W, Kyriazidis N, Cinquepalmi M, Lin BM, Modi R, et al. Changes in Electromyographic Amplitudes But Not Latencies Occur With Endotracheal Tube Malpositioning During Intraoperative Monitoring for Thyroid Surgery: Implications for Guidelines. *Laryngoscope* (2017) 127 (9):2182–8. doi: 10.1002/lary.26392
11. Zhang D, Wu CW, Wang T, Zhao Y, Kim HY, Pino A, et al. Drawbacks of Neural Monitoring Troubleshooting Algorithms in Transoral Endoscopic Thyroidectomy. *Langenbeck's Arch Surg* (2021). doi: 10.1007/s00423-021-02217-6
12. Brauckhoff K, Vik R, Sandvik L, Heimdal JH, Aas T, Biermann M, et al. Impact of EMG Changes in Continuous Vagal Nerve Monitoring in High-Risk Endocrine Neck Surgery. *World J Surg* (2016) 40(3):672–80. doi: 10.1007/s00268-015-3368-y
13. Mazzone S, Esposito A, Giacomarra V. Continuous Intraoperative Nerve Monitoring in Thyroid Surgery: Can Amplitude Be a Standardized Parameter? *Front Endocrinol* (2021) 12:873. doi: 10.3389/fendo.2021.714699

14. Wu CW, Chiang FY, Randolph GW, Dionigi G, Kim HY, Lin YC, et al. Feasibility of Intraoperative Neuromonitoring During Thyroid Surgery Using Transcartilage Surface Recording Electrodes. *Thyroid Off J Am Thyroid Assoc* (2018) 28(11):1508–16. doi: 10.1089/thy.2017.0680
15. Wu CW, Chiang FY, Randolph GW, Dionigi G, Kim HY, Lin YC, et al. Transcutaneous Recording During Intraoperative Neuromonitoring in Thyroid Surgery. *Thyroid Off J Am Thyroid Assoc* (2018) 28(11):1500–7. doi: 10.1089/thy.2017.0679
16. Zhao Y, Li C, Zhang D, Zhou L, Liu X, Li S, et al. Experimental Study of Needle Recording Electrodes Placed on the Thyroid Cartilage for Neuromonitoring During Thyroid Surgery. *Br J Surg* (2019) 106(3):245–54. doi: 10.1002/bjs.10994
17. Huang TY, Lin YC, Tseng HY, Kim HY, Dionigi G, Lu IC, et al. Full Percutaneous Intraoperative Neuromonitoring Technique in Remote Thyroid Surgery: Porcine Model Feasibility Study. *Head Neck* (2021) 43 (2):505–13. doi: 10.1002/hed.26500
18. Zhao Y, Zhang D, Zhou L, Li S, Wang T, Li F, et al. Proprieties of Adhesive Surface Arrays to Thyroid Cartilage for Recurrent Laryngeal Nerve Monitoring. *Ann Trans Med* (2021) 9(8):690. doi: 10.21037/atm-21-1229
19. Chiang F-Y, Lu IC, Chang P-Y, Dionigi G, Randolph GW, Sun H, et al. Comparison of EMG Signals Recorded by Surface Electrodes on Endotracheal Tube and Thyroid Cartilage During Monitored Thyroidectomy. *Kaohsiung J Med Sci* (2017) 33(10):503–9. doi: 10.1016/j.kjms.2017.06.014
20. Liddy W, Lawson BR, Barber SR, Kamani D, Shama M, Soylu S, et al. Anterior Laryngeal Electrodes for Recurrent Laryngeal Nerve Monitoring During Thyroid and Parathyroid Surgery: New Expanded Options for Neural Monitoring. *Laryngoscope* (2018) 128(12):2910–5. doi: 10.1002/lary.27362
21. Van Slycke S, Van Den Heede K, Magamadov K, Brusselaers N, Vermeersch H. New Placement of Recording Electrodes on the Thyroid Cartilage in Intra-Operative Neuromonitoring During Thyroid Surgery. *Langenbeck's Arch Surg* (2019) 404(6):703–9. doi: 10.1007/s00423-019-01825-7
22. Chiang FY, Wu CW, Chang PY, Wu SH, Chen HY, Lin YC, et al. Trans-Thyroid Cartilage Recording for Neural Monitoring of the Recurrent Laryngeal Nerve in Thyroid Surgery. *Laryngoscope* (2020) 130(4):E280–e3. doi: 10.1002/lary.28049
23. Jung SM, Tae K, Song CM, Lee SH, Jeong JH, Ji YB. Efficacy of Transcartilaginous Electrodes for Intraoperative Neural Monitoring During Thyroid Surgery. *Clin Exp otorhinolaryngol* (2020) 13(4):422–8. doi: 10.21053/ceo.2019.01529
24. Lee HS, Seo SG, Kim DY, Kim SW, Choi Y, Lee KD. Intraoperative Neuromonitoring Using a Single Transcartilage Needle Electrode During Thyroidectomy. *Laryngoscope* (2021) 131(2):448–52. doi: 10.1002/lary.28835
25. Li P, Liang QZ, Wang DL, Han B, Yi X, Wei W, et al. The Transcutaneous Electromyography Recording Method for Intraoperative Neuromonitoring of Recurrent Laryngeal Nerve During Minimally Invasive Parathyroidectomy. *Sci Rep* (2020) 10(1):7609. doi: 10.1038/s41598-020-64675-0
26. Lee HS, Oh J, Kim SW, Jeong YW, Wu CW, Chiang FY, et al. Intraoperative Neuromonitoring of Recurrent Laryngeal Nerve During Thyroidectomy With Adhesive Skin Electrodes. *World J Surg* (2020) 44(1):148–54. doi: 10.1007/s00268-019-05208-3
27. Türk Y, Kıvratma G, Özdemir M, İçöz G, Makay Ö. The Use of Thyroid Cartilage Needle Electrodes in Intraoperative Neuromonitoring During Thyroidectomy: A Case-Control Study. *Head Neck* (2021) 43(11):3287–93. doi: 10.1002/hed.26810
28. Huang TY, Kim HY, Dionigi G, Lu IC, Chang PY, Chiang FY, et al. Laryngeal Neural Monitoring During Pediatric Thyroid Cancer Surgery-Is Transcartilage Recording a Preferable Method? *Cancers (Basel)* (2021) 13 (16):4051. doi: 10.3390/cancers13164051
29. Shin SC, Sung ES, Kwon HK, Cheon YI, Lee M, Lee JC, et al. Investigation of Attachment Location of Adhesive Skin Electrodes for Intraoperative Neuromonitoring in Thyroid Surgery: Preclinical and Clinical Studies. *Surgery* (2021). doi: 10.1016/j.surg.2021.07.037
30. Iwata AJ, Liddy W, Barczynski M, Wu CW, Huang TY, Van Slycke S, et al. Superior Laryngeal Nerve Signal Attenuation Influences Voice Outcomes in Thyroid Surgery. *Laryngoscope* (2021) 131(6):1436–42. doi: 10.1002/lary.29413
31. Stack BC Jr, Twining C, Rastatter J, Angelos P, Baloch Z, Diercks G, et al. Consensus Statement by the American Association of Clinical Endocrinologists (Aace) and the American Head and Neck Society Endocrine Surgery Section (Ahns-Es) on Pediatric Benign and Malignant Thyroid Surgery. *Endocr Pract* (2020) 43(4):1027–42. doi: 10.1002/hed.26586
32. Schneider R, Machens A, Sekulla C, Lorenz K, Weber F, Dralle H. Twenty-Year Experience of Paediatric Thyroid Surgery Using Intraoperative Nerve Monitoring. *Br J Surg* (2018) 105(8):996–1005. doi: 10.1002/bjs.10792
33. Bergenfelz A, Salem AF, Jacobsson H, Nordenström E, Almquist M. Risk of Recurrent Laryngeal Nerve Palsy in Patients Undergoing Thyroidectomy With and Without Intraoperative Nerve Monitoring. *Br J Surg* (2016) 103 (13):1828–38. doi: 10.1002/bjs.10276
34. Staubitz JI, Watzka F, Poplawski A, Riss P, Clerici T, Bergenfelz A, et al. Effect of Intraoperative Nerve Monitoring on Postoperative Vocal Cord Palsy Rates After Thyroidectomy: European Multicentre Registry-Based Study. *BJS Open* (2020) 4(5):821–9. doi: 10.1002/bjs5.50310
35. Abdelhamid A, Aspinall S. Intraoperative Nerve Monitoring in Thyroid Surgery: Analysis of United Kingdom Registry of Endocrine and Thyroid Surgery Database. *Br J Surg* (2021) 108(2):182–7. doi: 10.1093/bjs/znaa081
36. Feng AL, Puram SV, Singer MC, Modi R, Kamani D, Randolph GW. Increased Prevalence of Neural Monitoring During Thyroidectomy: Global Surgical Survey. *Laryngoscope* (2020) 130(4):1097–104. doi: 10.1002/lary.28210
37. Dralle H, Sekulla C, Lorenz K, Brauckhoff M, Machens A. Intraoperative Monitoring of the Recurrent Laryngeal Nerve in Thyroid Surgery. *World J Surg* (2008) 32(7):1358–66. doi: 10.1007/s00268-008-9483-2
38. Wong KP. Non-Invasive Recording During Intra-Operative Neuro-Monitoring in Thyroid Surgery: Omitting Surface Electrode and Oversize Endotracheal Tube. *Gland Surg* (2019) 8(4):312–4. doi: 10.21037/gs.2018.10.07
39. Yang Y-C, Lin Y-T, Yu J, Chang H-T, Lu T-Y, Huang T-Y, et al. MXene Nanosheet-Based Microneedles for Monitoring Muscle Contraction and Electrostimulation Treatment. *ACS Appl Nano Mater* (2021) 4(8):7917–24. doi: 10.1021/acsanm.1c01237
40. Sung ES, Lee JC, Shin SC, Kwon HG, Kim MS, Kim DJ, et al. Development of a Novel Intraoperative Neuromonitoring System Using a Surface Pressure Sensor to Detect Muscle Movement: A Rabbit Model Study. *Clin Exp Otorhinolaryngol* (2019) 12(2):217–23. doi: 10.21053/ceo.2018.01207
41. Sung ES, Shin SC, Kwon HK, Kim J, Park DH, Choi SW, et al. Application of Novel Intraoperative Neuromonitoring System Using an Endotracheal Tube With Pressure Sensor During Thyroid Surgery: A Porcine Model Study. *Clin Exp Otorhinolaryngol* (2020) 13(3):291–8. doi: 10.21053/ceo.2019.01249
42. Sung ES, Lee JC, Shin SC, Kwon HK, Na HS, Park DH, et al. Development of a Novel Intraoperative Neuromonitoring System Using an Accelerometer Sensor in Thyroid Surgery: A Porcine Model Study. *Clin Exp Otorhinolaryngol* (2019) 12(4):420–6. doi: 10.21053/ceo.2019.00423
43. Kim DH, Lu N, Ma R, Kim YS, Kim RH, Wang S, et al. Epidermal Electronics. *Sci (New York NY)* (2011) 333(6044):838–43. doi: 10.1126/science.1206157

22

Improving Voice Outcomes after Thyroid Surgery and Ultrasound-Guided Ablation Procedures

Pia Pace-Asciak[1], *Jon O. Russell*[2] *and Ralph P. Tufano*[3]*

[1]*Department of Otolaryngology – Head and Neck Surgery, University of Toronto, Toronto, Canada,* [2]*Department of Otolaryngology – Head and Neck Surgery, Johns Hopkins University, Baltimore, Maryland, United States,* [3]*Sarasota Memorial Health Care System Multidisciplinary Thyroid and Parathyroid Center, Sarasota, Florida, United States*

Correspondence:
Ralph P. Tufano
Ralph-Tufano@smh.com

The field of endocrine surgery has expanded from the traditional open neck approach to include remote access techniques as well as minimally invasive approaches for benign and malignant thyroid nodules. In experienced hands and with careful patient selection, each approach is considered safe, however complications can and do exist. Post-operative dysphonia can have serious consequences to the patient by affecting quality of life and ability to function at work and in daily life. Given the significance of post-procedural dysphonia, we review the surgical and non-surgical techniques for minimizing and treating recurrent laryngeal nerve injury that can be utilized with the traditional open neck approach, remote access thyroidectomy, or minimally invasive thermal ablation.

Keywords: thyroid surgery, radiofrequency ablation, dysphonia, voice, vocal cord dysfunction

INTRODUCTION

Thyroid surgery has been performed for thousands of years and still remains one of the more common head and neck procedures (1). With the modernization of thyroid surgery, the mortality rate has significantly dropped to less than 1% compared to 40% when in 1850, the French Medical Society banned these operations (2). The open neck approach that Kocher fathered is still used today, while newer methods to address thyroid nodules have evolved to address specific shortcomings. Such methods involve accessing the thyroid remotely with an endoscope in order to avoid a neck incision, or by minimally invasive techniques such as thermal ablation to avoid removing the thyroid gland at all. Regardless of the surgical approach, complications still exist.

In the hands of an experienced and high volume thyroid surgeon, complication rates may vary by disease pathology. Intraoperative injury to the recurrent laryngeal nerve (RLN) is one of the dreaded complications that can occur with open surgical approaches and less commonly with thermal ablation. Symptoms of unilateral vocal cord paralysis may include hoarseness, choking, dysphagia, and dysphonia with unilateral vocal cord paralysis, or symptoms of airway obstruction and stridor with bilateral vocal cord paralysis (3–6). Changes in the quality of voice or swallowing can significantly diminish a patient's ability to work, socialize and perform many activities of daily living, thus emphasizing the importance of careful handling of the RLN (7, 8).

For open neck approaches to the thyroid, approximately 1 in 10 patients experience temporary RLN injury after surgery, with longer lasting permanent voice problems in up to 1 in 25 (9). Other contributing factors which may lead to temporary dysphonia post-surgery include laryngeal irritation, edema or injury from intubation. Injury to the external branch of the superior laryngeal nerve can also impair a patient's quality of life by reducing the pitch and projection of the voice (10). For thermal ablation, namely radiofrequency ablation (RFA), injury to the RLN can be temporary or less frequently permanent (11–13). Voice changes are less frequently noted (0.94%, 21/2245) in benign nodules treated with RFA compared with recurrent thyroid cancer (7.95%, 14/176) (11). The overall complication rate in RFA treated primary benign nodules is 2.11% compared with 10.98% for malignant thyroid nodules (11).

In this paper, we review the surgical and nonsurgical techniques for minimizing and treating post-operative dysphonia caused by an open approach or remote access thyroidectomy as well as minimally invasive thermal ablation (namely radiofrequency ablation). In addition, we review how intraoperative electromyographic (EMG) changes correlate to post-operative voice changes, and how to treat weakness of the recurrent laryngeal nerve.

PRACTICE RECOMMENDATIONS TO MINIMIZE DYSPHONIA POST THYROID SURGERY

Visualization of the Nerve

The gold standard approach for preventing inadvertent injury to the RLN during thyroid surgery has always been meticulous dissection of the nerve in order to visualize its entry into the cricothyroid joint and/or course (14). Many prospective studies have confirmed Lahey's observation in 1938 (15) that clear visualization of the RLN during thyroid surgery significantly lowers the incidence of nerve injury compared to surgery without visualization (16–20). Yet the best method to prevent nerve injury has been greatly debated. Even with a visually intact RLN, function can been compromised (21). Generally, the rate of RLN paralysis is low in experienced hands for open neck approaches (temporary injury 2%–8%, permanent in 0.5%–3%), however the rate tends to be higher for malignant thyroid disease, enlarged goiters, Graves' disease, re-operative cases, anatomic variability and surgeon's inexperience (22–24).

Most often, surgeons take a lateral approach for dissecting the thyroid in order to identify the RLN. Fixed landmarks, such as the cricothyroid joint, is a helpful guide for localizing the entry point of the RLN into the larynx. In certain situations a medial approach can be advantageous in cases with a nonrecurrent RLN, a large Tubercle of Zuckerkandl, or in cases with extrathyroidal extension of cancer along the distal RLN segment (with the exception of cricothyroid junction involvement), or large goiters (25). This approach allows for early and direct access to the RLN once the isthmus is divided and Berry's ligament is exposed (25). Care must be taken to avoid inadvertent injury when localizing the RLN with the medial approach since up to 80% of the time, the RLN is located superficial to Berry's ligament, and below it 15% of the time (26).

Intraoperative Nerve Monitoring

Over the past few decades, intraoperative nerve monitoring (IONM) has gained acceptance as an adjunct to nerve visualization during thyroid surgery and is used by most high volume thyroid surgeons in North America (27). The American Academy of Otolaryngology – Head and Neck Surgery guidelines have recommended its use, and it has become the standard of care at most institutions. Regardless of whether the surgeon has high-volume or low-volume experience, most would argue that IONM can aid the surgeon through difficult anatomical situations should the surgical field be impaired by bleeding, scarring or tumor infiltration that may complicate a clean dissection. However, IONM does not replace knowledge of the head and neck anatomy.

Whether IONM conveys a real advantage over no monitoring at all continues to be debated by endocrine surgeons (3, 14, 22, 23, 28–31). Barczynski et al. and others have demonstrated statistically lower rates for transient RLN paralysis with IONM compared with visualization alone (32). Whereas, Higgins et al., did not report a statistically significant difference in the overall incidence of true vocal fold palsy (3.52%) for IONM compared with (3.12%) for nerve identification alone (31). In a Cochrane analysis, the rates of permanent RLN palsy (RR 0.77, 95% CI 0.33 to 1.77; $P = 0.54$; 4 trials; 2895 nerves at risk; very low-certainty evidence) and transient RLN palsy (RR 0.62, 95% CI 0.35 to 1.08; $P = 0.09$; 4 trials; 2895 nerves at risk; very low-certainty evidence) when IONM was compared with nerve visualization alone did not conclude firm evidence showing an advantage or disadvantage for prevention of RLN injury (23). However, in Zheng's meta-analysis of over 12 different trials which included 36,487 participants, IONM was found to decrease the risk of transient RLN palsy, but had no significant effect on the permanent rate of injury (32).

The most widely available IONM system is one where two surface electrodes embedded in the endotracheal tube are positioned so they contact the vocal folds during intubation. This allows the surgeon to intermittently monitor the RLN or the vagus nerve with a handheld probe once the nerve has been surgically isolated (3, 27). This system is useful for confirming the localization of the RLN, for identifying whether there is a loss of signal from nerve injury, and to guide decision making for whether to stage the surgery in the case of an ipsilateral loss of signal during a bilateral procedure (3, 27, 33). Intermittent IONM has its limitations, namely the need to maintain constant contact with the surface electrodes on the endotracheal tube and the vocal folds to obtain an accurate EMG recording. Should the endotracheal tube shift during surgical manipulation, a false decrease or loss in the EMG signal can result. Once the surgery is in progress, it can be disruptive for the surgeon or the anesthetist to reposition the tube, particularly during remote access surgeries such as the transoral robotic approach (34). Various newer approaches have emerged to circumvent these limitations (33, 34).

Continuous IONM has evolved to circumvent the limitations of intermittent IONM so that nerve monitoring can occur continuously and in real time. It is beneficial for the early detection and prevention of thermal or traction injuries, thus allowing the surgeon to take immediate action if a change in the EMG is noted (28, 29). Some studies have noted improved outcomes with continuous monitoring relative to intermittent monitoring, which has spurred adoption in some centers (35). In a comparative study, Schneider et al., examined a total of 6029 patients, of whom 3139 underwent continuous and 2890 intermittent IONM (35). Continuous IONM independently reduced early postoperative vocal cord palsy 1.8-fold (OR 0.56) and permanent vocal cord palsy 29.4-fold (OR 0.034) compared with intermittent IONM (35). Early postoperative vocal cord palsies were 17.9-fold less likely to become permanent with continuous IONM than intermittent IONM, demonstrating the advantage for using continuous monitoring in the right clinical scenario (35).

Hemostasis with Energy Based Devices

With the modernization of thyroid surgery, advances have included the use of energy-based devices (EBD) as an extension from the "clamp-and-tie" technique that Theodore Kocher fathered in the 19th century. Today, hemostasis can be achieved in multiple ways: clamp-and-tie, electrocautery (monopoloar or bipolar), with hemostatic clips, and more advanced EBD that use thermal, ferromagnetic, or ultrasonic energy to ligate, seal and dissect tissue (36). Even though more advanced techniques with EBD have demonstrated reduced pain, wound drainage, decreased rates of neck hematoma and even hypocalcaemia (37–40), the results for EBD are inconsistent in terms of rates of RLN injury compared with conventional approaches (41, 42). Several studies have demonstrated that traction and thermal injury are the first and second most common causes of iatrogenic RLN injury during thyroidectomy (39, 43, 44). As one would expect, the use of EBDs can generate high temperatures that can spread to critical structures such as the RLN causing indirect thermal spread or direct thermal injury (36). Thus, various guidelines are published to ensure that surgeons maintain a safe distance between the activated EBD tip and the surrounding soft tissue (36). It is also recommended that enough time lapses for the tip or blade to cool sufficiently before using the device to dissect tissue or work close to the RLN.

Depending on whether monopolar electrocautery or bipolar cautery is used, a safe distance must be maintained in order to protect critical structures. Care should be taken when using monopolar electrocautery adjacent to the RLN given that thermal spread is diffuse. In a porcine model, Wu et al. demonstrated that an activation distance of 5 mm is required to maintain safety with a cooling time of 1 s for monopolar electrocautery set at 15 Watts (45). For bipolar cautery the recommendations differ since the current is confined to the tissue between the two arms of the tines (forcep-shaped electrode). Wu et al. reported an activation distance of 3 mm from critical structures with a 1 s cooling time set at 30 Watts (45). For advanced bipolar EBDs such as the LigaSure Small Jaw and Ligasure Exact Dissector, Dionigo et al, recommend a safe activation distance of 2 mm with a 2-second interval for cooling the instrument tip before further dissecting tissue (46). Similar distances are noted for EBDs that deliver energy in the form of ultrasonic vibrations (such as the Harmonic) or Ferromagnetic energy (47). Regardless of the EBD used, surgeons should be aware of the device specific recommended distance needed for a safe dissection. The perception of distance may be altered in remote access surgery where the surgical field is closed and visualized via endoscope compared with traditional open neck approaches but is key for minimizing thermal injury and for improving voice outcomes.

Thermal injury to the RLN is more detrimental to voice outcomes than mechanical injury cause by traction or compression. Studies have demonstrated that thermal injury can cause irreversible changes to the nerve, damaging the endoneurium with temperatures at little as 60 Celsius (48). Most EBDs reach temperatures that exceed 200 Celsius when they are activated, and more than 350 Celsius with monopolar electrocautery (36). Additional care should be taken to avoid inadvertent injury to nearby structures when operating in a wet surgical field, as high temperature steam can be generated if the EBD is activated (49). Furthermore, surgeons should be aware and cautious when using EBDs as dissectors post-activation particularly during endoscopic approaches where the field of view can be limited.

Despite meticulous dissection along tissue planes, a slow oozing type of bleeding can still occur often around neural structures that are nourished by smaller vessels. The use of clips, cautery or ties adjacent to the nerve can pose risk. For this reason, various hemostatic agents have been developed in the form of a gel or patch to help mitigate this risk of a hematoma and nerve injury with cauterization. The use of such hemostatic agents, such as topical gels and patches have been shown to be a safe practice and does not put the RLN at risk. In a meta-analysis comparing the use of a topical hemostatic patch or gel to conventional methods for hemostasis, no significant difference between groups (patch 95% CI, 0.28, 5.52; gel 95% CI, 0.20, 2.47) were found in terms of risk to RLN injury (50).

PRACTICE RECOMMENDATIONS TO MINIMIZE DYSPHONIA POST THERMAL ABLATION WITH RFA

The true rate of RLN injury post thermal ablation is not known since studies examining pre- and post-procedure laryngoscopy are lacking. However, the overall rate of transient or permanent voice change following RFA is 1.44% based on subjective voice assessment (11, 51).

Since RFA is done in an outpatient setting with local anesthesia, temporary voice changes can be noted either during radiofrequency ablation (RFA) or immediately after the procedure. The most important approach for mitigating this potential complication is to carefully map the location of the target nodule by ultrasound in relation to the "danger triangle"; which is localized posterior to the thyroid capsule and adjacent to the trachea where the RLN runs (52). The only study which specifically examined the effects of RFA along the posterior thyroid capsule is found in a recent prospective study. Sinclair et al. demonstrated in thirteen benign nodules that abutted the posterior thyroid capsule, that RFA could safety be performed at a power of up to 40 Watts without laryngeal adductor reflex (LAR) amplitude changes measured by continuous intraoperative neuromonitoring (CIONM) (13). No significant difference between pre- and postoperative laryngoscopy and voice assessments were noted, and after 12 month follow-up, regrowth was not noted at the posterior aspect of the nodule (13). For nodules that extend beyond the posterior thyroid capsule, or for nodules that lack a cuff of normal thyroid tissue, surgery should be considered instead of RFA due to the risk to the RLN and the lack of tissue to buffer thermal spread, especially if the nodule is malignant.

While RFA can be completed under general anesthesia with nerve monitoring, most operators feel that local sedation offers an improved safety profile. One of the benefits of an outpatient procedure is the real-time feedback that patients can give the operator in terms of pain control, change in voice or breathing. An important way to monitor for thermal damage to the RLN during ablation is to maintain communication with the patient during the procedure. Prior to the thermal ablation, perithyroidal lidocaine is injected around the anterior or superficial thyroid capsule to reduce pain. By avoiding anesthesia of the deeper tissues, if pain is experienced during the procedure, it can be an early sign of thermal propagation to the surrounding tissue and the electrode can be moved and then power can be reduced by 5 to 10 Watts before proceeding further (12, 53). If patients note changes to their voice immediately post-procedure, most often it is transient and can be treated with a short course of Prednisone during their recovery period. Furthermore, when using RFA to ablate bilateral thyroid nodules, care should be taken to monitor for voice changes to avoid bilateral RLN paresis. The operator should have a low threshold for staging bilateral procedures should dysphonia be noted during RFA.

Another useful approach for minimizing injury to the surrounding tissue (ie. RLN) prior to ablation is hydro-dissection with 5% dextrose solution along the plane between the target tumor and adjacent critical structures. This creates a thermal barrier as well as a "heat-sink effect" which allows for heat to escape during ablation (54). Dextrose solution is the fluid of choice since it is iso-molar (252 mOsmol/L) and non-ionic in composition, thus safer than normal saline which is anionic and able to conduct electricity. If thermal injury is suspected post-procedure, Lee et al. describe injecting cold 5% dextrose solution into the tracheoesophageal groove post-ablation as an effective method for cooling the tissues and for reducing heat conduction to surrounding structures (55). Compression of the neck is not recommended since it may enhance heat conduction to the surrounding tissue.

The safest technique described for performing RFA is the "moving shot technique", which involves alternating the position of the electrode in the nodule so each theoretical sub-unit is ablated. This limits the frictional heat generated from the electrode tip by intermittent active movement and limits the time of ablation for each subunit to a few seconds compared to a fixed approach used in organs such as the liver (54). By using the trans-isthmic approach, which refers to insertion of a RF electrode through the isthmus, this allows the operator to be able to pivot from a midline to lateral direction to access different angles depending on whether the nodule is situated in the right or left thyroid gland, and enables the operator to ensure that the contents of the "danger triangle" can be protected (54). By inserting the probe in the midline, it allows the operator to effectively monitor the electrode tip using ultrasound guidance and to stabilize the needle should a patient talk or cough during the procedure.

Although multiple sized electrodes are available for targeting different organs, it is important to use thyroid-dedicated internally cooled electrodes for RFA given the superficial and intricate anatomy of the thyroid and neck. Generally, for the thyroid, RFA consists of a 7-cm internally cooled electro (shaft length) with an 18 or 19-gauge active tip that measures either 5 mm, 7 mm, 10 mm or 15 mm) with typical workhorse tips sizes of 7 mm or 10 mm depending on the patient population (54, 56). Depending on where the nodule is located, small active tips (3.8 mm) can allow for a more precise treatment limiting collateral thermal spread to nearby structures (54).

CORRELATION BETWEEN INTRAOPERATIVE ELECTROPHYSIOLOGICAL CHANGE OF RLN/EBSLN AND VOICE IMPAIRMENT IN THYROID SURGERY

If a loss of signal or a decrease in the EMG amplitude is noted intraoperatively and equipment malfunction or neuromuscular blockage has been ruled out, careful stimulation of the nerve with the probe from distal (the laryngeal nerve entry site) to proximal is recommended to identify the site of neuropraxic injury. This is typically done for open neck procedures compared with closed remote access techniques. Generally, nerve injuries identified through intraoperative neural monitoring are divided into two types: Type I (segmental) or Type II (global) injury (27). Segmental injuries can be corrected if a section of the nerve is entrapped with a clip or a suture, however for global type injuries, where all segments are nonconductive, an intralaryngeal focus is more likely.

Several papers have looked at the correlation between intraoperative EMG responses and postoperative vocal cord mobility. The International Neural Monitoring Study Group Guideline describes an impending adverse EMG even defined as an amplitude decrease of >50% of the initial baseline value, and an adverse EMG event is defined as an amplitude of <100 uV (14, 27). A true negative test is one where the EMG response is within normal limits at the end of surgery with intact vocal cord mobility postoperatively. Several studies have demonstrated that when the EMG has a robust response at the end of surgery, intact post-operative vocal fold functioning (the negative predictive value) is more than 95% (57–64). In a more recent review, Schneider et al., describe an even higher NPV for RLN palsy (97.3%–99.8%) when intermittent, and continuous (99.8%–100%) IONM is used (64). In contrast, if a loss of signal is noted on EMG at the end of surgery combined with immediate post-operative vocal cord paralysis, the outcome is a true positive test (27). However, for PPV, the rate is more variable due to transient versus permanent paresis, with a range of 37.8%–80.5% for intermittent, and 99.8%–100% for continuous IONM (63, 64). These values still translate into excellent outcomes with low rates of post-operative vocal cord palsy in experienced surgical hands, with early transient palsy 0.8%–10.5% for intermittent, and 2.6%–2.9% for continuous IONM (64). For permanent palsy, the rates are lower (0.2%–1.5% for intermittent, and 0%–1.0% for continuous IONM) (64). As a general rule, if there is an intact IONM signal at the end of the case, any post-operative voice changes are unlikely to be related to permanent RLN dysfunction.

VOICE AND LARYNGEAL ASSESSMENT BEFORE AND AFTER THYROID SURGERY AND THERMAL ABLATION

It is standard of care to assess the patient's voice prior to thyroid surgery or thermal ablation to establish baseline function that can be compared post-surgically. As part of the history, patients should be asked about subjective changes in their pitch, loudness, quality or power of their voice (65). Validated standardized methods can also be employed, such as the Voice Handicap Index. This 30-item questionnaire determines the degree of voice impairment and has been used as a tool to determine pre- and postoperative voice status after thyroid surgery (66, 67). During physical exam, all patients with subjective voice changes should receive a preoperative glottic exam to ensure normal baseline glottic functioning. Approximately 1% of patients with benign thyroid disease have vocal fold paresis or paralysis and in up to 8% of patients with malignant thyroid disease who have not undergone prior thyroid, neck or chest surgery (68). Given that a preoperatively diagnosis for vocal fold paralysis is suspicious for thyroid cancer, such as finding may alter the surgeon's approach to surgical resection as well as how the patient is counselled preoperatively regarding expected voice outcomes.

The most commonly available method for examining the larynx is by flexible nasopharyngoscopy. More traditional methods involve the mirror exam, but have increasingly been replaced by flexible nasopharyngoscopy. Video-strobo-laryngoscopy (VSL) is another way to do a detailed functional examination of the larynx, however is less readily available except in more laryngology-based practices.

SPEECH THERAPY AND INJECTION LARYNGOPLASTY FOR POST-THYROID PROCEDURE DYSPHONIA (PTD)

When a patient presents with complains of breathiness, dyspnea and/or mild dysphagia post-thyroid surgery, and vocal fold immobility has been confirmed on flexible nasopharyngoscopy, several options that can be offered. The management of symptomatic patients post-thyroid surgery varies from patient to patient but can include speech therapy, vocal fold injection, thyroplasty, reconstructive approaches for unilateral vocal fold paralysis and tracheotomy for bilateral vocal fold paralysis (**Figure 1**).

The clinical practice guidelines for improving voice outcomes after thyroid surgery recommend that assessment of voice is done within 2 weeks to 2 months post-thyroid surgery by the surgeon (65). If voice changes are noted, a laryngeal mirror or flexible nasopharyngoscopy is done to document whether vocal fold paresis is present. If the surgeon does not have the equipment to assess the vocal folds, a referral is made to an Otolaryngologist – Head and Neck surgeon for further management. Once a diagnosis of unilateral vocal fold paresis

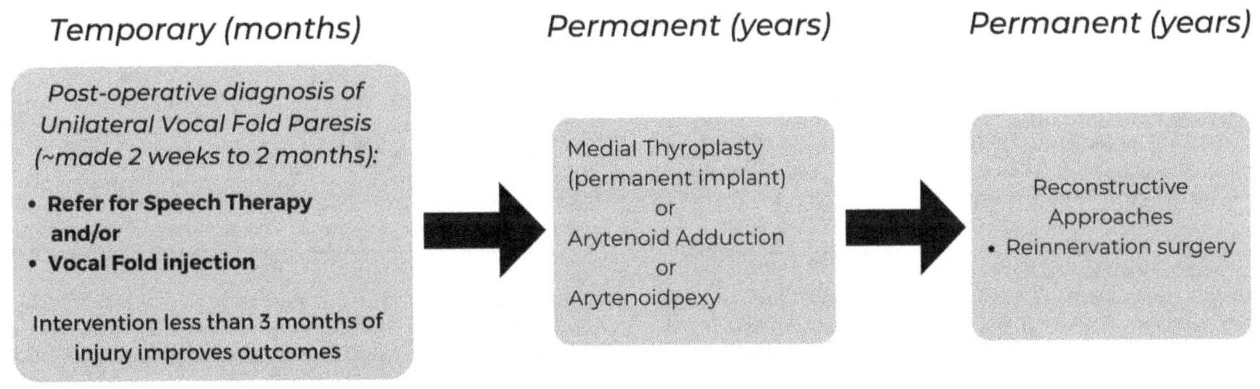

FIGURE 1 | Flow Chart summarizing the Management for Temporary and Permanent Post-Operative Dysphonia due to Unilateral Vocal Paresis.

is made or suspected, shared decision making with the patient regarding the next steps of management is made. Of note, the earlier the intervention with speech therapy and/or vocal fold injection (less than 3 months), the better the long-term outcomes in voice and swallowing for the patient (65).

Speech therapy focuses on rehabilitation of vocal fold approximation using behavioral approaches. The goal of voice therapy is to improve glottic closure by strengthening the intrinsic muscles of the larynx, rather than developing abdominal support for breathing and supraglottic hyperfunction (65). Procedural approaches include vocal fold injection, which is a temporary method to augment the immobile vocal fold to a more midline position. This outpatient procedure can improve laryngeal function by improving glottic closure during the recovery period, while also reducing the likelihood for permanent medialization laryngoplasty (69). In a retrospective review, Yung et al. demonstrated the benefit of temporary injection medialization in 19 patients with unilateral fold paresis compared with 35 patients who were managed conservatively (69). Those patients injected were significantly less likely to require permanent medialization laryngoplasty ($p = 0.0131$). In terms of the timing for injection medialization, Friedman et al., demonstrated the earlier the intervention, the better (70). In patients that had early injection medialization (less than 6 months from the time of injury to medialization), 62% (20/32) maintained an adequate voice obviating the need for open neck surgical reconstruction, whereas 100% (3/3) that underwent late injection (more than 6 months post paralysis) required surgical reconstruction ($P = 0.03$) (70).

For permanent unilateral vocal fold paralysis, medialization thyroplasty is an option to mobilize the vocal fold to a midline position through a small transcervical incision (71). Other permanent methods involve manipulating the laryngeal cartilage to perform an arytenoid adduction or arytenopexy (72, 73). These more advanced procedures involve an operating room setting and are generally done by surgeons with a laryngology based practice. Laryngeal reinnervation is another advanced procedure which is less commonly done, and typically performed by connecting the ansa cervicalis and the recipient RLN (74). Although there is a delay in voice improvement with this technique, it can partially improve the position of the vocal fold and provide bulk so long-term denervation atrophy of the laryngeal muscles is avoided (74). Often, the delay in voice improvement can be bridged with injection laryngoplasty. Depending on what was noted intraoperatively in terms of tumor involvement around the RLN, or transection of the nerve, decisions can be made to go directly to permanent solutions (such as medial thyroplasty, arytenoid adduction, arytenopexy or reinnervation surgery) if the nerve is deemed unlikely to recover.

CONCLUSION

Post-operative dysphonia has serious implications and consequences to patients, and thus, every effort should be taken to mitigate this complication. Various surgical and nonsurgical approaches can be taken reduce vocal fold injury during thyroid surgery as well as during thermal ablation. In symptomatic patients with RLN injury, various treatment options can be offered which range in behaviour therapy to more surgical type approaches to improve their quality of life.

AUTHOR CONTRIBUTIONS

PP-A contributed to the literature review and manuscript writing. JOR contributed to the revisions as well as the manuscript finalization. All authors contributed to the article and approved the submitted version.

REFERENCES

1. Haugen BR, Alexander EK, Bible KC, Doherty GM, Mandel SJ, Nikiforov YE, et al. 2015 American thyroid association management guidelines for adult patients with thyroid nodules and differentiated thyroid cancer: the american thyroid association guidelines task force on thyroid nodules and differentiated thyroid cancer. *Thyroid.* (2016) 26(1):1–133. doi: 10.1089/thy.2015.0020
2. Dorairajan N, Pradeep PV. Vignette thyroid surgery: a glimpse into its history. *Int Surg.* (2013) 98(1):70–5. doi: 10.9738/CC185.1
3. Schneider R, Randolph GW, Dionigi G, Wu CW, Barczynski M, Chiang FY, et al. International neural monitoring study group guideline 2018 part I: staging bilateral thyroid surgery with monitoring loss of signal. *Laryngoscope.* (2018) 128(Suppl 3):S1–S17. doi: 10.1002/lary.27359
4. Yu W-HV, Wu C-W. Speech therapy after thyroidectomy. *Gland Surg.* (2017) 6(5):501. doi: 10.21037/gs.2017.06.06
5. Borel F, Tresallet C, Hamy A, Mathonnet M, Lifante J-C, Brunaud L, et al. Self-assessment of voice outcomes after total thyroidectomy using the voice handicap index questionnaire: results of a prospective multicenter study. *Surgery.* (2020) 167(1):129–36. doi: 10.1016/j.surg.2019.05.090
6. Borel F, Christou N, Marret O, Mathonnet M, Caillard C, Bannani S, et al. Long-term voice quality outcomes after total thyroidectomy: a prospective multicenter study. *Surgery.* (2018) 163(4):796–800. doi: 10.1016/ j.surg.2017.09.023
7. Wilson JA, Deary IJ, Millar A, Mackenzie K. The quality of life impact of dysphonia. *Clin Otolaryngol Allied Sci.* (2002) 27(3):179–82. doi: 10.1046/j.1365-2273.2002.00559.x
8. Jones SM, Carding PN, Drinnan MJ. Exploring the relationship between severity of dysphonia and voice-related quality of life. *Clin Otolaryngol.* (2006) 31(5):411–7. doi: 10.1111/j.1749-4486.2006.01291.x
9. Jeannon JP, Orabi AA, Bruch GA, Abdalsalam HA, Simo R. Diagnosis of recurrent laryngeal nerve palsy after thyroidectomy: a systematic review. *Int J Clin Pract.* (2009) 63(4):624–9. doi: 10.1111/j.1742-1241.2008.01875.x
10. Roy N, Smith ME, Dromey C, Redd J, Neff S, Grennan D. Explorating the phonotory effets of external superior laryngeal nerve paralysis: an in vivo model. *Laryngoscope.* (2009) 119(4):816–26. doi: 10.1002/lary.20143
11. Chung SR, Suh CH, Baek JH, Park HS, Choi YJ, Lee JH. Safety of radiofrequency ablation of benign thyroid nodules and recurrent thyroid cancers: a systematic review and meta-analysis. *Int J Hyperthermia.* (2017) 33:920–30. doi: 10.1080/02656736.2017.1337936
12. Baek JH, Lee JH, Shung JY, Bae JI, Kim KT, Sim J, et al. Complications encountered in the treatment of benign thyroid nodules with US-guided

radiofrequency ablation: a multicenter study. Korean Society of Thyroid Radiology. *Radiology*. (2012) 262(1):335–42. doi: 10.1148/radiol.11110416

13. Sinclair CF, Tellez MJ, Pelaez-Cruz R, Diaz-Baamonde A, Ulkatan S. Continous neuromonitoring during radiofrequency ablation of benign thyroid nodules provides objective evidence of laryngeal nerve safety. *Am J Surg*. (2021) 222(2):354–60. doi: 10.1016/j.amjsurg.2020.12.033
14. Maneeprasopchoke P, Chongkolwatana C, Pongsapich W, Iwata AJ, Kamani D, Randolph GW. Intraoperative nerve monitoring in thyroid surgery: Analysis of recurrent laryngeal nerve identification and operative time. *Laryngoscope Investig Otolaryngol*. (2021) 6(2):354–61. doi: 10.1002/lio2.543
15. Lahey FH. Routine dissection and demonstration of recurrent laryngeal nerves in subtotal thyroidectomy. *Surg Gynecol Obstet*. (1938) 66:775–7.
16. Riddel VH. Injury to recurrent laryngeal nerves during thyroidectomy: a comparison between the results of identification and non-identification in 1022 nerves exposed to risk. *Lancet*. (1956) 29:638–41. doi: 10.1016/S0140-6736(56)92333-9
17. Jatzko GR, Lisborg PH, Muller MG, Wette VM. Recurrent nerve palsy after thyroid operations - principal nerve identification and a literature review. *Surgery*. (1994) 115:139–44.
18. Hermann M, Alk G, Roka R, Glaser K, Freissmuth M. Laryngeal recurrent nerve injury in surgery for benign thyroid disease: effect of the nerve dissection and impaction of individual surgeon in more than 27,000 nerves at risk. *Ann Surg*. (2002) 235:261–8. doi: 10.1097/00000658-200202000-00015
19. Steurer M, Passler C, Denk DM, Schneider B, Niederle B, Bigenzahn W. Advantages of recurrent laryngeal nerve identification in thyroidectomy and parathyroidectomy and the importance of preoperative and posteroperative laryngoscopic examination in more than 1000 nerves at risk. *Laryngoscope*. (2002) 112:124–33. doi: 10.1097/00005537-200201000-00022
20. Chiang FY, Wang LF, Huang YF, Lee KW, Kuo WR. Recurrent laryngeal nerve palpsy after thyroidectomy with routine identification of the recurrent laryngeal nerve. *Surgery*. (2005) 137:342–7. doi: 10.1016/j.surg.2004.09.008
21. Serpell JW, Phan D. Safety of total thyroidectomy. *ANZ J Surg*. (2007) 77(1–2):15–9. doi: 10.1111/j.1445-2197.2006.03897.x
22. Calò PG, Pisano G, Medas F, Pittau MR, Gordini L, Demontis R, et al. Identification alone versus intraoperative neuromonitoring of the recurrent laryngeal nerve during thyroid surgery: experience of 2034 consecutive patients. *Am J Otolaryngol Head Neck Surg*. (2014) 43:16. doi: 10.1186/1916-0216-43-16
23. Cirocchi R, Arezzo A, D'Andrea V, Abraha I, Popivanov GI, Avenia N, et al. Intraoperative neuromonitoring versus visual nerve identification for prevention of recurrent laryngeal nerve injury in adults undergoing thyroid surgery. *Cochrane Database Syst Rev*. (2019) 1:CD012483. doi: 10.1002/14651858.CD012483.pub2
24. Snyder SK, Sigmond BR, Lairmore TC, Govednik-Horny CM, Janicek AK, Jupiter DC. The long-term impact of routine intraoperative nerve monitoring during thyroid and parathyroid surgery. *Surgery*. (2013) 154(4):704–11; discussion 711–703. doi: 10.1016/j.surg.2013.06.039
25. Butskiy O, Chang BA, Luu K, McKenzie RM, Anderson DW. A systematic approach to the recurrent laryngeal nerve dissection at the cricothyroid junction. *J Otolaryngol Head Neck Surg*. (2018) 47(57):1–9. doi: 10.1186/s40463-018-0306-7
26. Henry BM, Sanna B, Graves MJ, Sanna S, Vikse J, Tomaszewska IM, et al. The Reliability of the tracheoesophageal groove and the Ligament of Berry as landmarks for identifying the Recurrent Laryngeal Nerve: a cadaveric study and meta-analysis. *BioMed Res Int*. (2017) 2017:1–11. doi: 10.1155/2017/4357591
27. Randolph GW, Dralle H, Abdullah H, Barczynski M, Bellantone R, Brauckhoff M, et al. International intraoperative monitoring study electrophysiologic recurrent laryngeal nerve monitoring during thyroid and parathyroid surgery: international standards guideline statement. *Laryngoscope*. (2011) 121(Suppl 1):S1–S16. doi: 10.1002/lary.21119
28. Phelan E, Schneider R, Lorenz K, Dralle H, Kamani D, Potenza A, et al. Continuous vagal IONM prevents recurrent laryngeal nerve paralysis by revealing initial EMG changes of impending neuropraxic injury: a prospective, multicenter study. *Laryngoscope*. (2014) 124(6):1498–505. doi: 10.1002/lary.24550
29. Dionigi G, Donatini G, Boni L, Rausei S, Rovera F, Tanda ML, et al. Continuous monitoring of the recurrent laryngeal nerve in thyroid surgery: a critical appraisal. *Int J Surg*. (2013) 11(Suppl):S44–6. doi: 10.1016/S1743-9191(13)60014-X
30. Sanabria A, Kowalski LP, Nixon I, Angelos P, Shaha A, Owen RP, et al. Methodological quality of systematic reviews of intraoperative neuromonitoring in thyroidectomy: a systematic review. *JAMA Otolaryngol Head Neck Surg*. (2019) 145:563–73. doi: 10.1001/jamaoto.2019.0092
31. Higgins TS, Gupta R, Ketcham AS, SataloK RT, Wadsworth JT, Sinacori JT. Recurrent laryngeal nerve monitoring versus identification alone on post-thyroidectomy true vocal fold palsy: a meta-analysis. *Laryngoscope*. (2011) 121(5):1009–17. doi: 10.1002/lary.21578
32. Zheng S, Xu Z, Wei Y, Zeng M, He J. Effect of intraoperative neuromonitoring on recurrent laryngeal nerve palsy rates after thyroid surgery - a meta-analysis. *J Formos Med Assoc*. (2013) 112(8):463–72. doi: 10.1016/j.jfma.2012.03.003
33. Sinclair CF, Tellez MJ, Ulkatan S. Continuous laryngeal adductor reflex versus intermittent nerve monitoring in neck endocrine surgery. *Laryngoscope*. (2020) 131:230–6. doi: 10.1002/lary.28710
34. Liu CH, Huang TY, Wu CW, Wang JJ, Wang F, Chan LP, et al. New developments in anterior laryngeal recording technique during neuromonitored thyroid and parathyroid surgery. *Front Endocrinol*. (2021) 12:763170. doi: 10.3389/fendo.2021.763170
35. Schneider R, Machens A, Sekulla C, Lorenz K, Elwerr M, Dralle H. Superiority of continuous over intermittent intraoperative nerve monitoring in preventing vocal cord palsy. *Br J Surg*. (2021) 108(5):566–73. doi: 10.1002/bjs.11901
36. Wang JJ, Huang TY, Wu CW, Lin YC, Tseng HY, Liu CH, et al. Improving voice outcomes after thyroid surgery - review of safety parameters for using energy-based devices near the recurrent laryngeal nerve. *Front Endocrinol*. (2021) 12:793431. doi: 10.3389/fendo.2021.793431
37. Moran K, Grigorian A, Elfenbein D, Schubl S, Jutric Z, Lekawa M, et al. Energy vessel sealant devices are associated with decreased risk of neck hematoma after thyroid surgery. *Updates Surg*. (2020) 72(4):1135–41. doi: 10.1007/s13304-020-00776-9
38. Canu GL, Medas F, Podda F, Tatti A, Pisano G, Erdas E, et al. Thyroidectomy with energy-based devices: surgical outcomes and complications—comparison between harmonic focus, ligasure small jaw and thunderbeat open fine jaw. *Gland Surg*. (2020) 9(3):721. doi: 10.21037/gs.2020.03.31
39. Dionigi G, Wu C-W, Kim H-Y, Liu X, Liu R, Randolph GW, et al. Safety of energy based devices for hemostasis in thyroid surgery. *Gland Surg*. (2016) 5(5):490. doi: 10.21037/gs.2016.09.01
40. Liu C-H, Wang C-C, Wu C-W, Lin Y-C, Lu I, Chang P-Y, et al. Comparison of surgical complications rates between ligasure small jaw and clamp-and tie hemostatic technique in 1,000 neuro-monitored Thyroidectomies. *Front Endocrinol*. (2021) 12:313. doi: 10.3389/fendo.2021.638608
41. Pacilli M, Tartaglia N, Gerundo A, Pavone G, Fersini A, Ambrosi A. Energy based vessel sealing devices in thyroid surgery: a systematic review to clarify the relationship with recurrent laryngeal nerve injuries. *Medicina*. (2020) 56(12):651. doi: 10.3390/medicina56120651
42. Garas G, Okabayashi K, Ashrafian H, Shetty K, Palazzo F, Tolley N, et al. Which hemostatic device in thyroid surgery? a network meta-analysis of surgical technologies. *Thyroid*. (2013) 23(9):1138–50. doi: 10.1089/ thy.2012.0588
43. Dionigi G, Wu CW, Kim HY, Rausei S, Boni L, Chiang FY. Severity of recurrent laryngeal nerve injuries in thyroid surgery. *World J Surg*. (2016) 40(6):1373–81. doi: 10.1007/s00268-016-3415-3
44. Dionigi G, Alesina PF, Barczynski M, Boni L, Chiang FY, Kim HY, et al. Recurrent laryngeal nerve injury in video-assisted thyroidectomy: lessons learned from neuromonitoring. *Surg Endosc*. (2012) 26(9):2601–8. doi: 10.1007/s00464-012-2239-y
45. Wu C-W, Huang T-Y, Chen H-C, Chen H-Y, Tsai T-Y, Chang P-Y, et al. Intra-operative neural monitoring of thyroid surgery in a porcine model. *JoVE*. (2019) 144:e57919. doi: 10.3791/57919
46. Dionigi G, Chiang FY, Kim HY, Randolph GW, Mangano A, Chang PY, et al. Safety of ligasure in recurrent laryngeal nerve dissection-porcine model using continuous monitoring. *Laryngoscope*. (2017) 127(7):1724–9. doi: 10.1002/lary.26271

47. Wu CW, Chai YJ, Dionigi G, Chiang FY, Liu X, Sun H, et al. Recurrent laryngeal nerve safety parameters of the H armonic focus during thyroid surgery: porcine model using continuous monitoring. *Laryngoscope.* (2015) 125(12):2838–45. doi: 10.1002/lary.25412
48. Lin YC, Dionigi G, Randolph GW, Lu IC, Chang PY, Tsai SY, et al. Electrophysiologic monitoring correlates of recurrent laryngeal nerve heat thermal injury in a porcine model. *Laryngoscope.* (2015) 125(8):E283–90. doi: 10.1002/lary.25362
49. Hayami M, Watanabe M, Mine S, Imamura Y, Okamura A, Yuda M, et al. Steam induced by the activation of energy devices under a wet condition may cause thermal injury. *Surg Endoscopy.* (2020) 34(5):2295–302. doi: 10.1007/s00464-019-07312-w
50. Khadra H, Bakeer M, Hauch A, Hu T, Kandil E. *Gland Surg.* (2018) 7(Suppl 1):S34–S41. doi: 10.21037/gs.2018.03.02
51. Orloff L, Noel JE, Stack Jr BC, Russell MD, Angelos P, Baek JH, et al. Radiofrequency ablation and related ultrasound-guided ablation technologies for for treatment of benign and malignant thyroid disease: An international multidisciplinary consensus statement of the American Head and Neck Society Endocrine Surgery Section with the Asia Pacific Society of Thyroid Surgery, Associazione Medici Endocrinologi, British Association of Endocrine and Thyroid Surgeons, Europoean Thyroid Association, Italian Thyroid Radiology, Latin American Thyroid Society and Thyroid Nodules Therapies Association. *Head & Neck.* (2021) 44(3): 633–660. doi: 10.1002/hed.26960
52. Ha EJ, Baek JH, Lee JH. Ultrasonography-based thyroidal and perithyroidal anatomy and its clinical significance. *Korean J Radiol.* (2015) 16:749–66. doi: 10.3348/kjr.2015.16.4.749
53. Park HS, Baek JH, Park AW, Chung SR, Choi YJ, Lee JH. Thyroid radiofrequency ablation: updates on innovative devices and techniques. *Korean J Radiol.* (2017) 18(4):615–23. doi: 10.3348/kjr.2017.18.4.615
54. Park HS, Baek JH, Choi YJ, Lee JH. Innovative techniques for image-guided ablation of benign thyrid nodules: combined ethanol and radiofrequency ablation. *Korean J Radiol.* (2017) 18(3):461–9. doi: 10.3348/kjr.2017.18.3.461
55. Lee MK, Baek JH, Chung SR, Choi YJ, Lee YM, Kim TY, et al. Effectiveness of injection cold 5% Dextrose into patients with nerve damage symptoms during thyroid Radiofrequency Ablation. *Endocrinol Metab.* (2020) 35:407–15. doi: 10.3803/EnM.2020.35.2.407
56. Jeong SY, Baek JH, Choi YJ, Lee JH. Ethanol and thermal ablation for malignant thyroid tumours. *Int J Hyperthermia.* (2017) 33:938–45 doi: 10.1080/02656736.2017.1361048
57. Tomoda C, Hirokawa Y, Uruno T, Takamura Y, Ito Y, Miya A, et al. Sensitivity and specificity of intraoperative recurrent laryngeal nerve stimulation test for predicting vocal cord palsy after thyroid surgery. *World J Surg.* (2006) 30:1230–3. doi: 10.1007/s00268-005-0351-z
58. Hamelmann WH, Meyer T, Timm S, Timmermann W. A critical estimation of intraoperative neuromonitoring (IONM) in thyroid surgery. *Zentralbl Chir.* (2002) 127:409–13. doi: 10.1055/s-2002-31982
59. Chan WF, Lang BH, Lo CY. The role of intraoperative neuromonitoring of recurrent laryngeal nerve during thyroidectomy: a comparative study on 1000 nerves at risk. *Surgery.* (2006) 140:866–72; discussion 872–873. doi: 10.1016/j.surg.2006.07.017
60. Thomusch O, Sekulla C, Machens A, Neumann HJ, Timmermann W, Dralle H. Validity of intraoperative neuromonitoring signals in thyroid surgery. *Langenbecks Arch Surg.* (2004) 389:499–503. doi: 10.1007/s00423-003-0444-9
61. Beldi G, Kinsbergen T, Schlumpf R. Evaluation of intraoperative recurrent nerve monitoring in thyroid surgery. *World J Surg.* (2004) 28:589–91. doi: 10.1007/s00268-004-7226-6
62. Hermann M, Hellebart C, Freissmuth M. Neuromonitoring in thyroid surgery: prospective evaluation of intraoperative electrophysiological responses for the prediction of recurrent laryngeal nerve injury. *Ann Surg.* (2004) 240:9–17. doi: 10.1097/01.sla.0000132260.34503.02
63. Dralle H, Sekulla C, Lorenz K, Brauckhoff M, Machens A. German IONM Study Group: Intraoperative monitoring of the recurrent laryngeal nerve and thyroid surgery. *World J Surg.* (2008) 32:1358–66. doi: 10.1007/s00268-008-9483-2
64. Schneider R, Machens A, Lorenz K, Dralle H. Intraoperative nerve monitoring in thyroid surgery – shifting current paradigms. *Gland Surg.* (2020) 9(Suppl 2):S120–8.
65. Chandrasekhar SS, Randolph GW, Seidman MD, Rosenfeld RM, Angelos P, Barkmeier-Kraemer J, et al. Clinical practice guideline: improving voice outcomes after thyroid surgery. *Otolaryngol Head Neck Surg.* (2013) 148(6S): S1–S37. doi: 10.1177/0194599813487301
66. Stojadinovic A, Henry LR, Howard RS, Gurevich-Uvena J, Makashay MJ, Coppit GL, et al. Prospective trial of voice outcomes after thyroidectomy: evaluation of patient-reported and clinician-determined voice assessments in identifying post-thyroidectomy dysphonia. *Surgery.* (2008) 143(6): 732–42. doi: 10.1016/j.surg.2007.12.004
67. Jacobson BH, Johnson A, Grywalski C, Silbergleit A, Jacobson G. The voice handicap index (VHI): development and validation. *Am J Speech Lang Pathol.* (1997) 6(3):66–70. doi: 10.1044/1058-0360.0603.66
68. Row-Jones JM, Leighton SEJ, Rosswick RO. Benign thyroid disease and vocal cord palsy. *Ann RCS Eng.* (1993) 75:241–4. PMID: 8379624 PMCID: PMC2497920.
69. Yung KC, Likhterov I, Courey MS. Effect of temporary vocal fold injection medialization on the rate of permanent medialization laryngoplasty in unilateral vocal fold paralysis patients. *Laryngoscope.* (2011) 121(10): 2191–4. doi: 10.1002/lary.21965
70. Friedman AD, Burns JA, Heaton JT, Zeitels SM. Early versus late injection medialization for unilateral vocal cord paralysis. *Laryngoscope.* (2010) 120 (10):2191–4. doi: 10.1002/lary.21097
71. Isshiki N, Okamura H, Ishikawa T. Thyroplasty type I (lateral compression) for dysphonia due to vocal cord paralysis or atrophy. *Acta Otolaryngol.* (1975) 80(5–6):465–73. doi: 10.3109/00016487509121353
72. Isshiki N, Tanabe M, Sawada M. Arytenoid adduction for unilateral vocal cord paralysis. *Arch Otolaryngol.* (1978) 104(10):555–8. doi: 10.1001/archotol.1978.00790100009002
73. Zeitels SM, Mauri M, Dailey SH. Adduction arytenopexy for vocal fold paralysis: indications and technique. *J Laryngol Otol.* (2004) 118(7):508–16. doi: 10.1258/0022215041615263
74. Aynehchi BB, McCoul ED, Sundaram K. Systematic review of laryngeal reinnervation techniques. *Otolaryngol Head Neck Surg.* (2010) 143(6): 749–59. doi: 10.1016/j.otohns.2010.09.031

23

Resistance to Thyroid Hormone Beta: A Focused Review

Theodora Pappa[1] *and Samuel Refetoff*[2*]

[1] *Division of Endocrinology, Diabetes and Hypertension, Brigham and Women's Hospital, Boston, MA, United States,*
[2] *Departments of Medicine, Pediatrics and Committee on Genetics, The University of Chicago, Chicago, IL, United States*

***Correspondence:**
Samuel Refetoff
refetoff@uchicago.edu

Resistance to thyroid hormone (RTH) is a clinical syndrome defined by impaired sensitivity to thyroid hormone (TH) and its more common form is caused by mutations in the *thyroid hormone receptor beta (THRB)* gene, termed RTHβ. The characteristic biochemical profile is that of elevated serum TH levels in absence of thyrotropin suppression. Although most individuals are considered clinically euthyroid, there is variability in phenotypic manifestation among individuals harboring different *THRB* mutations and among tissue types in the same individual due in part to differential expression of the mutant TRβ protein. As a result, management is tailored to the specific symptoms of TH excess or deprivation encountered in the affected individual as currently there is no available therapy to fully correct the TRβ defect. This focused review aims to provide a concise update on RTHβ, discuss less well recognized associations with other thyroid disorders, such as thyroid dysgenesis and autoimmune thyroid disease, and summarize existing evidence and controversies regarding the phenotypic variability of the syndrome. Review of management addresses goiter, attention deficit disorder and "foggy brain". Lastly, this work covers emerging areas of interest, such as the relevance of variants of unknown significance and novel data on the epigenetic effect resulting from intrauterine exposure to high TH levels and its transgenerational inheritance.

Keywords: resistance to thyroid hormone, thyroid hormone receptor, variant of unknown significance, autoimmune thyroid disease, thyroid dysgenesis, epigenetic effect

INTRODUCTION

The term resistance to thyroid hormones (RTH) refers to the clinical syndrome of reduced sensitivity to thyroid hormones (TH) first described in 1967 (1) and until recently it was synonymous with mutations in the *thyroid hormone receptor beta (THRB)* gene. In the past decade, mutations in the *THRA* gene, as well as genetic defects involving TH cell transport and metabolism were added to those of defects of TH action, broadening our understanding of impaired TH sensitivity (2–4).

This mini-review is dedicated to RTH due to mutations in *THRB* gene producing RTHβ, having as a signature elevated serum free iodothyronines levels but non-suppressed thyrotropin (TSH) in the absence of other conditions that may produce some of the characteristic test abnormalities. It focuses on emerging concepts, unusual associations and controversies involving diagnosis and management, while providing a succinct overview of RTHβ covered in most medicine and specialty textbooks (5, 6).

OVERVIEW OF RTHβ

As most neonatal screening programs are based on TSH measured in dry blood spots, the precise incidence of RTHβ is unknown. Surveys of 80,884 and 74,992 newborns using TSH and T_4 measurements identified 2 and 4 infants with *THRB* gene mutations indicating a prevalence of 1 in 40,000 and 1 in 19,000 live births respectively (7, 8). Frequency among sexes is equal, whereas prevalence may vary somewhat among ethnic groups. The inheritance of RTHβ is typically autosomal dominant. This is explained by the formation of dimers between the mutant and normal (wild-type; WT) TH receptor (TR) interfering with the function of the WT TRβ. Since the first description of a *THRB* gene missense mutation causing RTHβ (9), 236 different mutations in 805 families have been identified. They are located in the functional areas of the ligand (T_3)-binding domain and adjacent hinge region (10). In 14% of individuals manifesting the RTHβ phenotype no *THRB* mutations were identified. Rarely familial, they may be caused by mosaicism (11), whereas it has been postulated that mutations in enhancers, repressors or cofactors may be responsible for this subgroup of RTHβ (12).

The distinctive biochemical feature of RTHβ is high serum free iodothyronine levels (principally free T_4) with normal or high TSH concentration. This discrepant correlation has brought the term "inappropriate TSH secretion". Its wide use is deplorable as in fact the degree of TSH secretion is appropriate for the reduced sensitivity of the hypothalamic-pituitary axis to TH. Individuals with RTHβ maintain a nearly euthyroid state compensated by the high TH level in concert with the tissue expression level of the mutant receptor. Thus, features of TH deficiency and excess may co-exist, producing sinus tachycardia in the heart expressing mainly the WT TRα and goiter by TSH stimulation, as the pituitary expresses mainly TRβ including the mutant form. Visual disorders may also be present due to retinal photoreceptor dysfunction (13). Serum TSH determination remains the most sensitive test to determine reduced sensitivity to TH. In contrast, serum markers of TH action on peripheral tissues, such as cholesterol, creatine kinase, alkaline phosphatase, osteocalcin and sex hormone-binding globulin are less reliable, unless they are measured before and after administration of T_3 (14).

After excluding assay interference as a cause of discrepant thyroid function tests (15), the principal other condition to be considered in the differential diagnosis of RTHβ is TSH secreting pituitary adenoma (TSH-oma), particularly in the absence of family history. Thus, testing of first-degree relatives is helpful and cost effective. Characteristics of a TSH-oma include failure to suppress TSH after the administration of supra-physiologic doses of T_3, failure to normally stimulate TSH with TSH releasing hormone (TRH) (although exceptions of TSH-omas with TSH response to TRH have been reported), elevated sex hormone binding globulin levels and increased ratio of pituitary α glycoprotein relative to TSH (16). Co-secretion of growth hormone and prolactin and abnormal pituitary imaging on computerized tomography or magnetic resonance imaging are important diagnostic findings. However, incidental pituitary lesions may be found in up to 24% of patients with RTHβ (15), thus increasing the complexity in differential diagnosis and the value of hormonal investigation and dynamic testing. Conditions that increase the serum iodothyronine levels in the absence of thyrotoxicosis must be considered, including familial dysalbuminemic hyperthyroxinemia (FDH). In a recent study of Khoo et al., the presence of the albumin mutation R218H in FDH interfered with the measurements of free T_4 and T_3 by automated immunometric assays leading to misdiagnosis of FDH as RTHβ or TSH secreting tumor (17). The diagnosis of RTHβ becomes quite challenging in the presence of concomitant thyroid pathology, a subject addressed in greater detail below. Caution should be exercised in the reduction of TH levels with antithyroid medication and ablative therapies (radioactive iodine or surgery) as it leads to difficulty in the subsequent treatment of hypothyroidism.

COMBINED RTHβ AND THYROID DYSGENESIS

The diagnosis of RTHβ is challenging and its management complicated when it co-exists with other disorders, such as congenital hypothyroidism (CH) and thyroid dysgenesis. Children with RTHβ commonly have short stature, goiter and learning difficulties (14) and in association with CH will present high serum TSH and may exhibit hypothyroid symptoms when treated with standard levothyroxine doses. Five reports of RTHβ with CH due to ectopic thyroid tissue have been reported (18–22). Of note, the case reported by Guo et al., had a lingual thyroid with a typical RTHβ phenotype but no detectable mutations in the *THRB* gene (21).

Persistent serum TSH elevation is frequently encountered during the early treatment of CH despite reaching serum T_4 level in the upper limit of normal. This has been attributed to a delayed maturation of the T_4 mediated feedback control of TSH (23). Defining the cause of persistent TSH elevation and addressing it appropriately is of paramount importance, as undertreatment may adversely impact growth and mental development. When non-compliance and suboptimal treatment are excluded by measurement of serum T_4 and T_3, suspicion for co-existence of RTHβ should be raised and, when confirmed, treatment with supraphysiologic doses of levothyroxine aims to bring the serum TSH to near normal while following growth, bone maturation and cognitive development. When RTHβ and ectopic thyroid tissue co-exist, another reason to aim at TSH suppression is to prevent thyroid tissue expansion in anatomic locations, such as the base of the tongue, that may cause dysphonia and hemoptysis.

AUTOIMMUNE THYROID DISEASE AND RTHβ

Autoimmune thyroid disease (AITD) is a common thyroid condition affecting the general population and its coexistence with RTHβ has been considered incidental (24, 25). However, in a study of 330 individuals with RTHβ and 92 unaffected first-degree relatives, subjects with RTHβ had an over 2-fold higher frequency of positive thyroid auto-antibodies (26), suggesting that this association is not coincidental. A proposed pathophysiologic mechanism by the group of Gavin et al. invoked chronic stimulation of intrathyroidal lymphocytes by elevated TSH in RTHβ leading to pro-inflammatory cytokine production and thyrocyte destruction (27). Yet, in the study of Barkoff et al., the prevalence of AITD by age group was not influenced by the TRβ genotype which argues against high TSH being the cause of AITD (26).

Previous studies have shown that TH activates the immune system by acting on thymic epithelial cells and by direct effect on neutrophils, natural killer cells, macrophages and dendritic cells (28, 29). TH augments dendritic cell maturation and induces pro-inflammatory and cytotoxic responses. Given that dendritic cells are involved in the pathogenesis of AITD (30, 31), this might be a pathway mediating the association between RTHβ and AITD.

VARIABILITY IN RTHβ MANIFESTATION

RTHβ manifestations can be variable in tissue expression and in severity. The terms "generalized", "isolated pituitary" and "peripheral tissue" resistance have been used to describe different clinical manifestations of RTHβ suggesting tissue variability in the resistance to TH. The term generalized resistance to TH (GRTH) was applied to most patients with RTHβ that appear to maintain a euthyroid state whereas pituitary resistance to TH (PRTH) referred to patients with RTHβ that have symptoms of thyroid excess in peripheral tissues or demonstrate changes in peripheral tissue markers compatible to TH action without significant suppression of TSH (32). A single patient with presumed isolated peripheral RTH (PRTH) was reported, in whom administration of high dose of liothyronine (L-T_3) suppressed serum TSH but elicited no clinical signs of TH excess (33). Subsequently shown not to have a *THRB* gene mutation, this case likely represents acquired reduced sensitivity to TH through deiodinase-3 induced hormone inactivation. The clinical spectrum in RTHβ is quite broad and overlapping, even among carriers of the same *THRB* mutation and within the same family, suggesting that the classifications of generalized and pituitary RTHβ are rather semantics to describe a varying range of clinical signs and symptoms resulting from altered sensitivity to TH (34–36).

In some instances, the variability in the severity of the resistance to TH is readily explained on the basis of the character and position of the genetic defect. Homozygous *THRB* mutations are clinically more severe as they lack a WT TRβ and they interfere with the function of the WT TRα through heterodimerization (37, 38). Frame-shift mutations, producing a nonsense extension of the TRβ carboxyl terminus, interfere not only with ligand binding but also with interaction of the cofactors (39). Similarly, mutations with near normal ligand-biding can interfere with function through impaired binding to DNA (R243Q/W) (40, 41) and others (L454V and R383H) have altered binding to coactivators or corepressors (32, 42, 43) leading as in the case of R429Q (44) to more prominent suppression of TSH through predominant effect on genes negatively regulated by TH. Alberobello et al. (45) showed that when a single nucleotide polymorphism located in an intronic enhancer was associated with R338W, it produced pituitary specific over-expression of the mutant TRβ2 receptor illustrating the role of regulatory regions in tissue specific manifestation of RTHβ.

Differences in the level of expression of the mutant *THRB* allele relative to the WT in germline transmitted RTHβ have been shown in fibroblasts (46), but this was not found in another study (47). However, variable tissue expression of a mutant TRβ does occur in *de-novo* mutations resulting in mosaicism (11). The latter can also explain the failure to identify a *THRB* gene mutation in individuals with classical presentation of RTHβ when the only DNA source was circulating leukocytes. Finally, dramatic differences in phenotype observed among members of a family with the same *THRB* gene mutation have remained unexplained despite extensive genetic *in vivo* and *in vitro* functional studies (48).

CURRENT AND FUTURE TREATMENT APPROACHES

No specific therapy to fully correct the TRβ defect is currently available. Based on the mechanism producing the defect, it is clear that developing mutation-specific ligands would abrogate the dominant negative effect of the mutant TRβs, allowing the WT TRβ to elicit T_3 mediated thyroid hormone action. In 2005, the laboratory of the chemist John Kho synthesized TH analogues able to abrogate the dominant negative effect of the TRβ mutants R2320C, R230H and R316H when tested *in vitro* (49). More recently Yao et al. (50) showed that roxadustat, a drug used to treat anemia of renal failure, had 3- to 5-fold higher binding to the TRβ mutants V264D, H435L and R438H than T_3. However, none of these agonists have been tested *in vivo*. Similarly, the development of cell and tissue-specific TH antagonists could reduce the cardiotoxic effects of high serum TH levels acting on the WT TRα predominantly expressed in the heart. Therefore, as of this writing, management of TRβ is tailored to the individuals' symptoms resulting either from tissue TH excess or deprivation. Goiter, hyperactivity and mental "clouding" are clinical features that benefit from judicious treatment with L-T_3 without inducing side effects from TH excess.

Goiter is frequently observed in individuals with RTHβ but is usually of little consequence. However, in the occasion of larger symptomatic goiter, a surgical approach is usually ineffective, as goiter tends to re-occur. Therefore, it is logical to target TSH suppression to inhibit thyroid gland growth (51). An approach of administering supraphysiologic doses of T_3 every other day (250 μg in the case of TRβ R243Q) was successful in drastically reducing goiter size in a young patient without inducing thyrotoxic symptoms, as serum T_3 rapidly declined reaching levels lower than baseline before the ingestion of the next L-T_3 dose (52). The rationale is to deliver a large dose of the short lived L-T_3 to achieve very high peak serum level suppressing the TSH below 0.1 mIU/L to inhibit thyrocyte growth without sustaining elevated TH levels long enough to cause thyrotoxic symptoms (52). Thyroid nodules are quite prevalent in the general population and thus may occasionally co-exist with RTHβ. Although the majority of thyroid nodules are benign and do not require surgical management, there are few reported cases of papillary thyroid carcinoma in patients with RTHβ. In these cases, thyroidectomy and radioactive iodine ablation to prevent disease recurrence result in lifelong levothyroxine replacement therapy, and in RTHβ persistently high serum TSH. Although the outcomes in the reported cases were fortunately not unfavorable, levothyroxine therapy is challenging and supraphysiologic doses are often needed to maintain serum TSH in lowest tolerable level (53). Alternative options to consider include 3,3,5-triiodothyroacetic acid (Triac), a thyroid hormone analogue with thyromimetic effects on pituitary and liver tissue that may be used to suppress TSH, combination of levothyroxine with beta-blocker to alleviate tachycardia along with calcium and vitamin D supplementation to prevent bone loss acceleration. Lastly, surveillance strategy may be considered for occult, micro-papillary thyroid carcinomas with low potential for aggressive progression.

Attention deficit disorder (ADHD), reported in 48-83% of individuals with RTHβ, is treated using conventional drugs. When such medications are ineffective, treatment with L-T_3 was found beneficial in reducing impulsivity in 5 of 8 and hyperactivity in 4 of 7 individuals with RTHβ and ADHD but not in individuals with ADHD only (54). Every-other-day L-T_3 therapy was also effective to improve the insomnia and hyperactivity in a young child with severe RTHβ phenotype intolerant to daily L-T_4 therapy (55).

The success of treatment with intermittent high dose L-T_3 in improving brain function seems to be linked to the reduction of serum T_4, a hormone more readily available to the brain which expresses predominantly TRα, providing a thyrotoxic local environment. This would be the rationale to consider block-and-replace strategy, proposed by Dr. Alexandra Dumitrescu, and used by the senior author to ameliorate "foggy brain" and anxiety occasionally reported by RTHβ patients, whereas beta blockade may be employed to help with tachycardia.

Lastly, Triac with higher affinity than T_3 for several TRβ mutants may be used to diminish the dominant negative effect of a TRβ mutation. Further, though its short half-life, Triac can effectively reduce TSH with lesser thyromimetic effect on peripheral tissues (56). Triac therapy has been used in few RTHβ cases and was found beneficial in partially alleviating thyrotoxic symptoms including tachycardia, excessive perspiration, attention deficit disorders, as well as goiter. This was the case in patients harboring mutations in the ligand binding domain (residues 310-353 and 429-460), whereas two cases with mutations in the hinge region were refractory to Triac (56, 57). Notably, in a pediatric case of a homozygous *R243Q* mutation with features of thyrotoxicosis and early dilated cardiomyopathy, combination of Triac with methimazole resulted in reduction of thyroid hormones levels and normal TSH accompanied by lower basal metabolic rate and improved growth and cardiac function (58).

A summary of recommendations to guide clinical management of subjects with RTHβ is presented in **Figure 1**.

THE IMPACT OF *TRβ* VARIANTS OF UNKNOWN SIGNIFICANCE

The development of next generation sequencing (NGS) and its increased availability in clinical practice leads to identification of variants of unknown significance (VUS). These include variants of the *THRB* gene not previously reported to be associated with RTHβ. The interpretation of such genetic reports, particularly missense mutations, poses a problem to the practicing physicians; how to explain the findings to the patient and how to proceed with future care. *In vitro* functional analyses of VUS are not commercially available and results cannot be deduced with certainty even when they are.

THRB gene mutations are clustered in three regions of the ligand-binding domain of the TRβ. Yet a major region devoid of mutation ("cold area") contains CG-dinucleotides which are mutagenic hot spots. Artificial mutations created in these CGs produced TRβs weak in dominant negative effect explaining the failure to identify mutations in this region of the receptor (59). This is explained by the fact that the same region is included in the dimerization domain. This region originally encompassed codons 348-437. Later, with the identification of *THRB* gene mutations causing RTHβ, the "cold region" was narrowed down to encompass codons 384-425 (32, 60). Within this region, 12 variants (P384L, G385R, L386V, E390D, R391K, D397G, S398G, N408S, H413D, V414M, K420R, and V425L) were reported in the gnomAD database without information regarding clinical phenotype (61). Although most variants are considered benign based on *in silico* prediction algorithms, conflicting predictions were made for the P384L, D397G and K420R variants and the G385R variant was considered damaging (62). Recently, a 48 year-old patient with AITD, treated with levothyroxine, was found to have high free T_4 with non-suppressed TSH. A mutant TRβ G385E was identified and reported as VUS. Family screening uncovered the same mutation in relatives with normal thyroid function, suggesting that this mutation may not be responsible for the abnormal thyroid pattern (63). Similarly, the G339S variant was identified in a family with AITD after an individual was misdiagnosed with RTHβ, but the same variant was then found in several family members with normal thyroid function, making it unlikely for the G339S variant to be causally related to a RTHβ phenotype (24).

The above paradigms illustrate that *in silico* prediction algorithms may not always be reliable when studying the functional relevance of VUS. Genotype-phenotype co-segregation among family members is useful in characterizing the functional impact of *THRB* mutations. Computational resources that factor in protein specific functional domains may have some predictive functional relevance of VUS but should not be the basis guiding clinical decision making.

EPIGENETIC EFFECT OF RTHβ AND ITS TRANSGENERATIONAL INHERITANCE

The first body of evidence on fertility and pregnancy outcome in RTHβ came from studies in a large Azorean kindred harboring the

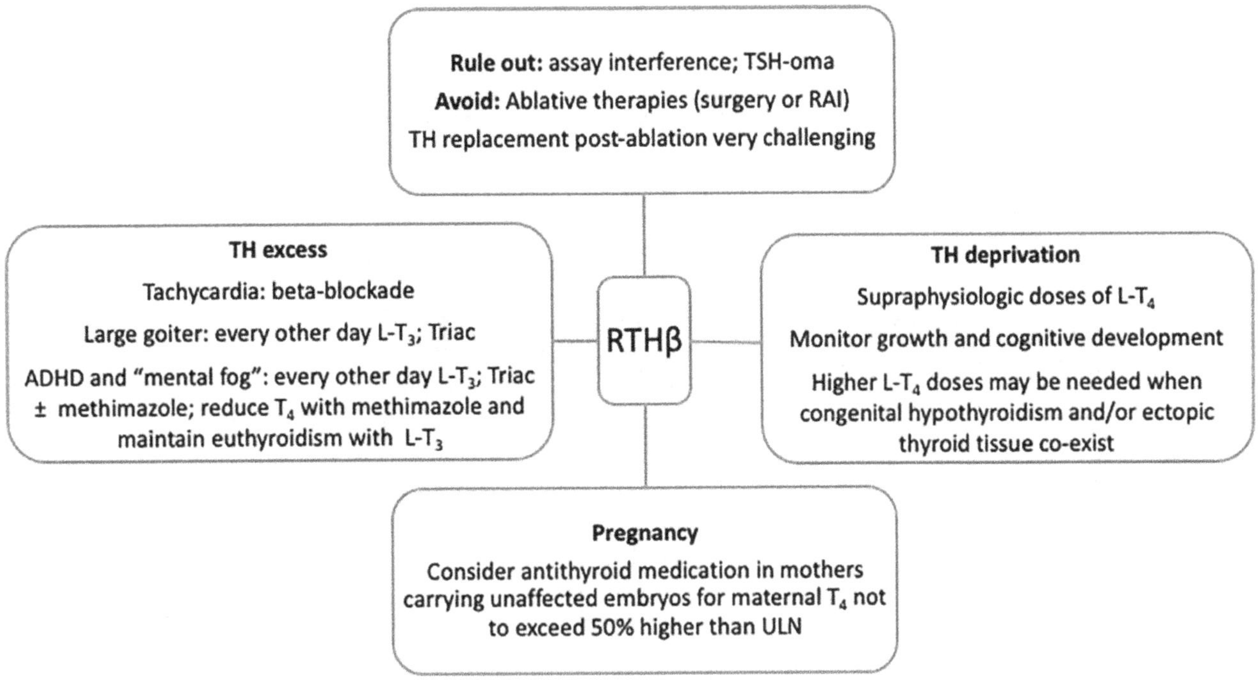

FIGURE 1 | Summary of recommendations to guide clinical management of RTHβ. RAI, radioactive iodine; ADHD, attention deficit and hyperactivity disorder; TH, thyroid hormones; ULN, upper limit of normal.

R243Q mutation. Fertility was not affected and, contrary to women with thyrotoxicosis, RTHβ did not produce an increase in premature labor, stillbirth or pre-eclampsia, jn agreement with the women's euthyroid state despite elevated TH levels (64). However, a significantly higher rate of early miscarriages was observed in women with RTHβ compared to spouses of males with RTHβ or unaffected first-degree relatives independent of maternal age and parity. Furthermore, a tendency was seen for these women to miscarry unaffected fetuses rather than fetuses with RTHβ, suggesting that the miscarriages occurred due to fetal exposure to incongruent high TH levels. In addition, unaffected newborns of mothers with RTHβ had significantly lower birth weight and suppressed TSH at birth compared to offspring of unaffected mothers, arguing that they were exposed in a hypercatabolic intrauterine environment of high TH concentration, whereas infants with RTHβ were protected from the toxic effect of TH excess. Of note, when women with RTHβ carrying unaffected fetuses were given antithyroid medication to avoid free T_4 levels 20% higher than the upper limit of normal, the birth weight and TSH levels at birth of their offspring was similar to infants with RTHβ (65).

In a subsequent study, the long-term effect of intrauterine exposure to high TH levels was examined in WT members of the Azorean kindred. Specifically, the study involved unaffected offspring of mothers with RTHβ and offspring of unaffected mothers, whose fathers had RTHβ, as well as mice mimicking the human phenotype. Unaffected humans and WT mice born to mothers with RTHβ and exposed to high TH levels *in utero* developed reduced central sensitivity to thyroid hormone (RSTH), that persisted during adulthood (66) (**Figure 2**). Increased expression of deiodinase 3, the enzyme that inactivates TH, was found in the pituitaries of the WT mice born to dams with RTHβ (66). This effect was found to be transmitted by male descendants but not in female with likewise RSTH (67). Although the exact mechanism of this transgenerational epigenetic inheritance is not fully characterized, it is thought to involve possible modulation of the imprinted deiodinase 3 gene that regulates local TH availability at a tissue specific level. It remains unclear whether prolonged exposure to high TH levels could have similar implications in adult life. This deserves further investigation as such a finding would have implications in the management of larger populations, such as individuals on long term TSH suppressive levothyroxine therapy for differentiated thyroid cancer.

DISCUSSION–CONCLUSIONS

The diagnosis of RTHβ is challenging and the main condition in the differential diagnosis is TSH-oma. Diagnosis and management of RTHβ are more challenging when other thyroid disorders co-exist, such as CH and ectopic thyroid tissue. More recently, an association has been described between RTHβ and AITD. Although the causal relation remains unclear, proposed pathophysiologic mechanisms include TSH or TH induced stimulation of pro-inflammatory and cytotoxic responses. The observed variability in clinical manifestation of RTHβ can be explained by the type of genetic defect, e.g. homo- *vs* hetero-zygosity, frameshift *vs* insertion/deletion, mutations with predominantly TRβ2 mediated action, mosaicism, and the tissue specific variability in TRβ expression, e.g. heart and brain *vs* pituitary and liver. Management is tailored to

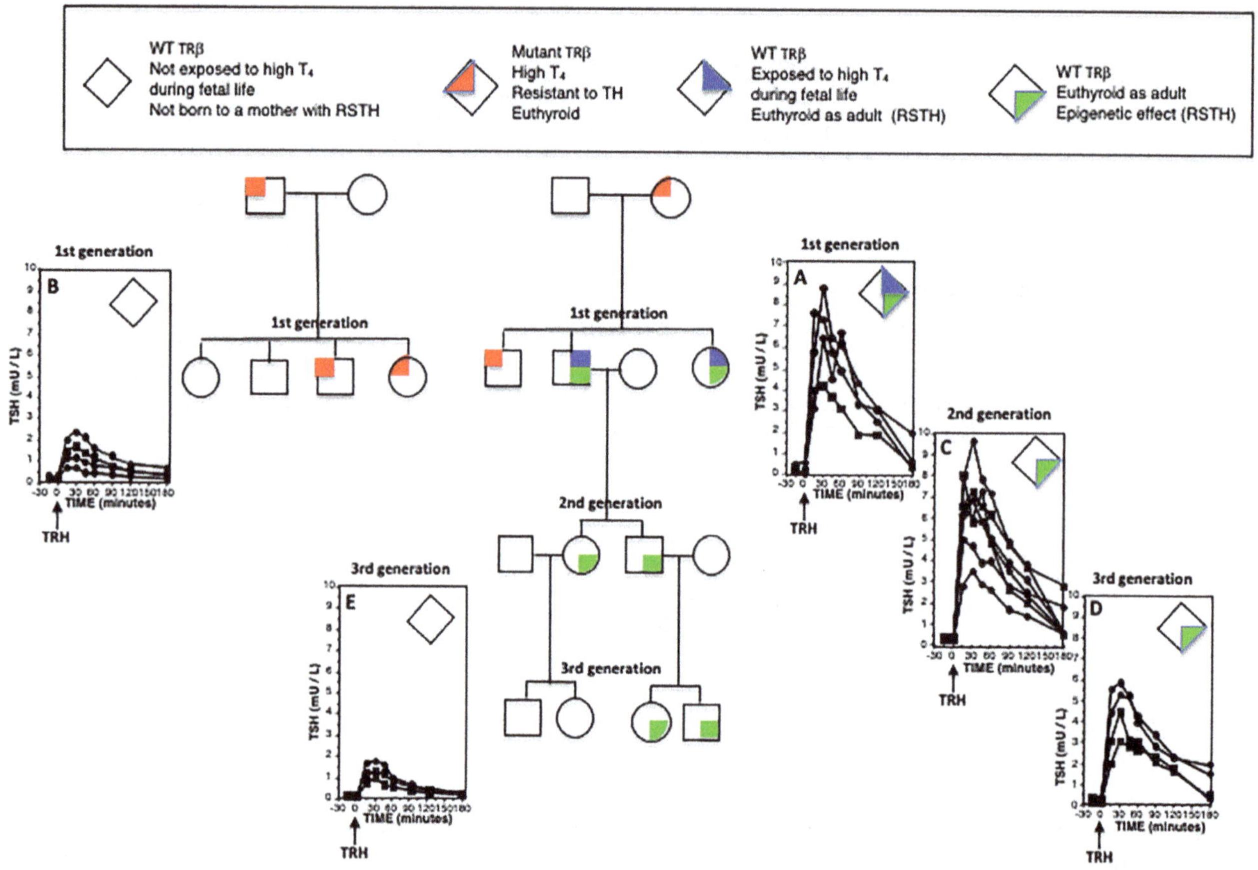

FIGURE 2 | Epigenetic effect of RTHβ and its transgenerational inheritance across the male line. Individuals were given 25 μg L-T_3 twice daily for three days. They were then injected intravenously with 200 μg of thyrotropin releasing hormone (TRH) and samples of blood were obtained at the indicated times for the measurement of serum TSH. Plotted on the graphs are results from female (circles) and males (squares). Increased peak responses in **(A, C, D)**, as compared to those of **(B, E)** indicate reduced sensitivity to thyroid hormone (RSTH). While this epigenetic effect of exposure to high TH levels during fetal life **(A)** is transmitted to both sexes, it is inherited along male line only **(C, D)** but not the female line **(E)**.

control symptoms arising from tissue specific excess or lack of TH. In small case series treatment with every-other-day L-T_3 was beneficial in improvement of goiter and ADHD symptoms. When RTHβ co-exists with CH, supraphysiologic doses of L-T_4 are needed to achieve normal bone and cognitive development. The advances in NGS have led to increasing frequency of VUS identification, where there may be limited data on their functional relevance beyond *in silico* prediction models. Caution should be exercised as to not guide clinical decision making based on computational resources and utilize information from genotype-phenotype co-segregation in family members. Transgenerational studies in humans and mice provide evidence of an epigenetic effect induced by RTHβ, by *in utero* exposure of WT fetuses to high TH concentration. The resulting reduced sensitivity to TH shows transgenerational inheritance across the male but not the female line and is thought to be mediated *via* modulation of deiodinase 3, that regulates local TH availability.

The advances in our knowledge on RTHβ raise novel questions about TH action outside the hypothalamus-pituitary-thyroid axis and the emerging concepts on epigenetic effect of RTHβ need to be explored further, as they may have implications in larger populations, such as patients with thyroid cancer on long term TSH suppression therapy with TH.

AUTHOR CONTRIBUTIONS

TP and SR designed and wrote this manuscript and both conceptually contributed to this work. All authors contributed to the article and approved the submitted version.

FUNDING

This work was supported in part by grant DK15070 from the National Institutes of Health. The content is solely the responsibility of the authors and does not necessarily represent the official views of the National Institute of Diabetes and Digestive and Kidney Diseases or the National Institutes of Health. TP is supported by the NIH T32 grant 5T32HL007609-33.

REFERENCES

1. Refetoff S, DeWind LT, DeGroot LJ. Familial syndrome combining deaf-mutism, stuppled epiphyses, goiter and abnormally high PBI: possible target organ refractoriness to thyroid hormone. *J Clin Endocrinol Metab* (1967) 99:768–70. doi: 10.1210/jcem-27-2-279
2. Refetoff S, Bassett JH, Beck-Peccoz P, Bernal J, Brent G, Chatterjee K, et al. Classification and proposed nomenclature for inherited defects of thyroid hormone action, cell transport, and metabolism. *Thyroid* (2014) 3:7–9. doi: 10.1089/thy.2013.3393.nomen
3. Refetoff S, Bassett JH, Beck-Peccoz P, Bernal J, Brent G, Chatterjee K, et al. Classification and proposed nomenclature for inherited defects of thyroid hormone action, cell transport, and metabolism. *J Clin Endocrinol Metab* (2014) 99:768–70. doi: 10.1210/jc.2013-3393
4. Refetoff S, Bassett JH, Beck-Peccoz P, Bernal J, Brent G, Chatterjee K, et al. Classification and proposed nomenclature for inherited defects of thyroid hormone action, cell transport, and metabolism. *Eur Thyroid J* (2014) 3:7–9. doi: 10.1159/000358180
5. Dumitrescu AM, Korwutthikulrangsri M, Refetoff S. Impaired Sensituvito to ThyrHormaone: Defects of Transport, Metabolism and Action (Capter 64). In: LE Braverman, DS Cooper, PA Kopp, editors. *Werner & Ingbar's The Thyroid: A Fundamental and Clinical Text.* PA, USA: Lippincott, Williams & Wilkins Philadelphia (2021). p. 868–907.
6. Gurnell M, Visser TJ, Beck-Peccoz P, Chatterjee VK. Resistance to Thyroid Hormone. In: JL Jameson, LJ DeGroot, editors. *Endocrinology Adult and Pediatric.* Philadelphia: Endocrinology Adult and Pediatric Elsevier Saunders (2016). p. 1648–65.
7. Lafranchi SH, Snyder DB, Sesser DE, Skeels MR, Singh N, Brent GA, et al. Follow-up of newborns with elevated screening T4 concentrations. *J Pediatr* (2003) 143:296–301. doi: 10.1067/S0022-3476(03)00184-7
8. Vela A, Perez-Nanclares G, Rios I, Rica I, Portillo N, Castano L, et al. Spanish Group for the Study of, Thyroid hormone resistance from newborns to adults: a Spanish experience. *J Endocrinol Invest* (2019) 42:941–9. doi: 10.1007/s40618-019-1007-4
9. Sakurai A, Takeda K, Ain K, Ceccarelli P, Nakai A, Seino S, et al. Generalized resistance to thyroid hormone associated with a mutation in the ligand-binding domain of the human thyroid hormone receptor beta. *Proc Natl Acad Sci U S A* (1989) 86:8977–81. doi: 10.1073/pnas.86.22.8977
10. Pappa T, Refetoff S. Human Genetics of Thyroid Hormone Receptor Beta: Resistance to Thyroid Hormone Beta (RTHbeta). *Methods Mol Biol* (2018) 1801:225–40. doi: 10.1007/978-1-4939-7902-8_18
11. Mamanasiri S, Yesil S, Dumitrescu AM, Liao XH, Demir T, Weiss RE, et al. Mosaicism of a thyroid hormone receptor-beta gene mutation in resistance to thyroid hormone. *J Clin Endocrinol Metab* (2006) 91:3471–7. doi: 10.1210/jc.2006-0727
12. Reutrakul S, Sadow PM, Pannain S, Pohlenz J, Carvalho GA, Macchia PE, et al. Search for abnormalities of nuclear corepressors, coactivators, and a coregulator in families with resistance to thyroid hormone without mutations in thyroid hormone receptor beta or alpha genes. *J Clin Endocrinol Metab* (2000) 85:3609–17. doi: 10.1210/jcem.85.10.6873
13. Campi I, Cammarata G, Bianchi Marzoli S, Beck-Peccoz P, Santarsiero D, Dazzi D, et al. Retinal Photoreceptor Functions Are Compromised in Patients With Resistance to Thyroid Hormone Syndrome (RTHbeta). *J Clin Endocrinol Metab* (2017) 102:2620–7. doi: 10.1210/jc.2016-3671
14. Refetoff S, Weiss RE, Usala SJ. The syndromes of resistance to thyroid hormone. *Endocr Rev* (1993) 14:348–99. doi: 10.1210/edrv-14-3-348
15. Campi I, Covelli D, Moran C, Fugazzola L, Cacciatore C, Orlandi F, et al. The Differential Diagnosis of Discrepant Thyroid Function Tests: Insistent Pitfalls and Updated Flow-Chart Based on a Long-Standing Experience. *Front Endocrinol (Lausanne)* (2020) 11:432. doi: 10.3389/fendo.2020.00432
16. Macchia E, Lombardi M, Raffaelli V, Piaggi P, Macchia L, Scattina I, et al. Clinical and genetic characteristics of a large monocentric series of patients affected by thyroid hormone (Th) resistance and suggestions for differential diagnosis in patients without mutation of Th receptor beta. *Clin Endocrinol (Oxf)* (2014) 81:921–8. doi: 10.1111/cen.12556
17. Khoo S, Lyons G, Solomon A, Oddy S, Halsall D, Chatterjee K, et al. Familial dysalbuminemic hyperthyroxinemia confounding management of coexistent autoimmune thyroid disease. *Endocrinol Diabetes Metab Case Rep* (2020) 2020. doi: 10.1530/EDM-19-0161
18. Grasberger H, Ringkananont U, Croxson M, Refetoff S. Resistance to thyroid hormone in a patient with thyroid dysgenesis. *Thyroid* (2005) 15:730–3. doi: 10.1089/thy.2005.15.730
19. Nakajima Y, Yamada M, Horiguchi K, Satoh T, Hashimoto K, Tokuhiro E, et al. Resistance to thyroid hormone due to a novel thyroid hormone receptor mutant in a patient with hypothyroidism secondary to lingual thyroid and functional characterization of the mutant receptor. *Thyroid* (2010) 20:917–26. doi: 10.1089/thy.2009.0389
20. Heather N, Hall K, Neas K, Potter H, Wiltshire E. Growth and development in a child with resistance to thyroid hormone and ectopic thyroid gland. *Pediatrics* (2012) 129:e817–20. doi: 10.1542/peds.2011-0634
21. Guo ML, Zheng X, Yang LX, Qiu YL, Cheng L, Ma SG. Coexistence of resistance to thyroid hormone and ectopic thyroid: ten-year follow-up. *Arch Endocrinol Metab* (2016) 60:601–4. doi: 10.1590/2359-3997000000214
22. Zhou Z, Yang C, Lv F, Liu W, Yan S, Zang H, et al. Novel THRB mutation analysis in congenital hypothyroidism with thyroid dysgenesis. *J Cell Biochem* (2018) 119:9474–82. doi: 10.1002/jcb.27264
23. Fisher DA, Schoen EJ, La Franchi S, Mandel SH, Nelson JC, Carlton EI, et al. The hypothalamic-pituitary-thyroid negative feedback control axis in children with treated congenital hypothyroidism. *J Clin Endocrinol Metab* (2000) 85:2722–7. doi: 10.1210/jcem.85.8.6718
24. Larsen CC, Dumitrescu A, Guerra-Arguero LM, Gallego-Suarez C, Vazquez-Mellado A, Vinogradova M, et al. Incidental identification of a thyroid hormone receptor beta (THRB) gene variant in a family with autoimmune thyroid disease. *Thyroid* (2013) 23:1638–43. doi: 10.1089/thy.2013.0174
25. Shiwa T, Oki K, Awaya T, Nakanishi S, Yamane K. Resistance to thyroid hormone accompanied by Graves' disease. *Intern Med* (2011) 50:1977–80. doi: 10.2169/internalmedicine.50.4904
26. Barkoff MS, Kocherginsky M, Anselmo J, Weiss RE, Refetoff S. Autoimmunity in patients with resistance to thyroid hormone. *J Clin Endocrinol Metab* (2010) 95:3189–93. doi: 10.1210/jc.2009-2179
27. Gavin C, Meggison H, Ooi TC. Proposing a causal link between thyroid hormone resistance and primary autoimmune hypothyroidism. *Med Hypotheses* (2008) 70:1024–8. doi: 10.1016/j.mehy.2007.08.015
28. Fabris N, Mocchegiani E, Mariotti S, Pacini F, Pinchera A. Thyroid function modulates thymic endocrine activity. *J Clin Endocrinol Metab* (1986) 62:474–8. doi: 10.1210/jcem-62-3-474
29. Villa-Verde DM, Defresne MP, Vannier-dos-Santos MA, Dussault JH, Boniver J, Savino W. Identification of nuclear triiodothyronine receptors in the thymic epithelium. *Endocrinology* (1992) 131:1313–20. doi: 10.1210/endo.131.3.1505466
30. Ganesh BB, Cheatem DM, Sheng JR, Vasu C, Prabhakar BS. GM-CSF-induced CD11c+CD8a–dendritic cells facilitate Foxp3+ and IL-10+ regulatory T cell expansion resulting in suppression of autoimmune thyroiditis. *Int Immunol* (2009) 21:269–82. doi: 10.1093/intimm/dxn147
31. Montesinos MDM, Pellizas CG. Thyroid Hormone Action on Innate Immunity. *Front Endocrinol (Lausanne)* (2019) 10:350. doi: 10.3389/fendo.2019.00350
32. Safer JD, O'Connor MG, Colan SD, Srinivasan S, Tollin SR, Wondisford FE. The thyroid hormone receptor-beta gene mutation R383H is associated with isolated central resistance to thyroid hormone. *J Clin Endocrinol Metab* (1999) 84:3099–109. doi: 10.1210/jc.84.9.3099
33. Kaplan MM, Swartz SL, Larsen PR. Partial peripheral resistance to thyroid hormone. *Am J Med* (1981) 70:1115–21. doi: 10.1016/0002-9343(81)90885-8
34. Pohlenz J, Wirth S, Winterpacht A, Wemme H, Zabel B, Schonberger W. Phenotypic variability in patients with generalised resistance to thyroid hormone. *J Med Genet* (1995) 32:393–5. doi: 10.1136/jmg.32.5.393
35. Beck-Peccoz P, Chatterjee VK. The variable clinical phenotype in thyroid hormone resistance syndrome. *Thyroid* (1994) 4:225–32. doi: 10.1089/thy.1994.4.225
36. Toumba M, Neocleous V, Fanis P, Tanteles GA, Kyriakidou-Himonas M, Picolos M. Phenotype variability and different genotype of four patients with thyroid hormone resistance syndrome due to variants in the THRB gene. *Hippokratia* (2019) 23:135–9.
37. Ferrara AM, Onigata K, Ercan O, Woodhead H, Weiss RE, Refetoff S. Homozygous thyroid hormone receptor beta gene mutations in resistance

to thyroid hormone: Three new cases and review of the literature. *J Clin Endocrinol Matab* (2012) 97:1328–36. doi: 10.1210/jc.2011-2642
38. Yen PM, Sugawara A, Refetoff S, Chin WW. New insights on the mechanism (s) of the dominant negative effect of mutant thyroid hormone receptor in generalized resistance to thyroid hormone. *J Clin Invest* (1992) 90:1825–31. doi: 10.1172/JCI116058
39. Wu SY, Cohen RN, Simsek E, Senses DA, Yar NE, Grasberger H, et al. A novel thyroid Hormone receptor-beta mutation that fails to bind nuclear receptor corepressor in a patient as an apparent cause of severe, predominantly pituitary resistance to thyroid hormone. *J Clin Endocrinol Metab* (2006) 91:1887–95. doi: 10.1210/jc.2005-2428
40. Yagi H, Pohlenz J, Hayashi Y, Sakurai A, Refetoff S. Resistance to thyroid hormone caused by two mutant thyroid hormone receptor ß, R243Q and R243W, with marked impairment of function that cannot be explained by altered in-vitro 3,5,3'-triiodothyronine binding affinity. *J Clin Endocrinol Metab* (1997) 82:1608–14. doi: 10.1210/jc.82.5.1608
41. Safer JD, Cohen RN, Hollenberg AN, Wondisford FE. Defective release of corepressor by hinge mutants of the thyroid hormone receptor found in patients with resistance to thyroid hormone. *J Biol Chem* (1998) 273:30175–82. doi: 10.1074/jbc.273.46.30175
42. Collingwood TN, Rajanayagam O, Adams M, Wagner R, Cavaillès V, Kalkhoven E, et al. A natural transactivation mutation in the thyroid hormone ß receptor: Impaired interaction with putative transcriptional mediators. *Proc Natl Acad Sci USA* (1997) 94:248–53. doi: 10.1073/pnas.94.1.248
43. Clifton-Bligh RJ, de Zegher F, Wagner RL, Collingwood TN, François I, Van Helvoirt M, et al. A novel mutation (R383H) in resistance to thyroid hormone syndrome predominantly impairs corepressor release and negative transcriptional regulation. *Mol Endocrinol* (1998) 12:609–21. doi: 10.1210/mend.12.5.0113
44. Machado DS, Sabet A, Santiago LA, Sidhaye AR, Chiamolera MI, Ortiga-Carvalho TM, et al. A thyroid hormone receptor mutation that dissociates thyroid hormone regulation of gene expression *in vivo*. *Proc Natl Acad Sci U S A* (2009) 106:9441–6. doi: 10.1073/pnas.0903227106
45. Alberobello AT, Congedo V, Liu H, Cochran C, Skarulis MC, Forrest D, et al. An intronic SNP in the thyroid hormone receptor beta gene is associated with pituitary cell-specific over-expression of a mutant thyroid hormone receptor beta2 (R338W) in the index case of pituitary-selective resistance to thyroid hormone. *J Transl Med* (2011) 9:144. doi: 10.1186/1479-5876-9-144
46. Mixson AJ, Hauser P, Tennyson G, Renault JC, Bodenner DL, Weintraub BD. Differential expression of mutant and normal beta T3 receptor alleles in kindreds with generalized resistance to thyroid hormone. *J Clin Invest* (1993) 91:2296–300. doi: 10.1172/JCI116458
47. Hayashi Y, Janssen OE, Weiss RE, Murata Y, Seo H, Refetoff S. The relative expression of mutant and normal thyroid hormone receptor genes in patients with generalized resistance to thyroid hormone determined by estimation of their specific messenger ribonucleic acid products. *J Clin Endocrinol Metab* (1993) 76:64–9. doi: 10.1210/jcem.76.1.8421105
48. Fujisawa H, Gagne J, Dumitrescu AM, Refetoff S. Very Severe Resistance to Thyroid Hormone beta in One of Three Affected Members of a Family with a Novel Mutation in the THRB Gene. *Thyroid* (2019) 29:1518–20. doi: 10.1089/thy.2019.0095
49. Shi Y, Ye H, Link KH, Putnam MC, Hubner I, Dowdell S, et al. Mutant-selective thyromimetics for the chemical rescue of thyroid hormone receptor mutants associated with resistance to thyroid hormone. *Biochemistry* (2005) 44:4612–26. doi: 10.1021/bi0482349
50. Yao B, Wei Y, Zhang S, Tian S, Xu S, Wang R, et al. Revealing a Mutant-Induced Receptor Allosteric Mechanism for the Thyroid Hormone Resistance. *iScience* (2019) 20:489–96. doi: 10.1016/j.isci.2019.10.002
51. Weiss RE, Dumitrescu A, Refetoff S. Approach to the patient with resistance to thyroid hormone and pregnancy. *J Clin Endocrinol Metab* (2010) 95:3094–102. doi: 10.1210/jc.2010-0409
52. Anselmo J, Refetoff S. Regression of a large goiter in a patient with resistance to thyroid hormone by every other day treatment with triiodothyronine. *Thyroid* (2004) 14:71–4. doi: 10.1089/105072504322783876
53. Unluturk U, Sriphrapradang C, Erdogan MF, Emral R, Guldiken S, Refetoff S, et al. Management of differentiated thyroid cancer in the presence of resistance to thyroid hormone and TSH-secreting adenomas: a report of four cases and review of the literature. *J Clin Endocrinol Metab* (2013) 98:2210–7. doi: 10.1210/jc.2012-4142
54. Weiss RE, Stein MA, Refetoff S. Behavioral effects of liothyronine (L-T3) in children with attention deficit hyperactivity disorder in the presence and absence of resistance to thyroid hormone. *Thyroid* (1997) 7:389–93. doi: 10.1089/thy.1997.7.389
55. Maruo Y, Mori A, Morioka Y, Sawai C, Mimura Y, Matui K, et al. Successful every-other-day liothyronine therapy for severe resistance to thyroid hormone beta with a novel THRB mutation; case report. *BMC Endocr Disord* (2016) 16:1. doi: 10.1186/s12902-015-0081-7
56. Groeneweg S, Peeters RP, Visser TJ, Visser WE. Therapeutic applications of thyroid hormone analogues in resistance to thyroid hormone (RTH) syndromes. *Mol Cell Endocrinol* (2017) 458:82–90. doi: 10.1016/j.mce.2017.02.029
57. Anzai R, Adachi M, Sho N, Muroya K, Asakura Y, Onigata K. Long-term 3,5,3'-triiodothyroacetic acid therapy in a child with hyperthyroidism caused by thyroid hormone resistance: pharmacological study and therapeutic recommendations. *Thyroid* (2012) 22:1069–75. doi: 10.1089/thy.2011.0450
58. Moran C, Habeb AM, Kahaly GJ, Kampmann C, Hughes M, Marek J, et al. Homozygous Resistance to Thyroid Hormone beta: Can Combined Antithyroid Drug and Triiodothyroacetic Acid Treatment Prevent Cardiac Failure? *J Endocr Soc* (2017) 1:1203–12. doi: 10.1210/js.2017-00204
59. Hayashi Y, Sunthornthepvarakul T, Refetoff S. Mutations of CpG dinucleotides located in the triiodothyronine (T3)-binding domain of the thyroid hormone receptor (TR) beta gene that appears to be devoid of natural mutations may not be detected because they are unlikely to produce the clinical phenotype of resistance to thyroid hormone. *J Clin Invest* (1994) 94:607–15. doi: 10.1172/JCI117376
60. Menzaghi C, Di Paola R, Corrias A, Einaudi S, Trischitta V, De Sanctis C, et al. T426I a new mutation in the thyroid hormone receptor beta gene in a sporadic patient with resistance to thyroid hormone and dysmorphism. Mutations Brief no. 192. *Online Hum Mutat* (1998) 12:289.
61. Lek M, Karczewski KJ, Minikel EV, Samocha KE, Banks E, Fennell T, et al. Analysis of protein-coding genetic variation in 60,706 humans. *Nature* (2016) 536:285–91. doi: 10.1038/nature19057
62. Concolino P, Costella A, Paragliola RM. Mutational Landscape of Resistance to Thyroid Hormone Beta (RTHbeta). *Mol Diagn Ther* (2019) 23:353–68. doi: 10.1007/s40291-019-00399-w
63. Korwutthikulrangsri M, Dosiou C, Dumitrescu AM, Refetoff S. A Novel G385E Variant in the Cold Region of the T3-Binding Domain of Thyroid Hormone Receptor Beta Gene and Investigations to Assess Its Clinical Significance. *Eur Thyroid J* (2019) 8:293–7. doi: 10.1159/000503860
64. Anselmo J, Cao D, Karrison T, Weiss RE, Refetoff S. Fetal loss associated with excess thyroid hormone exposure. *JAMA* (2004) 292:691–5. doi: 10.1001/jama.292.6.691
65. Pappa T, Anselmo J, Mamanasiri S, Dumitrescu AM, Weiss RE, Refetoff S. Prenatal Diagnosis of Resistance to Thyroid Hormone and Its Clinical Implications. *J Clin Endocrinol Metab* (2017) 102:3775–82. doi: 10.1210/jc.2017-01251
66. Srichomkwun P, Anselmo J, Liao XH, Hones GS, Moeller LC, Alonso-Sampedro M, et al. Fetal Exposure to High Maternal Thyroid Hormone Levels Causes Central Resistance to Thyroid Hormone in Adult Humans and Mice. *J Clin Endocrinol Metab* (2017) 102:3234–40. doi: 10.1210/jc.2017-00019
67. Anselmo J, Scherberg NH, Dumitrescu AM, Refetoff S. Reduced Sensitivity to Thyroid Hormone as a Transgenerational Epigenetic Marker Transmitted Along the Human Male Line. *Thyroid* (2019) 29:778–82. doi: 10.1089/thy.2019.0080

24

Improving Voice Outcomes after Thyroid Surgery – Review of Safety Parameters for using Energy-Based Devices near the Recurrent Laryngeal Nerve

Jia Joanna Wang[1,2], *Tzu-Yen Huang*[1,3], *Che-Wei Wu*[1,4], *Yi-Chu Lin*[1], *Hsin-Yi Tseng*[1], *Cheng-Hsin Liu*[1,2], *I-Cheng Lu*[5], *Pi-Ying Chang*[6], *Hui-Chun Chen*[7], *Hsiu-Ya Chen*[8], *Gianlorenzo Dionigi*[9,10], *Feng-Yu Chiang*[11,12] *and Ling-Feng Wang*[1*]

[1] *Department of Otorhinolaryngology-Head and Neck Surgery, International Thyroid Surgery Center, Kaohsiung Medical University Hospital, Kaohsiung Medical University, Kaohsiung, Taiwan,* [2] *Department of Otolaryngology-Head and Neck Surgery, Kaohsiung Municipal Siaogang Hospital, Kaohsiung Medical University, Kaohsiung, Taiwan,* [3] *Department of Biological Science and Technology, National Yang Ming Chiao Tung University, Hsinchu, Taiwan,* [4] *Center for Liquid Biopsy and Cohort Research, and Faculty of Medicine, College of Medicine, Kaohsiung Medical University, Kaohsiung, Taiwan,* [5] *Department of Anesthesiology, Kaohsiung Municipal Siaogang Hospital, Kaohsiung Medical University, Kaohsiung, Taiwan,* [6] *Department of Anesthesiology, Kaohsiung Municipal Tatung Hospital, Kaohsiung Medical University, Kaohsiung, Taiwan,* [7] *Department of Nursing, Kaohsiung Medical University Hospital, Kaohsiung, Taiwan,* [8] *Department of Anesthesiology, Kaohsiung Medical University Hospital, Kaohsiung, Taiwan,* [9] *Division of General Surgery, Endocrine Surgery Section, Istituto Auxologico Italiano IRCCS, Milan, Italy,* [10] *Department of Pathophysiology and Transplantation, University of Milan, Milan, Italy,* [11] *Department of Otolaryngology-Head and Neck Surgery, E-Da Hospital, Kaohsiung, Taiwan,* [12] *School of Medicine, College of Medicine, I-Shou University, Kaohsiung, Taiwan*

***Correspondence:**
Ling-Feng Wang
lifewang@kmu.edu.tw

Technological advances in thyroid surgery have rapidly increased in recent decades. Specifically, recently developed energy-based devices (EBDs) enable simultaneous dissection and sealing tissue. EBDs have many advantages in thyroid surgery, such as reduced blood loss, lower rate of post-operative hypocalcemia, and shorter operation time. However, the rate of recurrent laryngeal nerve (RLN) injury during EBD use has shown statistically inconsistent. EBDs generate high temperature that can cause iatrogenic thermal injury to the RLN by direct or indirect thermal spread. This article reviews relevant medical literatures of conventional electrocauteries and different mechanisms of current EBDs, and compares two safety parameters: safe distance and cooling time. In general, conventional electrocautery generates higher temperature and wider thermal spread range, but when applying EBDs near the RLN adequate activation distance and cooling time are still required to avoid inadvertent thermal injury. To improve voice outcomes in the quality-of-life era, surgeons should observe safety parameters and follow the standard procedures when using EBDs near the RLN in thyroid surgery

Keywords: energy-based devices, safety parameter, recurrent laryngeal nerve, thyroid surgery, voice

INTRODUCTION

Thyroidectomy is one of the most common head and neck surgeries. In the United States, more than 150,000 thyroidectomies were performed annually, and the case number of thyroid surgery is increasing each year (1). Specific challenges of thyroid surgery include the complex vascularization of anatomy, the proximity of the operating field to the recurrent laryngeal nerve (RLN), and the need to preserve the parathyroid gland. Therefore, thorough hemostasis is essential for avoiding further complications after thyroid surgery (2).

The "clamp-and-tie" technique was first introduced by Theodor Kocher in the 19th century. Since then, until the 1980s, clamp-and-tie, suture-ligation, electrocautery (monopolar or bipolar) and hemostatic clips have been widely adopted for hemostatic use in thyroid surgery (1, 3, 4). However, one of the most important technological advances in thyroid surgery occurred three decades ago: the introduction of energy-based devices (EBDs). Although the specific purpose of using EBDs in thyroid surgery is to achieve hemostasis, the mechanism through which EBDs achieve hemostasis differs from one devices to another (3).

Recent studies indicate that EBDs are used in 65.7% of thyroidectomy patients (1). Reported intraoperative advantages of EBDs include considerably decreased operative time, incision length and blood loss. Other clinically significant advantages of EBDs over conventional techniques include the superior postoperative outcomes of EBDs, e.g., reduced pain, wound drainage, neck hematoma, and hypocalcemia (1, 2, 5, 6).

In terms of RLN safety, however, EBDs have not proven superior to conventional devices used for thyroid surgery. For example, reported rates of RLN injury showed statistically inconsistent between EBDs and conventional devices (7). In fact, one 10-year meta-analysis reported that EBD use was associated with higher RLN paralysis rates (3). In another study, clinical outcomes of thyroidectomy were compared between 11,355 thyroidectomy patients treated with EBDs and a control group treated without EBDs. Compared to the non-EBD group, the EBD group had a significantly higher rate of hoarseness. However, the rate of severe hoarseness was significantly higher in the non-EBD group (1, 8, 9).

In another study, Liu et al. reported that the RLN palsy rate did not significantly differ between an EBD group and a clamp-and-tie group. However, the nerve injury mechanisms are significantly differed between the two groups. No patients in the clamp-and-tie group had thermal injury, whereas one-third of patients in the EBD group suffered thermal injury caused by lateral thermal spread in palsied RLNs (6).

INTRAOPERATIVE NEUROMONITORING AND RLN THERMAL INJURY CAUSED BY EBDs

Intraoperative injury to the RLN can cause vocal cord paralysis. Symptoms may include hoarseness, choking, dysphagia and dysphonia in unilateral vocal cord paralysis, in addition, difficulty breathing may occur in cases of bilateral vocal cord paralysis (10–13). To reduce this major cause of morbidity after thyroid surgery, visual identification of RLN is the standard practice, and IONM facilitates this procedure (10, 14–16). Use of IONM not only enables the surgeons to evaluate RLN function in real time, but also to assess the mechanism of an impending or actual RLN injury and the appropriate surgical procedure for preventing or treating the injury (17–21). By elucidating the mechanism of iatrogenic RLN injury with IONM, many studies noted that traction and thermal injury are the first and second most common causes of RLN injury during thyroidectomy (5, 17, 22). Most intraoperative thermal injuries to the RLN result from thermal spread during use of high-temperature electrocautery devices and EBDs. Tissue contraction during EBD activation increases the risk of thermal injury because it reduces the distance from the RLN at which an EBD can be safely used (6). Thermal injury to the RLN often occurs unexpectedly when an EBD is activated or used for dissection. This type of injury usually is not only severe but irreversible (17).

In addition to the conventional uses of EBDs for tissue sealing, cutting, and hemostasis, surgeons have recently begun using EBDs for grasping and dividing tissue when dissection is performed near the RLN or even in direct contact with the RLN, especially in endoscopic procedures. As a results of technological advances in EBDs and the growing acceptance of surgical applications of EBDs, the increased incidence of thermal injury has emerged one of the main adverse events in thyroid surgery (23). Direct thermal burn injury can occur during or after activation of an EBD when the temperature of the blade is still high. Such injuries result from inadvertent contact between the blade and the skin or surrounding soft tissue, especially the RLN (24). Unlike direct thermal injury to the RLN, an indirect thermal injury to the RLN, which results from lateral thermal spread, is rarely visible to the naked eye. Therefore, animal experiments by using continuous IONM are needed for objective evaluation of the electrophysiology of RLN thermal injury and for establishing guidelines for safe use of EBDs, including minimum cooling time and safe distance between the EBD tip and the skin or surrounding soft tissue (**Figure 1**) (25, 26).

ANIMAL STUDIES IN EBD SAFETY

Studies of EBD safety in the literature are typically performed in two stages: activation studies and cooling studies. Activation studies assess the distance from the RLN at which an EBD can be safely used without causing thermal injury; cooling studies assess the time (after activation) needed for the EBD tip or blade to cool sufficiently for use of the EBD in performing a dissection close to or in contact with the RLN (**Figure 2**).

Activation Studies

The EBD is typically applied to RLN soft tissue at a distance starting from 5 mm and gradually decreased to 0 mm. Real-time

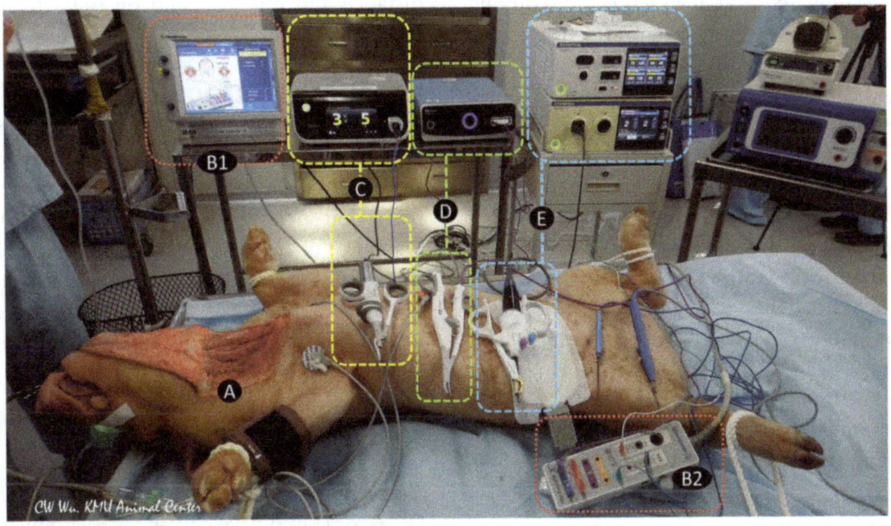

FIGURE 1 | Animal models of continuous intraoperative neuromonitoring (cIONM) provide an objective platform for optimizing the safety parameters for various energy-based devices used for hemostasis and dissection near the recurrent laryngeal nerve (RLN) during thyroid surgery. **(A)** Preparation of porcine animal model by transverse incision and flap formation in neck skin. **(B1)** IONM monitoring system used for recording, monitoring, and analyzing real-time changes in laryngeal EMG. **(B2)** IONM interface box for connecting recording, stimulation, and ground electrodes. **(C)** Ultrasonic energy based device and energy generator. **(D)** Advanced biopolar energy based device and energy platform. **(E)** Hybrid energy based device (ultrasonic and bipolar energy) and multifunctional platform.

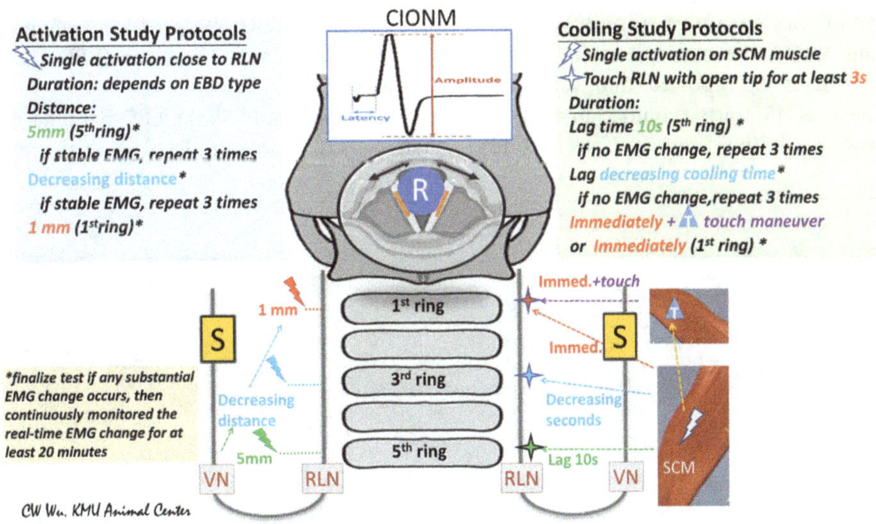

FIGURE 2 | Flowchart of study protocols for using energy-based devices (EBDs). **(Left)** Activation Study Protocols: Tests were performed from the proximal to distal segments of the RLN. The distance from the tip of the EBD to the RLN was measured. In this study, the first test was performed at a distance of 5 mm from the fifth tracheal ring. If the EMG remained stable after three tests, further tests were performed at a shorter distance. If the EMG remained stable after repeated tests, further tests were performed at a distance of 1 mm or with the EBD tip in direct contact with the RLN. **(Right)** Cooling Study Protocol: Tests were performed on the RLN from the proximal to distal segment. After a single EBD activation on the SCM muscle, the operator touched the RLN with the tip of the open blade after varying cooling times. The fifth tracheal ring was touched after a cooling time of 10 seconds. If EMG remained stable in three tests, tests proceeded from the proximal RLN (fifth tracheal ring, green cross) to the distal RLN (first tracheal ring, red cross) after progressively decreasing cooling times. *asterisk: If a substantial EMG change was noted, the RLN experiment was considered complete, and EMG was continuously monitored for at least 20 minutes. T, touch maneuver: cooling by quickly touching surrounding tissue. S, Stimulation electrode for automatic periodic stimulation (APS) of vagus nerve (VN); R, Recording electrode on endotracheal tube for recording electromyography (EMG) signals evoked by vocal cord movement (black arrow); cIONM, continuous intraoperative neuromonitoring; RLN, recurrent laryngeal nerve; VN, vagus nerve; EBD, energy-based device; SCM, sternocleidomastoid; EMG, electromyography.

electrophysiologic electromyography (EMG) information is continuously recorded, compared and analyzed during varying durations of activation and under varying power settings. If a substantial EMG change occurs after any test, the RLN experiment is stopped, and real-time EMG is continuously recorded for 20 to 60 minutes to determine whether the injury is reversible (**Figure 2**, left) (5, 25, 27).

Cooling Studies

After activation of the EBD on the sternocleidomastoid (SCM) muscle, surgeons touches the tip on the RLN after 10 seconds of waiting and cooling, then the cooling time gradually decreases to 0 seconds and observes the EMG for adverse changes. The "muscle touch maneuver" can be performed by touching the EBD tip/blade to the surrounding tissue right after activation. This maneuver offers ideal cooling effect by reducing the temperature immediately (**Figure 2**, right) (25).

ELECTROCAUTERIES AND ENERGY-BASED DEVICES

Monopolar Electrocautery

Electrocautery equipment is most commonly used in conventional thyroidectomy. In a monopolar electrocautery, current from the probe electrode passes through the patient to a return pad. This equipment is known for its lateral and vertical transmission and diffusion of electrical power into surrounding tissue. Since monopolar electrocautery rapidly generates temperatures exceeding 350°C, thermal spread in tissues is problematic (27–29). Wu et al. reported that safe use of monopolar electrocautery at 15 watts requires an activation distance of 5 mm and a cooling time of 1 second (25). However, the optimal safety parameters (i.e., activation distance and time) depend on the activation power use to on the tissue.

Bipolar Electrocautery

In bipolar electrocautery, current only passes through tissue between two arms of a forceps-shaped electrode. Bipolar electrocautery is performed at a temperature significantly lower than that of monopolar electrocautery, and showed little difference of Celsius degree when compare to advanced bipolar EBDs (e.g., Ligasure) (28). An animal study indicated that, the safety parameters for bipolar electrocautery performed at 30 watts are an activation distance of 3 mm and a cooling time of 1 second (25).

Advanced Bipolar EBDs

LigaSure, an advanced bipolar EBD, can seal vessels up to 7 mm in diameter (30, 31). The Ligasure Small Jaw (LSJ) and Ligasure Exact Dissector (LED) have curved jaws with bilateral symmetric blades coated with anti-adherent material to enable their use in performing fine-manipulation tasks (**Figure 3**). Reports of experiments performed using infrared cameras or thermosensors indicate that both devices operate at a temperature below 100°C (32–34).

LigaSure Small Jaw (LSJ) (Medtronic, Minneapolis, MN, USA)

The LSJ has an activation button with tactile feedback and a 16.5 mm long curved tip. According to Dionigi et al, the safe activation distance is 2 mm, and a 2-second interval or muscle touch maneuver is required for cooling (31).

LigaSure Exact Dissector (LED) (Medtronic, Minneapolis, MN, USA)

Compared to LSJ, the LED has a narrower jaw (2 mm) and a longer seal (20.6 mm). For sealing, the required activation time is

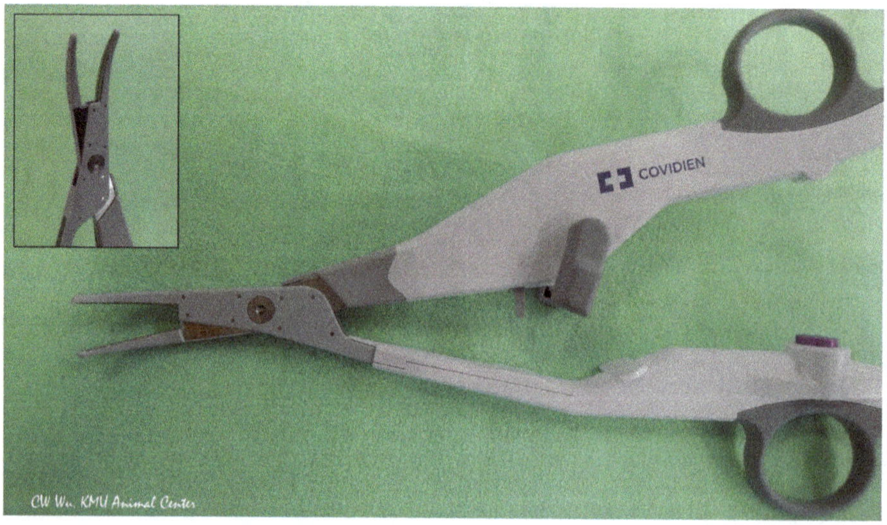

FIGURE 3 | The LigaSure Exact Dissector (LED) (Medtronic, Mineapolis, MN, USA) is an advanced bipolar energy based device commonly used for open thyroid surgery. The finely curved symmetrical jaws have an anti-adherent nano-coating.

2 to 4 seconds, which is shorter than that of LSJ. In Huang et al. study, the safe activation distance was 1 mm, and the cooling study revealed no adverse EMG events after a 2-second cooling interval or after muscle touch maneuver (35).

Ultrasonic EBDs

Ultrasonic EBDs deliver energy in the form of ultrasonic vibrations, which enable simultaneous cutting and coagulation. When a Harmonic device is used for transecting and sealing tissue, contact between the blade and the tissue pad of the device causes a rapid temperature increase.(**Figure 4**) A Harmonic device can seal vessels up to 7 mm in diameter. Notably, ultrasonic EBDs such as the Harmonic enable sealing at lower temperatures compared to monopolar electrocautery equipment (30, 36).

Harmonic Focus (HF) (Ethicon, Johnson and Johnson, Cincinnati, OH, USA)

The activation study in Wu et al. revealed no adverse EMG event at an activation distance of 1 mm and an activation time between 3 and 10 seconds. At a distance of 0 mm, EMG was stable in the first 3 seconds, but adverse EMG events occurred when activation time reached 4 seconds or longer. The cooling study revealed no adverse EMG event after a 10-second cooling period. When muscle touch maneuver was used for cooling, no adverse EMG events occurred after a 2-second cooling time (37).

Harmonic Focus+ (HF+) (Ethicon, Johnson and Johnson, Cincinnati, OH, USA)

Unlike the HF, the HF+ has Adaptive Tissue Technology, which increases precision in delivery of energy and reduces the time required for the device to reach its operating temperature (36). In the study, the HF+ did not cause significant thermal damage to the RLN at an activation distance of 1mm or even when the non-acting blade was activated while in direct contact with the nerve in the dry field. However, activation at a distance of 1 mm increased latency in some nerves whereas activation in direct contact revealed decreased amplitude in some nerves. In both cases, EMG changes recovered to baseline within 5-6 minutes (27).

Harmonic ACE (Ethicon, Johnson and Johnson, Cincinnati, OH, USA)

The Harmonic ACE is applicable in both endoscopic and open surgery. The device, 23cm length, 5.5mm diameter, can rotate 360 degrees. Kim et al. reported no adverse EMG events within 25 seconds after activation at a distance of 4 mm. At activation distances of 1-3 mm, however, shrinkage occurred in adjacent tissue within 6 to 25 seconds after activation. In some patients, activation resulted in adverse EMG events (38).

Harmonic ACE+ (Ethicon, Johnson and Johnson, Cincinnati, OH, USA)

The Adaptive Tissue Technology used in the HF+ is also used in the Harmonic ACE+. This technology theoretically reduces thermal spread and transection time. Experiments showed that Harmonic ACE+ did not cause adverse EMG events within 20 seconds after activation at a distance of 1 mm from the RLN. When the HA+ was activated in direct contact with the RLN, however, adverse EMG events occurred after 6 seconds of activation (38).

Sonicision (Medtronic, Minneapolis, MN, USA)

Sonicision is an ultrasonic EBD that can perform vessel sealing and dissection in surgery. The device is cordless, which increases mobility and convenience. Since the device is available in lengths ranging from 13 to 48 cm, it can be used in either endoscopic or open surgery. According to Hayami et al., Sonicision can be safely used at a distance of 1 mm from the RLN (39).

Hybrid EBDs (Ultrasonic and Bipolar EBDs)

Thunderbeat (TB) (Olympus Co Inc, Tokyo, Japan)

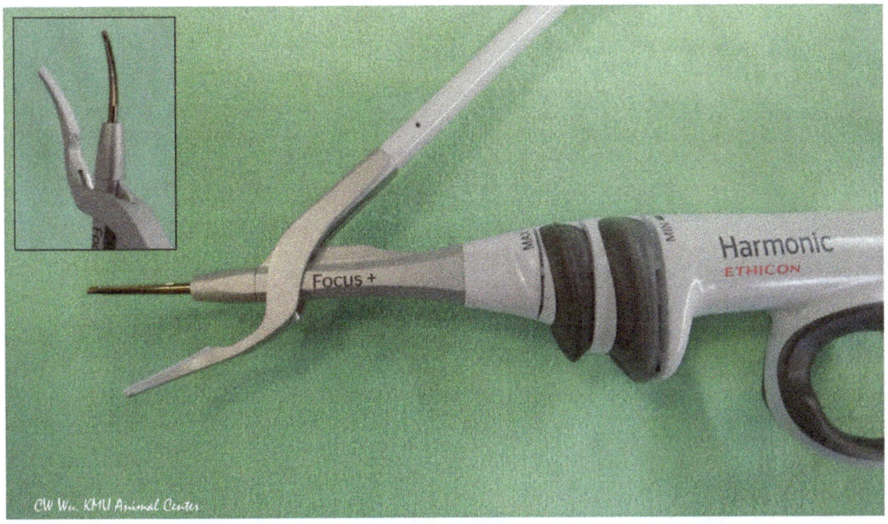

FIGURE 4 | Ultrasonic energy based device. Harmonic Focus+ (HF+) (Ethicon, Johnson and Johnson, Cincinnati, OH, USA). The HF+ is widely used in open thyroid surgery. Its curved and tapered tip has bare blades on one side and a non-active tissue pad on the opposite side.

The TB integrates both ultrasonic and advanced bipolar energy. The curved probe is composed of aluminum and has a thin profile to aid release of residual heat after activation (**Figure 5**). Surgeons can use TB to coagulate, dissect and cut blood vessels 5-7 mm in diameter (4, 33). In Kwak et al. study, no adverse EMG events occurred when the TB was activated for less than 10 seconds at distances of 3 mm from the RLN. However, when the TB was activated for 8 seconds at a distance of 2 mm from the RLN, amplitude decreased (4).

Ferromagnetic EBDs

Ferromagnetic EBDs are recently developed devices that enable hemostasis and dissection during thyroid surgery. Ferromagnetic EBDs generate pure thermal energy in response to a rapidly alternating magnetic field (40, 41).

FMwand (Domain Surgical, Salt Lake City, Utah)

The FMwand is a hemostatic dissecting scalpel with a dissecting loop. In Huang et al. study, no adverse EMG events occurred at distances of 2 mm or longer. Additionally, the cooling study revealed no adverse EMG events after a 1-second interval or after muscle touch maneuver (40).

FMsealer (Domain Surgical, Salt Lake City, Utah)

The FMsealer is a vessel sealing instrument that can seal vessels up to 7 mm in diameter. Compared to ultrasonic devices, FMsealer has a significantly lower peak temperature (92.1°C) and enables faster transection of tissue bundles (41). In their activation study, Huang et al. reported that the safe distance is 2 mm for a single 3-second activation. No adverse EMG events occurred after a 3-second cooling time or after muscle touch maneuver (40).

DISCUSSION

Thyroid surgery is one of the most commonly performed endocrine surgical procedures, the risk of complications is high due to the anatomical structure and physiological function of the RLN. Symptoms after thyroid surgery may include dysphagia, dysphonia, aspiration, choking, and even dyspnea (10–13). The management of symptomatic patients varied case by case, from voice therapy, vocal fold injection, thyroplasty to tracheotomy. It is noteworthy that patients who underwent thyroidectomy without RLN injury may also suffered from dysphonia and dysphagia. However, most of the symptoms are transient with good prognosis (9, 11–13). Avoiding iatrogenic RLN injury is essential for voice and swallowing outcomes after thyroid surgery. Impaired RLN function and vocal fold movement are problematic complications that may lead to medicolegal litigation after thyroid surgery in the quality-of-life era (8, 9, 42, 43).

Because they are ideal for dissection and provide a hemostatic effect, EBDs are currently used in more than 60% of thyroid surgeries (1). However, the high temperatures generated by EBD blades raise the risk of unexpected iatrogenic RLN thermal injury. This article reviewed recently published medical literature relevant to safety parameters for EBD use in thyroid surgery. For various EBDs, **Table 1** summarizes the recent literature on optimal activation distances in terms of safety and cooling time. Surgeons should be familiar with the safety parameters of an EBD before using it in thyroid surgery and should follow standard procedures for hemostasis and dissection near the RLN to prevent iatrogenic RLN thermal injury and to improve the voice outcomes of patients.

TABLE 1 | Summary of safety parameters of EBDs near the RLN during thyroid surgery.

Device/Generator (Power)	Activation distance (activation time)	Cooling time	Reference (all by porcine model)
Monopolar Electrocautery (15W)	5 mm (1 sec)	1 sec	(25)
Bipolar Electrocautery (30W)	3 mm (1 sec)	1 sec	(25)
Advanced Bipolar Energy Based Device			
LigaSure Small Jaw (LSJ)/ ForceTriad energy platform (level2)	2 mm (2-4 sec)	2 sec or muscle touch (immediately)	(31)
LigaSure Exact Dissector (LED)/ ValleylabTM LS10 energy platform	1 mm (2-4 sec)	2 sec or muscle touch (immediately)	(35)
Ultrasonic Energy BasedDevice			
Harmonic Focus (HF)/ Ethicon Endo-Surgery Generator G11(level5)	1 mm (3-10 sec)	10 sec or muscle touch(2 sec)	(37)
Harmonic Focus+ (HF+)/ Ethicon Endo-Surgery Generator G11(level5)	1 mm (4.7 ± 1.1sec)		(27)
Harmonic ACE/ Ethicon Endo-Surgery Generator G11(level5)	4 mm (10-25 sec)		(38)
Harmonic ACE+/ Ethicon Endo-Surgery Generator G11(level5)	1 mm (5-20 sec)		(38)
Sonicision/ maximum power mode (55 kHz)	1mm (1.5-2 sec)		(39)
Hybrid Energy Based Device (Ultrasonic and Bipolar Energy)			
Thunderbeat (TB)	3 mm (10 sec)		(4)
Ferromagnetic Energy Based Device			
FMwand/ FMX G1 Generator (Max45)	2 mm (3 sec)	1 sec or muscle touch (immediately)	(35)
FMsealer/ FMX G1 Generator (Max3)	2 mm (3 sec)	1 sec or muscle touch (immediately)	(35)

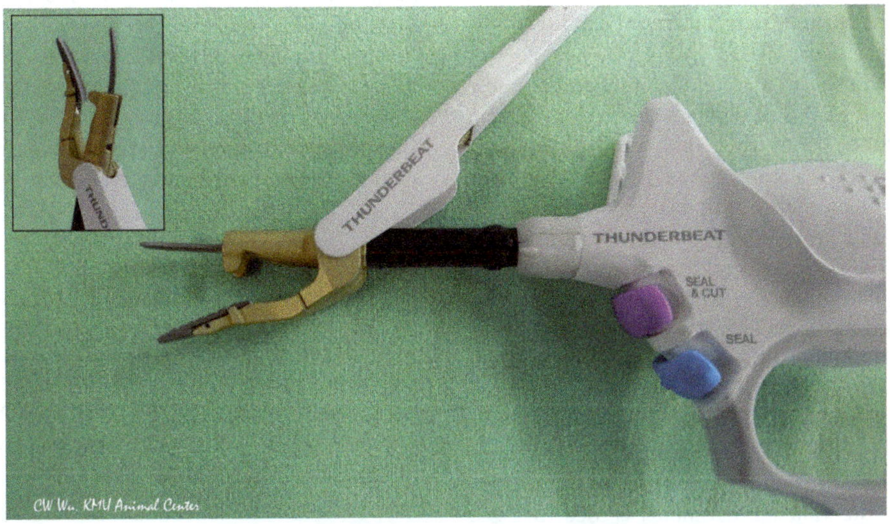

FIGURE 5 | Hybrid energy based device (ultrasonic and bipolar energy). The Thunderbeat Open Fine Jaw (TB; Olympus Co Inc, Tokyo, Japan) has a thin, curved probe for fine dissection. The counter jaw enables its use for grasping tissue. The aluminum coating dissipates residual heat.

In the past two decades, IONM use in thyroid surgery has become well established and is increasingly accepted worldwide. Additionally, many studies have reported that continuous IONM by periodic vagal stimulation can be useful in high-risk procedure and enables corrective action to prevent RLN traction injuries (44–46). Unlike traction injury, however, thermal injury often occurs suddenly and unexpectedly. Since IONM may be inapplicable for early detection and prevention of thermal injuries, safe use of EBDs is more important than using IONM to identify thermal injuries retrospectively.

Recent experimental and clinical studies indicate that thermal injury to the RLN is more severe than mechanical injury (i.e., injury caused by traction, compression, etc.) to the RLN because thermal injury tends to cause irreversible changes in nerve function (17, 19). Additionally, visual identification of a thermal injury to the RLN is often difficult, and lateral thermal spread can occur even when the heat source does not make direct contact with the nerve (31, 37). Protein denaturation and RLN injuries occur at a temperature of 60°C (47). Thermal stimuli applied to the RLN at temperatures over 60°C can cause permanent functional damage to the endoneurium (19). Since most EBDs reach temperatures exceeding 60°C after activation, surgeons must carefully consider the risk of endoneurium injury, regardless of the EBD type used. Maximum activation temperatures of ultrasonic EBDs and hybrid devices (e.g. TB) may exceed 200°C, only lower to monopolar electrocautery which have a higher maximum activation temperature (> 350°C) (28, 29, 33, 39). Advanced bipolar EBDs, bipolar electrocautery and FMsealer have maximum activation temperatures ranging from 80 to 100°C (33, 41, 48). Therefore, surgeons should remain cognizant that using EBDs for dissection near the RLN can potentially cause thermal injury of varying severity, especially during endoscopic procedures in which the surgical field is limited and the EBDs is commonly used for dissection.

Different EBDs deliver energy through different mechanisms, and the high temperature generated by an EBD may not be proportional to the activation distance (32). Recent studies also indicate that advanced bipolar devices induce greater thermal spread compared to ultrasonic devices. However, the temperature of adjacent tissue affected by thermal spread reportedly remains below 30°C, which would not substantially change EMG (39, 48).

Notably, Hayami et al. argued that activating EBDs in the wet condition (e.g., after exposure to liquid content from tissue) generates high-temperature steam. Since the steam, hyperthermal liquid, or smog may cause thermal injury to the RLN, caution should be taken when operate in specific condition, and increasing the activation distance is essential (49, 50).

Long duration of EBDs use may cause tissue shrinkage or thermal injury (38). Temperatures potentially generated by EBDs increase as activation time increases. Heat production is slower in ultrasonic EBDs compared to electrocautery equipment. Ultrasonic EBDs, temperatures may reach 150 to 200°C when activation time exceeds 10 seconds (29, 33, 39).

Similarly, advanced bipolar EBDs reach much higher temperatures after a double activation compared to a single activation. Consequently, thermal injuries may occur when an advanced bipolar EBDs is not allowed to cool between activations (35).

For some EBDs, data for cooling time were unavailable and were not included in **Table 1**. Experiments using infrared cameras and thermo-sensors had elucidated this issue. According to the literature, the time required for ultrasonic EBDs to cool to 60°C is almost two-fold longer than that for advanced bipolar EBDs (32–34). The surgeons may opt to perform muscle touch maneuver if the surgeons concludes that the long cooling time for an EBD during surgery would raise the risk of an extended surgical time. For ultrasonic EBDs, the recommended minimum duration of the muscle touch maneuver is 2 seconds (37).

This article reviewed relevant medical literature on the safety parameters for use of EBDs in thyroid surgery, including minimum safe distance from the RLN and the cooling duration of EBDs. Applying continuous IONM in animal experiments is an ideal method to establish the safety parameters of newly launched EBDs (51). Notably, all reviewed studies were animal studies, and all used porcine models of the RLN since experimentally inducing RLN injury in a human patient would violate ethical guidelines. Recommended distances for safe use of EBDs slightly differed among some studies, possibly due to differences in the mechanical properties of tissue specimens (e.g. wet versus dry condition), differences in experimental animal species, and differences in instrument settings and methodologies. Neural and tissue characteristics may differ even when the same animal model is used (37, 49). Therefore, data obtained in animal experiments should be applied cautiously to human patients (30). Future large observational clinical studies are needed for further verification of the findings of this study.

CONCLUSION

In conclusion, energy-based device (EBD) in thyroidectomy yields many superior outcomes, including considerable reduction of operative time, incision length, blood loss, and post-operative pain. One major advantage is significantly lowered rate of postoperative neck hematoma and postoperative hypocalcemia. To avoid an inadvertent iatrogenic RLN thermal injury caused by EBDs, standard procedures for safe use of these advanced medical devices must be developed and implemented. Many studies agree that animal models are ideal for experiments in continuous IONM because they provide objective data that can be used for electrophysiological evaluation of RLN thermal injury and for development of safety parameters for newly developed EBDs.

In general, conventional electrocautery generates higher temperature and wider thermal spread range, but when applying EBDs near the RLN adequate activation distance and cooling time are still required to avoid inadvertent thermal injury. Understanding EBD safety parameters and following standard procedures for using EBDs in thyroid surgery can improve safety and surgical outcomes, especially in voice quality and vocal cord mobility.

AUTHOR CONTRIBUTIONS

JJ-W, TY-H, and CW-W conceived and designed the study. Administrative support was obtained by CH-L, LF-W. Provision of study materials by IC-L, PY-C, HC-C, HY-C, HY-T, YC-L and G-D. had collected and assembled the data. Data analysis and interpretation was done by FY-C, TY-H, CW-W. All authors were participated in manuscript writing and final approval of manuscript.

FUNDING

This study was supported by grants from Kaohsiung Medical University Hospital (KMUH109-9M44), Kaohsiung Municipal Siaogang Hospital/Kaohsiung Medical University Research Center grants (KMHK-DK (C)110009, I-109-04, H-109-05, I-108-02) and Ministry of Science and Technology (MOST 108-2628-B-037-006, MOST 109-2628-B-037-014, MOST 110-2314-B-037-104-MY2, MOST 110-2314-B-037-120), Taiwan.

ACKNOWLEDGMENTS

The authors would like to thank all authors of the papers included in this study, as well as participants in the contributing studies.

REFERENCES

1. Moran K, Grigorian A, Elfenbein D, Schubl S, Jutric Z, Lekawa M, et al. Energy Vessel Sealant Devices Are Associated With Decreased Risk of Neck Hematoma After Thyroid Surgery. *Updates Surg* (2020) 72(4):1135–41. doi: 10.1007/s13304-020-00776-9
2. Canu GL, Medas F, Podda F, Tatti A, Pisano G, Erdas E, et al. Thyroidectomy With Energy-Based Devices: Surgical Outcomes and Complications—Comparison Between Harmonic Focus, Ligasure Small Jaw and Thunderbeat Open Fine Jaw. *Gland Surg* (2020) 9(3):721. doi: 10.21037/gs.2020.03.31
3. Garas G, Okabayashi K, Ashrafian H, Shetty K, Palazzo F, Tolley N, et al. Which Hemostatic Device in Thyroid Surgery? A Network Meta-Analysis of Surgical Technologies. *Thyroid* (2013) 23(9):1138–50. doi: 10.1089/thy.2012.0588
4. Kwak HY, Dionigi G, Kim D, Lee HY, Son GS, Lee JB, et al. Thermal Injury of the Recurrent Laryngeal Nerve by THUNDERBEAT During Thyroid Surgery: Findings From Continuous Intraoperative Neuromonitoring in a Porcine Model. *J Surg Res* (2016) 200(1):177–82. doi: 10.1016/j.jss.2015.06.066
5. Dionigi G, Wu C-W, Kim H-Y, Liu X, Liu R, Randolph GW, et al. Safety of Energy Based Devices for Hemostasis in Thyroid Surgery. *Gland Surg* (2016) 5(5):490. doi: 10.21037/gs.2016.09.01
6. Liu C-H, Wang C-C, Wu C-W, Lin Y-C, Lu I, Chang P-Y, et al. Comparison of Surgical Complications Rates Between Ligasure Small Jaw and Clamp-and-Tie Hemostatic Technique in 1,000 Neuro-Monitored Thyroidectomies. *Front Endocrinol* (2021) 12:313. doi: 10.3389/fendo.2021.638608
7. Pacilli M, Tartaglia N, Gerundo A, Pavone G, Fersini A, Ambrosi A. Energy Based Vessel Sealing Devices in Thyroid Surgery: A Systematic Review to Clarify the Relationship With Recurrent Laryngeal Nerve Injuries. *Medicina* (2020) 56(12):651. doi: 10.3390/medicina56120651
8. Huang T-Y, Yu W-HV, Chiang F-Y, Wu C-W, Fu S-C, Tai A-S, et al. How the Severity and Mechanism of Recurrent Laryngeal Nerve Dysfunction During Monitored Thyroidectomy Impact on Postoperative Voice. *Cancers* (2021) 13 (21):5379. doi: 10.3390/cancers13215379
9. Christakis I, Klang P, Talat N, Galata G, Schulte K-M. Long-Term Quality of Voice Is Usually Acceptable After Initial Hoarseness Caused by a Thyroidectomy or a Parathyroidectomy. *Gland Surg* (2019) 8(3):226. doi: 10.21037/gs.2018.09.02

10. Schneider R, Randolph GW, Dionigi G, Wu CW, Barczynski M, Chiang FY, et al. International Neural Monitoring Study Group Guideline 2018 Part I: Staging Bilateral Thyroid Surgery With Monitoring Loss of Signal. *Laryngoscope* (2018) 128 Suppl 3:S1–17. doi: 10.1002/lary.27359
11. Yu W-HV, Wu C-W. Speech Therapy After Thyroidectomy. *Gland Surg* (2017) 6(5):501. doi: 10.21037/gs.2017.06.06
12. Borel F, Tresallet C, Hamy A, Mathonnet M, Lifante J-C, Brunaud L, et al. Self-Assessment of Voice Outcomes After Total Thyroidectomy Using the Voice Handicap Index Questionnaire: Results of a Prospective Multicenter Study. *Surgery* (2020) 167(1):129–36. doi: 10.1016/j.surg.2019.05.090
13. Borel F, Christou N, Marret O, Mathonnet M, Caillard C, Bannani S, et al. Long-Term Voice Quality Outcomes After Total Thyroidectomy: A Prospective Multicenter Study. *Surgery* (2018) 163(4):796–800. doi: 10.1016/j.surg.2017.09.023
14. Wu CW, Dionigi G, Barczynski M, Chiang FY, Dralle H, Schneider R, et al. International Neuromonitoring Study Group Guidelines 2018: Part II: Optimal Recurrent Laryngeal Nerve Management for Invasive Thyroid Cancer-Incorporation of Surgical, Laryngeal, and Neural Electrophysiologic Data. *Laryngoscope* (2018) 128 Suppl 3:S18–s27. doi: 10.1002/lary.27360
15. Wu CW, Randolph GW, Barczyński M, Schneider R, Chiang FY, Huang TY, et al. Training Courses in Laryngeal Nerve Monitoring in Thyroid and Parathyroid Surgery- the INMSG Consensus Statement. *Front Endocrinol (Lausanne)* (2021) 12:705346. doi: 10.3389/fendo.2021.705346
16. Feng AL, Puram SV, Singer MC, Modi R, Kamani D, Randolph GW. Increased Prevalence of Neural Monitoring During Thyroidectomy: Global Surgical Survey. *Laryngoscope* (2020) 130(4):1097–104. doi: 10.1002/lary.28210
17. Dionigi G, Wu CW, Kim HY, Rausei S, Boni L, Chiang FY. Severity of Recurrent Laryngeal Nerve Injuries in Thyroid Surgery. *World J Surg* (2016) 40(6):1373–81. doi: 10.1007/s00268-016-3415-3
18. Wu CW, Lee KD, Tae K, Ji YB, Kim SU, Lee HS, et al. Recurrent Laryngeal Nerve (RLN) Injury in Thyroid Surgery: Lessons Learned From the Intraoperative Neural Monitoring (IONM). *Int J Head Neck Sci* (2017) 1 (1):19–26. doi: 10.6696/IJHNS.2017.0101.04
19. Wu CW, Dionigi G, Sun H, Liu X, Kim HY, Hsiao PJ, et al. Intraoperative Neuromonitoring for the Early Detection and Prevention of RLN Traction Injury in Thyroid Surgery: A Porcine Model. *Surgery* (2014) 155(2):329–39. doi: 10.1016/j.surg.2013.08.015
20. Randolph GW, Dralle H, Abdullah H, Barczynski M, Bellantone R, Brauckhoff M, et al. Electrophysiologic Recurrent Laryngeal Nerve Monitoring During Thyroid and Parathyroid Surgery: International Standards Guideline Statement. *Laryngoscope* (2011) 121 Suppl 1:S1–16. doi: 10.1002/lary.21119
21. Chiang FY, Lu IC, Kuo WR, Lee KW, Chang NC, Wu CW. The Mechanism of Recurrent Laryngeal Nerve Injury During Thyroid Surgery–the Application of Intraoperative Neuromonitoring. *Surgery* (2008) 143(6):743–9. doi: 10.1016/j.surg.2008.02.006
22. Dionigi G, Alesina PF, Barczynski M, Boni L, Chiang FY, Kim HY, et al. Recurrent Laryngeal Nerve Injury in Video-Assisted Thyroidectomy: Lessons Learned From Neuromonitoring. *Surg Endosc* (2012) 26(9):2601–8. doi: 10.1007/s00464-012-2239-y
23. Dionigi G. Energy Based Devices and Recurrent Laryngeal Nerve Injury: The Need for Safer Instruments. *Langenbecks Arch Surg* (2009) 394(3):579–80; author reply 81-6. doi: 10.1007/s00423-008-0454-8
24. Lee E, Tong JY, Pasick LJ, Benito DA, Joshi A, Thakkar PG, et al. Complications Associated With Energy-Based Devices During Thyroidectomy From 2010–2020. *World J Otorhinolaryngology-Head Neck Surg* (2021). doi: 10.1016/j.wjorl.2021.04.008
25. Wu C-W, Huang T-Y, Chen H-C, Chen H-Y, Tsai T-Y, Chang P-Y, et al. Intra-Operative Neural Monitoring of Thyroid Surgery in a Porcine Model. *JoVE* (2019) 144):e57919. doi: 10.3791/57919
26. Wu C-W, Randolph GW, Lu I-C, Chang P-Y, Chen Y-T, Hun P-C, et al. Intraoperative Neural Monitoring in Thyroid Surgery: Lessons Learned From Animal Studies. *Gland Surg* (2016) 5(5):473–80. doi: 10.21037/gs.2016.09.06
27. Chávez KV, Barajas EM, Soroa F, Gamboa-Dominguez A, Ordóñez S, Pantoja JP, et al. Safety Assessment of the Use of Ultrasonic Energy in the Proximity of the Recurrent Laryngeal Nerve in a Porcine Model. *Am J Surg* (2018) 215 (1):186–90. doi: 10.1016/j.amjsurg.2017.04.013
28. Sutton P, Awad S, Perkins A, Lobo D. Comparison of Lateral Thermal Spread Using Monopolar and Bipolar Diathermy, the Harmonic Scalpel™ and the Ligasure™. *J Br Surg* (2010) 97(3):428–33. doi: 10.1002/bjs.6901
29. Kinoshita T, Kanehira E, Omura K, Kawakami K, Watanabe Y. Experimental Study on Heat Production by a 23.5-Khz Ultrasonically Activated Device for Endoscopic Surgery. *Surg Endoscopy* (1999) 13(6):621–5. doi: 10.1007/s004649901055
30. Bakkar S, Papavramidis TS, Aljarrah Q, Materazzi G, Miccoli P. Energy-Based Devices in Thyroid Surgery—An Overview. *Gland Surg* (2020) 9(Suppl 1):S14. doi: 10.21037/gs.2019.08.05
31. Dionigi G, Chiang FY, Kim HY, Randolph GW, Mangano A, Chang PY, et al. Safety of Ligasure in Recurrent Laryngeal Nerve Dissection-Porcine Model Using Continuous Monitoring. *Laryngoscope* (2017) 127(7):1724–9. doi: 10.1002/lary.26271
32. Smith CT, Zarebczan B, Alhefdhi A, Chen H. Infrared Thermographic Profiles of Vessel Sealing Devices on Thyroid Parenchyma. *J Surg Res* (2011) 170 (1):64–8. doi: 10.1016/j.jss.2011.03.005
33. Seehofer D, Mogl M, Boas-Knoop S, Unger J, Schirmeier A, Chopra S, et al. Safety and Efficacy of New Integrated Bipolar and Ultrasonic Scissors Compared to Conventional Laparoscopic 5-Mm Sealing and Cutting Instruments. *Surg Endoscopy* (2012) 26(9):2541–9. doi: 10.1007/s00464-012-2229-0
34. Kim FJ, Chammas M, Gewehr E, Morihisa M, Caldas F, Hayacibara E, et al. Temperature Safety Profile of Laparoscopic Devices: Harmonic ACE (ACE), Ligasure V (LV), and Plasma Trisector (PT). *Surg endoscopy* (2008) 22 (6):1464–9. doi: 10.1007/s00464-007-9650-9
35. Huang T-Y, Lin Y-C, Tseng H-Y, Dionigi G, Kim H-Y, Lu I-C, et al. Safety of Ligasure Exact Dissector in Thyroidectomy With Continuous Neuromonitoring: A Porcine Model. *Gland Surg* (2020) 9(3):702. doi: 10.21037/gs.2020.03.17
36. Broughton D, Welling AL, Monroe EH, Pirozzi K, Schulte JB, Clymer JW. Tissue Effects in Vessel Sealing and Transection From an Ultrasonic Device With More Intelligent Control of Energy Delivery. *Med Devices* (2013) 6:151. doi: 10.2147/MDER.S51663
37. Wu CW, Chai YJ, Dionigi G, Chiang FY, Liu X, Sun H, et al. Recurrent Laryngeal Nerve Safety Parameters of the H Armonic F Ocus During Thyroid Surgery: Porcine Model Using Continuous Monitoring. *Laryngoscope* (2015) 125(12):2838–45. doi: 10.1002/lary.25412
38. Kim HK, Chai YJ, Lee HY, Kim HY, Dionigi G. Comparing the Safety of Harmonic ACE and ACE+ Around the Recurrent Laryngeal Nerve in Swine Models. *Ann Surg Treat Res* (2018) 94(6):285–90. doi: 10.4174/astr.2018.94.6.285
39. Hayami M, Watanabe M, Mine S, Imamura Y, Okamura A, Yuda M, et al. Lateral Thermal Spread Induced by Energy Devices: A Porcine Model to Evaluate the Influence on the Recurrent Laryngeal Nerve. *Surg Endoscopy* (2019) 33(12):4153–63. doi: 10.1007/s00464-019-06724-y
40. Huang TY, Lin YC, Tseng HY, Dionigi G, Kim HY, Chai YJ, et al. Safety Parameters of Ferromagnetic Device During Thyroid Surgery: Porcine Model Using Continuous Neuromonitoring. *Head Neck* (2020) 42(10):2931–40. doi: 10.1002/hed.26334
41. Chen J, Jensen CR, Manwaring PK, Glasgow RE. Validation of a Laparoscopic Ferromagnetic Technology-Based Vessel Sealing Device and Comparative Study to Ultrasonic and Bipolar Laparoscopic Devices. *Surg Laparoscopy Endoscopy* (2017) 27(2):e12. doi: 10.1097/SLE.0000000000000385
42. Dralle H, Lorenz K, Machens A. Verdicts on Malpractice Claims After Thyroid Surgery: Emerging Trends and Future Directions. *Head Neck* (2012) 34(11):1591–6. doi: 10.1002/hed.21970
43. Gualniera P, Scurria S, Mondello C, Asmundo A, Sapienza D, Gianlorenzo D. Narrative Review of Proving the Causal Link of Recurrent Laryngeal Nerve Injury and Thyroidectomy: A Medico Legal Appraisal. *Gland Surg* (2020) 9 (5):1564–72. doi: 10.21037/gs-20-203
44. Dionigi G, Donatini G, Boni L, Rausei S, Rovera F, Tanda ML, et al. Continuous Monitoring of the Recurrent Laryngeal Nerve in Thyroid Surgery: A Critical Appraisal. *Int J Surg* (2013) 11(Suppl)1:S44–6. doi: 10.1016/S1743-9191(13)60014-X
45. Schneider R, Przybyl J, Hermann M, Hauss J, Jonas S, Leinung S. A New Anchor Electrode Design for Continuous Neuromonitoring of the Recurrent Laryngeal Nerve by Vagal Nerve Stimulations. *Langenbecks Arch Surg* (2009) 394(5):903–10. doi: 10.1007/s00423-009-0503-y

46. Phelan E, Schneider R, Lorenz K, Dralle H, Kamani D, Potenza A, et al. Continuous Vagal IONM Prevents Recurrent Laryngeal Nerve Paralysis by Revealing Initial EMG Changes of Impending Neuropraxic Injury: A Prospective, Multicenter Study. *Laryngoscope* (2014) 124(6):1498–505. doi: 10.1002/lary.24550
47. Lin YC, Dionigi G, Randolph GW, Lu IC, Chang PY, Tsai SY, et al. Electrophysiologic Monitoring Correlates of Recurrent Laryngeal Nerve Heat Thermal Injury in a Porcine Model. *Laryngoscope* (2015) 125(8): E283–E90. doi: 10.1002/lary.25362
48. Hruby GW, Marruffo FC, Durak E, Collins SM, Pierorazio P, Humphrey PA, et al. Evaluation of Surgical Energy Devices for Vessel Sealing and Peripheral Energy Spread in a Porcine Model. *J Urol* (2007) 178(6):2689–93. doi: 10.1016/j.juro.2007.07.121
49. Hayami M, Watanabe M, Mine S, Imamura Y, Okamura A, Yuda M, et al. Steam Induced by the Activation of Energy Devices Under a Wet Condition may Cause Thermal Injury. *Surg Endoscopy* (2020) 34(5):2295–302. doi: 10.1007/s00464-019-07312-w
50. Yu X, Liu C, Yan M, Gong W, Wang Y. Hyperthermal Liquid, Spray, and Smog may be Potential Risk Factors for Recurrent Laryngeal Nerve Thermal Injury During Thyroid Surgeries. *Endocrine* (2021) 72(1):198–207. doi: 10.1007/s12020-020-02451-w
51. Prasad A, Durrant J, Smeak DD, Newman JG. The Thermal Safety Profile of a New Bipolar Vessel Sealing Device for Thyroid Surgery. *Surg Technol Int* (2021) 39:sti39/1501. doi: 10.52198/21.STI.39.SO1501

25

Novel Approaches for Treating Autonomously Functioning Thyroid Nodules

*Pia Pace-Asciak, Jon O. Russell, Mohammad Shaear and Ralph P. Tufano**

Division of Otolaryngology-Head and Neck Surgery, Johns Hopkins University, Baltimore, MD, United States

Correspondence:
Ralph P. Tufano
rtufano@jhmi.edu

Benign thyroid nodules are exceedingly common in the adult population. Only a small percentage of nodules are toxic or autonomously functioning thyroid nodules (AFTNs). The options clinicians have for treating the symptoms of hyperthyroidism include anti-thyroidal medications, radioactive iodine, or surgery. Depending on the patient population treated, these options may not be suitable or have inherent risks that are undesirable to the patient. On the other hand, untreated hyperthyroidism can lead to osteoporosis, atrial fibrillation, emotional lability, and neurological consequences. Thus, we present a review of two novel safe and effective approaches for treating AFTN; one surgical (transoral endoscopic thyroid surgery) and one non-surgical (radiofrequency ablation), as a means for expanding our treatment armamentarium.

Keywords: benign thyroid nodules, toxic nodules, transoral endoscopic thyroidectomy, radiofrequency ablation, hyperthyroidism

INTRODUCTION

Benign thyroid nodules (BTNs) are generally asymptomatic but can cause symptoms due to size or autonomous function. The frequency of incidental nodules is common in the adult population and can be found on high resolution ultrasound anywhere from 19 to 68%, with a higher proportion in females and the elderly (1). Over time, about 5–10% thyroid nodules can undergo progressive development to become autonomously functioning thyroid nodules (AFTNs) and secrete an abnormally higher amount of thyroid hormone. This may be more common in iodine deficient parts of the world (2, 3). AFTN is the second most common cause of hyperthyroidism, which occur more commonly in older women as these nodules degenerate with age (2).

Accompanying symptoms of hyperthyroidism can be overt or mild depending on the severity and include anxiety, emotional lability, weakness, tremor, palpitations, heat intolerance, increased perspiration, and weight loss despite a normal or increased appetite (4). Untreated hyperthyroidism can have deleterious effects on the cardiovascular and neurologic system, while also increasing the risk of osteoporosis and fractures (3, 4).

For decades, clinicians have treated the symptoms of hyperthyroidism with anti-thyroid drugs (ATDs) such as Methimazole or Propylthioruacil, Radioactive iodine ablation (RAI), or Surgery (4). Each treatment has unique risks, and the treatment therefore should be tailored to meet the needs of the patient population being treated. ATDs are commonly used to decrease thyroid hormone production and are useful in the short term, but they are not as definitive as surgery or radioactive iodine ablation (RAI) (3). Moreover, RAI may not be suitable in young women of child-bearing age, or patients who may not wish to endure the possibility of hypothyroidism (3). Surgery is a definitive intervention, but not all patients with AFTN are eligible for thyroid surgery or want surgery. While each of these strategies is appropriate for some patients, the inherent risks and limitations of each leave some patients seeking a more definitive option with more limited risks. In an age where there is a push towards 'personalized medicine', we review two recent advancements for the treatment of AFTN which may potentially broaden the surgical and non-surgical options for patients.

TRANSORAL ENDOSCOPIC THYROID SURGERY VESTIBULAR APPROACH

For decades, surgical resection of the affected lobe or the whole thyroid using a mid-transcervical incision has been the primary surgical approach for AFTNs. Surgery is rarely the first option offered to patients in the Western Hemisphere (3). However, surgery is recognized as a safe and definitive option for the treatment of AFTN (3). Surgical removal of an AFTN is effective in alleviating the pressure from the trachea while also normalizing thyroid function. However, surgery is not without risk, and may be elevated in older patients (5). Potential surgical complications include the presence of a life-long visible scar despite having benign disease, recurrent laryngeal nerve injury, and temporary or permanent hypocalcemia (6, 7). Additionally, thyroid lobectomy has the 5–49% chance of leading to postoperative hypothyroidism (8–11).

Novel minimally invasive techniques have emerged over the years to avoid the need for a traditional mid-cervical scar. Transoral endoscopic thyroidectomy vestibular approach (TOETVA) has gained favor because it allows remote access to the thyroid through an incision in the mucosa of the lower lip, avoiding the need for any kind of visible scar in the neck (12). Other remote access techniques include the retroauricular approach, trans-axillary technique, and bilateral axillo-breast approach (13–16). To date, none of these other approaches have become common in the West, while TOETVA is becoming relatively popular due to broad operative indications, wide eligibility and applicability for patients with benign or malignant disease, and even with a BMI greater than 30 (17–19). Although TOETVA has longer operative time when compared to the conventional open technique, patient satisfaction and cosmesis are superior with TOETVA (20, 21).

TOETVA evolved from a sublingual incision to a small incision in the oral vestibule (12, 18). In the initial series of TOETVA, Anuwong et al. found TOETVA to be safe, efficacious, with quick recovery and a superior cosmetic outcome (12). The momentum for this novel approach gained favor among international circles, and several trials have reproduced the safety and efficacy of TOETVA in Asia, Europe, and the United States (18, 22–29). When compared to open surgical approaches, TOETVA has reliably demonstrated similar rates of postoperative infection, reduced pain, safety, and a similar complication profile to open techniques (recurrent laryngeal nerve injury and hypoparathyroidism) (17, 22, 25, 26, 30)

Surgical removal of AFTN is a recognized indication for TOETVA (31). Due to the novelty of this approach and low incidence of AFTN, the data regarding resection for AFTN is limited. There are no published studies specifically looking at the outcome of TOETVA in AFTN alone; rather toxic nodules are likely grouped into 'benign thyroid disease' in the literature (23, 25, 32, 33) or TOETVA is compared to the open approach in patients with Graves disease (34). Given that one of the largest published series demonstrated a similar safety and complication rate for TOETVA compared to the traditional open approach, one can assume that the rate of success for treatment in AFTN would be similar to the open surgical open (22, 34). Luo et al. describe their case series of 204 patients; however, only one patient in their series demonstrated hyperthyroidism secondary to a secreting nodule as part of the 'benign nodule' category (35). Future studies would need to address this aspect directly.

TOETVA has been shown to be a safe approach with minimal complications. Russell et al.'s analysis of literature yielded 689 cases whereby TOETVA outcomes were evaluated, and articles using robotic or floor of mouth techniques were excluded. Of the 689 cases that underwent TOETVA, there were no published cases of RLN injury or permanent hypoparathyroidism, and only one report of a hematoma (0.1%) (32, 36). Technique-specific complications, such as mental nerve injury and related hypoesthesia, CO2 embolism, and neck infection were extremely limited, with no cases of permanent mental nerve injury or CO2 embolism and only one case of neck infection (0.1%). Given that access is through an intraoral incision, perioperative antibiotic treatment is recommended to avoid potential infection. Furthermore, surgeons should be aware of the rare but potential complication of CO2 insufflation. CO2 embolism has been reported in four other cases where other transoral techniques were employed as well (two *via* a floor of mouth technique and two *via* the transoral vestibular approach) (37–39). Finally, 683/689 (99%) cases were completed *via* TOETVA without conversion to another technique. Five cases reported excessive bleeding that could not be controlled *via* TOETVA, and one case reported excessive tumor size with evidence of pretracheal nodal metastasis (32, 36).

Other smaller technique-specific complications are related to thinning of the skin or perforation of the skin flap in three cases (0.4%) resulting in a skin burn. In terms of postoperative pain control, some reports show TOETVA to be superior compared with the open thyroidectomy, but in our experience, pain control is relatively equal (22, 32, 34, 36).

For benign thyroid disease, the benefits of TOETVA may not be limited to cosmesis alone. From a surgical point of view, the birds-eye view magnifies the operative view and gives excellent visualization of the RLN and its insertion site. This allows for access to a favorable dissection plane centrally and bilaterally, providing a view that is familiar to most endocrine surgeons (25). The magnified view also enhances visualization of the parathyroid glands, allowing for their preservation and may reduce the risk of temporary postoperative hypocalcemia that can occur 14–40% of patients when accessing the central neck (40). Furthermore, even though the endoscopic approach affords a narrow working space, TOETVA provides a birds-eye view that enables the surgeon to have meticulous control of bleeding (12). While these theoretical benefits remain unproven, early evidence suggests that TOETVA is not inferior to the traditional surgical approach while offering improved cosmesis.

As with any new technique, there is a learning curve associated with implementing and refining the endoscopic approach which leads to longer operative times. Various authors have noted similar learning curves (22, 35, 41). As this technique becomes readily available at institutions, and surgeons become facile with this approach, it will likely become more available. There are very few barriers to adopting this technique since laparoscopic equipment is readily available at most institutions. Utilizing this novel approach adds very little extra cost making this approach accessible to motivated surgeons that wish to add TOETVA to their surgical armamentarium (42).

NON-SURGICAL APPROACH: RADIOFREQUENCY ABLATION

Radiofrequency ablation (RFA) is a novel minimally invasive approach that is a potential alternative to surgery for treating symptomatic benign nodules (43) as well as AFTN (44). This approach eliminates the need for a general anesthetic, an incision, radioactive iodine, or prolonged ATD treatment, making it an attractive non-surgical option. With the use of local anesthesia, the RFA probe is introduced into the midline of the anterior neck at the level of the isthmus, and the nodule is approached using the moving shot technique under ultrasound guidance (45). This causes tissue necrosis and fibrosis by introducing a high frequency alternating current, which raises tissue temperatures to 60 to 100 C (46). Over time, there is progressive shrinkage of the ablated nodule. In benign nodules, the volume of the nodule is thought to decrease between 50 and 80% for most patients, although this is operator and tumor dependent (47, 48).

RFA has been offered to patients internationally since 2000 and has been used to treat primary and metastatic tumors of the liver, lung, bone, and kidney and to ablate aberrant conduction pathways in the heart (49–53). More recently, RFA has been applied to the head and neck, particularly for thyroid nodules. While the early results have been promising internationally, there is little North American data (47, 48, 54–61). The current international recommendations for treating benign thyroid nodules include patients who are symptomatic or those who have a disfiguring goiter or a nodule that exceeds 2 cm, or if an AFTN is present (43, 44, 57). Prior to RFA treatment of AFTN, confirmation that the nodule is benign on at least one US-guided FNA or core biopsy is recommended, unless there are concerning features on ultrasound in which case two biopsies should be obtained (43, 44). Nodules that are benign on FNA but that have suspicious US features (EU-TIRADS 5), the latest European Thyroid Association Guidelines strongly recommend (moderate quality evidence) against thyroid ablation to avoid potential delay in treatment of a malignant lesion (62).

RFA has shown excellent efficacy and safety in the management of cosmesis related concerns and pressure symptoms (47, 48, 54–61, 63, 64). In a systematic review and meta-analysis of RFA in benign nodules, a pooled proportion of 2.38% for overall RFA complications was noted (95% CI: 1.42–3.34%), with 1.35% for major complications (95% CI: 0.89–1.81%) and no evidence of any life-threatening complications. The most common complaint post treatment was transient or rarely permanent voice changes (35/2,421). Nodule rupture, permanent hypothyroidism 6 months after treatment, and transient brachial plexus injury was only found in one patient out of 2,421 patients (65). Minor complications included pain during or after the procedure (16/2421), hematoma which disappeared after 1–2 weeks (25/2,421), vomiting (9/2,421), skin burns (six patients had first degree burns and 1 patient had second degree burn which recovered after a month) and transient thyroiditis (one patient three months after the treatment) (65). Furthermore, various studies have shown that the volume of a benign symptomatic thyroid nodule can be reduced by more than 50%, and up to 75–97% in long-term follow-ups (60, 66, 67).

The American Thyroid Association Guidelines outline that surgery or radioactive iodine (RAI) are effective for the treatment of AFTN (1, 3). These two options are not always acceptable for patients since RAI involves receiving radiation which is controversial in women of childbearing age, or for patients reluctant to endure the long-term risks associated with radiation (3). Additionally, both treatments have potential complications such as hypothyroidism. Even with lobectomy, surgery confers roughly a 30% chance of hypothyroidism, which is generally avoided in RFA-treated patients (10, 11, 68). RFA may gain favor with patients wishing to avoid developing hypothyroidism (55, 57, 58, 69–71).

Many trials have demonstrated the efficacy and safety of treating AFTN with RFA (55, 57, 58, 69–71). In a large multicenter trial, Sung JY et al. demonstrated improved symptoms of hyperthyroidism along with normalized TSH levels in 81.8% of study patients without the development of hypothyroidism post RFA (35, 69). In a systematic review, more than 50% of patients after RFA could discontinue their anti-hyperthyroid medications after RFA (44, 46). Additionally, patients that received RFA found significant improvement in their compressive symptoms due to the reduced nodule volume (mean volume reduction ratio, 81.7% during the mean follow-up period of 19.9 months). No major complications were reported in this trial; however, in previous trials, the most common complication reported was temporary pain (55, 57, 58, 63). Progression of hypothyroidism, if any, after treatment may be better explained by the progression of autoimmune thyroiditis associated with preexisting thyroid antibodies.

In a recent systematic review and meta-analysis, Cesareo et al. demonstrated moderate efficacy of RFA in AFTN (72). The overall rate of patients with TSH normalization or scintigraphically proven efficacy was about 60%, with a volume reduction of 79% found 1 year later in RFA treated AFTN (72). Bernardi et al. demonstrated that 50% of patients with AFTN treated with RFA withdrew their ATD after 12 months (70), which is similar to Deandrea (55) and Faggiano (73) who reported normalized thyroid function in 40% of patients after 12 months. However, Cervelli et al. demonstrated a greater volume reduction rate of 76% with a 91% TSH normalization at 12-month follow-up in AFTN treated with RFA (74). Even though there is heterogeneity between studies, and patients were only followed for 12 months, longer follow-up is warranted as well as how to achieve a predictable response rate with discontinuation of ATD after one session of RFA. It is also possible that these findings represent technical differences in the procedure, as it may be assumed that there is a learning curve with this procedure. Nevertheless, it is apparent that, while many patients benefit in the short term, a sizeable component may need additional treatment.

The success rate of RFA is greater when the volume of the AFTN is relatively small in size. Cesareo et al. compared the reduction between medium sized nodules (18 ml) and smaller sized nodules (5 ml), euthyroidism was achieved 86% in small nodules *vs.* 45% in medium size nodules (75). Similarly, Cappelli et al. report a volume reduction rate of 73% with TSH normalization in 94% of patients treated with RFA with nodules an average of 7 ml (76). An earlier study by Lim et al. confirmed that larger nodules (>20 ml) required repeat RFA treatment compared with smaller nodules to achieve a similar volume reduction in during 4 year follow-up (77). This work has improved our understanding of how to counsel patients with AFTN.

Since the Korean Guidelines in 2012, the consensus for RFA of AFTN has evolved. In line with the Korean Guidelines, the Italian Minimally Invasive Treatment of the Thyroid (MITT) group have advised clinicians to offer RFA as first line treatment in non-functioning nodules. However for AFTN, RFA is best reserved as second line treatment in patients who refuse conventional therapy or when it is contraindicated (75, 78). RFA can be considered as primary treatment for small sized AFTN (average 5 ml) since an optimal response (symptom improvement and TSH normalization) is noted when the nodule is reduced in size by more than 80% (72, 75).

Key factors that affect the therapeutic response of RFA on AFTN have been debated. Baek et al., demonstrated the importance of nodule vascularity on ultrasound for normalization in TSH and volume reduction (67), while Bernardi et al. found the percentage of volume reduction at 12 months correlated with the therapeutic response (70). Whereas, Cesareo et al.'s work demonstrates the importance of the size of nodule prior to RFA and the volume reduction after 12 months (75).

Localization of the nodule with ultrasound is also key in determining whether partial or complete ablation can be achieved, particularly if the nodule is adjacent to the trachea or recurrent laryngeal nerve. Ideally, complete ablation is preferred to avoid nodule regrowth. The moving shot technique is the standard approach that is used in conjunction with ultrasound for real time surveillance of nearby structures (43, 45). As with any awake technique, patient comfort is key in order to avoid patient movement which could result in injury to one of the neighboring structures. Light sedation can overcome this potential risk and ease patient comfort along with local anesthetic. Finally, the proficiency of the operator is important since there is a learning curve associated with complete removal of tissue to avoid recurrence of an untreated remnant. Tracing the residual viable area of the nodule by ultrasound (usually isoechoic and on the periphery of the ablation zone) can be helpful to predict regrowth and the area to target for reablation (79).

Single-session RFA has shown significant volume and symptom reduction (43, 45, 47, 48, 55–57, 66, 70, 72, 73, 76). Progressive reduction in the volume of treated nodules occurs incrementally over time, with reports ranging from 50 to 80% after 6 months and 79 to 90% after 2 years follow-up (55, 57, 70, 72). Previous studies report a mean number of RFA treatment sessions to be 1.8–2.2 (one to six sessions) for AFTN (58, 66). Previous reports show that single session RFA allowed withdrawal of ATD in 22–57% of patients (55, 70, 72), with one report showing 100% in pre-toxic nodules and 53% in toxic nodules (57). Other reports show a reduced dose of Methimazole after RFA in 78% of patients (55). The improvement in thyroid function is seen over time after RFA treatment, with up to 57% remission 12 months after the procedure (70, 72). However, other studies have demonstrated a tendency for regrowth after 2 to 3 years follow-up in non-functioning nodules (77, 79). The number of required treatments or how often nodules require RFA treatments still needs to be determined, especially when treating AFTNs. However, the pre-treatment nodule volume seems to play a key role in volume reduction and discontinuation of ATD. Currently, the Korean Guidelines suggest that follow-up should be based on TSH post RFA treatment of the AFTN. This will determine whether the patient's antithyroidal medications can be stopped or if they require another treatment with RFA.

Imaging such as ultrasound examination and a thyroid scan with scintigraphy can also be helpful to know whether RFA was successful. Previous studies show post-treatment, scintigraphy demonstrated the majority of hot nodules (45–80%) became cold or normal, while 20.4–56% nodules had decreased uptake but still remained as hot nodules (58, 66). After treatment, evaluation *via* ultrasound should be done to ensure the absence of potential early complications from the procedure, such as an evolving hematoma, burns or damage to the thyroid capsule (62). On ultrasound, changes in the size, volume, intranodular vascularity and echogenicity are assessed (43). On ultrasound, the ablated area appears as a mildly hypoechoic and inhomogenous zone, with scattered hyperechoic spots due to tissue vaporization compared with the non-treated tissue (43, 62, 80). Color Doppler mapping of the treated areas are devoid of vascular signals (62, 80). If a patient is still symptomatic, the nodule can be assessed for persistent vascularity as a potential source for regrowth (81). The wide range of therapeutic effects of RFA may be attributed to remaining thyroid tissue left at the margin of the nodule. The best modality for detecting intranodular vascularity is contrast-enhanced ultrasound since color-Doppler is not as sensitive to detect small vessels and slow blood flow (43). Repeat RFA can be considered after 3 months from the first treatment because the most change is seen within the first 3 months (43, 69).

Given the potential for long-term cardiovascular mortality in the setting of untreated hyperthyroidism, the need for multiple treatments for patients treated with RFA does pose a theoretical risk that must be discussed appropriately (3, 57, 58, 70, 82). As newer evidence emerges, hopefully RFA will become standard of care. However, currently the Korean guidelines as well as the Italian MITT group discussed above take a more cautious tone when discussing the role of RFA in managing AFTN (43).

CONCLUSION

AFTN are benign nodules with multiple treatment options. TOETVA and RFA are two novel treatments that may be safe and effective in the treatment of symptomatic benign thyroid nodules and could be applied to AFTN. TOETVA offers a surgical approach with the removal of the thyroid gland which avoids a cervical scar and is definitive, whereas RFA offers a non-surgical approach for patients who wish to avoid surgery altogether or are poor surgical candidates. Because there is risk associated with multiple rounds of treatment, it may not be appropriate for all patients and international guidelines suggest exercising caution (43). Each of these approaches may be appropriate in the right clinical setting.

AUTHOR CONTRIBUTIONS

PP-A reviewed the literature and wrote the paper. JR was involved with the writing and editing as well as the key concepts behind the paper. MS was involved with reviewing/editing the paper. RT was involved with editing as well as the key concepts behind the paper. All authors contributed to the article and approved the submitted version.

REFERENCES

1. Haugen BR, Alexander EK, Bible KC, Doherty GM, Mandel SJ, Nikiforov YE, et al. 2015 American Thyroid Association Management Guidelines for Adult patients with Thyroid Nodules and Differentiated Thyroid Cancer: The American Thyroid Association Guidelines Task Force on Thyroid Nodules and Differentiated Thyroid Cancer. *Thyroid* (2016) 26(1):1–133. doi: 10.1089/thy.2015.0020
2. Hollowell JG, Staehling NW, Flanders WD, Hannon WH, Gunter EW, Spencer CA, et al. Serum TSH, T(4), and thyroid antibodies in the United States population (1988 to 1994): National Health and Nutrition Examination Survey (NHANES III). *J Clin Endocrinol Metab* (2002) 87:489. doi: 10.1210/jcem.87.2.8182
3. Ross DS, Burch HB, Cooper DS, Greenlee MC, Laurberg P, Maia AL, et al. 2016 American Thyroid Association Guidelines for diagnosis and management of hyperthyroidism and other causes of thyrotoxicosis. *Thyroid* (2016) 26(10):1343–421. doi: 10.1089/thy.2016.0229
4. Nordyke RA, Gilbert FIJr, Harada AS. Graves' disease. Influence of age on clinical findings. *Arch Intern Med* (1988) 148:626. doi: 10.1001/archinte.148.3.626
5. Sosa JA, Mehta PJ, Wang TS, Boudourakis L, Roman SA. A population-based study of outcomes from thyroidectomy in aging Americans: at what cost? *J Am Coll Surg* (2008) 206:1097–105. doi: 10.1016/j.jamcollsurg.2007.11.023
6. Vashishta R, Mahalingam-Dhingra A, Lander L, Shin EJ, Shah RK. Thyroidectomy outcomes: a national perspective. *Otolaryngol Head Neck Surg* (2012) 147:1027–34. doi: 10.1177/0194599812454401
7. Liao D, Ishii LE, Chen LW, Chen J, Juarez M, Darrach HM, et al. Transoral Neck Surgery Prevents Attentional Bias Towards the Neck Compared to Open Neck Surgery. *Laryngoscope* (2019) 00:1–6. doi: 10.1002/lary.28305
8. Farkas EA, King TA, Bolton JS, Fuhrman GM. A comparison of total thyroidectomy and lobectomy in the treatment of dominant thyroid nodules. *Am Surgeon* (2002) 68:678–82; discussion 82-3.
9. Wormald R, Sheahan P, Rowley S, Rizkalla H, Toner M, Timon C. Hemithyroidectomy for benign thyroid disease: who needs follow-up for hypothyroidism? *Clin Otolaryngol: Off J ENT-UK* (2008) 33:587–91. doi: 10.1111/j.1749-4486.2008.01794.x
10. McHenry CR, Slusarczyk SJ. Hypothyroidism following hemithyroidectomy: incidence, risk factors, and management. *Surgery* (2000) 128:994–8. doi: 10.1067/msy.2000.110242
11. Vaiman M, Nagibin A, Hagag P, Kessler A, Gavriel H. Hypothyroidism following partial thyroidectomy. *Otolaryngol - Head Neck Surgery* (2008) 138:98–100. doi: 10.1016/j.otohns.2007.09.015
12. Anuwong A. Transoral endoscopic thyroidectomy vestibular approach: a series of the first 60 human cases. *World J Surg* (2016) 40(3):491–7. doi: 10.1007/s00268-015-3320-1
13. Choe J-H, Kim SW, Chung K-W, Park KS, Han W, Noh D-Y, et al. Endoscopic thyroidectomy using a new bilateral axillo-breast approach. *World J Surg* (2007) 31(3):601–6. doi: 10.1007/s00268-006-0481-y
14. Kang S-W, Jeong JJ, Yun J-S, Sung TY, Lee SC, Lee YS, et al. Robot-assisted endoscopic surgery for thyroid cancer: experience with the first 100 patients. *Surg Endosc* (2009) 23(11):2399–406. doi: 10.1007/s00464-009-0366-x
15. Terris DJ, Singer MC, Seybt MW. Robotic facelift thyroidectomy: II. Clinical feasibility and safety: Robotic Facelift Thyroidectomy. *Laryngoscope* (2011) 121(8):1636–41. doi: 10.1002/lary.21832
16. Tae K, Ji YB, Song CM, Ryu J. Robotic and Endoscopic Thyroid Surgery: Evolution and Advances. *Clin Exp Otorhinolaryngol* (2019) 12(1):1–11. doi: 10.21053/ceo.2018.00766
17. Grogan R, Suh I, Chomsky-Higgins K, Alsafran S, Vasilious E, Razavi CR, et al. Patient Eligibility for Transoral Endocrine Surgery Procedures in the United States. *JAMA Netw Open* (2019) 2(5):1–9. doi: 10.1001/jamanetworkopen.2019.4829
18. Russell JO, Clark J, Noureldine SI, Anuwong A, Al Khadem MG, Yub Kim H, et al. Transoral thyroidectomy and parathyroidectomy—a North American series of robotic and endoscopic transoral approaches to the central neck. *Oral Oncol* (2017) 71:75–80. doi: 10.1016/j.oraloncology.2017.06.001
19. Tai DKC, Kim HY, Park D, You J, Kim HK, Russell JO, et al. Obesity may not affect outcomes of transoral robotic thyroidectomy: subset analysis of 304 patients. *Laryngoscope* (2019) 130(5):1343–8. doi: 10.1002/lary.28239 2019;00, 1-6.
20. Jackson NR, Yao L, Tufano RP, Kandil EH. Safety of robotic thyroidectomy approaches: Meta-analysis and systematic review: Safety Comparison of Robotic Thyroidectomy: Meta-Analysis. *Head Neck* (2014) 36(1):137–43. doi: 10.1002/hed.23223
21. Sun GH, Peress L, Pynnonen MA. Systematic review and meta-analysis of robotic vs conventional thyroidectomy approaches for thyroid disease. *Otolaryngol Head Neck Surg Off J Am Acad Otolaryngol Head Neck Surg* (2014) 150(4):520–32. doi: 10.1177/0194599814521779
22. Anuwong A, Ketwong K, Jitpratoom P, Sasanakietkul T, Duh Q-Y. Safety and outcomes of the transoral endoscopic thyroidectomy vestibular approach. *JAMA Surg* (2018) 153(1):21–7. doi: 10.1001/jamasurg.2017.3366
23. Fernandez Ranvier GF, Menkat A, Guevara DE, Llorente PM, Vidal Fortuny J, Sneider M, et al. International Multi-Institutional experience with the Transoral Endoscopic ThryoidectomyThyroidectomy Vestibular Approach.

J Laparoendoscopic Adv Surg Techniques (2020) 30(3):1–6. doi: 10.1089/lap.2019.0645

24. Le QV, Ngo DQ, Tran TD, Ngo QX. Transoral Endoscopic Thyroidectomy Vestibular Approach: An Initial Experience in Vietnam. *Surg Laparosc Percutan Tech* (2020) 6;00:00:1–5. doi: 10.1097/SLE.0000000000000764
25. Razavi CR, Khadem MGA, Fondong A, Clark JH, Richmon JD, Tufano RP, et al. Early outcomes in transoral vestibular thyroidectomy: Robotic versus endoscopic techniques. *Head Neck* (2018) 40(10):2246–53. doi: 10.1002/hed.25323
26. Perez-Soto RH, Ponce de Leon-Ballesteros G, Montalvo-Hernandez J, Sierra-Salazar M, Pantoja Millan JP, Herrera-Hernandez MF, et al. Transoral Endoscopic Thyroidectomy by Vestibular Approach – Initial Experience and Comparative Analysis in the First Reported Mexican Cohort. *J Laparoendoscopic Adv Surg Tech A* (2019) 29(12):1526–31. doi: 10.1089/lap.2019.0537
27. Park JO, Anuwong A, Kim MR, Sun DI, Kim MS. Transoral endoscopic thyroid surgery in a Korean population. *Surg Endosc* (2019) 33(7):2104–13. doi: 10.1007/s00464-018-6481-9
28. Dionigi G, Bacuzzi A, Lavazza M, Inversini D, Pappalardo V, Boni L, et al. Transoral endoscopic thyroidectomy via vestibular approach: operative steps and video. *Gland Surg Dec* (2016) 5(6):625–7. doi: 10.21037/gs.2016.12.05
29. Anuwong A, Sasanakietkul T, Jitpratoom P, Ketwong K, Kim HY, Dionigi G, et al. Transoral endoscopic thyroidectomy vestibular approach (TOETVA): indications, techniques and results. *Surg Endosc* (2018) 32(1):456–65. doi: 10.1007/s00464-017-5705-8
30. Sun H, Zheng H, Wang X, Zeng Q, Wang P, Wang Y, et al. Comparison of transoral endoscopic thyroidectomy vestibular approach, total endoscopic thyroidectomy via areola approach, and conventional thyroidectomy: a retrospective analysis of safety, trauma, and feasibility of central neck dissection in the treatment of papillary thyroid carcinoma. *Surg Endoscopy* (2020) 34:268–74. doi: 10.1007/s00464-019-06762-6
31. James BC, Angelos P, Grogan RH. Transoral endocrine surgery: Considerations for adopting a new technique. *Surg Oncol* (2020) 25:1–5. doi: 10.1002/jso.25953
32. Russell JO, Razavi CR, Shaear M, Chen LW, Lee AH, Ranganath R, et al. Transoral Vestibular Thyroidectomy: Current State of Affairs and Considerations for the Future. *J Clin Endocrinol Metab* (2019) 104(9):3779–84. doi: 10.1210/jc.2019-00116
33. Russell JO, Razavi CR, Garstka ME, Chen LW, Vasiliou E, Kang SW, et al. Remote-Access Thyroidectomy: A Multi-Institutional North American Experience with Transaxillary, Robotic Facelift, and Transoral Endoscopic Vestibular Approaches. *J Am Coll Surg* (2019) 228(4):516–22. doi: 10.1016/j.jamcollsurg.2018.12.005
34. Jitpratoom P, Ketwong K, Sasanakietkul T, Anuwong A. Transoral endoscopic thyroidectomy vestibular approach (TOETVA) for Graves' disease: a comparison of surgical results with open thyroidectomy. *Gland Surg* (2016) 5(6):546–52. doi: 10.21037/gs.2016.11.04
35. Luo JH, Xiang C, Wang P, Wang Y. The Learning curve for transoral endoscopic thyroid surgery: A single surgeon's 204 case experience. *J Laparendosc Adv Surg Tech A* (2020) 30(2):163–9. doi: 10.1089/lap.2019.0560
36. Russell JO, Sahi ZT, Shaear M, Razavi C, Ali K, Tufano RP. Transoral thyroid and parathyroid surgery via the vestibular approach – a 2020 update. *Gland Surg* (2020) 9(2):409–16. doi: 10.21037/gs.2020.03.05
37. Fu J, Luo Y, Chen Q, Lin F, Hong X, Kuang P, et al. Transoral endoscopic thyroidectomy: review of 81 cases in a single institute. *J Laparoendosc Adv Surg Tech A* (2018) 28(3):286–91. doi: 10.1089/lap.2017.0435
38. Tae K, Lee DW, Song CM, Ji YB, Park JH, Kim DS, et al. Early experience of transoral thyroidectomy: comparison of robotic and endoscopic procedures. *Head Neck* (2019) 41(3):730–8. doi: 10.1002/hed.25426
39. Russell JO, Vasiliou E, Razavi CR, Prescott JD, Tufano RP. Letter to the editor regarding "carbon dioxide embolism during transoral robotic thyroidectomy: a case report. *Head Neck* (2019) 41(3):830–1. doi: 10.1002/hed.25500
40. Razavi C, Fondong A, Tufano RP, Russell JO. Central neck dissection via the transoral approach. *Ann Thyroid* (2017) 2(5):1–10. doi: 10.21037/aot.2017.10.02
41. Razavi C, Vasiliou E, Tufano RP, Russell JO. Learning curve for Transoral Endoscopic Thyroid Lobectomy. *Otolaryng Head Neck Surg* (2018) 159 (4):625–9. doi: 10.1177/0194599818795881
42. Zhang D, Park D, Sun H, Anuwong A, Tufano RP, Kim HY, et al. Indications, benefits and risks of transoral thyroidectomy. *Best Pract Res Clin Endocrinol Metab* (2019) 33(4):101280. doi: 10.1016/j.beem.2019.05.004
43. Kim JH, Baek JH, Lim HK, Ahn HS, Baek SM, Choic YJ, et al. 2017 Thyroid Radiofrequency Ablation Guideline: Korean Society of Thyroid Radiology. *Thyroid* (2018) 19(4):632–55. doi: 10.3348/kjr.2018.19.4.632
44. Garberoglio R, Aliberti C, Appetecchia M, Attard M, Boccuzzi G, Boraso F, et al. Radiofrequency ablation for thyroid nodules: which indications? The first Italian opinion statement. *J Ultrasound* (2015) 18(4):423–30. doi: 10.1007/s40477-015-0169-y
45. Huh JY, Baek JH, Choi H, Kim JK, Lee JH. Symptomatic benign thyroid nodules: efficacy of additional radiofrequency ablation treatment sessions – prospective randomized study. *Radiology* (2012) 263(3):909–16. doi: 10.1148/radiol.12111300
46. Fuller CW, Nguyen SA, Lohia S, Gillespie MB. 2014 Radiofrequency ablation for treatment of benign thyroid nodules: systematic review. *Laryngoscope* (2014) 124(1):346–53. doi: 10.1002/lary.24406
47. Jeong WK, Baek JH, Rhim H, Kim YS, Kwak MS, Jeong HJ, et al. Radiofrequency ablation of benign thyroid nodules: safety and imaging follow-up in 236 patients. *Eur Radiol* (2008) 18(6):1244–50. doi: 10.1007/s00330-008-0880-6
48. Jung SL, Baek JH, Lee JH, Shong YK, Sung JY, Kim KS, et al. Efficacy and safety of radiofrequency ablation for benign thyroid nodules: a prospective multicenter study. *Korean J Radiol Jan-Feb* (2018) 19(1):167–74. doi: 10.3348/kjr.2018.19.1.167
49. Hall WH, McGahan JP, Link DP, deVere White RW. Combined embolization and percutaneous radiofrequency ablation of a solid renal tumor. *Am J Roentgenol* (2000) 174:3. doi: 10.2214/ajr.174.6.1741592
50. Steinke K. Radiofrequency ablation of pulmonary tumours: current status. *Cancer Imaging* (2008) 8:27–35. doi: 10.1102/1470-7330.2008.0008
51. McGahan JP, Browning PD, Brock JM, Tesluk H. Hepatic ablation using radiofrequency electrocautery. *Invest Radiol* (1990) 25(3):267–70. doi: 10.1097/00004424-199003000-00011
52. Rosenthal DJ, Hornicek FJ, Wolfe MW, Jennings LC, Gebhardt MC, Mankin HJ. Percutaneous radiofrequency coagulation of osteoid osteoma compared with operative treatment. *J Bone Joint Surg* (1998) 80(6):815–21. doi: 10.2106/00004623-199806000-00005
53. Sousa J, el-Atassi R, Rosenheck S, Calkins H, Langberg J, Morady F. Radiofrequency catheter ablation of the atrioventricular junction from the left ventricle. *Circulation* (1991) 84(2):567–71. doi: 10.1161/01.cir.84.2.567
54. Mauri G, Cova L, Monaco CG, Sconfienza LM, Corbetta S, Benedini S, et al. Benign thyroid nodules treatment using percutaneous laser ablation (PLA) and radiofrequency ablation (RFA). *Int J Hyperthermia* (2017) 33(3):295–9. doi: 10.1080/02656736.2016.1244707
55. Deandrea M, Limone P, Basso E, Mormile A, Ragazzoni F, Gamarra E, et al. US-guided percutaneous radiofrequency thermal ablation for the treatment of solid benign hyperfunctioning or compressive thyroid nodules. *Ultrasound Med Biol* (2008) 34(5):784–91. doi: 10.1016/j.ultrasmedbio.2007.10.018
56. Kim YS, Rhim H, Tae K, Park DW, Kim ST. Radiofrequency ablation of benign cold thyroid nodules: initial clinical experience. *Thyroid* (2006) 16 (4):361–7. doi: 10.1089/thy.2006.16.36
57. Spiezia S, Garberoglio R, Milone F, Ramundo V, Caiazzo C, Assanti AP, et al. Thyroid nodules and related symptoms are stably controlled two years after radiofrequency thermal ablation. *Thyroid Mar* (2009) 19(3):219–25. doi: 10.1089/thy.2008.0202
58. Baek JH, Jeong HJ, Kim YS, Kwak MS, Lee D. Radiofrequency ablation for an autonomously functioning thyroid nodule. *Thyroid* (2008) 18:675–6. doi: 10.1089/thy.2007.0274
59. Baek JH, Kim YS, Lee D, Huh JY, Lee JH. Benign predominantly solid thyroid nodules: prospective study of efficacy of sonographically guided radiofrequency ablation versus control condition. *AJR Am J Roentgenol* (2010) 194:1137–42. doi: 10.2214/AJR.09.3372
60. Lee JH, Kim YS, Lee D, Choi H, Yoo H, Baek JH. Radiofrequency ablation (RFA) of benign thyroid nodules in patients with incompletely resolved clinical problems after ethanol ablation (EA). *World J Surg* (2010) 34 (7):1488–93. doi: 10.1007/s00268-010-0565-6
61. Sung JY, Kim YS, Choi H, Lee JH, Baek JH. Optimum first-line treatment technique for benign cystic thyroid nodules: ethanol ablation or

radiofrequency ablation? *AJR Am J Roentgenol* (2011) 196(2):W210–4. doi: 10.2214/AJR.10.5172

62. Papini E, Monpeyssen H, Frasoldati A, Hegedus L. 2020 European Thyroid Association Clinical Practice Guideline for the Use of Image-Guided Ablation in Benign Thyroid Nodules. *Eur Thyroid J* (2020) 9:172–85. doi: 10.1159/000508484
63. Hamidi O, Callstrom MR, Lee RA, Dean D, Castro MR, Morris JC, et al. Outcomes of Radiofrequency Ablation Therapy for Large Benign Thyroid Nodules: A Mayo Clinic Case series. *Mayo Clin Proc Aug* (2018) 93(8):1018–25. doi: 10.1016/j.mayocp.2017.12.011
64. Tang X, Cui D, Chi J, Wang Z, Wang T, Zhai B, et al. Evaluation of the safety and efficacy of radiofrequency ablation for treating benign thyroid nodules. *J Cancer* (2017) 8(5):754–60. doi: 10.7150/jca.17655
65. Chung SR, Suh CH, Baek JH, Park HS, Choi YJ, Lee JH. Safety of radiofrequency ablation of benign thyroid nodules and recurrent thyroid cancers: a systematic review and meta-analysis. *Int J Hyperthermia* (2017) 33:920–30. doi: 10.1080/02656736.2017.1337936
66. Sung JY, Baek JH, Kim KS, Lee D, Yoo H, Kim JK, et al. Single-session treatment of benign cystic thyroid nodules with ethanol versus radiofrequency ablation: a prospective randomized study. *Radiology* (2013) 269(1):293–300. doi: 10.1148/radiol.13122134
67. Baek JH, Moon WJ, Kim YS, Lee JH, Lee D. Radiofrequency ablation for the treatment of autonomously functioning thyroid nodules. *World J Surg* (2009) 33:1971–7. doi: 10.1007/s00268-009-0130-3
68. Ha EJ, Baek JH, Lee JH, Sung JY, Lee D, Kim JK, et al. Radiofrequency ablation of benign thyroid nodules does not affect thyroid function in patients with previous lobectomy. *Thyroid* (2013) 23(3):289–93. doi: 10.1089/thy.2012.0171
69. Sung JY, Baek JH, Jung SL, Kim KS, Lee D, Kim WB, et al. Radiofrequency ablation for autonomously functioning thyroid nodules: a multicenter study. *Thyroid* (2015) 25:112–7. doi: 10.1089/thy.2014.0100
70. Bernardi S, Stacul F, Michelli A, Giudici F, Zuolo G, de Manzini N, et al. 12-month efficacy of a single radiofrequency ablation on autonomously functioning thyroid nodules. *Endocrine* (2017) 57(3):402–8. doi: 10.1007/s12020-016-1174-4
71. Che Y, Jin S, Shi C, Wang L, Zhang X, Li Y, et al. Treatment of benign thyroid nodules: comparison of surgery with radiofrequency ablation. *AJNR Am J Neuroradiol* (2015) 36(7):1321–5. doi: 10.3174/ajnr.A4276
72. Cesareo R, Palermo A, Benvenuto D, Cella E, Pasqualini V, Bernardi S, et al. Efficacy of radiofrequency ablation in autonomous functioning thyroid nodules. A systematic review and meta-analysis. *Rev Endocrine Metab Disord* (2019) 20(1):37–44. doi: 10.1007/s11154-019-09487-y
73. Faggiano A, Ramundo V, Assanti AP, Fonderico F, Macchia PE, Misso C, et al. Thyroid nodules treated with percutaneous radiofrequency thermal ablation: a comparative study. *J Clin Endocrinol Metab* (2012) 97:4439–45. doi: 10.1210/jc.2012-2251
74. Cervelli R, Mazzeo S, Boni G, Boccuzzi A, Bianchi F, Brozzi F, et al. Comparison between radioiodine therapy and single-session radiofrequency ablation of autonomously functioning thyroid nodules: a retrospective study. *Clin Endocrinol* (2019) 90:608–16. doi: 10.1111/cen.13938
75. Cesareo R, Naciu AM, Iozzino M, Pasqualini V, Simeoni C, Casini A, et al. Nodule size as predictive factor of efficacy of radiofrequency ablation in treating autonomously functioning thyroid nodules. *Int J Hyperthermia* (2018) 34:617–23. doi: 10.1080/02656736.2018.1430868
76. Cappelli C, Franco F, Pirola I, Gandossi E, Marini F, Di Lodovico E, et al. Radiofrequency ablation of functioning and non-functioning thyroid nodules: a single institution 12-month survey. *J Endocrinol Invest* (2020) 43:477–82. doi: 10.1007/s40618-019-01132-4
77. Lim HK, Lee JH, Ha EJ, Sung JY, Kim JK, Baek JH. Radiofrequency ablation of benign non-functioning thyroid nodules: 4 year follow-up results for 111 patients. *Eur Radiol* (2013) 23:1044–9. doi: 10.1007/s00330-012-2671-3
78. Cesareo R, Palermo A, Pasqualini V, et al. Radiofrequency Ablation on Autonomously Functioning Thyroid Nodules: A Critical Appraisal and Review of the Literature. *Front Endocrinol* (2020) 22:317. doi: 10.3389/fendo.2020.00317
79. Sim JS, Baek JH, Lee J, Cho W, Jung SI. Radiofrequency ablation of benign thyroid nodules: depicting early sign of regrowth by calculating vital volume. *Int J Hyperthermia* (2017) 33(8):905–10. doi: 10.1080/02656736.2017.1309083
80. Papini E, Pacella CM, Misischi I, Guglielmi R, Bizzarri G, Dossing H, et al. The advent of ultrasound-guided ablation techniques in nodular thyroid disease: towards a patient-tailored approach. *Best Pract Res Clin Endocrinol Metab* (2014) 28(4):601–18. doi: 10.1016/j.beem.2014.02.004
81. Baek JH. Radiofrequency ablation of thyroid and parathyroid nodules. In: T Clark, T Sabharwak, editors. *Interventional radiology techniques in ablation, 1st ed.* London: Springer (2013). p. 53–72.
82. Sandrock D, Olbricht T, Emrich D, Benker G, Reinwein D. Long-term follow-up in patients with autonomous thyroid adenoma. *Acta Endocrinol (Copenh)* (1993) 128(1):51–5. doi: 10.1530/acta.0.1280051

26

Outcomes of Minimally Invasive Thyroid Surgery

Lisa H. de Vries[1†], *Dilay Aykan*[1†], *Lutske Lodewijk*[1], *Johanna A. A. Damen*[2], *Inne H. M. Borel Rinkes*[1] *and Menno R. Vriens*[1*]

[1] *Department of Surgical Oncology and Endocrine Surgery, University Medical Center Utrecht, Utrecht, Netherlands,* [2] *Julius Center for Health Sciences and Primary Care, University Medical Center Utrecht, Utrecht University, Utrecht, Netherlands*

***Correspondence:**
Menno R. Vriens
Mvriens@umcutrecht.nl

†*These authors have contributed equally to this work and share first authorship*

Purpose: Conventional thyroidectomy has been standard of care for surgical thyroid nodules. For cosmetic purposes different minimally invasive and remote-access surgical approaches have been developed. At present, the most used robotic and endoscopic thyroidectomy approaches are minimally invasive video assisted thyroidectomy (MIVAT), bilateral axillo-breast approach endoscopic thyroidectomy (BABA-ET), bilateral axillo-breast approach robotic thyroidectomy (BABA-RT), transoral endoscopic thyroidectomy *via* vestibular approach (TOETVA), retro-auricular endoscopic thyroidectomy (RA-ET), retro-auricular robotic thyroidectomy (RA-RT), gasless transaxillary endoscopic thyroidectomy (GTET) and robot assisted transaxillary surgery (RATS). The purpose of this systematic review was to evaluate whether minimally invasive techniques are not inferior to conventional thyroidectomy.

Methods: A systematic search was conducted in Medline, Embase and Web of Science to identify original articles investigating operating time, length of hospital stay and complication rates regarding recurrent laryngeal nerve injury and hypocalcemia, of the different minimally invasive techniques.

Results: Out of 569 identified manuscripts, 98 studies met the inclusion criteria. Most studies were retrospective in nature. The results of the systematic review varied. Thirty-one articles were included in the meta-analysis. Compared to the standard of care, the meta-analysis showed no significant difference in length of hospital stay, except a longer stay after BABA-ET. No significant difference in incidence of recurrent laryngeal nerve injury and hypocalcemia was seen. As expected, operating time was significantly longer for most minimally invasive techniques.

Conclusions: This is the first comprehensive systematic review and meta-analysis comparing the eight most commonly used minimally invasive thyroid surgeries individually with standard of care. It can be concluded that minimally invasive techniques do not lead to more complications or longer hospital stay and are, therefore, not inferior to conventional thyroidectomy.

Keywords: minimally invasive video assisted thyroidectomy (MIVAT), bilateral axillo-breast approach endoscopic thyroidectomy (BABA-ET), bilateral axillo-breast approach robotic thyroidectomy (BABA-RT), transoral endoscopic thyroidectomy *via* vestibular approach (TOETVA), retro-auricular endoscopic thyroidectomy (RA-ET), retro-auricular robotic thyroidectomy (RA-RT), gasless transaxillary endoscopic thyroidectomy (GTET), robot assisted transaxillary surgery (RATS)

INTRODUCTION

During the last century the number of detected thyroid nodules has increased significantly. At present, nearly 5% of the female population has a thyroid nodule (1). For thyroid nodules that require surgery, conventional thyroidectomy has been standard of care (2). The extent of surgery varies from lobectomy to total thyroidectomy. Due to new diagnostic techniques to detect small malignant lesions and better surveillance, the number of thyroidectomies performed has increased substantially (3). Conventional thyroidectomy provides excellent exposure of the thyroid but leaves the patient with a visible scar in the lower region of the neck. Since most patients with a thyroid nodule are young women, different techniques have emerged to avoid a potentially disfiguring scar (2).

The first innovative thyroid technique was the endoscopic thyroidectomy, first performed in 1997 by Huscher (4). Two years later Miccoli performed the first minimally invasive video assisted thyroidectomy (MIVAT) (5). In the following years different types of endoscopic remote access techniques were introduced. Of the many endoscopic remote access techniques, the gasless transaxillary endoscopic thyroidectomy (GTET), bilateral axillo-breast approach (BABA), retro-auricular (RA) facelift approach, and transoral endoscopic thyroidectomy *via* vestibular approach (TOETVA) are the most commonly used techniques today (6). To date TOETVA, as shown in **Figure 1**, is the only technique performed without cutaneous scars (9). In 2007, the Da Vinci robotic platform, was first used for robot-assisted transaxillary surgery (RATS) by Chung et al. (10). Since then, bilateral axillo-breast and RA approaches have also been developed for the Da Vinci system (10).

In this systematic review, the MIVAT, TOETVA, transaxillary, bilateral axillo-breast and retro-auricular techniques are compared regarding operating time, hospital stay and complications.

METHODS

Search Strategy

This systematic review was reported according to Preferred Reporting Items for Systematic Reviews and Meta-Analysis guidelines (PRISMA). Eligible studies were identified using Medline, Embase and Web of Science on 11 November 2020. There was no limitation to language or publication date during the search. Combinations of the following keywords and its synonyms were used in the search: "robotic thyroidectomy", "endoscopic thyroidectomy", "thyroid surgery", "RATS", "TOETVA", "BABA", "MIVAT", "facelift" and "outcome". In addition, reference lists of included studies were carefully analyzed for related studies. The full search can be found in the **Supplementary Material**.

Study Selection

Studies were included that reported total operating time, length of hospital stay, outcomes including transient/permanent recurrent laryngeal nerve (RLN) palsy and/or transient/permanent hypocalcemia; and were either a (non-)randomized controlled trial, controlled clinical trial or observational study. Studies with and without control groups were included. Only studies published as original articles and written in English were included. Exclusion criteria were preclinical studies, (systematic) reviews, guidelines, case reports, publications in abstract form only, editorials, letters or conference proceedings.

The titles and abstracts were reviewed by one author (DA) and discussed with another author (LHdV). This was followed by full-text review of potentially eligible studies. Disagreements were discussed and solved with help of a third reviewer (LL) when necessary.

Quality Analysis of the Studies

Non-randomized and observational studies were assessed using the MINORS checklist, while randomized controlled studies were assessed using the Cochrane risk of bias tool (11, 12).

Data Extraction

For each study included in the final analysis, the following data was extracted: title, study design, author, year of publication,

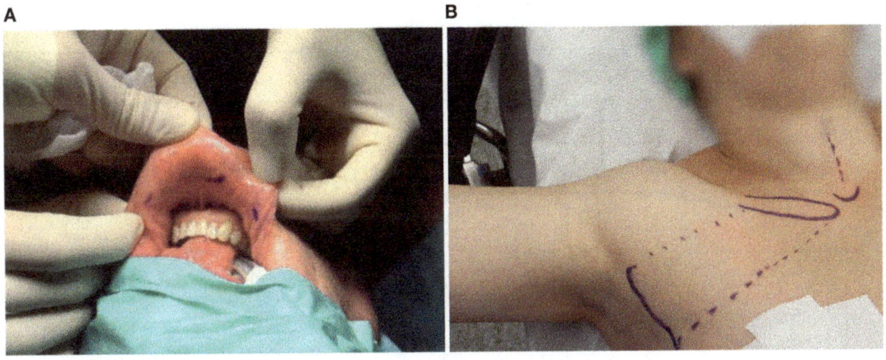

FIGURE 1 | Preoperatively marked patients who will undergo **(A)** TOETVA (7). Three incisions will be made in the oral vestibule, one for the camera and two laterally for dissection and coagulation instruments; and **(B)** RATS (8). The incision site is marked laterally. The dotted lines mark the borders of the surgical working space.

geographic location, number of patients, patients' age, gender, surgical approach, type of procedure, total operating time, hospital stay, transient RLN palsy (defined as hoarseness <6 months), permanent RLN palsy (hoarseness >6 months), transient hypocalcemia (defined as hypoparathyroidism <6 months) and permanent hypocalcemia (hypoparathyroidism >6 months). In most studies, hypoparathyroidism was defined as a reduction in serum iPTH and/or iCa concentration below the normal limit, with or without hypocalcemic symptoms. Due to heterogeneous reporting on cosmetic results, cosmetic satisfaction could not be analyzed in this study.

Both the mean and median were extracted from the articles, if available. Some articles reported results on partial, subtotal or total thyroidectomy; some studies reported results combining multiple extents of surgeries. Means were noted with SD and medians with ranges, if provided in the original article. To provide an impression of operating time and length of hospital stay, the median and interquartile range (IQR) was calculated per technique. This was done using the overall mean per article. The same was done for the incidence of RLN injury and hypocalcemia, using the percentage per article. Articles that described the mean operating time for both partial and total thyroidectomy were included to assess median overall operating time.

Statistical Analysis

Only studies comparing a minimal invasive technique to conventional thyroidectomy (standard of care) were included in the meta-analysis, studies without control arms were therefore not included. Data was analyzed using Review Manager software, version 5.0 (Cochrane Collaboration, Oxford, UK). Standardized mean difference (SMD) was calculated for continues variables and odds ratio (OR) for the dichotomous variables, including 95% confidence intervals (CI). The Mantel-Haenszel method for pooling was used in case of multiple odds ratios close to one and even sample sizes in both arms. In plots with zero events in one arm without one of these characteristics Peto's method was used (13). I^2 above 50% was considered substantial heterogeneity. A random effects model was used for all analyses. P <0.05 was considered to be statistically significant.

RESULTS

Study Characteristics

A flowchart of study selection is shown in **Figure 2**. A total of 569 articles were retrieved from the databases. Four additional references were found through the reference lists. After duplication removal 409 articles were left. All 409 articles were screened, and 280 articles were excluded based on the abstract, leaving 129 eligible articles. After reading the full text, 31 additional articles were excluded. Ninety-eight articles were included in the qualitative analysis (2, 14–110). Among the 98 articles, there were five randomized studies, one non-randomized study and 92 observational studies. Twenty-one

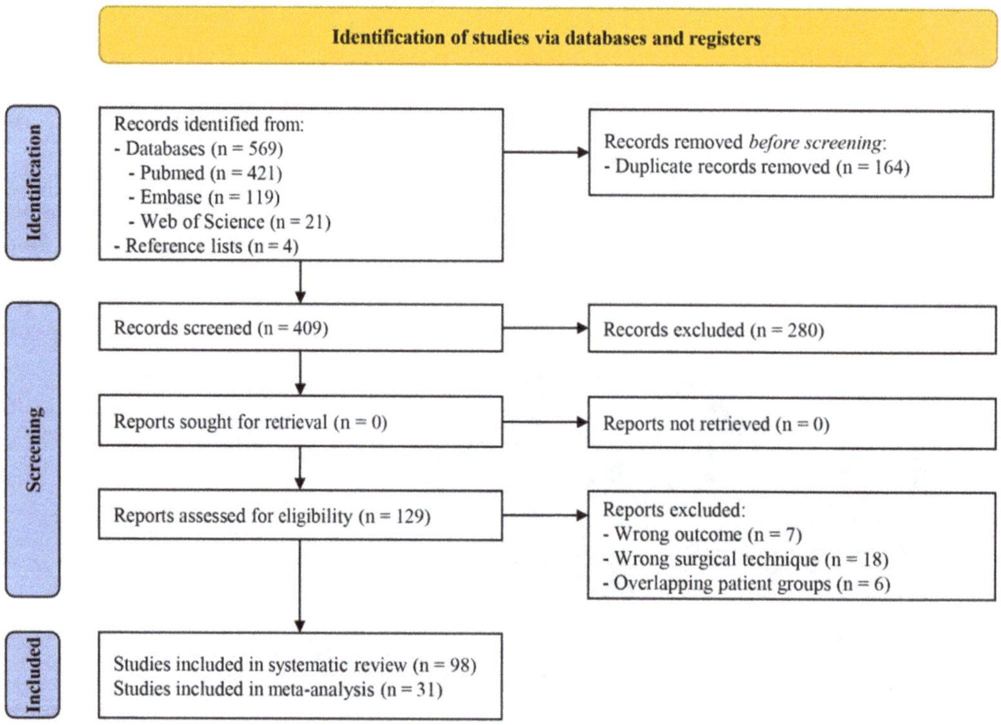

FIGURE 2 | Flowchart of study selection using PRISMA 2020 flow diagram.

studies were conducted in North America, three in South America, 11 in Europa, one in Africa and 62 in Asia. Study characteristics are shown in **Supplementary Table 1**.

A total of 25,373 participants were included. Median age was 44 years. The vast majority of patients were female. Sample sizes ranged from five to 5,000 participants.

Thirteen articles described the bilateral axillo-breast approach endoscopic thyroidectomy (BABA-ET) in a total number of 1,567 patients, whilst the bilateral axillo-breast approach robotic thyroidectomy (BABA-RT) was described in 15 articles and included 1,498 patients. Eighteen articles described the results of the MIVAT in 4,180 patients. Fourteen articles described the TOETVA in 802 patients. There were five articles that conducted thyroidectomy through the retro-auricular endoscopic approach (RA-ET) in 89 patients. The retro-auricular robotic approach (RA-RT) included 55 patients in two articles. The GTET was described in ten papers and involved 2,017 patients. Thirty articles described the RATS and included the most patients, 15,165 in total.

Quality of Included Studies

All included studies were considered high quality. Full quality assessment can be found in **Supplementary Tables 2, 3**.

Operating Time

The mean or median operating times per study are shown in **Supplementary Table 4**. The median operating times including IQR per technique are shown in **Table 1A**. The median operating time of conventional thyroidectomy was 105.5 minutes. For all minimally invasive techniques, the median operating time was longer than the standard of care, with the exception of the MIVAT, which required 74.3 minutes.

The meta-analysis displayed in **Figure 3** showed a significantly longer operating time for the BABA-ET, BABA-RT, MIVAT (lobectomy), TOETVA, RATS techniques in comparison to standard of care. Operating times for the MIVAT (total thyroidectomy) and GTET were not significantly different compared to standard of care.

Hospital Stay

Mean or median length of hospital stay per study is shown in **Supplementary Table 4**. The median length of hospital stay including IQR per technique is shown in **Table 1B**. A median hospital stay of approximately three days was reported for all techniques including the standard of care, except for the RA-ET and MIVAT which had a median hospital stay of 4.5 and 1.9 days, respectively. Length of hospital stay was not reported for the RA-RT.

The meta-analysis presented in **Figure 4** showed a significantly longer length of hospital stay for the BABA-ET compared to the standard of care. For all other minimally invasive techniques, no significant difference was seen compared to standard of care.

Transient RLN Injury

Results on transient RLN injury can be found in **Supplementary Table 4** per study and in **Table 2A** per technique. The median

TABLE 1 | Operating time and length of hospital stay.

A.	Median	Minimum	Q1	Q3	Maximum	IQR	No. of patients
Operating time in minutes							
BABA-ET (16, 33, 34, 36, 65, 66, 69, 80, 85, 103)	154.2	109.3	128.9	165.3	238.2	36.4	1,416
BABA-RT (22, 29, 31, 32, 51, 63, 66, 68, 69, 79, 90)	190.5	118.8	165.1	206.0	290.6	40.9	1,169
MIVAT (26, 39, 46, 47, 62, 73, 86, 87, 98, 99, 110)	74.3	41.0	66.4	91.3	222.5	24.9	3,463
TOETVA (14, 17, 19, 23, 50, 61, 93, 96, 102, 104, 107)	152.0	97.0	121.0	196.1	216.7	75.1	590
RA-ET (17, 25, 27, 35, 92)	143.0	123.4	127.2	148.5	152.0	21.3	89
RA-RT (17, 101)	179.1	167.1	NA	NA	191.0	NA	55
GTET (2, 28, 40, 41, 55, 64, 73, 76, 81)	166.8	129.8	140.6	189.1	297.5	48.6	882
RATS (15, 20, 24, 28, 37, 45, 48, 49, 56, 57, 59, 60, 67, 72, 75, 76, 78, 86, 89, 94, 95)	141.5	101.1	123.2	178.0	232.0	54.8	13,357
Standard of care (2, 14–16, 20, 22, 31, 32, 36, 45, 48, 51, 52, 55, 61, 64, 69, 72, 89, 93, 105, 110)	105.5	70.8	86.1	123.5	156.2	37.4	2,150
B.	**Median**	**Minimum**	**Q1**	**Q3**	**Maximum**	**IQR**	**No. of patients**
Length of hospital stay in days							
BABA-ET (16, 34, 36, 65, 66, 69, 80, 85, 103, 109)	3.1	2.5	3.0	4.3	6.9	1.3	1,353
BABA-RT (22, 29–32, 51, 63, 66, 68, 69, 74, 109)	3.6	2.9	3.2	4.0	5.1	0.8	1,256
MIVAT (38, 39, 42, 62, 73, 86, 87, 99, 105, 110)	1.9	0.0	1.4	2.7	4.7	1.3	2,937
TOETVA (14, 18, 19, 43, 50, 61, 91, 93, 104, 106, 107)	3.6	0.8	2.3	4.3	5.4	2.0	740
RA-ET (25, 27, 35, 92)	4.5	2.5	3.2	5.6	5.9	2.4	84
RA-RT (101)	NA	NA	NA	NA	NA	NA	0
GTET (2, 28, 55, 73, 76, 79, 84)	3.4	2.2	2.6	5.0	6.5	2.4	1,167
RATS (15, 20, 24, 28, 48, 49, 56, 59, 60, 67, 70, 72, 75, 76, 78, 81, 83, 84, 86, 89, 94, 95)	2.9	0.0	1.2	3.3	5.1	2.1	14,232
Standard of care (2, 14–16, 20, 21, 30, 32, 48, 51, 55, 58, 64, 66, 72, 79, 89, 93, 105, 106, 110)	3.1	0.0	1.0	3.6	5.5	2.6	2,250

Q1, first quartile; Q3, third quartile; IQR, interquartile range; NA, not applicable.

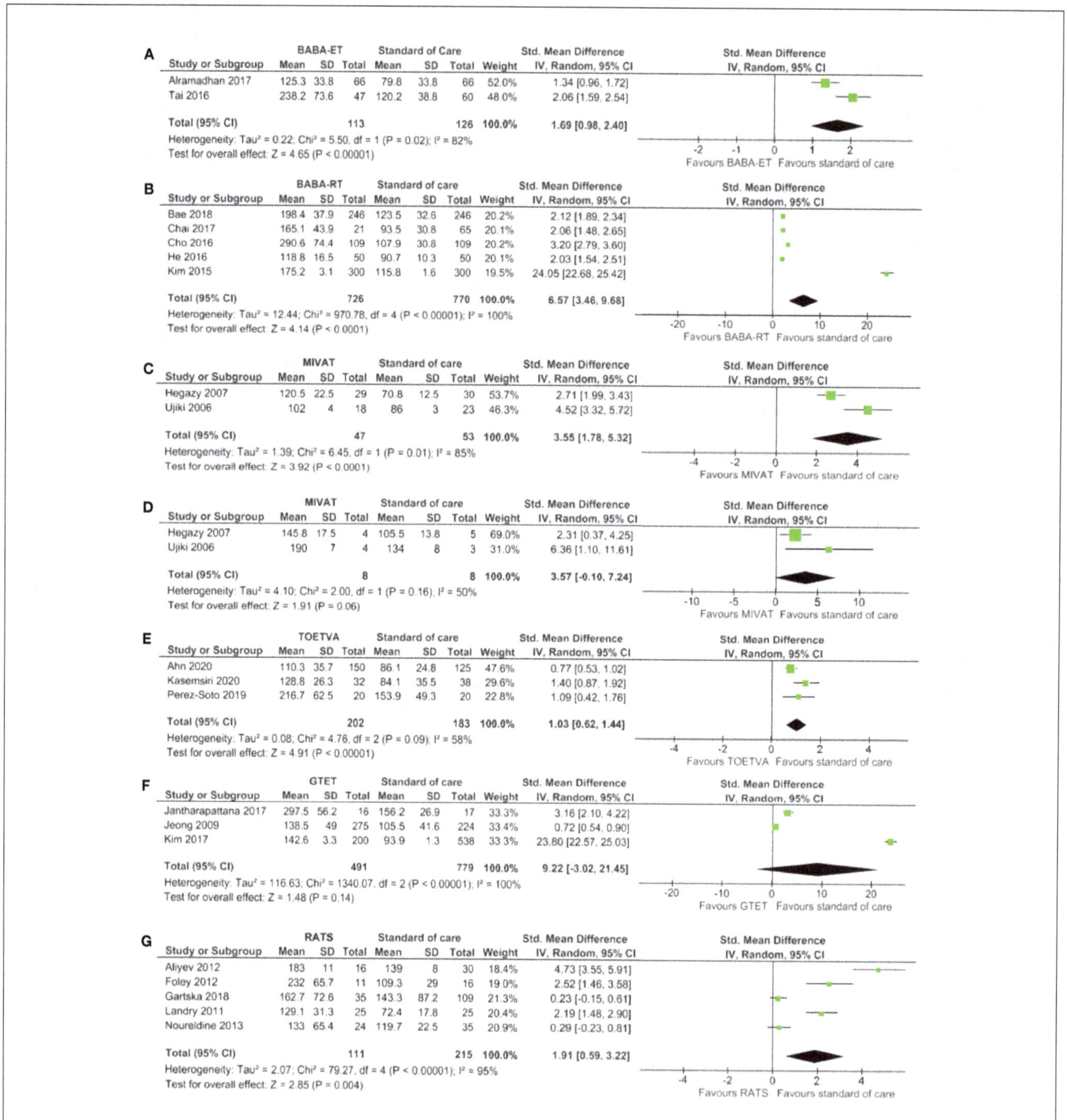

FIGURE 3 | Forest plots of operating time for **(A)** BABA-ET, **(B)** BABA-RT, **(C)** MIVAT lobectomy, **(D)** MIVAT total thyroidectomy, **(E)** TOETVA, **(F)** GTET and **(G)** RATS.

incidence of transient RLN injury after BABA-ET (3.7% of 1,491 patients), BABA-RT (3.0% of 1,554 patients), MIVAT (2.5% of 1,727 patients), TOETVA (4.0% of 736 patients) and RATS (3.3% of 15,780) was comparable to the standard of care, which was 3.3% of 2,908 patients. The median incidence of RLN injury was higher in RA-RT and GTET patients (5.0% of 20 patients and 5.3% of 1,921 patients, respectively) and lower after RA-ET (1.1% of 84 patients).

As shown in **Figure 5**, the meta-analysis showed no significant difference between the minimally invasive techniques and the standard of care considering transient RLN injury.

Permanent RLN Injury

Permanent RLN injury results are shown in **Supplementary Table 4** per study and in **Table 2B** per technique. The median incidence of permanent RLN injury was 0.4% in 2,970 standard

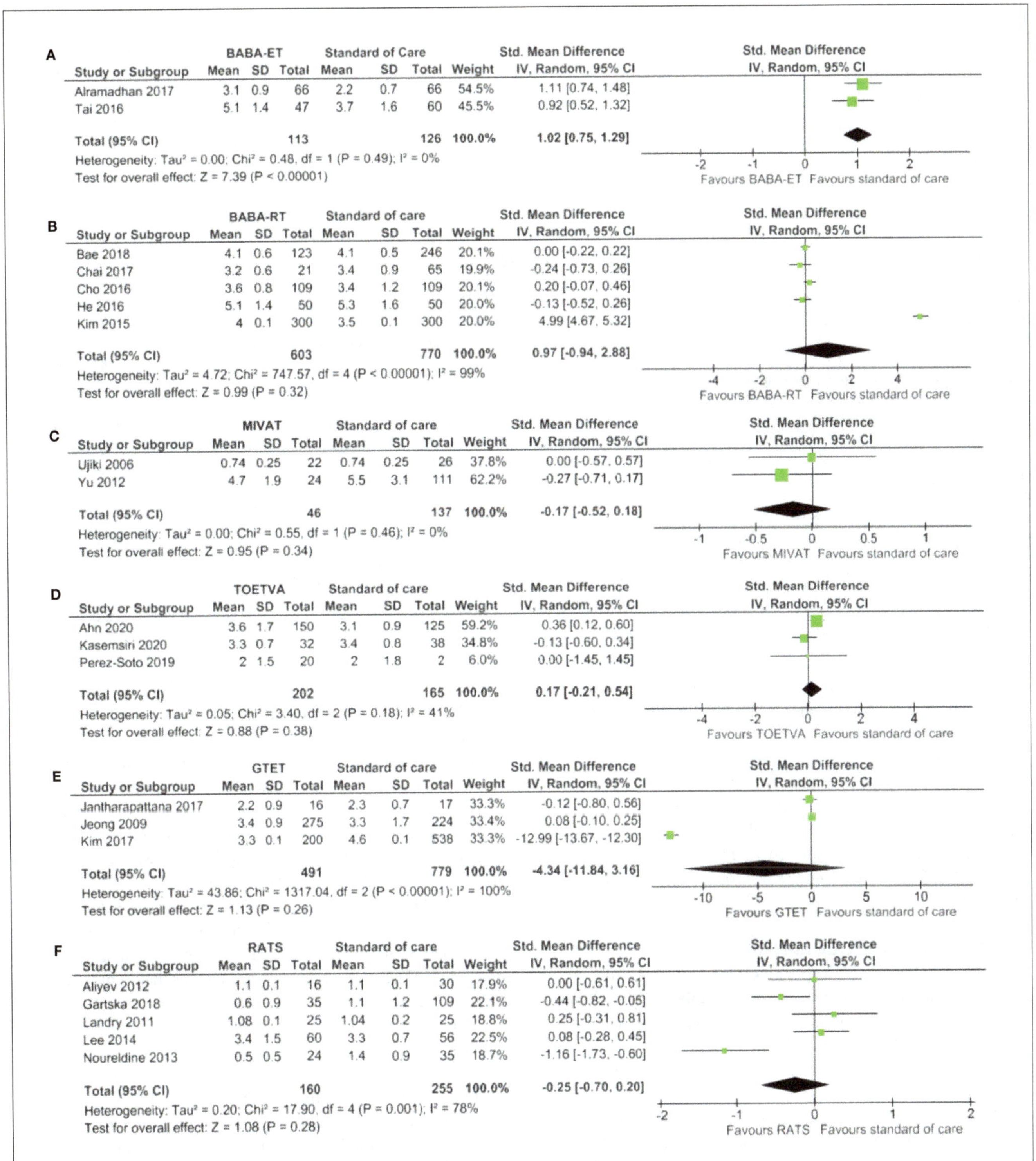

FIGURE 4 | Forests plots of hospital stay for **(A)** BABA-ET, **(B)** BABA-RT, **(C)** MIVAT, **(D)** TOETVA, **(E)** GTET and **(F)** RATS.

of care patients and was comparable for all minimally invasive techniques, ranging from 0.0% to 0.4%.

Figure 6 shows the meta-analysis, which confirmed no significant difference for the BABA-ET, BABA-RT, MIVAT, TOETVA, GTET and RATS compared to the standard of care.

Transient Hypocalcemia

Results on the incidence of transient hypocalcemia can be found in **Supplementary Table 4** per study and in **Table 3A** per technique. The median incidence of transient hypocalcemia seemed to vary between techniques. Transient hypocalcemia

TABLE 2 | Incidence of recurrent laryngeal nerve injury.

A.	Median	Minimum	Q1	Q3	Maximum	IQR	No. of cases	No. of patients
Transient recurrent laryngeal nerve injury in %								
BABA-ET (16, 33, 34, 36, 54, 65, 66, 69, 80, 85, 103, 109)	3.7	0.0	1.4	7.3	28.0	5.9	162	1,491
BABA-RT (21, 22, 29–32, 51, 63, 66, 68, 69, 74, 79, 90, 109)	3.0	0.0	2.0	6.4	19.0	4.4	77	1,554
MIVAT (26, 38, 39, 42, 44, 45, 52, 62, 71, 73, 86, 98, 99, 105, 110)	2.5	0.0	1.7	4.2	17.0	2.5	86	1,727
TOETVA (14, 18, 19, 23, 43, 61, 91, 93, 102, 106, 107)	4.0	0.0	3.1	7.1	12.5	4.0	32	736
RA-ET (25, 27, 35, 92)	1.1	0.0	0	6.6	11.1	6.6	3	84
RA-RT (101)	5.0	NA	NA	NA	NA	NA	1	20
GTET (28, 40, 41, 55, 59, 64, 73, 76, 81, 84)	5.3	0.0	3.1	6.3	15.0	3.2	85	1,921
RATS (20, 24, 28, 37, 45, 48, 49, 56, 57, 59, 60, 67, 72, 75–78, 81–84, 86, 89, 94, 95, 97, 100)	3.3	0.0	1.8	6.0	20.5	4.2	456	15,780
Standard of care (2, 14, 16, 20, 22, 31, 32, 36, 45, 48, 51, 52, 54, 55, 61, 64, 68, 72, 77, 81, 82, 89, 90, 93, 103, 105, 110)	3.3	0.0	0.0	8.8	19.5	8.8	172	2,908
B.	**Median**	**Minimum**	**Q1**	**Q3**	**Maximum**	**IQR**	**No. of cases**	**No. of patients**
Permanent recurrent laryngeal nerve injury in %								
BABA-ET (16, 34, 36, 54, 65, 66, 69, 80, 85, 103, 109)	0.0	0.0	0.0	2.1	4.3	2.1	15	1,385
BABA-RT (21, 22, 29–32, 51, 63, 66, 68, 69, 74, 79, 90, 109)	0.0	0.0	0.0	0.7	0.9	0.7	5	1,554
MIVAT (26, 38, 39, 42, 44, 46, 52, 62, 71, 73, 86–88, 98, 99, 105, 110)	0.0	0.0	0.0	1.5	2.9	1.5	45	4,129
TOETVA (14, 18, 19, 23, 43, 61, 91, 93, 96, 102, 106, 107)	0.0	0.0	0.0	1.1	3.1	1.1	6	756
RA-ET (25, 27, 35, 92)	0.0	0.0	0.0	0.0	0.0	0.0	0	84
RA-RT (101)	0.0	NA	NA	NA	NA	NA	0	20
GTET (28, 40, 41, 55, 59, 64, 73, 76, 81, 84)	0.4	0.0	0.0	1.6	6.3	1.6	11	2,033
RATS (20, 24, 28, 37, 48, 49, 56, 57, 59, 60, 67, 72, 75, 76, 78, 83, 84, 86, 89, 94, 95, 97, 100, 108)	0.1	0.0	0.0	0.5	1.3	0.5	59	15,756
Standard of care (2, 14, 16, 20, 22, 31, 32, 36, 48, 51, 52, 54, 55, 61, 64, 68, 72, 88–90, 93, 103, 105, 108, 110)	0.4	0.0	0.0	0.9	4.0	0.9	26	2,970

Q1, first quartile; Q3, third quartile; IQR, interquartile range; NA, not applicable.

occurred in 17.1% of 3,157 patients after standard of care, which was similar to the incidence after RATS (18.4% of 7,002 patients). The median incidence was lower after BABA-ET, MIVAT, TOETVA, RA-ET and GTET (14.0% of 1,208 patients, 5.6% of 3,588 patients, 7.1% of 644 patients, 0.0% of 84 patients and 3.3% of 1,020 patients, respectively) and higher after BABA-RT and RA-RT (21.6% of 1,171 patients and one of three patients, respectively).

The meta-analysis is displayed in **Figure 7** and showed no significant difference between the minimally invasive techniques and standard of care.

Permanent Hypocalcemia

Results on permanent hypocalcemia can be found in in **Supplementary Table 4** per study and in **Table 3B** per technique. The median incidence of permanent hypocalcemia after standard of care was 1.5% of 3,024 patients. The median incidence was lower for all other minimally invasive techniques and varied between 0.0% and 1.3%.

The meta-analysis in **Figure 8**, showed no significant difference in incidence of transient hypocalcemia after BABA-ET, BABA-RT, MIVAT, TOETVA, GTET and RATS compared to the standard of care.

DISCUSSION

This systematic review and meta-analysis shows that minimally invasive techniques are not inferior to cervical thyroidectomy with regards to length of hospital stay, transient RLN injury, permanent RLN injury, transient hypocalcemia and permanent hypocalcemia. Prior to this study, multiple systematic reviews have been published regarding either the robotic thyroidectomy techniques or endoscopic thyroidectomy techniques (111–119). However, these systematic reviews combine the different types of techniques. In this systematic review and meta-analysis all minimally invasive techniques were analyzed independently. To the best of our knowledge, this is the largest and most comprehensive systematic review and meta-analysis comparing the eight widely used robotic and endoscopic thyroidectomy techniques.

While the results of our systematic review suggest that the MIVAT is the only minimally invasive technique with a shorter operating time than standard of care, the meta-analysis showed that all techniques, except the GTET have a longer operating time than standard of care. This is to be expected since the docking of the robot platform is time consuming, and in some techniques a subcutaneous route to the thyroid needs to be developed. This longer operating time for the endoscopic and robotic surgical techniques is in concordance with the findings of two other meta-analyses (117, 119).

To provide an overview of the operating time and length of hospital stay, the median overall operating time and hospital stay were calculated. Many studies did not provide the percentage of total thyroidectomies or lobectomies. This makes interpretation of median operating time and length of hospital stay not reliable. The meta-analysis revealed that there was no significant difference regarding the length of hospital stay, between the minimally invasive techniques compared to standard of care, with the exception of shorter hospital stay after BABA-ET. In other studies, also no significant difference was found between the minimally invasive techniques and the conventional approach

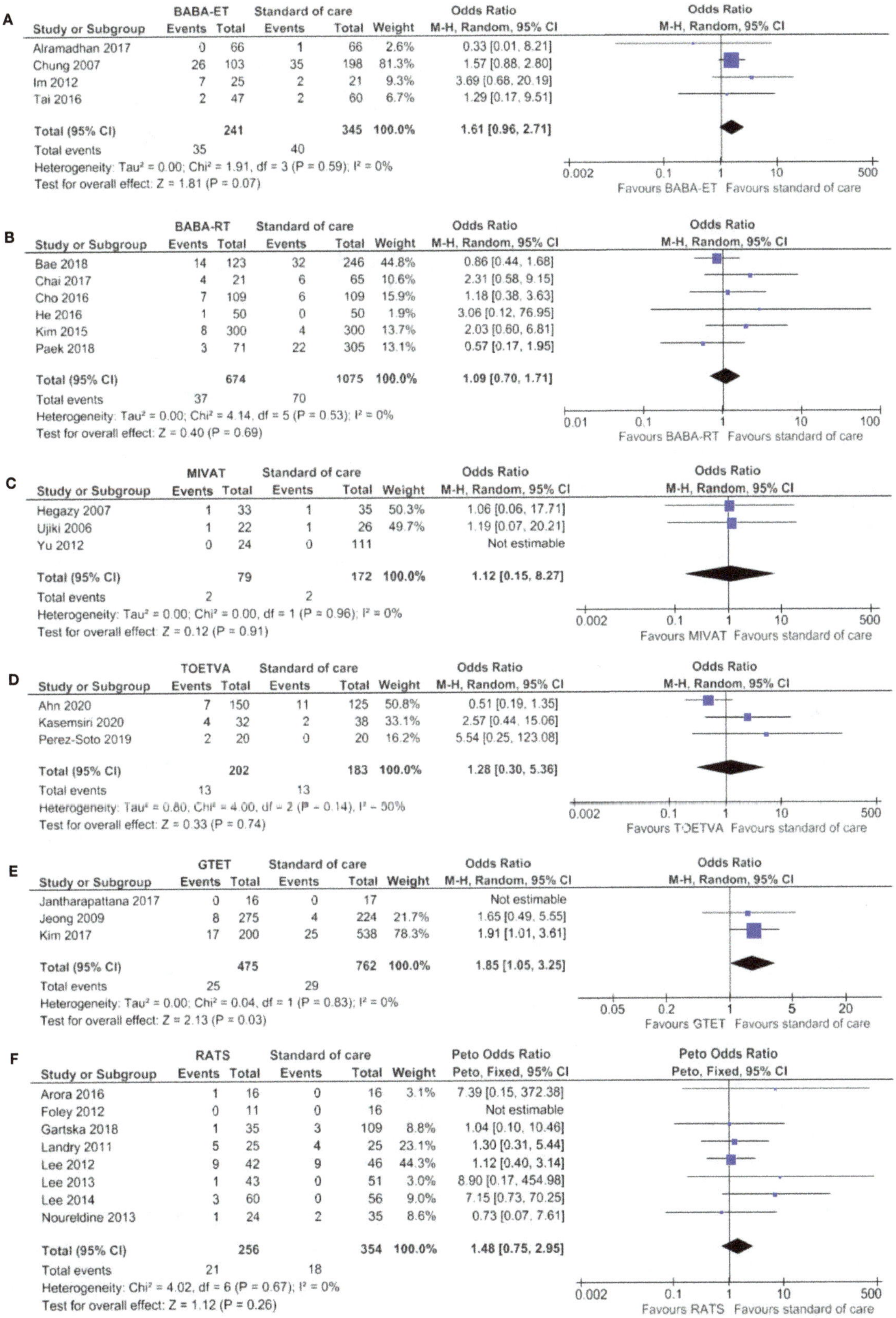

FIGURE 5 | Forests plots of transient recurrent laryngeal nerve injury for **(A)** BABA-ET, **(B)** BABA-RT, **(C)** MIVAT, **(D)** TOETVA, **(E)** GTET and **(F)** RATS.

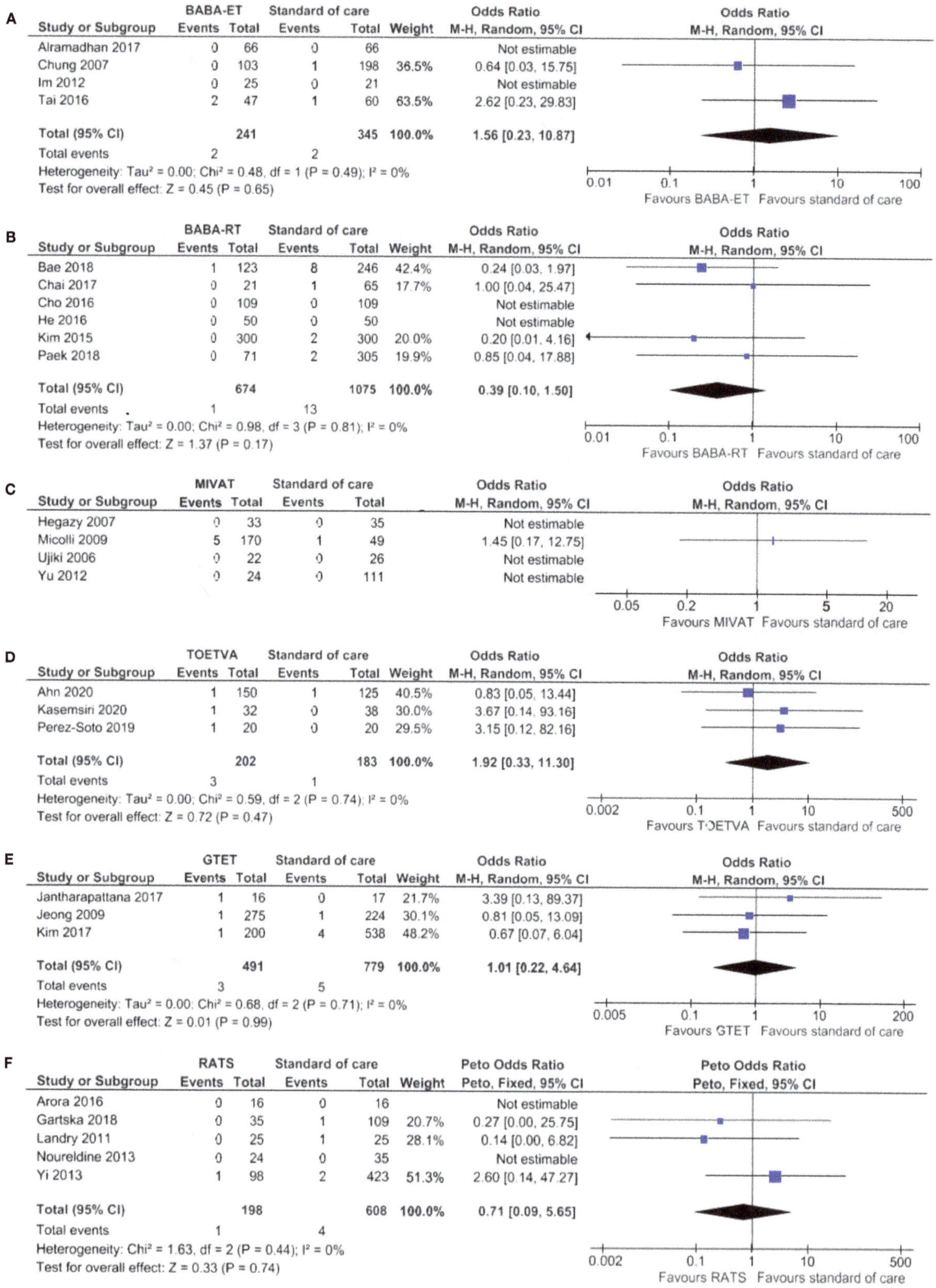

FIGURE 6 | Forests plots of permanent recurrent laryngeal nerve injury for **(A)** BABA-ET, **(B)** BABA-RT, **(C)** MIVAT, **(D)** TOETVA, **(E)** GTET and **(F)** RATS.

TABLE 3 | Incidence of hypocalcemia.

A.	Median	Minimum	Q1	Q3	Maximum	IQR	No. of cases	No. of patients
Transient hypocalcemia in %								
BABA-ET (16, 33, 34, 36, 53, 54, 65, 66, 69, 80, 85, 103, 109)	14.0	0.0	3.3	28.2	46.2	24.9	259	1,208
BABA-RT (21, 22, 29–32, 51, 63, 66, 68, 69, 74, 79, 90, 109)	21.6	2.8	10.8	31.7	38.6	20.9	283	1,171
MIVAT (26, 38, 39, 42, 44, 46, 47, 52, 62, 71, 73, 87, 98, 99, 110)	5.6	0.0	3.0	10.0	23.4	7.0	231	3,588
TOETVA (14, 18, 19, 43, 91, 93, 102, 106, 107)	7.1	0.0	4.0	21.3	50.0	17.3	64	644
RA-ET (25, 27, 35, 92)	0.0	0.0	0.0	2.8	5.8	2.8	1	84
RA-RT (101)	33.3	NA	NA	NA	NA	NA	1	3
GTET (28, 40, 41, 55, 59, 64, 73, 76, 84)	3.3	0.0	0.0	26.7	33.3	26.7	95	1,020
RATS (15, 24, 28, 37, 45, 48, 49, 56, 57, 59, 60, 67, 70, 75, 76, 78, 81–84, 89, 94, 95, 97, 100, 108)	18.4	0.0	8.3	39.9	51.7	31.7	2,239	7,002
Standard of care (14–16, 22, 31, 32, 36, 45, 48, 51, 52, 54, 55, 64, 68, 81, 82, 89, 90, 93, 103, 107, 110)	17.1	0.0	4.5	34.0	44.6	29.5	631	3,157
B.	**Median**	**Minimum**	**Q1**	**Q3**	**Maximum**	**IQR**	**No. of cases**	**No. of patients**
Permanent hypocalcemia in %								
BABA-ET (16, 34, 36, 54, 65, 66, 69, 80, 85, 103, 109)	1.3	0.0	0.0	2.1	4.2	2.1	25	1,048
BABA-RT (21, 22, 29–32, 51, 63, 66, 68, 69, 74, 79, 90, 109)	0.9	0.0	0.0	1.7	4.8	1.7	13	1,171
MIVAT (26, 38, 39, 46, 52, 62, 71, 73, 87, 88, 98, 99, 105, 110)	0.0	0.0	0.0	0.0	0.4	0.4	23	3,402
TOETVA (14, 18, 19, 43, 91, 93, 102, 106, 107)	0.0	0.0	0.0	0.7	5.0	0.7	2	644
RA-ET (25, 27, 35, 92)	0.0	0.0	0.0	0.0	0.0	0.0	0	84
RA-RT (101)	0.0	NA	NA	NA	NA	NA	0	3
GTET (28, 40, 41, 55, 59, 64, 73, 76, 84)	0.0	0.0	0.0	0.7	2.7	0.7	4	1,020
RATS (24, 28, 37, 45, 48, 49, 56, 57, 59, 60, 67, 70, 75, 76, 78, 81–84, 89, 94, 95, 97, 100, 108)	0.0	0.0	0.0	0.1	3.1	0.1	45	6,986
Standard of care (14, 16, 22, 31, 32, 36, 45, 48, 51, 52, 54, 55, 64, 68, 88–90, 93, 103, 105, 108, 110)	1.5	0.0	0.0	3.2	6.7	3.2	57	3,024

Q1, first quartile; Q3, third quartile; IQR, interquartile range; NA, not applicable.

(112, 114, 116, 117, 119). However, length of hospital stay is not a good metric to assess the best thyroidectomy approach, since it is mostly determined by local prevailing hospital protocols rather than outcome of surgery.

The systematic review showed that the RA-RT and GTET patients had more transient RLN injury compared to the standard of care, while the incidence was lower or comparable after the other techniques. The meta-analysis showed that for the BABA-ET, BABA-RT, RATS, MIVAT and TOETVA no significant difference was found in transient RLN injury when compared to the cervical thyroidectomy. Results from the systematic review regarding the permanent RLN injury showed that the BABA-ET and MIVAT were the only two techniques with more permanent RLN injuries than the standard of care. The meta-analysis, however, showed that none of the minimally invasive technique had a statistically significant difference with the standard of care. Other meta-analyses also found no significant difference in RLN injury (112, 114, 119).

Risk of hypocalcemia is largely influenced by the surgical extent. However, in most articles it was not clearly stated whether hypocalcemia was reported for all surgical extents or solely for total thyroidectomy. Results from this systematic review regarding transient hypocalcemia differed between the techniques. It seemed that the BABA-ET, MIVAT, TOETVA, RA-ET and GTET led to fewer transient hypocalcemia cases than the standard of care. The meta-analysis showed no statistically significant difference between standard of care and minimally invasive techniques. The systematic review showed that all minimally invasive techniques had less cases of permanent hypocalcemia than the standard of care. The meta-analysis showed no significant difference between the minimally invasive techniques and standard of care considering permanent hypocalcemia. Other meta-analyses also found no statistical difference in hypocalcemia between minimally invasive techniques and conventional thyroidectomy (112, 117, 119). Only Jiang et al. reported a lower incidence of hypocalcemia after the endoscopic technique (116). The RA-ET and RA-RT could not be included in the meta-analysis, because of lacking control arms. Therefore the results of RA-ET and RA-RT are solely based on the systematic review.

Minimally invasive techniques can also be used to perform completion thyroidectomies in patients who have undergone minimally invasive thyroid surgery before. Of the studies included in this article, completion thyroidectomy was described by eight studies, using all mentioned techniques except the RA-ET and RA-RT (31, 34, 41, 43, 46, 57, 65, 89). Moreover, several other studies described the safety and feasibility of minimally invasive techniques for the completion thyroidectomy, showing the vast range of application of these techniques (65, 120–122). It is advised to either perform re-operation within two weeks after initial surgery or after two to three months to minimize complications due to adhesions (57, 65, 120).

This systematic review has few limitations. First, there were only a few randomized studies included. The majority of the articles are retrospective in nature, which may have led to selection and reporting bias. Furthermore, only the studies with control groups, a minority of the articles, could be included in the meta-analysis. Lastly, the incidence of permanent RLN injury and permanent hypocalcemia was low in all groups, which made it difficult to show differences between standard of care and minimally invasive techniques.

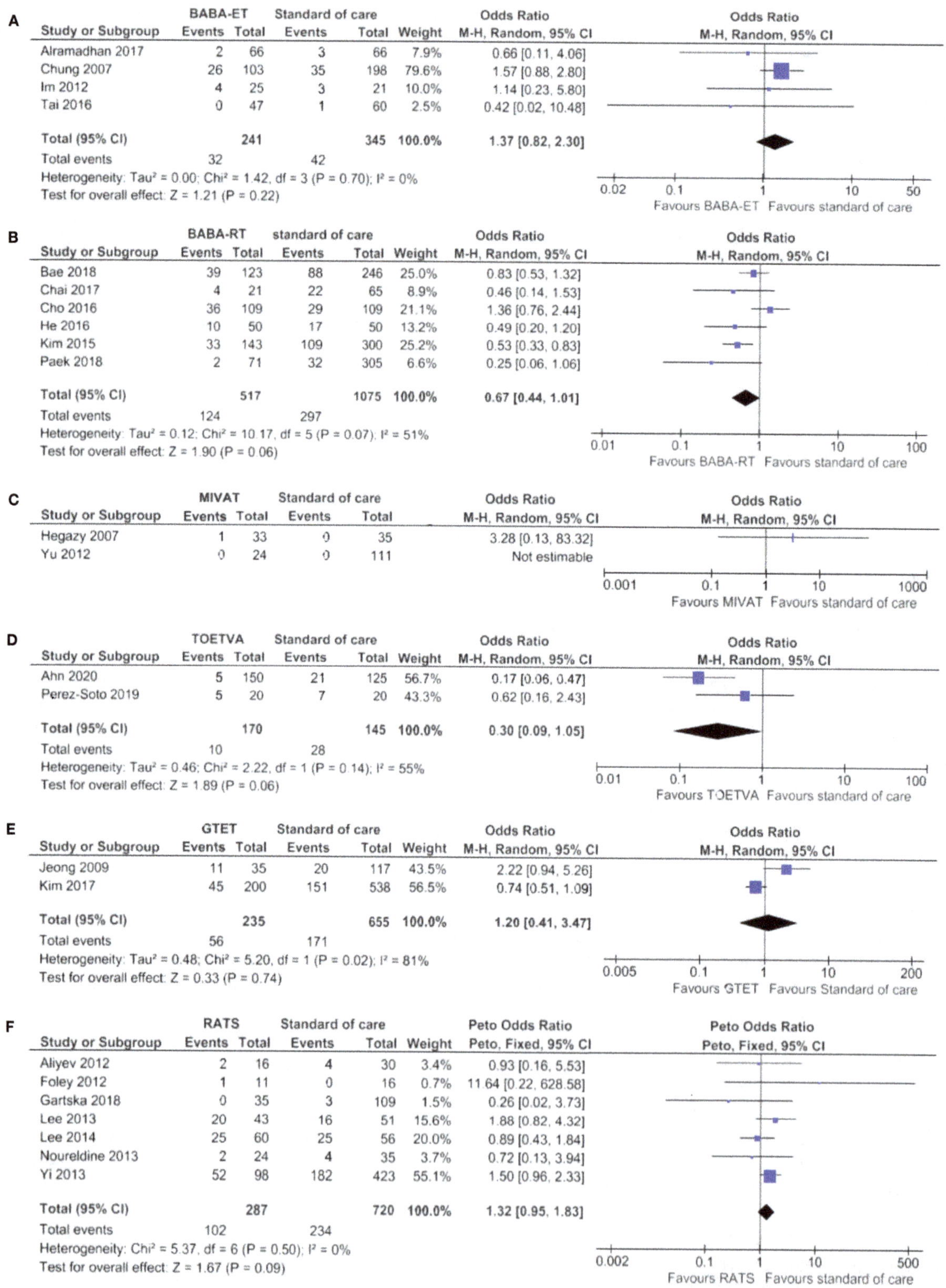

FIGURE 7 | Forests plots of transient hypocalcemia for **(A)** BABA-ET, **(B)** BABA-RT, **(C)** MIVAT, **(D)** TOETVA, **(E)** GTET and **(F)** RATS.

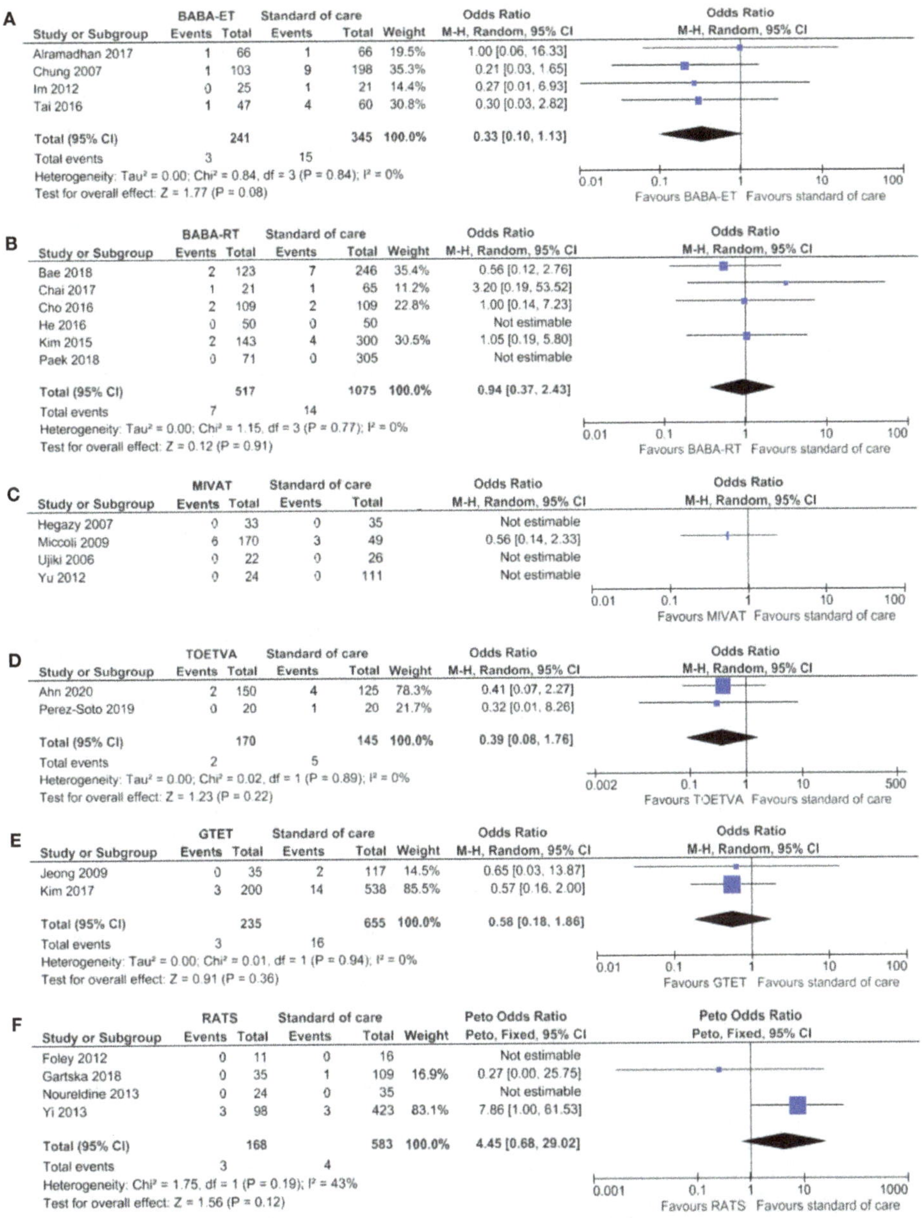

FIGURE 8 | Forests plots of permanent hypocalcemia for **(A)** BABA-ET, **(B)** BABA-RT, **(C)** MIVAT, **(D)** TOETVA, **(E)** GTET and **(F)** RATS.

Previous meta-analyses included mainly studies from Asia (112, 115, 116). Strength of our paper is the inclusion of studies from North America and European countries, in addition to the previously reported Asian articles. Therefore, our results are also applicable to Western populations.

CONCLUSION

This study provides a comprehensive review on the most used minimally invasive thyroid surgical techniques. From the systematic review and meta-analysis, it can be concluded that for selected patients, these modern techniques are not inferior to standard of care and are a safe alternative, with the advantage of avoiding a potentially disfiguring scar in the neck.

AUTHOR CONTRIBUTIONS

All authors listed have made a substantial, direct, and intellectual contribution to the work and approved it for publication.

REFERENCES

1. Haugen BR, Alexander EK, Bible KC, Doherty GM, Mandel DJ, Nikiforov YE. 2015 American Thyroid Association Management Guidelines for Adult Patients With Thyroid Nodules and Differentiated Thyroid Cancer. The American Thyroid Association Guidelines Task Force on Thyroid Nodules and Differentiated Thyroid Cancer. *Thyroid* (2016) 26:1–133. doi: 10.1089/thy.2015.0020
2. Jantharapattana K. Transaxillary Gasless Endoscopic Thyroidectomy Versus Conventional Open Thyroidectomy: A Randomized Study. *Eur Arch Otorhinolaryngol* (2017) 274:495–500. doi: 10.1007/s00405-016-4242-8
3. Vaccarella S, Franceschi S, Bray F, Wild CP, Plummer M, Dal Maso L. Worldwide Thyroid Cancer Epidemic? The Increasing Impact of Overdiagnosis. *N Engl J Med* (2016) 375:614–7. doi: 10.1056/NEJMp1604412
4. Huscher CS, Chiodini S, Napolitano C, Recher A. Endoscopic Right Thyroid Lobectomy. *Surg Endosc* (1997) 11:877. doi: 10.1007/s004649900476
5. Miccoli P, Berti P, Conte M, Bendinelli C, Marcocci C. Minimally Invasive Surgery for Thyroid Small Nodules: Preliminary Report. *J Endocrinol Invest* (1999) 22:849–51. doi: 10.1007/BF03343657
6. Tae K, Ji YB, Song CM, Ryu J. Robotic and Endoscopic Thyroid Surgery: Evolution and Advances. *Clin Exp Otorhinolaryngol* (2019) 12:1–11. doi: 10.21053/ceo.2018.00766
7. Vriens MR, Borel Rinkes IHM. TOETVA: Schildklierchirurgie Zonder Blijvend Litteken [TOETVA: Thyroid Surgery Without Permanent Scar]. *Ned Tijdschr Geneeskd* (2019) 163:D3397. doi: 10.21037/gs.2018.02.01
8. Vriens MR, Kist JW, Lodewijk L, van Hillegersberg R, Borel Rinkes IHM. Robotgeassisteerde Transaxillaire Schildklieroperatie [Robot-Assisted Transaxillary Thyroid Surgery]. *Ned Tijdschr Geneeskd* (2013) 157(28):A5841.
9. Luna-Ortiz K, Gómez-Pedraza A, Anuwong A. Lessons Learned From the Transoral Endoscopic Thyroidectomy With Vestibular Approach (TOETVA) for the Treatment of Thyroid Carcinoma. *Ann Surg Oncol* (2020) 27:1356–60. doi: 10.1245/s10434-019-07899-3
10. Chang E, Kim HY, Koh YW, Chung WY. Overview of Robotic Thyroidectomy. *Gland Surg* (2017) 6:218–28. doi: 10.21037/gs.2017.03.18
11. Slim K, Nini E, Forestier D, Kwiatkowski F, Panis Y, Chipponi J. Methodological Index for Non-Randomized Studies (Minors): Development and Validation of a New Instrument. *ANZ J Surg* (2003) 73(9):712–6. doi: 10.1046/j.1445-2197.2003.02748.x
12. Higgins JPT, Savović J, Page MJ, Elbers RG, Sterne JAC. Chapter 8: Assessing Risk of Bias in a Randomized Trial. In: JPT Higgins, J Thomas, J Chandler, M Cumpston, T Li, MJ Page and VA Welch, editors. *Cochrane Handbook for Systematic Reviews of Interventions, Version 6.2 (Updated February 2021).* Chichester (UK): Cochrane (2021). Available at: www.training.cochrane.org/handbook.
13. Deeks JJ, Higgins JPT, Altman DG. Chapter 10: Analysing Data and Undertaking Meta-Analyses. In: JPT Higgins, J Thomas, J Chandler, M Cumpston, T Li, MJ Page and VA Welch, editors. *Cochrane Handbook for Systematic Reviews of Interventions, Version 6.2 (Updated February 2021).* Chichester (UK): Cochrane (2021). Available at: www.training.cochrane.org/handbook.
14. Ahn JH, Yi JW. Transoral Endoscopic Thyroidectomy for Thyroid Carcinoma: Outcomes and Surgical Completeness in 150 Single-Surgeon Cases. *Surg Endosc* (2020) 34:861–7. doi: 10.1007/s00464-019-06841-8
15. Aliyev S, Taskin HE, Agcaoglu O, Aksoy E, Milas M, Siperstein A, et al. Robotic Transaxillary Total Thyroidectomy Through a Single Axillary Incision. *Surgery* (2013) 153:705–10. doi: 10.1016/j.surg.2012.10.013
16. Alramadhan M, Choe JH, Lee JH, Kim JH, Kim JS. Propensity Score-Matched Analysis of the Endoscopic Bilateral Axillo-Breast Approach (BABA) Versus Conventional Open Thyroidectomy in Patients With Benign or Intermediate Fine-Needle Aspiration Cytology Results, a Retrospective Study. *Int J Surg* (2017) 48:9–15. doi: 10.1016/j.ijsu.2017.09.077
17. Alshehri M, Mohamed HE, Moulthrop T, Kandil E. Robotic Thyroidectomy and Parathyroidectomy: An Initial Experience With Retroauricular Approach. *Head Neck* (2017) 39:1568–72. doi: 10.1002/hed.24794
18. Anuwong A. Transoral Endoscopic Thyroidectomy Vestibular Approach: A Series of the First 60 Human Cases. *World J Surg* (2016) 40:491–7. doi: 10.1007/s00268-015-3320-1
19. Anuwong A, Sasanakietkul T, Jitpratoom P, Ketwong K, Kim HY, Dionigi G, et al. Transoral Endoscopic Thyroidectomy Vestibular Approach (TOETVA): Indications, Techniques and Results. *Surg Endosc* (2018) 32:456–65. doi: 10.1007/s00464-017-5705-8
20. Arora A, Garas G, Sharma S, Muthuswamy K, Budge J, Palazzo F, et al. Comparing Transaxillary Robotic Thyroidectomy With Conventional Surgery in a UK Population: A Case Control Study. *Int J Surg* (2016) 27:110–7. doi: 10.1016/j.ijsu.2016.01.071
21. Bae DS, Suh BJ, Park JK, Koo do H. Technical, Oncological, and Functional Safety of Bilateral Axillo-Breast Approach (BABA) Robotic Total Thyroidectomy. *Surg Laparosc Endosc Percutan Tech* (2016) 26:253–8. doi: 10.1097/SLE.0000000000000262
22. Bae DS, Koo do H. A Propensity Score-Matched Comparison Study of Surgical Outcomes in Patients With Differentiated Thyroid Cancer After Robotic Versus Open Total Thyroidectomy. *World J Surg* (2019) 43:540–51. doi: 10.1007/s00268-018-4802-8
23. Bakkar S, Al Hyari M, Naghawi M, Corsini C, Miccoli P. Transoral Thyroidectomy: A Viable Surgical Option With Unprecedented Complications-A Case Series. *J Endocrin* (2018) 41(7):809–13. doi: 10.1007/s40618-017-0808-6
24. Ban EJ, Yoo JY, Kim WW, Son HY, Park S, Lee SH, et al. Surgical Complications After Robotic Thyroidectomy for Thyroid Carcinoma: A Single Center Experience With 3,000 Patients. *Surg Endosc* (2014) 28:2555–63. doi: 10.1007/s00464-014-3502-1
25. Ban MH, Chang JW, Kim WS, Byeon HK, Koh YQ, Park JH. Minimal Endoscope-Assisted Thyroidectomy Through a Retroauricular Approach: An Evolving Solo Surgery Technique. *Surg Laparosc Endosc Percutan Tech* (2016) 26:e109–12. doi: 10.1097/SLE.0000000000000353
26. Bellotti C, Capponi MG, Cinquepalmi M, Castagnola G, Marchetta S, Mallozzi F, et al. MIVAT: The Last 2 Years Experience, Tips and Techniques After More Than 10 Years. *Surg Endosc* (2018) 32:2340–4. doi: 10.1007/s00464-017-5929-7
27. Byeon HK, Holsinger FC, Tufano RP, Park JH, Sim NS, Kim WS, et al. Endoscopic Retroauricular Thyroidectomy: Preliminary Results. *Surg Endosc* (2016) 30:355–65. doi: 10.1007/s00464-015-4202-1
28. Cabot JC, Lee CR, Brunaud L, Kleiman DA, Chung WY, Fahey TJ, et al. Robotic and Endoscopic Transaxillary Thyroidectomies may be Cost Prohibitive When Compared to Standard Cervical Thyroidectomy: A Cost Analysis. *Surgery* (2012) 152:1016–24. doi: 10.1016/j.surg.2012.08.029
29. Chae S, Min SY, Park WS. Comparison Study of Robotic Thyroidectomies Through a Bilateral Axillo-Breast Approach and a Transoral Approach. *J Laparoendosc Adv Surg Tech A* (2020) 30:175–82. doi: 10.1089/lap.2019.0585
30. Chai YJ, Kim HY, Kim HK, Jun SH, Dionigi G, Anuwong A, et al. Comparative Analysis of 2 Robotic Thyroidectomy Procedures: Transoral Versus Bilateral Axillo-Breast Approach. *Head Neck* (2018) 40:886–92. doi: 10.1002/hed.25034
31. Chai YJ, Suh H, Woo JW, Yu HW, Song RY, Kwon H, et al. Surgical Safety and Oncological Completeness of Robotic Thyroidectomy for Thyroid Carcinoma Larger Than 2 Cm. *Surg Endosc* (2017) 31:1235–40. doi: 10.1007/s00464-016-5097-1
32. Cho JN, Park WS, Min SY, Han SA, Song JW. Surgical Outcomes of Robotic Thyroidectomy vs. Conventional Open Thyroidectomy for Papillary Thyroid Carcinoma. *World J Surg Oncol* (2016) 14:181. doi: 10.1186/s12957-016-0929-y
33. Choe JH, Kim SW, Chung KW, Park KS, Han W, Noh DY, et al. Endoscopic Thyroidectomy Using a New Bilateral Axillo-Breast Approach. *World J Surg* (2007) 31:601–6. doi: 10.1007/s00268-006-0481-y
34. Choi Y, Lee KE, Chung KW, Kim SW, Choe JH, Koo do H, et al. Endoscopic Thyroidectomy *via* Bilateral Axillo-Breast Approach (BABA): Review of 512 Cases in a Single Institute. *Surg Endosc* (2012) 26:948–55. doi: 10.1007/s00464-011-1973-x
35. Chung EJ, Park MW, Cho JG, Baek SK, Kwon SY, Woo JS, et al. A Prospective 1-Year Comparative Study of Endoscopic Thyroidectomy *via* a Retroauricular Approach Versus Conventional Open Thyroidectomy at a Single Institution. *Ann Surg Oncol* (2015) 22:3014–21. doi: 10.1245/s10434-014-4361-7
36. Chung YS, Choe JH, Kang KH, Kim SW, Chung KW, Park KS, et al. Endoscopic Thyroidectomy for Thyroid Malignancies: Comparison With

Conventional Open Thyroidectomy. *World J Surg* (2007) 31:2302–8. doi: 10.1007/s00268-007-9117-0
37. Ciabatti PG, Burali G, D'Ascanio L. Single-Incision Robot-Assisted Transaxillary Surgery for Early-Stage Papillary Thyroid Cancer. *Ann Otol Rhinol Laryngol* (2012) 121:811–5. doi: 10.1177/000348941212101207
38. Dedivitis RA, Guimarães AV. Preliminary Results From Minimally Invasive Video-Assisted Thyroidectomy. *Sao Paulo Med J* (2005) 123:298–9. doi: 10.1590/S1516-31802005000600011
39. Dobrinja C, Trevisan G, Makovac P, Liguori G. Minimally Invasive Video-Assisted Thyroidectomy Compared With Conventional Thyroidectomy in a General Surgery Department. *Surg Endosc* (2009) 23:2263–7. doi: 10.1007/s00464-008-0303-4
40. Duncan TD, Rashid Q, Speights F, Ejeh I. Endoscopic Transaxillary Approach to the Thyroid Gland: Our Early Experience. *Surg Endosc* (2007) 21:2166–71. doi: 10.1007/s00464-007-9325-6
41. Duncan TD, Rashid Q, Speights F, Ejeh I. Transaxillary Endoscopic Thyroidectomy: An Alternative to Traditional Open Thyroidectomy. *J Natl Med Assoc* (2009) 101:783–7. doi: 10.1016/S0027-9684(15)31006-3
42. Fan Y, Guo B, Guo S, Kang J, Wu B, Zhang P, et al. Minimally Invasive Video-Assisted Thyroidectomy: Experience of 300 Cases. *Surg Endosc* (2010) 24:2393–400. doi: 10.1007/s00464-010-0960-y
43. Fernandez Ranvier G, Meknat A, Guevara DE, Llorente PM, Vidal Fortuny J, Sneider M, et al. International Multi-Institutional Experience With the Transoral Endoscopic Thyroidectomy Vestibular Approach. *J Laparoendosc Adv Surg Tech A* (2020) 30:278–83. doi: 10.1089/lap.2019.0645
44. Fík Z, Astl J, Zábrodský M, Lukeš P, Merunka I, Betka J, et al. Minimally Invasive Video-Assisted Versus Minimally Invasive Nonendoscopic Thyroidectomy. *BioMed Res Int* (2014) 2014:45017. doi: 10.1155/2014/450170
45. Foley CS, Agcaoglu O, Siperstein AE, Berber E. Robotic Transaxillary Endocrine Surgery: A Comparison With Conventional Open Technique. *Surg Endosc* (2012) 26:2259–66. doi: 10.1007/s00464-012-2169-8
46. Frank E, Park J, Simantal A Jr, Vuong C, Liu Y, Kwon D, et al. Minimally Invasive Video-Assisted Thyroidectomy: Almost a Decade of Experience at an Academic Center. *Am Surg* (2016) 82:949–52. doi: 10.1177/000313481608201019
47. Gagner M, Inabnet WB. Endoscopic Thyroidectomy for Solitary Thyroid Nodules. *Thyroid* (2001) 11:161–3. doi: 10.1089/105072501300042848
48. Garstka M, Mohsin K, Ali DB, Shalaby H, Ibraheem K, Farag M, et al. Well-Differentiated Thyroid Cancer and Robotic Transaxillary Surgery at a North American Institution. *J Surg Res* (2018) 228:170–8. doi: 10.1016/j.jss.2018.03.030
49. Giulianotti PC, Addeo P, Buchs NC, Ayloo SM, Bianco FM. Robotic Thyroidectomy: An Initial Experience With the Gasless Transaxillary Approach. *J Laparoendosc Adv Surg Tech A* (2012) 22:387–91. doi: 10.1089/lap.2010.0380
50. Guo F, Wang W, Zhu X, Xiang C, Wang P, Wang Y. Comparative Study Between Endoscopic Thyroid Surgery via the Oral Vestibular Approach and the Areola Approach. *J Laparoendosc Adv Surg Tech A* (2020) 30:170–4. doi: 10.1089/lap.2019.0562
51. He QQ, Zhu J, Zhuang DY, Fan ZY, Zheng LM, Zhou P, et al. Comparative Study Between Robotic Total Thyroidectomy With Central Lymph Node Dissection *via* Bilateral Axillo-Breast Approach and Conventional Open Procedure for Papillary Thyroid Microcarcinoma. *Chin Med J* (2016) 129:2160–6. doi: 10.4103/0366-6999.189911
52. Hegazy MA, Khater AA, Setit AE, Amin MA, Kotb SZ, El shafei MA, et al. Minimally Invasive Video-Assisted Thyroidectomy for Small Follicular Thyroid Nodules. *World J Surg* (2007) 31:1743–50. doi: 10.1007/s00268-007-9147-7
53. Hur SM, Kim SH, Lee SK, Kim WW, Choe JH, Lee JE, et al. New Endoscopic Thyroidectomy With the Bilateral Areolar Approach: A Comparison With the Bilateral Axillo-Breast Approach. *Surg Laparosc Endosc Percutan Tech* (2011) 21:219–24. doi: 10.1097/SLE.0b013e3182239989
54. Im HJ, Koo do H, Paeng JC, Lee KE, Chung YS, Lim I, et al. Evaluation of Surgical Completeness in Endoscopic Thyroidectomy Compared With Open Thyroidectomy With Regard to Remnant Ablation. *Clin Nucl Med* (2012) 37:148–51. doi: 10.1097/RLU.0b013e3182335fdc
55. Jeong JJ, Kang SW, Yun JS, Sung TY, Lee SC, Lee YS, et al. Comparative Study of Endoscopic Thyroidectomy Versus Conventional Open Thyroidectomy in Papillary Thyroid Microcarcinoma (PTMC) Patients. *J Surg Oncol* (2009) 100:477–80. doi: 10.1002/jso.21367
56. Kandil E, Winters R, Aslam R, Friedlander P, Bellows C. Transaxillary Gasless Robotic Thyroid Surgery With Nerve Monitoring: Initial Two Experince in a North American Center. *Minim Invasive Ther Allied Technol* (2012) 21:90–5. doi: 10.3109/13645706.2011.561862
57. Kandil EH, Noureldine SI, Yao L, Slakey DP. Robotic Transaxillary Thyroidectomy: An Examination of the First One Hundred Cases. *J Am Coll Surg* (2012) 214:558–64. doi: 10.1016/j.jamcollsurg.2012.01.002
58. Kang SW, Jeong JJ, Yun JS, Sung TY, Lee SC, Lee YS, et al. Gasless Endoscopic Thyroidectomy Using Trans-Axillary Approach; Surgical Outcome of 581 Patients. *Endocr J* (2009) 56:361–9. doi: 10.1507/endocrj.K08E-306
59. Kang SW, Lee SC, Lee SH, Lee KY, Jeong JJ, Lee YS, et al. Robotic Thyroid Surgery Using a Gasless, Transaxillary Approach and the Da Vinci S System: The Operative Outcomes of 338 Consecutive Patients. *Surgery* (2009) 146:1048–55. doi: 10.1016/j.surg.2009.09.007
60. Kang SW, Park JH, Jeong JS, Lee CR, Park S, Lee SH, et al. Prospects of Robotic Thyroidectomy Using a Gasless, Transaxillary Approach for the Management of Thyroid Carcinoma. *Surg Laparosc Endosc Percutan Tech* (2011) 21:223–9. doi: 10.1097/SLE.0b013e3182266f31
61. Kasemsiri P, Trakulkajornsak S, Bamroong P, Mahawerawat K, Piromchai P, Ratanaanekchai T. Comparison of Quality of Life Between Patients Undergoing Trans-Oral Endoscopic Thyroid Surgery and Conventional Open Surgery. *BMC Surg* (2020) 20:18. doi: 10.1186/s12893-020-0685-3
62. Kim AJ, Liu JC, Ganly I, Kraus DH. Minimally Invasive Video-Assisted Thyroidectomy 2.0: Expanded Indications in a Tertiary Care Cancer Center. *Head Neck* (2011) 33:1557–60. doi: 10.1002/hed.21633
63. Kim EB, Cho JW, Lee YM, Sung TY, Yoon JH, Chung KW, et al. Postsurgical Outcomes and Surgical Completeness of Robotic Thyroid Surgery: A Single Surgeon's Experience on 700 Cases. *J Laparoendosc Adv Surg Tech A* (2018) 28:540–5. doi: 10.1089/lap.2017.0597
64. Kim EY, Lee KH, Park YL, Park CH, Lee CR, Jeong JJ, et al. Single-Incision, Gasless, Endoscopic Trans-Axillary Total Thyroidectomy: A Feasible and Oncologic Safe Surgery in Patients With Papillary Thyroid Carcinoma. *J Laparoendosc Adv Surg Tech A* (2017) 27:1158–64. doi: 10.1089/lap.2016.0669
65. Kim SJ, Lee KE, Choe JH, Lee J, Koo do H, Oh SK, et al. Endoscopic Completion Thyroidectomy by the Bilateral Axillo-Breast Approach. *Surg Laparosc Endosc Percutan Tech* (2010) 20:312–6. doi: 10.1097/SLE.0b013e3181f195fc
66. Kim SK, Woo JW, Park I, Lee JH, Choe JH, Kim JH, et al. Propensity Score-Matched Analysis of Robotic Versus Endoscopic Bilateral Axillo-Breast Approach (BABA) Thyroidectomy in Papillary Thyroid Carcinoma. *Langenbeck's Arch Surg* (2017) 402:243–50. doi: 10.1007/s00423-016-1528-7
67. Kim W, Kim K, Kim M, Choi J, Lee C, Lee J, et al. Yonsei Experience of 5,000 Transaxillary Robotic Thyroidectomies. *World J Surg* (2018) 42:393–401. doi: 10.1007/s00268-017-4209-y
68. Kim WW, Jung JH, Park HY. A Single Surgeon's Experience and Surgical Outcomes of 300 Robotic Thyroid Surgeries Using a Bilateral Axillo-Breast Approach. *J Surg Oncol* (2015) 111:135–40. doi: 10.1002/jso.23793
69. Kim WW, Kim JS, Hur SM, Kim SH, Lee SK, Choi JH, et al. Is Robotic Surgery Superior to Endoscopic and Open Surgeries in Thyroid Cancer? *World J Surg* (2011) 35:779–84. doi: 10.1007/s00268-011-0960-7
70. Kuppersmith RB, Holsinger FC. Robotic Thyroid Surgery: An Initial Experience With North American Patients. *Laryngoscope* (2011) 121:521–6. doi: 10.1002/lary.21347
71. Lai SY, Walvekar RR, Ferris RL. Minimally Invasive Video-Assisted Thyroidectomy: Expanded Indications and Oncologic Completeness. *Head Neck* (2008) 30:1403–7. doi: 10.1002/hed.20883
72. Landry CS, Grubbs EG, Warneke CL, Ormond M, Chua C, Lee JE, et al. Robot-Assisted Transaxillary Thyroid Surgery in the United States: Is it Comparable to Open Thyroid Lobectomy? *Ann Surg Oncol* (2012) 19:1269–74. doi: 10.1245/s10434-011-2075-7
73. Lang BH, Wong KP. A Comparison of Surgical Morbidity and Scar Appearance Between Gasless, Transaxillary Endoscopic Thyroidectomy (GTET) and Minimally Invasive Video-Assisted Thyroidectomy (VAT). *Ann Surg Oncol* (2013) 20:646–52. doi: 10.1245/s10434-012-2613-y

74. Lee HY, Yang IS, Hwang SB, Lee JB, Bae JW, Kim HY. Robotic Thyroid Surgery for Papillary Thyroid Carcinoma: Lessons Learned From 100 Consecutive Surgeries. *Surg Laparosc Endosc Percutan Tech A* (2015) 25:27–32. doi: 10.1097/SLE.0b013e3182a2b0ae
75. Lee J, Kang SW, Jung JJ, Choi UJ, Yun JH, Nam KH, et al. Multicenter Study of Robotic Thyroidectomy: Short-Term Postoperative Outcomes and Surgeon Ergonomic Considerations. *Ann Surg Oncol* (2011) 18:2538–47. doi: 10.1245/s10434-011-1628-0
76. Lee J, Lee JH, Nah KY, Soh EY, Chung WY. Comparison of Endoscopic and Robotic Thyroidectomy. *Ann Surg Oncol* (2011) 18:1439–46. doi: 10.1245/s10434-010-1486-1
77. Lee J, Na KY, Kim RM, Oh Y, Lee JH, Lee J, et al. Postoperative Functional Voice Changes After Conventional Open or Robotic Thyroidectomy: A Prospective Trial. *Ann Surg Oncol* (2012) 19:2963–70. doi: 10.1245/s10434-012-2253-2
78. Lee J, Yun JH, Nam KH, Choi UJ, Chung WY, Soh EY. Perioperative Clinical Outcomes After Robotic Thyroidectomy for Thyroid Carcinoma: A Multicenter Study. *Surg Endosc* (2011) 25:906–12. doi: 10.1007/s00464-010-1296-3
79. Lee KE, Koo do H, Kim SJ, Lee J, Park KS, Oh SK, et al. Outcomes of 109 Patients With Papillary Thyroid Carcinoma Who Underwent Robotic Total Thyroidectomy With Central Node Dissection *via* the Bilateral Axillo-Breast Approach. *Surgery* (2010) 148:1207–13. doi: 10.1016/j.surg.2010.09.018
80. Lee MC, Park H, Choi IJ, Lee BC, Lee GH. Comparative Study of a Gasless Transaxillary Approach Versus a Bilateral Axillo-Breast Approach for Endoscopic Thyroidectomy in a Single Institute. *Head Neck* (2014) 36:702–8. doi: 10.1002/hed.23349
81. Lee S, Kim HY, Lee CR, Park S, Son H, Kang SW, et al. A Prospective Comparison of Patient Body Image After Robotic Thyroidectomy and Conventional Open Thyroidectomy in Patients With Papillary Thyroid Carcinoma. *Surgery* (2014) 156:117–25. doi: 10.1016/j.surg.2014.02.007
82. Lee S, Lee CR, Lee SC, Park S, Kim HY, Son H, et al. Surgical Completeness of Robotic Thyroidectomy: A Prospective Comparison With Conventional Open Thyroidectomy in Papillary Thyroid Carcinoma Patients. *Surg Endosc* (2014) 28:1068–75. doi: 10.1007/s00464-013-3303-y
83. Lee S, Rye HR, Park JH, Kim KH, Kang SW, Jeong JJ, et al. Excellence in Robotic Thyroid Surgery: A Comparative Study of Robot-Assisted Versus Conventional Endoscopic Thyroidectomy in Papillary Thyroid Microcarcinoma Patients. *Ann Surg* (2011) 253:1060–6. doi: 10.1097/SLA.0b013e3182138b54
84. Lee YM, Yi O, Sung TY, Chung KW, Yoon JH, Hong SJ. Surgical Outcomes of Robotic Thyroid Surgery Using a Double Incision Gasless Transaxillary Approach: Analysis of 400 Cases Treated by the Same Surgeon. *Head Neck* (2014) 36:1413–9. doi: 10.1002/hed.23472
85. Liu SYW, Wong SKH, Chiu PWY, Ng EKW, Liu SY-W, Wong SK-H, et al. Endoscopic Thyroid Lobectomy Using Bilateral Axillo-Breast Approach: Surgical Techniques and Outcomes. *Surg Pract* (2015) 19:128–32. doi: 10.1111/1744-1633.12124
86. Materazzi G, Fregoli L, Manzini G, Baggiani A, Miccoli M, Miccoli P. Cosmetic Result and Overall Satisfaction After Minimally Invasive Video-Assisted Thyroidectomy (MIVAT) Versus Robot-Assisted Transaxillary Thyroidectomy (RATT): A Prospective Randomized Study. *World J Surg* (2014) 38:1282–8. doi: 10.1007/s00268-014-2483-5
87. Miccoli P, Biricotti M, Matteucci V, Ambrosini CE, Wu J, Materazzi G. Minimally Invasive Video-Assisted Thyroidectomy: Reflections After More Than 2400 Cases Performed. *Surg Endosc* (2016) 30:2489–95. doi: 10.1007/s00464-015-4503-4
88. Miccoli P, Pinchera A, Materazzi G, Biagini A, Berti P, Faviana P, et al. Surgical Treatment of Low- and Intermediate-Risk Papillary Thyroid Cancer With Minimally Invasive Video-Assisted Thyroidectomy. *J Clin Endocrinol Metab* (2009) 94:1618–22. doi: 10.1210/jc.2008-1418
89. Noureldine SI, Jackson NR, Tufano RP, Kandil E. A Comparative North American Experience of Robotic Thyroidectomy in a Thyroid Cancer Population. *Langenbecks Arch Surg* (2013) 398:1069–74. doi: 10.1007/s00423-013-1123-0
90. Paek SH, Kang KH, Park SJ. A Comparison of Robotic Versus Open Thyroidectomy for Papillary Thyroid Cancer. *Surg Laparosc Endosc Percutan Tech* (2018) 28:170–3. doi: 10.1097/SLE.0000000000000529
91. Park JO, Anuwong A, Kim MR, Sun DI, Kim MS. Transoral Endoscopic Thyroid Surgery in a Korean Population. *Surg Endosc* (2019) 33:2104–13. doi: 10.1007/s00464-018-6481-9
92. Park JO, Kim SY, Chun BJ, Joo YH, Cho JH, Park YH, et al. Endoscope-Assisted Facelift Thyroid Surgery: An Initial Experience Using a New Endoscopic Technique. *Surg Endosc* (2015) 29:1469–75. doi: 10.1007/s00464-014-3826-x
93. Pérez-Soto SH, Ponce de León-Ballesteros G, Montalvo-Hernández J, Sierra-Salazar M, Pantoja Millán JP, Herrera-Hernández MF, et al. Transoral Endoscopic Thyroidectomy by Vestibular Approach-Initial Experience and Comparative Analysis in the First Reported Mexican Cohort. *J Laparoendosc Adv Surg Tech A* (2019) 29:1526–31. doi: 10.1089/lap.2019.0537
94. Piccoli M, Mullineris B, Gozzo D, Colli G, Pecchini F, Nigro C, et al. Evolution Strategies in Transaxillary Robotic Thyroidectomy: Considerations on the First 449 Cases Performed. *J Laparoendosc Adv Surg Tech A* (2019) 29:433–40. doi: 10.1089/lap.2019.0021
95. Prete FP, Marzaioli R, Lattarulo S, Paradies D, Barile G, D'Addetta MV, et al. Transaxillary Robotic-Assisted Thyroid Surgery: Technique and Results of a Preliminary Experience on the Da Vinci Xi Platform. *BMC Surg* (2019) 18:19. doi: 10.1186/s12893-019-0473-0
96. Razavi CR, Khadem MGA, Fondong A, Clark JH, Richmon JD, Tufano RP, et al. Early Outcomes in Transoral Vestibular Thyroidectomy: Robotic Versus Endoscopic Techniques. *Head Neck* (2018) 40:2246–53. doi: 10.1002/hed.25323
97. Ryu HR, Kang SW, Lee SH, Rhee KY, Jeong JJ, Nam KH, et al. Feasibility and Safety of a New Robotic Thyroidectomy Through a Gasless, Transaxillary Single-Incision Approach. *J Am Coll Surg* (2010) 211:e13–9. doi: 10.1016/j.jamcollsurg.2010.05.021
98. Schabram J, Vorländer C, Wahl RA. Differentiated Operative Strategy in Minimally Invasive, Video-Assisted Thyroid Surgery Results in 196 Patients. *World J Surg* (2004) 28:1282–6. doi: 10.1007/s00268-004-7681-0
99. Shan YZ, Zhou LM, Yu ZF, Wang SG, Gao GL, Shen Y, et al. Comparison Between Transareola Singlesite Endoscopic Thyroidectomy and Minimally Invasive Video-Assisted Thyroidectomy. *J Int Med Res* (2012) 40:2213–9. doi: 10.1177/030006051204000619
100. Stang MT, Yip L, Wharry L, Bartlett DL, McCoy KL, Carty SE. Gasless Transaxillary Endoscopic Thyroidectomy With Robotic Assistance: A High-Volume Experience in North America. *Thyroid* (2018) 28:1655–61. doi: 10.1089/thy.2018.0404
101. Sung ES, Ji YB, Song CM, Yun BR, Chung WS, Tae K. Robotic Thyroidectomy: Comparison of a Postauricular Facelift Approach With a Gasless Unilateral Axillary Approach. *Otolaryngol Head Neck Surg* (2016) 154:997–1004. doi: 10.1177/0194599816636366
102. Tae K, Lee DW, Song CM, Ji YB, Park JH, Kim DS, et al. Early Experience of Transoral Thyroidectomy: Comparison of Robotic and Endoscopic Procedures. *Head Neck* (2019) 41:730–8. doi: 10.1002/hed.25426
103. Tai DKC, Chick W-K, Chan PCM, Lau C-H, Tang DLC. Experience of Endoscopic Thyroidectomy in a Single-Centre Institution. *Surg Pr* (2016) 20:161–5. doi: 10.1111/1744-1633.12216
104. Tesseroli MAS, Spagnol M, Sanabria Á. Transoral Endoscopic Thyroidectomy by Vestibular Approach (TOETVA): Initial Experience in Brazil. *Rev Col Bras Cir* (2018) 45:e1951. doi: 10.1590/0100-6991e-20181951
105. Ujiki MB, Sturgeon C, Denham D, Yip L, Angelos P. Minimally Invasive Video-Assisted Thyroidectomy for Follicular Neoplasm: Is There an Advantage Over Conventional Thyroidectomy? *Ann Surg Oncol* (2006) 13:182–6. doi: 10.1245/ASO.2006.03.057
106. Wang Y, Zhang Z, Zhao Q, Xie Q, Yan H, Yu X, et al. Transoral Endoscopic Thyroid Surgery *via* the Tri-Vestibular Approach With a Hybrid Space-Maintaining Method: A Preliminary Report. *Head Neck* (2018) 40:1774–9. doi: 10.1002/hed.25157
107. Yi JW, Yoon SG, Kim HS, Yu HW, Kim SJ, Chai YJ, et al. Transoral Endoscopic Surgery for Papillary Thyroid Carcinoma: Initial Experiences of a Single Surgeon in South Korea. *Ann Surg Treat Res* (2018) 95:73–9. doi: 10.4174/astr.2018.95.2.73
108. Yi O, Yoon JH, Lee YM, Sung TY, Chung KW, Kim TY, et al. Technical and Oncologic Safety of Robotic Thyroid Surgery. *Ann Surg Oncol* (2013) 20:1927–33. doi: 10.1245/s10434-012-2850-0

109. Yoo H, Chae BJ, Park HS, Kim KH, Kim SH, Song BJ, et al. Comparison of Surgical Outcomes Between Endoscopic and Robotic Thyroidectomy. *J Surg Oncol* (2012) 105:705–8. doi: 10.1002/jso.22106
110. Yu JJ, Bao SL, Yu SL, Zhang DQ, Loo WT, Chow LW, et al. Minimally Invasive Video-Assisted Thyroidectomy for the Early-Stage Differential Thyroid Carcinoma. *J Transl Med* (2012) 10:S13. doi: 10.1186/1479-5876-10-S1-S13
111. Liu J, Song T, Xu M. Minimally Invasive Video-Assisted Versus Conventional Open Thyroidectomy: A Systematic Review of Available Data. *Surg Today* (2012) 42:848–56. doi: 10.1007/s00595-012-0130-z
112. Pan J, Zhou H, Zhao X, Ding H, Wei L, Qin L, et al. Robotic Thyroidectomy Versus Conventional Open Thyroidectomy for Thyroid Cancer: A Systematic Review and Meta-Analysis. *Surg Endosc* (2017) 31:3985–4001. doi: 10.1007/s00464-017-5433-0
113. Jackson N, Yao L, Tufano R, Kandil E. Safety of Robotic Thyroidectomy Approaches: Meta-Analysis and Systematic Review. *Head Neck* (2013) 36:137–43. doi: 10.1002/hed.23223
114. Sun G, Peress L, Pynnonen M. Systematic Review and Meta-Analysis of Robotic vs Conventional Thyroidectomy Approaches for Thyroid Disease. *Otolaryngol Head Neck Surg* (2014) 150:520–32. doi: 10.1177/0194599814521779
115. Kandil E, Hammad A, Walvekar R, Hu T, Masoodi H, Mohamed S, et al. Robotic Thyroidectomy Versus Nonrobotic Approaches. *Surg Innov* (2015) 23:317–25. doi: 10.1177/1553350615613451
116. Jiang WJ, Yan PJ, Zhao CL, Si MB, Tian W, Zhang YI, et al. Comparison of Total Endoscopic Thyroidectomy With Conventional Open Thyroidectomy for Treatment of Papillary Thyroid Cancer: A Systematic Review and Meta-Analysis. *Surg Endosc* (2020) 34:1891–903. doi: 10.1007/s00464-019-07283-y
117. Chen C, Huang S, Huang A, Jia Y, Wang J, Mao M, et al. Total Endoscopic Thyroidectomy Versus Conventional Open Thyroidectomy in Thyroid Cancer: A Systematic Review and Meta-Analysis. *Ther Clin Risk Manag* (2018) 14:2349–61. doi: 10.2147/TCRM.S183612
118. Lang B, Wong C, Tsang J, Wong K. A Systematic Review and Meta-Analysis Comparing Outcomes Between Robotic-Assisted Thyroidectomy and Non-Robotic Endoscopic Thyroidectomy. *J Surg Res* (2014) 191:389–98. doi: 10.1016/j.jss.2014.04.023
119. Xing Z, Qiu Y, Abuduwaili M, Xia B, Fei Y, Zhu J, et al. Surgical Outcomes of Different Approaches in Robotic Assisted Thyroidectomy for Thyroid Cancer: A Systematic Review and Bayesian Network Meta-Analysis. *Int J Surg* (2021) 89:105941. doi: 10.1016/j.ijsu.2021.105941
120. Wu YJ, Chi SY, Chan YC, Chou FF, Wee SY, Wu KT. Scarless Completion Thyroidectomy After Initial Transoral Approach for Differentiated Thyroid Cancer: How and When to Start? *Surg Laparosc Endosc Percutan Tech* (2021). doi: 10.1097/SLE.0000000000000933
121. Kwak J, Kim SJ, Xu Z, Lee K, Ahn JH, Yu HW, et al. Robotic Completion Thyroidectomy *via* the Bilateral Axillo-Breast Approach. *J Clin Med* (2021) 10:1707. doi: 10.3390/jcm10081707
122. Razavi CR, Tufano RP, Russell JO. Completion Thyroidectomy *via* the Transoral Endoscopic Vestibular Approach. *Gland Surg* (2018) 7:S77–9. doi: 10.21037/gs.2018.02.01

Permissions

All chapters in this book were first published by Frontiers; hereby published with permission under the Creative Commons Attribution License or equivalent. Every chapter published in this book has been scrutinized by our experts. Their significance has been extensively debated. The topics covered herein carry significant findings which will fuel the growth of the discipline. They may even be implemented as practical applications or may be referred to as a beginning point for another development.

The contributors of this book come from diverse backgrounds, making this book a truly international effort. This book will bring forth new frontiers with its revolutionizing research information and detailed analysis of the nascent developments around the world.

We would like to thank all the contributing authors for lending their expertise to make the book truly unique. They have played a crucial role in the development of this book. Without their invaluable contributions this book wouldn't have been possible. They have made vital efforts to compile up to date information on the varied aspects of this subject to make this book a valuable addition to the collection of many professionals and students.

This book was conceptualized with the vision of imparting up-to-date information and advanced data in this field. To ensure the same, a matchless editorial board was set up. Every individual on the board went through rigorous rounds of assessment to prove their worth. After which they invested a large part of their time researching and compiling the most relevant data for our readers.

The editorial board has been involved in producing this book since its inception. They have spent rigorous hours researching and exploring the diverse topics which have resulted in the successful publishing of this book. They have passed on their knowledge of decades through this book. To expedite this challenging task, the publisher supported the team at every step. A small team of assistant editors was also appointed to further simplify the editing procedure and attain best results for the readers.

Apart from the editorial board, the designing team has also invested a significant amount of their time in understanding the subject and creating the most relevant covers. They scrutinized every image to scout for the most suitable representation of the subject and create an appropriate cover for the book.

The publishing team has been an ardent support to the editorial, designing and production team. Their endless efforts to recruit the best for this project, has resulted in the accomplishment of this book. They are a veteran in the field of academics and their pool of knowledge is as vast as their experience in printing. Their expertise and guidance has proved useful at every step. Their uncompromising quality standards have made this book an exceptional effort. Their encouragement from time to time has been an inspiration for everyone.

The publisher and the editorial board hope that this book will prove to be a valuable piece of knowledge for researchers, students, practitioners and scholars across the globe.

List of Contributors

Zhen Liu, Run-sheng Ma, Tao Wang, Dao-hong Zuo and De-tao Yin
Department of Thyroid Surgery, The First Affiliated Hospital of Zhengzhou University, He'nan, China

Jun-li Jia
Department of Respiratory, The First Affiliated Hospital of Zhengzhou University, He'nan, China

Hiroo Masuoka and Akira Miyauchi
Department of Surgery, Kuma Hospital Center for Excellence in Thyroid Care, Kobe, Japan

How-Yun Ko and Cheng-Hsun Chuang
Department of Otorhinolaryngology-Head and Neck Surgery, International Thyroid Surgery Center, Kaohsiung Medical University Hospital, Kaohsiung Medical University, Kaohsiung, Taiwan

Jia Joanna Wang and Ning-Chia Chang
Department of Otorhinolaryngology-Head and Neck Surgery, International Thyroid Surgery Center, Kaohsiung Medical University Hospital, Kaohsiung Medical University, Kaohsiung, Taiwan
Department of Otorhinolaryngology-Head and Neck Surgery, Kaohsiung Municipal Siaogang Hospital, Faculty of Medicine, College of Medicine, Kaohsiung Medical University, Kaohsiung, Taiwan

I-Cheng Lu
Department of Anesthesiology, Kaohsiung Municipal Siaogang Hospital, Kaohsiung Medical University Hospital, Kaohsiung Medical University, Kaohsiung, Taiwan
Faculty of Medicine, College of Medicine, Kaohsiung Medical University, Kaohsiung, Taiwan

Pi-Ying Chang
Department of Anesthesiology, Kaohsiung Municipal Tatung Hospital, Kaohsiung Medical University Hospital, Faculty of Medicine, College of Medicine, Kaohsiung Medical University, Kaohsiung, Taiwan

Gregory W. Randolph
Division of Thyroid and Parathyroid Endocrine Surgery, Department of Otolaryngology—Head and Neck Surgery, Massachusetts Eye and Ear Infirmary, Harvard Medical School, Boston, MA, United States

Gianlorenzo Dionigi
Department of Pathophysiology and Transplantation, Faculty of Medicine and Surgery, University of Milan, Milan, Italy
Division of General Surgery, Endocrine Surgery Section, Istituto Auxologico Italiano IRCCS (Istituto di ricovero e cura a carattere scientifico), Milan, Italy

Jing Ye, Jia-Wei Feng, Wan-Xiao Wu, Jun Hu, Li-Zhao Hong and Yong Jiang
Department of Thyroid Surgery, The Third Affiliated Hospital of Soochow University, Changzhou First People's Hospital, Changzhou, China

An-Cheng Qin
The Affiliated Suzhou Hospital of Nanjing Medical University, Suzhou Municipal Hospital, Suzhou, China

Wei-Hai Shi
The Affiliated Hospital of Nanjing Medical University, Changzhou Second People's Hospital, Changzhou, China

Shuting Zhu
Department of Ultrasound, The First Medical Center of Chinese People's Liberation Army (PLA) General Hospital, Beijing, China

Qingxuan Wang
Department of Thyroid Surgery, The First Affiliated Hospital of Wenzhou Medical University, Wenzhou, China

Danni Zheng and Cong Jin
Department of Breast Surgery, The First Affiliated Hospital of Wenzhou Medical University, Wenzhou, China

Lei Zhu
Thyroid Surgery Department, The Fifth Hospital Affiliated to Wenzhou Medical University, Lishui Central Hospital, Lishui, China

Zheng Zhou
Department of Head and Neck Surgery, Bengbu Medical College Graduate School, Anhui, China

Shiying Xu
Zhejiang Chinese Medical University, The Second Clinical Medical, Hangzhou, China

Binbin Shi
Department of Medical Ultrasound, the First Affiliated Hospital of Wenzhou Medical University, Wenzhou, China

Guowan Zheng
Department of Head and Neck Surgery, Otolaryngology & Head and Neck Center, Cancer Center, Zhejiang Provincial People's Hospital (Affiliated People's Hospital, Hangzhou Medical College), Hangzhou, China
Key Laboratory of Endocrine Gland Diseases of Zhejiang Province, Hangzhou, China

Yefeng Cai
Department of Thyroid Surgery, The First Affiliated Hospital of Wenzhou Medical University, Wenzhou, China
Department of Head and Neck Surgery, Otolaryngology & Head and Neck Center, Cancer Center, Zhejiang Provincial People's Hospital (Affiliated People's Hospital, Hangzhou Medical College), Hangzhou, China
Key Laboratory of Endocrine Gland Diseases of Zhejiang Province, Hangzhou, China

Zeyu Zhang, Botao Sun, Hui Ouyang, Rong Cong, Fada Xia and Xinying Li
Department of Thyroid Surgery, Xiangya Hospital, Central South University, Changsha, China

Hsiao-Yu Huang and Chien-Chung Wang
Department of Otolaryngology-Head and Neck Surgery, E-Da Hospital, Kaohsiung, Taiwan

Ching-Feng Lien, Chih-Chun Wang, Tzer-Zen Hwang and Feng-Yu Chiang
Department of Otolaryngology-Head and Neck Surgery, E-Da Hospital, Kaohsiung, Taiwan
School of Medicine, College of Medicine, I-Shou University, Kaohsiung, Taiwan

Yu-Chen Shih
Department of Otolaryngology, E-Da Cancer Hospital, Kaohsiung, Taiwan

Fang Dong, Lin Zhou, Shuntao Wang, Chunping Liu and Wei Shi
Department of Breast and Thyroid Surgery, Union Hospital, Tongji Medical College, Huazhong University of Science and Technology, Wuhan, China

Jinqian Mao
Department of Vascular Surgery, Union Hospital of Tongji Medical College, Huazhong University of Science and Technology, Wuhan, China

Zipeng Wang, Gongbo Du, Shuo Li, Yihao Liu, Hanlin Sun and Qungang Chang
Department of Thyroid Surgery, The First Affiliated Hospital of Zhengzhou University, Zhengzhou, China

Hanyin Zhang
Department of Dermatology, First Affiliated Hospital of Zhengzhou University, Zhengzhou, China

Detao Yin
Department of Thyroid Surgery, The First Affiliated Hospital of Zhengzhou University, Zhengzhou, China
Engineering Research Center of Multidisciplinary Diagnosis and Treatment of Thyroid Cancer of Henan Province, Zhengzhou, China
Key Medicine Laboratory of Thyroid Cancer of Henan Province, Zhengzhou, China

Yan-Rong Li, Feng-Hsuan Liu, Szu-Tah Chen and Miaw-Jene Liou
Division of Endocrinology and Metabolism, Department of Internal Medicine, Linkou Chang Gung Memorial Hospital, Taoyuan, Taiwan
College of Medicine, Chang Gung University, Taoyuan, Taiwan

Wei-Yu Chou, Wai-Kin Chan and Jui-Hung Sun
Division of Endocrinology and Metabolism, Department of Internal Medicine, Linkou Chang Gung Memorial Hospital, Taoyuan, Taiwan

Kai-Lun Cheng
Department of Medical Imaging, Chung Shan Medical University Hospital, Taichung, Taiwan
School of Medical Imaging and Radiological Sciences, Chung Shan Medical University, Taichung, Taiwan

Shanwen Chen, Dong Wang, Jianxin Qiu, Yehai Liu and Yi Zhao
Department of Otorhinolaryngology-Head and Neck Surgery, The First Affiliated Hospital of Anhui Medical University, Hefei, China

Xing Yu, Yong Wang and Ping Wang
Department of Thyroid Surgery, The Second Affiliated Hospital, Zhejiang University School of Medicine, Hangzhou, China

Yuancong Jiang, Yujun Li, Qionghua He, Lei Pan and Peifeng Zhu
College of Medicine, Zhejiang University, Hangzhou, China

Alessia Dolci, Maura Arosio and Rita Indirli
Endocrinology Unit, Fondazione IRCCS Cà Granda Ospedale Maggiore Policlinico, Milan, Italy
Department of Clinical Sciences and Community Health, University of Milan, Milan, Italy

Giovanni Genovese and Angelo Valerio Marzano
Dermatology Unit, Fondazione IRCCS Ca' Granda Ospedale Maggiore Policlinico, Milan, Italy
Department of Pathophysiology and Transplantation, University of Milan, Milan, Italy

Federica Derlino
Dermatology Unit, Department of Health Sciences, ASST Santi Paolo e Carlo, University of Milan, Milan, Italy

Chiung-Dan Hsu
Department of Anesthesiology, Kaohsiung Municipal Siaogang Hospital, Kaohsiung Medical University Hospital, Kaohsiung Medical University, Kaohsiung, Taiwan

Sheng-Hua Wu
Faculty of Medicine, College of Medicine, Kaohsiung Medical University, Kaohsiung, Taiwan
Department of Anesthesiology, Kaohsiung Municipal Ta-Tung Hospital, Kaohsiung Medical University Hospital, Kaohsiung Medical University, Kaohsiung, Taiwan

How-Yun Ko
Department of Otorhinolaryngology, Kaohsiung Medical University Hospital, Kaohsiung Medical University, Kaohsiung, Taiwan

Young Jun Chai
Department of Surgery, Seoul National University College of Medicine, Seoul Metropolitan Government—Seoul National University Boramae Medical Center, Transdisciplinary Department of Medicine & Advanced Technology, Seoul National University Hospital, Seoul, South Korea

Yi-Wei Kuo
Department of Anesthesiology, Kaohsiung Medical University Hospital, Kaohsiung Medical University, Kaohsiung, Taiwan

Richard Wahl
Internal Medicine (Department of Endocrinology and Diabetology, Angiology, Nephrology and Clinical Chemistry), University of Tuebingen, Tuebingen, Germany

Eleonore Fröhlich
Internal Medicine (Department of Endocrinology and Diabetology, Angiology, Nephrology and Clinical Chemistry), University of Tuebingen, Tuebingen, Germany
Center for Medical Research, Medical University Graz, Graz, Austria

Tzu-Yen Huang
International Thyroid Surgery Center, Department of Otolaryngology-Head and Neck Surgery, Kaohsiung Medical University Hospital, Faculty of Medicine, College of Medicine, Kaohsiung Medical University, Kaohsiung, Taiwan
Department of Biological Science and Technology, National Yang Ming Chiao Tung University, Hsinchu, Taiwan
Department of Biological Science and Technology, National Chiao Tung University, Hsinchu, Taiwan

Wing-Hei Viola Yu and Yi-Chu Lin
International Thyroid Surgery Center, Department of Otolaryngology-Head and Neck Surgery, Kaohsiung Medical University Hospital, Faculty of Medicine, College of Medicine, Kaohsiung Medical University, Kaohsiung, Taiwan

Che-Wei Wu
International Thyroid Surgery Center, Department of Otolaryngology-Head and Neck Surgery, Kaohsiung Medical University Hospital, Faculty of Medicine, College of Medicine, Kaohsiung Medical University, Kaohsiung, Taiwan
Department of Otolaryngology-Head and Neck Surgery, Kaohsiung Municipal Siaogang Hospital, Kaohsiung Medical University Hospital, Faculty of Medicine, College of Medicine, Kaohsiung Medical University, Kaohsiung, Taiwan

Shih-Chen Fu and An-Shun Tai
Institute of Statistics, National Yang Ming Chiao Tung University, Hsinchu, Taiwan
Institute of Statistics, National Chiao Tung University, Hsinchu, Taiwan

Ka-Wo Lee
International Thyroid Surgery Center, Department of Otolaryngology-Head and Neck Surgery, Kaohsiung Medical University Hospital, Faculty of Medicine, College of Medicine, Kaohsiung Medical University, Kaohsiung, Taiwan
Department of Otolaryngology-Head and Neck Surgery, Kaohsiung Municipal Tatung Hospital, Kaohsiung Medical University Hospital, Faculty of Medicine, College of Medicine, Kaohsiung Medical University, Kaohsiung, Taiwan

Sheng-Hsuan Lin
Institute of Statistics, National Yang Ming Chiao Tung University, Hsinchu, Taiwan
Institute of Statistics, National Chiao Tung University, Hsinchu, Taiwan
Institute of Data Science and Engineering, National Yang Ming Chiao Tung University, Hsinchu, Taiwan
Institute of Data Science and Engineering, National Chiao Tung University, Hsinchu, Taiwan

Stephen H. LaFranchi
Department of Pediatrics, Doernbecher Children's Hospital, Oregon Health & Sciences University, Portland, OR, United States

Li-Jen Liao
Department of Otolaryngology Head and Neck Surgery, Far Eastern Memorial Hospital, Taipei, Taiwan
Department of Electrical Engineering, Yuan Ze University, Taoyuan, Taiwan

Chi-Te Wang
Department of Otolaryngology Head and Neck Surgery, Far Eastern Memorial Hospital, Taipei, Taiwan
Department of Electrical Engineering, Yuan Ze University, Taoyuan, Taiwan
Department of Special Education, University Of Taipei, Taipei, Taiwan

Cheng-Hsin Liu and Jia Joanna Wang
International Thyroid Surgery Center, Department of Otolaryngology-Head and Neck Surgery, Kaohsiung Medical University Hospital, Faculty of Medicine, College of Medicine, Kaohsiung Medical University, Kaohsiung, Taiwan
Department of Otolaryngology-Head and Neck Surgery, Kaohsiung Municipal Siaogang Hospital, Kaohsiung Medical University Hospital, Faculty of Medicine, College of Medicine, Kaohsiung Medical University, Kaohsiung, Taiwan

Ling-Feng Wang
International Thyroid Surgery Center, Department of Otolaryngology-Head and Neck Surgery, Kaohsiung Medical University Hospital, Faculty of Medicine, College of Medicine, Kaohsiung Medical University, Kaohsiung, Taiwan
Center for Liquid Biopsy and Cohort Research, Faculty of Medicine, College of Medicine, Kaohsiung Medical University, Kaohsiung, Taiwan

Leong-Perng Chan
International Thyroid Surgery Center, Department of Otolaryngology-Head and Neck Surgery, Kaohsiung Medical University Hospital, Faculty of Medicine, College of Medicine, Kaohsiung Medical University, Kaohsiung, Taiwan
Center for Liquid Biopsy and Cohort Research, Faculty of Medicine, College of Medicine, Kaohsiung Medical University, Kaohsiung, Taiwan
Department of Otolaryngology-Head and Neck Surgery, Kaohsiung Municipal Tatung Hospital, Kaohsiung Medical University Hospital, Faculty of Medicine, College of Medicine, Kaohsiung Medical University, Kaohsiung, Taiwan

Pia Pace-Asciak
Department of Otolaryngology - Head and Neck Surgery, University of Toronto, Toronto, Canada
Division of Otolaryngology-Head and Neck Surgery, Johns Hopkins University, Baltimore, MD, United States

Jon O. Russell
Department of Otolaryngology - Head and Neck Surgery, Johns Hopkins University, Baltimore, Maryland, United States

Ralph P. Tufano
Sarasota Memorial Health Care System Multidisciplinary Thyroid and Parathyroid Center, Sarasota, Florida, United States
Division of Otolaryngology-Head and Neck Surgery, Johns Hopkins University, Baltimore, MD, United States

Theodora Pappa
Division of Endocrinology, Diabetes and Hypertension, Brigham and Women's Hospital, Boston, MA, United States

Samuel Refetoff
Departments of Medicine, Pediatrics and Committee on Genetics, The University of Chicago, Chicago, IL, United States

Hsin-Yi Tseng
Department of Otorhinolaryngology-Head and Neck Surgery, International Thyroid Surgery Center, Kaohsiung Medical University Hospital, Kaohsiung Medical University, Kaohsiung, Taiwan

Hui-Chun Chen
Department of Nursing, Kaohsiung Medical University Hospital, Kaohsiung, Taiwan

Hsiu-Ya Chen
Department of Anesthesiology, Kaohsiung Medical University Hospital, Kaohsiung, Taiwan

Yasser Ali Hakami
Obesity, Endocrine and Metabolism Center, King Fahad Medical City, Riyadh, Saudi Arabia

Jon O. Russell and Mohammad Shaear
Division of Otolaryngology-Head and Neck Surgery, Johns Hopkins University, Baltimore, MD, United States

Lisa H. de Vries, Dilay Aykan, Lutske Lodewijk, Inne H. M. Borel Rinkes and Menno R. Vriens
Department of Surgical Oncology and Endocrine Surgery, University Medical Center Utrecht, Utrecht, Netherlands

Johanna A. A. Damen
Julius Center for Health Sciences and Primary Care, University Medical Center Utrecht, Utrecht University, Utrecht, Netherlands

Index

www.ingramcontent.com/pod-product-compliance
Lightning Source LLC
LaVergne TN
LVHW060534210926
848485LV00005B/1198
* 9 7 8 1 6 4 6 4 7 5 1 9 3 *